Medical
Genetics

Notice

Medical Genetics

AN INTEGRATED APPROACH

G. Bradley Schaefer, MD

Professor of Genetics and Pediatrics
University of Arkansas for Medical Sciences
Arkansas Children's Hospital
Little Rock, Arkansas

James N. Thompson, Jr., PhD

David Ross Boyd Professor
Department of Biology
University of Oklahoma
Norman, Oklahoma

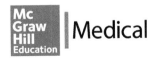

New York Chicago San Francisco Athens London Madrid
Mexico City Milan New Delhi Singapore Sydney Toronto

Medical Genetics: An Integrated Approach

1 2 3 4 5 6 7 8 9 0   CTP/CTP   18 17 16 15 14 13

ISBN 978-0-07-166438-7
MHID 0-07-166438-6

This book was set in Times LT Std by Cenveo® Publisher Services.
The editors were Michael Weitz and Peter J. Boyle.
The production supervisor was Catherine H. Saggese.
Project management was provided by Harleen Chopra, Cenveo Publisher Services.
The designer was Elise Lansdon.
China Translation & Printing Services, Ltd., was printer and binder.

This book was printed on acid-free paper.

Library of Congress Cataloging-in-Publication Data

Schaefer, G. Bradley.
    Medical genetics / G. Bradley Schaefer, James N. Thompson Jr.
            p. ; cm.
    Includes bibliographical references and index.
    ISBN-13: 978-0-07-166438-7 (soft cover : alk. paper)
    ISBN-10: 0-07-166438-6 (soft cover : alk. paper)
    I. Thompson, James N.   II. Title.
    [DNLM: 1. Genetics, Medical.   2. Cytogenetics.   3. Genetic Phenomena—genetics.   4. Genetic Techniques.   QZ 50]
    RB155
    616′.042—dc23

                                                                    2013011825

McGraw-Hill Education books are available at special quantity discounts to use as premiums and sales promotions, or for use in corporate training programs. To contact visit the Contact Us pages at mhprofessional.com.

DEDICATION

To my wife, Becky. She has been my encourager, listening ear and motivator throughout the entirety of this project. Hopefully she gets more out of this than just a free copy of the book. — **G. Bradley Schaefer**

To my mother, Jean, and my sister, Lisa. Their patient encouragement helped make this an especially rewarding project. In addition, with his excellent work ethic and sense of humor, working with my longtime friend and colleague, Brad Schaefer, could not have been more enjoyable. — **James N. Thompson, Jr.**

Contents

Preface ix

Acknowledgments x

1 Genetics: Unity and Diversity 1

2 Information Flow and Levels of Regulation 17

3 The Organization of Development 49

4 The Structure and Function of Genes 77

5 Clinical Cytogenetics 99

6 Mendelian Genetics: Patterns of Gene Transmission 139

7 Mutation 165

8 Metabolism 183

9 Family History and Pedigree Analysis 201

10 Multifactorial Inheritance and Gene × Environment Interactions 213

11 Genetic Testing and Screening 229

12 Atypical Modes of Inheritance 249

13 Disorders of Organelles 269

14 Genetic Therapeutics 297

15 Population Genetics and Genetic Diversity 309

16 Of Fruit Flies, Mice, and Patients: Tying It All Together 325

Key Genetic Diseases, Disorders, and Syndromes 341

Glossary 343

Answers to Board-Format Practice Questions 357

Index 365

Preface

Genetics in medicine. Genetics and medicine. The genetics of medicine. All of these reflect slightly different aspects of the integration of basic genetic principles into the practice of medicine. The genetic "revolution" that has occurred over the past 20 years has thrust clinical genetics into the mainstream of medical practice. No longer is genetics a small, poorly understood discipline tucked away in the department of pediatrics or obstetrics. Rather, every component of health care delivery requires at least a working knowledge of core genetic principles. This fact is directly reflected in changes in medical school curricula, board questions, and continuing medical education. While the vast majority of medical students will not go on to specialize in medical genetics, all of them will need to know much about genetic concepts and principles—more, perhaps, than some would like. Still, there truly is not a discipline in all of medicine that does not use genetic principles, genetic information, and genetic techniques in the practice of its field. Thus, a textbook in medical genetics must of necessity be broad and inclusive in the scope of material covered. The principles must be unifying and globally applicable. There must be sufficient detail to guide the student to successful completion of the curriculum at his/her respective medical school and to pass all three steps of the United States Medical Licensing Examination (USMLE). Most importantly, it should be a resource that students can use throughout their medical school years and beyond to refer to when questions arise during the times of residency and practice as a professional.

One caveat needs to be mentioned. The rapid pace at which genetic information is changing will require frequent and periodic updates to the information base. The printed textbook will require electronic augmentation for this generation of learners and updates to keep up with the dizzying pace of additional genetic knowledge. Any updates will be available at **http://www.langetextbooks.com/.**

This book utilizes an integrated approach to medical genetics by combining a tailored introduction to essential general genetics and up-to-date coverage of medical genetics following the curriculum recommended by the Association of Professors of Human Genetics and Medical Genetics and by the American Society of Human Genetics Guidelines. Core genetic principles are reviewed with an emphasis on mechanisms and unifying concepts.

One of the great challenges of teaching medical genetics is the tremendous diversity found in the educational background of entering medical students. Over the past decade, medical schools have purposefully sought a more diversified group of applicants. While this diversity definitely provides a more interesting—and fun—group of students, it presents a major challenge in teaching "medicine" and medical genetics in particular. One student in the class may have just finished a doctorate degree in molecular genetics while a classmate may have a liberal arts background and have taken only the minimal amount of required science courses for admission and to attain a decent score on the MCATs. Instructors can assume a student's motivation and intelligence, but undergraduate background diversity means that they cannot necessarily assume specific prior science knowledge.

With this in mind, we have organized each chapter in this book into three distinct parts:

1. background and systems integration
2. medical genetics, and
3. case study applications.

The background and systems portion contain the basic genetic principles needed to understand the medical application. This information is available for any student needing to refresh themselves on the principles—or in some cases to learn it for the first time. This information draws upon principles that would have been covered in an undergraduate genetics course and utilizes abundant graphics and tabular information. It emphasizes the "why" and "how" of these principles to hopefully address the common concern voiced by many medical students, "Why do I need to know this. I'm going to be a _____." For the student with a stronger background in genetics, this section may be easily skipped; each part of the chapter is written as a stand-alone component. The "meat" of each chapter is in the second (medical genetics) part. This part contains all of the pertinent information to build a strong knowledge base for being successful on all three steps of the USMLE. The third part uses case study examples to emphasize the direct application of these facts and principles to patient care.

This book is written as a narrative that develops with subsequent chapters building upon the foundation laid by the previous chapters. Thus, the whole "story" of medical genetics could be read from cover to cover if so desired. Alternatively, each chapter is also organized to stand alone and can be accessed for specific references and topics.

As the readers work their way through the book they should be on the lookout for several recurring themes. Woven throughout the details of each chapter are the basic themes of medical genetics. Some of the most important themes to observe include:

- Genotype to phenotype correlation(s)—the need to correlate clinical observations with information obtained by laboratory genetic techniques
    - what is a phenotype?
    - levels of describing a phenotype.
    - defining endophenotypes as a critical strategy for therapy.
- Pathogenesis—how do changes in genes translate into human medical conditions?
- Variability (expanded phenotypes).

- Genetic/etiologic heterogeneity–the rule, not the exception.

Without a doubt a working knowledge of genetic principles will be a necessity for all practicing health care providers regardless of their chosen specialty. We hope that you have as much fun reading this text as we did writing it. Nothing would thrill us more than to know that you took something from this book and applied it directly to your practice.

Best wishes.

G. Bradley Schaefer, MD
James N. Thompson, Jr., PhD
October 2013

Acknowledgments

I would like to express my sincere thanks to the many people who walked through the writing of this book with me. My partners, colleagues, and office were simply selfless in allowing me time off and away to write. My family and friends were so patient in listening to my angst as I often stalled in the process. I would particularly like to thank our accomplished group of medical reviewers. Their comments, insight and suggestions were invaluable:

Celia Kaye, MD, PhD
University of Colorado (Denver) School of Medicine
Denver, Colorado

Nancy Mendelsohn, MD
Children's Hospitals and Clinics of Minnesota
Minneapolis, Minnesota

Sonja A. Rasmussen, MD, MS
Centers for Disease Control and Prevention
Atlanta, Georgia

Angela Scheuerle, MD
Medical City Hospital
Dallas, Texas

— G. Bradley Schaefer

I, too, owe a debt of gratitude to the reviewers who made many constructive recommendations to improve this book and to my family and friends who supported and encouraged me during the project. In addition, I thank the many students over the years who have asked questions that made me think about concepts in a new way and who encouraged my work through their individual successes. The changing face of a science like medical genetics leads us all to continue being students.

——**James N. Thompson, Jr.**

chapter 1

Genetics: Unity and Diversity

CHAPTER SUMMARY

If asked for one phrase to define the theme of this text on medical genetics, it might be "the cascade of consequences." This is a major departure from the simple view that a gene causes a trait. Traits can be appearance, behavior, or body chemistry. For much of recent history, and certainly in common discussion, one imagines that a gene has a simple and direct effect on a character. For example, one might say that albinism is caused by the "a" gene (Figure 1-1). While this view is not quite wrong, the reality is both more complex and more interesting. There is in fact an intricate interaction among genes, hormones, enzymes, membrane receptors, neuron networks, and so on that creates a maze of connections that prescribes our individual functional and developmental path. Many of these pathways and interactions are shared by even distantly related animals. There is both unity and diversity in the genetics of life.

Part 1: Background and Systems Integration

Conception. Development. Birth. Growth. Maturity. Old age. A familiar pattern. A physician's role may have begun months before birth in prenatal care of the mother or may focus decades later when the patient is elderly. But the genetic encyclopedia the patient is drawing from was written at fertilization and will be expressed progressively from the embryo to old age. Deoxyribonucleic acid (DNA) codes for proteins and for various kinds of ribonucleic acid (RNA) made in the many cell types of the body. It can dictate much about an individual's physical abilities and limitations. But it is not a static information resource. Throughout life it changes by mutation and by processes that reduce or block the use of various gene sequences. In addition, environmental factors can influence epigenetic processes, the subsequent chemical interactions that cascade from an initial gene action to have major effects both early and late in life.

With the possible exception of identical twins, each of us begins with a unique genotype that defines our individual biochemistry and form. We recognize that uniqueness in ourselves. We take individuality for granted. Now, as a physician, reflect that perspective on a patient. Clearly, understanding the physiological consequences of a treatment is critical to the medical outcome. But patients come from a diverse human population. Not everyone responds in the same way to any given drug. Normally effective dosages of a prescription medicine might have little effect on some and potentially life-threatening side effects on others. A study cited by National Institute of Health (NIH) (1998) found that 2.2 million serious cases of adverse drug reactions had occurred in 1 year and resulted in over 100,000 deaths. That makes adverse reactions to properly prescribed medications one of the leading causes of death in the United States. For that reason, research in biomedical technology is exploring ways to profile a person's unique genotype to aid in defining biochemical variables that affect individual treatment outcomes. Medicine does not need to take a "one size fits all" approach. Because of our biological diversity, future medical practice will increasingly rely on new insights from genetics and molecular biology.

Yet, human genetic diversity is not uniformly distributed. The same is true in populations of essentially all animals and plants. Due to historical sharing of ancestral lineages, the genetic makeup of human population groups can differ in medically important ways. For example, lactose intolerance is common in people of many African, Asian, Native American, Middle Eastern, and other heritages. But lactose tolerance is typical in those of European and some African ancestries. One hypothesis points to the fact that those with lactose tolerance share a tradition of pastoralism and dependence on milk products. (Throughout this book we will discuss other examples of medically-relevant population genetic diversity.)

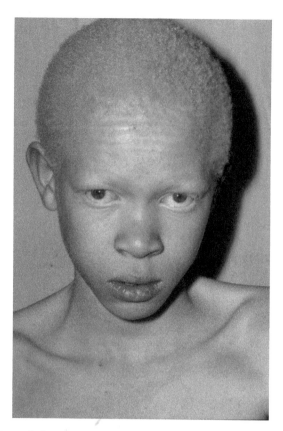

Figure 1-1. Albinism can be traced to homozygosity for a recessive mutation in the pathway for biosynthesis of melanin pigment. (Reprinted with permission from Kelly AP and Taylor ST. *Dermatology for Skin of Color*. New York: McGraw-Hill, 2009, Fig. 47-1.)

Some genetic variation is normal, but not all genetic changes are benign. Major gene mutations or chromosome structural changes can cause severe alterations in development and even death. The challenge for physicians is to understand the range of genetic variability among patients. Genetics and molecular biology can be tools for diagnosis and can offer clues to the most appropriate treatment choice. Genetic resources and the technologies of molecular biology are changing medicine in fundamental ways, and the consequences of that change will have both biomedical and bioethical implications for the future practice of every physician.

The Origin of Life

The unity of life is reflected in its origin. We do not know what that origin was, and alternative explanations do not need to be mutually exclusive. In reality, it is not possible to test directly any hypothesis of events that happened in the distant past. It is possible, however, to test the current environment for principles of evolutionary science, i.e. the change in living systems over time. While these investigations will never establish the origin of life with unambiguous certainty, they do have direct implications for existing biologic organisms.

Genetics is a scientific discipline, which delimits the structure of its hypotheses in an easily recognized fashion. Its data are limited to observations that can be made about the current physical universe and to hypotheses that can be falsified by observation and experimentation. Since the purpose of the present discussion is to explore how possible scientific models of an origin of life might shed light on the unifying concepts of inheritance and gene expression, our focus will be on scientific tests of competing hypotheses regarding the unity among present-day living organisms.

Strong evidence for the unity of life comes from molecular conservation that is from organic molecules that have not changed or that have changed only a small amount from one organism to others that are distantly related. For example, all living organisms share an essentially identical genetic code, like a shared alphabet among languages. Other forms of a genetic code could theoretically be just as efficient. But the same one is used by all. This supports the conclusion that current living forms, from bacteria and viruses to higher plants and humans, share an information storage ancestry. Still, the evidence goes far beyond a common genetic code. Many protein compositions are highly conserved among diverse taxonomic groups. Not surprisingly, the strongest similarities are in proteins that contribute to fundamental structures, such as the histones that compose the globular protein complexes, the nucleosomes, that bind DNA into chromosomes (Figure 1-2). A shared biological ancestry has broad implications for biology in general and for medicine in particular. What we can learn from one organism can help us understand the others.

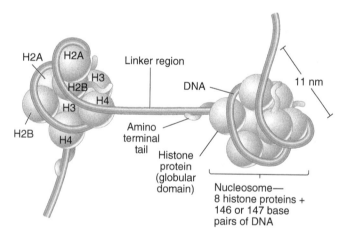

Figure 1-2. A nucleosome is an octomer of histone proteins H2A, H2B, H3, and H4. Its overall positive charge covalently binds to the negatively charged DNA molecule. Together with histone H1 and some non-histone proteins that act as linkers, the nucleosomes help compact DNA into the organized higher-order folds of the chromosome. Nucleosomes can also have general gene regulation effects. In the sea urchin and other advanced animals, the genes for these histones are even arranged in a repeated linear order: spacer–H2A–spacer–H3–spacer–H2B–spacer–H4–spacer–H1–spacer. (Reprinted with permission from Brooker RJ: *Genetics: Analysis and Principles*, 3rd ed. New York: McGraw-Hill, 2008, Fig. 10-14A).

RNA and the "RNA World"

Deoxyribonucleic acid is the hereditary macromolecule in most life forms, but it was likely not the first. There is strong theoretical and experimental evidence in support of the hypothesis that ribonucleic acid (RNA) formed first. Both DNA and RNA are composed of chains of monomers called nucleotides. As we will see in more detail later, RNA plays a central role in the synthesis of proteins. But it can also have a catalytic function, like that of enzymes (protein catalysts). Catalytic RNA molecules, called ribozymes, can make complementary copies of other short RNAs in addition to producing proteins.

The synthesis of RNA and proteins by self-replicating or catalytic RNA is likely to have been error-prone. The diverse products of such "mutation" events could differ in their successful competition for monomers like amino acids and RNA nucleotides. The performance quality of their products would also vary. This is raw material for natural selection on the molecular scale. RNA can also serve as the template for the creation of DNA strands in a process now used by some RNA viruses to make DNA copies during cell infection. In its complementary double-stranded structure, DNA has the advantage of high molecular stability and an efficient mechanism of accurate duplication. Once in operation, natural selection would favor the improvement of replication and error-correction capabilities, and these are now among the most highly conserved proteins across the taxonomic spectrum. Such a sequence of events leaves RNA, more specifically messenger RNA (mRNA), as the intermediate in the flow of genetic information from the DNA of the nucleus, through the mRNA transcripts created from spliced RNA, to the protein products (Figure 1-3). On that stable foundation, increasingly complex cell structures and activities are possible.

Ribozymes still play critical roles in the cell. Among other things, they assist in splicing nucleotides out of the initial RNA transcript. Variations in splicing contribute to the wide array of protein products that can come from a single active gene. In later sections we will explore the consequences of both normal splicing variation and the disease states that can arise from ribozyme activity. Practical applications are also on the horizon. Artificially engineered ribozymes can identify and break a specific type of mRNA and prevent expression of its coded protein. Targeting RNAs of a pathogen like HIV thus offers a potential molecular therapy.

Biogenesis and the Cell Theory

Life forms are united by a small set of principles that describe the flow of information required to create each type of organism. Even prokaryotes, simple cells like bacteria that lack a defined nucleus and other membranous organelles, are governed by many of the same processes as found in more complex organisms, including humans. Biogenesis is the principle that all life forms come from reproduction by earlier life forms. Although abiogenesis, the spontaneous creation of a living system under appropriate conditions, must have occurred at the end of the prebiotic world, spontaneous generation of

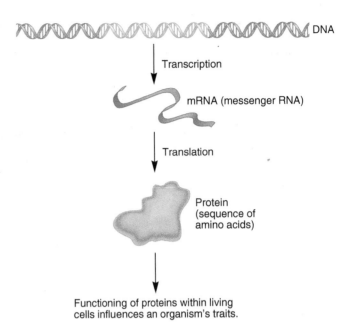

Figure 1-3. The flow of genetic information. The sequence of DNA nucleotides is transcribed into a complementary sequence of RNA nucleotides (transcription). The RNA is processed and transported out of the nucleus where it is translated into a sequence of amino acids, the protein product, on ribosomes in the cytoplasm (translation). The "RNA World" hypothesis is that this information flow began with catalytic RNA coding for protein synthesis. DNA and transcription came later. (Reprinted with permission from Brooker RJ: *Genetics: Analysis and Principles*, 3rd ed. New York: McGraw-Hill, 2008, Fig. 1-6.)

life no longer occurs. Even if a complex molecule happens to form spontaneously today, the oxidizing atmosphere will soon break its chemical bonds or an organism will eat it as food. There is no longer enough time for complex molecules to accumulate in necessary combinations to create a novel living structure.

A related principle is that cells are the fundamental building blocks of life. Technical advances have pushed forward the boundaries of knowledge by increasing the quality of observations that can be made about the natural world. Anton van Leeuwenhoek and others in the seventeenth century began the development of microscopes, and Robert Hooke was the first to report using a magnifying device to see cell structure in a section of cork. This is one of many examples where an invention opens a previously unknown domain to study. Building from Hooke's discovery and the confirming observations by others, Matthias Schleiden (1838) and Theodor Schwann (1839) independently presented the first clear statement of the Cell Theory, the principle that all organisms are composed of cells.

Although the study of genetics often tends to focus on the organization and use of encoded information in the nucleus, an understanding of the "cascade of consequences" to come from the nucleus requires knowledge about other cell organelles, about membrane structure, and about the molecular components of the cytoplasmic domain. Genetics is only important in its functional context—what does genetically-encoded

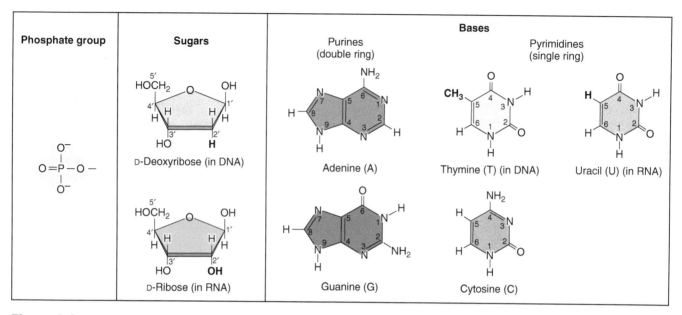

Figure 1-4. Components of DNA and RNA nucleotides. Deoxyribose sugar differs from ribose in the absence of oxygen ("deoxy") on the 2′carbon. Adenine, guanine, and cytosine are found in both DNA and RNA, but uracil replaces thymine in RNA. (Reprinted with permission from Brooker RJ: *Genetics: Analysis and Principles*, 3rd ed. New York: McGraw-Hill, 2008.)

information do? The unity of life is reflected in the great similarity in cell structures among organisms. For that reason, studies of model organisms, especially animal models, will be called upon frequently to clarify mechanisms at work in human development and disease.

The Molecular Basis of Inheritance

For much of their history, two threads—transmission genetics and molecular genetics—were separate pursuits. Transmission genetics is concerned with the way traits are combined and passed among generations of offspring. Molecular genetics explores the biochemical basis of a trait's expression.

The difference between organic and inorganic molecules was recognized by the early 1800s, and by about 1830 three major classes of organic molecules had been distinguished chemically: carbohydrates, lipids, and proteins. But one key class of organic molecules, nucleic acid, was not discovered until 1868 when Friedrich Miescher isolated a phosphorus-rich organic molecule from white blood cell (WBC) nuclei. Initially named "nuclein," it was later found to have organic acid characteristics and renamed "nucleic acid." Thus the discovery of what would turn out to be the molecule of inheritance did not occur until after Gregor Mendel published his *Experiments on Plant Hybridization* (1866) and Charles Darwin published *On the Origin of Species by Natural Selection* (1859). The discovery of nucleic acid was more than a decade after Florence Nightingale began critical reforms in hygiene and patient care in the Crimean War that led to the modern nursing profession (1854). Modern genetics has matured within a very brief historical time frame. Its practical applications to medicine are even younger.

Like protein, nucleic acids are polymeric chains of subunits. The nucleic acid subunits are nucleotides, each composed of a 5-carbon sugar, a phosphoric acid group, and a nitrogenous base (Figure 1-4). There are two classes of nucleic acids. DNA nucleotides contain the 5-carbon sugar deoxyribose (thus, DNA); RNA contains ribose (ribonucleic acid). Both classes of nucleic acid have four different nitrogenous bases, two purines and two pyrimidines. The sequence of nitrogenous bases gives these molecules their coding capability.

Carbons of the sugar are numbered clockwise in the nucleotide (Figure 1-5). The nitrogenous base is attached to the 1′ carbon and the phosphate group to the 5′ carbon. During synthesis of a new strand, nucleotides are linked together by attaching a new nucleotide to the 3′ carbon of the existing strand (Figure 1-6). RNA remains single-stranded, although regions will fold to produce complex three-dimensional patterns that are important to its function. DNA, on the other

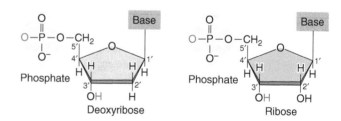

Figure 1-5. Nucleotides of DNA and RNA. The atoms shown in red are removed when nucleotides are linked together by phosphodiester bonds to form a single strand. (Reprinted with permission from Brooker RJ: *Genetics: Analysis and Principles*, 3rd ed. New York: McGraw-Hill, 2008.)

Figure 1-6. A single strand of deoxyribose nucleotides. A phosphodiester bond joins the 3′ carbon of one nucleotide to the phosphate group of the next nucleotide. During synthesis, nucleotides are added at the 3′ end, as shown by the direction of the arrow. At the top end is the most distal 5′ carbon, and the 3′ carbon is the open attachment site at the other end. This 5′ to 3′ directionality plays a critical role in DNA replication and in translation during protein synthesis. (Reprinted with permission from Brooker RJ: *Genetics: Analysis and Principles*, 3rd ed. New York: McGraw-Hill, 2008.)

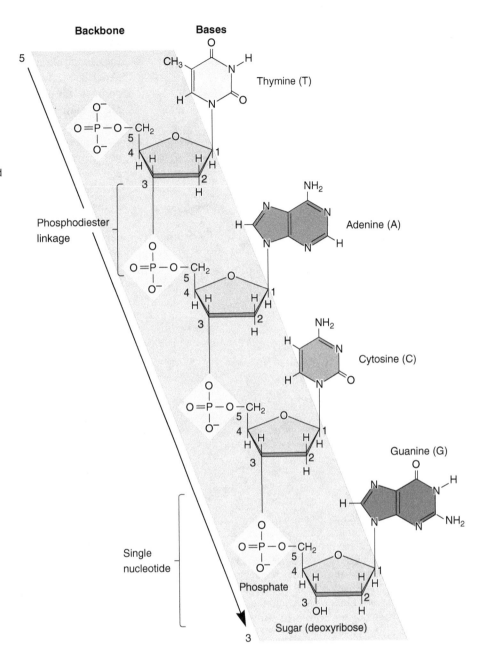

hand, is a double-stranded molecule that is produced when one strand, the template, binds sequentially with a complementary nucleotide during synthesis of a new strand (Figure 1-7). When there is the purine adenine (A) on the template, a thymine (T) pyrimidine is linked into the growing strand, and vice versa. When there is the purine guanine (G), the pyrimidine cytosine (C) is attached. This creates a double-stranded DNA molecule (Figure 1-8) connected by large numbers of hydrogen bonds. In Chapter 2 we will discuss the replication of DNA in more detail and explore how the sequence of nucleotides is used to encode the information for creating defined protein sequences. But clearly the sequence of nucleotides is the key. Learning about that sequence and its biomedical importance is a primary goal of genome studies like the Human Genome Project.

The Genome

The term "genome" refers to the genetic information needed to code for the biochemical processes and development of an individual. Most of this genetic information is in the "nuclear genome," but some resides in copies of the "mitochondrial genome" in the cytoplasm. In green plants there is also the "chloroplast genome." Unless otherwise noted, however, we will use "nuclear genome" and "genome" interchangeably.

Genome can also be defined in terms of the nucleotide content of an individual's DNA. That is different from the first definition, because not all nucleotide regions are translated into biochemical products. When looking at the complete nucleotide sequence, therefore, comparisons of genome size and information content may not match very closely.

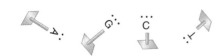

Nucleotides

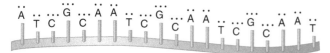

Single strand

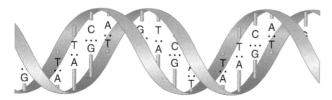

Double helix

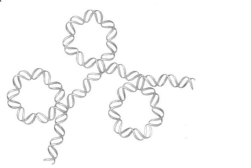

Three-dimensional structure

Figure 1-7. The DNA molecule is a double helix, produced when a single strand of nucleotides serves as the template for synthesis of a new complementary strand. Stable pairings occur between adenine and thymine with two hydrogen bonds (shown by the pair of dots) and between guanine and cytosine with three hydrogen bonds. This double-stranded DNA molecule then binds with nucleosomes and other proteins into the three-dimensional coils of a chromosome. (Reprinted with permission from Brooker RJ: *Genetics: Analysis and Principles*, 3rd ed. New York: McGraw-Hill, 2008.)

True, bacterial genomes are smaller than those of eukaryotes. But among eukaryotes, there is no direct correlation between the genetic complexity of an organism and the amount of DNA or the number of chromosomes it carries. Many cellular and biochemical processes are held in common. Comparisons include these many genetic similarities and thereby tend to overshadow the smaller number of genes that may account for even large phenotypic differences. The same is true of the amount of DNA. Only about 2% or 3% of the DNA in a human nucleus codes for proteins. With that insight, one can appreciate why the DNA amounts in different species can vary a lot without marked effects on the array of protein products.

About 20,000 to 22,000 genes are required by a human during a lifespan. That is about the same as the 25,300 in *Arabidopsis thaliana*, the mustard grass, which serves as an important genetic model for plant species. Even the fruit fly,

Drosophila melanogaster, is estimated to have only about 13,600 genes. An explanation of how complicated cell activity and developmental processes can be controlled by so few genes had to wait on the results of genome mapping. But it is perhaps less difficult to appreciate why the numbers of genes are so similar. Consider the similarities among organisms at the cellular level where so many life functions are shared.

Chromosome numbers among species are even less diagnostic. Apparently simple animals often have many more chromosomes than the 23 pairs found in humans (Figure 1-9).

Chromosomes are simply the structures that carry subsets of the genome of a species during cell division. But within a single individual, a change in chromosome structure or number can alter their genome information content significantly and have severe, even fatal, consequences.

Each chromosome is made up of only one very long double-stranded DNA molecule. Each gene in the nuclear genome is arranged linearly along the DNA molecule of one of its chromosomes. We can therefore describe the information content of each kind of chromosome as a "linkage group." Ignoring the relatively neutral Y chromosome found only in males, there are 23 linkage groups in humans. If we assume 22,000 genes in the human genome, there must be about 1000 genes per average linkage group. In reality, however, both genes and chromosomes differ a lot in size. Some chromosomes are long and carry more genes. Others are quite small.

One copy of each linkage group, the "haploid" chromosome number (n), will be contributed by the egg nucleus (n = 23), and the other haploid set of each linkage group (n = 23) will be

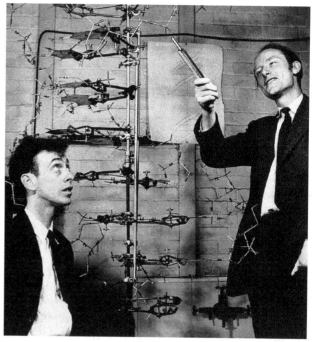

(a)

Figure 1-8. (a) Watson and Crick with a model of DNA. (b) Representation of exact spacing in a DNA double helix (a: Reprinted with permission from Hartwell LH, et al. *Genetics: From Genes to Genomes.* 4th ed. New York: McGraw-Hill, 2010.)

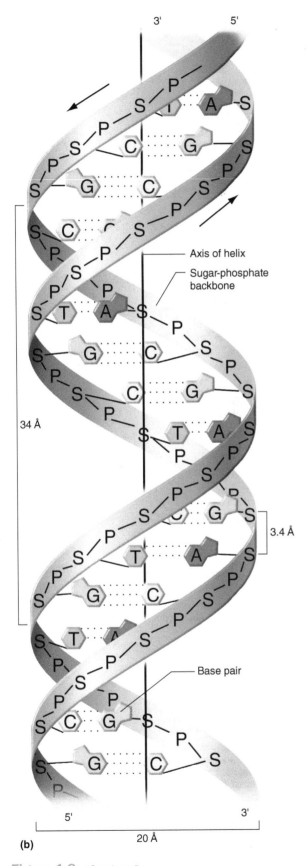

Axis of helix

Sugar-phosphate backbone

34 Å

3.4 Å

Base pair

5'   3'

(b)

20 Å

Figure 1-8. (*Continued*)

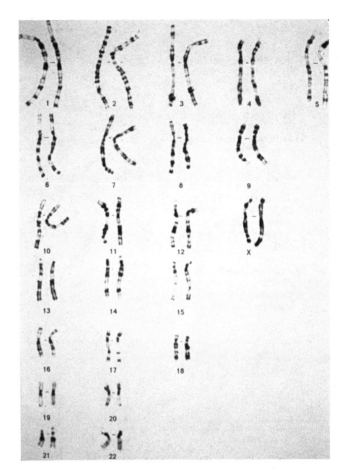

Figure 1-9. A karyotype, or chromosome picture, showing the 22 pairs of chromosomes plus two X chromosomes. This karyotype was, therefore, produced from a normal female. The 46 chromosomes make up the diploid (2n) composition of a human somatic cell. (Reproduced with permission of Warren G. Sanger, PhD, University of Nebraska Medical Center, Omaha, Nebraska.)

contributed by the sperm. Fertilization establishes the diploid (2n) genetic makeup of the individual's unique genotype. After fertilization, each of the 46 chromosomes will be duplicated and distributed to the resulting daughter cells in each cycle of cell division. Thus each adult cell retains two copies of each linkage group, with the exception of the single X chromosome found in a male (its partner is the single Y chromosome).

There is some overlap among the terms employed to describe genetic makeup. This can be confusing. One way to clarify the relationships is to recognize that some terms refer to a concrete structure and others are more abstract. Haploid (n) or diploid (2n) chromosome number is concrete. We can fix and stain dividing cell nuclei and then count chromosomes to produce a picture, the karyotype. "Linkage group," on the other hand, is an abstract reference to the individual DNA content of each different kind of chromosome. One can list the genes that are located on a given chromosome, such as chromosome 4 (Figure 1-10). Whether one is talking about the haploid or diploid set of chromosome 4s, the genetic content remains the same.

"Haploid" refers to a cell with one copy of that genetic content, or linkage group. "Diploid" is a cell with two. Similarly, since the term "genome" refers to content, it indicates

DNA, the molecule of life

Trillions of cells

Each cell contains:

- 46 human chromosomes, found in 23 pairs

- 2 m of DNA

- Approximately 3 billion DNA base pairs per set of chromosomes, containing the bases A, T, G, and C

- Approximately 20,000 to 25,000 genes code for proteins that perform most life functions

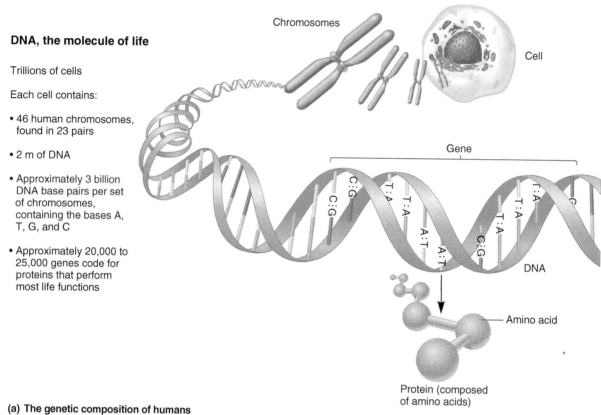

(a) The genetic composition of humans

Chromosome 4

Huntington disease
Wolf-Hirschhorn syndrome
PKU due to dihydropteridine
  reductase deficiency

MPS 1 (Hurler and Scheie syndromes)
Mucopolysaccharidosis I

Periodontitis, juvenile
Dysalbuminemic hyperzincemia
Dysalbuminemic hyperthyroxinemia
Analbuminemia

Hereditary persistence of alpha-fetoprotein
AFP deficiency, congenital
Piebaldism

Dentinogenesis imperfecta-1

Polycystic kidney disease, adult, type II
Mucolipidosis II
Mucolipidosis III

Severe combined immunodeficiency due
  to IL2 deficiency
Rieger syndrome

C3b inactivator deficiency
Aspartylglucosaminuria
Williams-Beuren syndrome, type II
Sclerotylosis
Anterior segment
  mesenchymal dysgenesis

Dysfibrinogenemia, gamma types
Hypofibrinogenemia, gamma types

Pseudohypoaldosteronism
Hepatocellular carcinoma

Dysfibrinogenemia, alpha types
Amyloidosis, hereditary renal
Dysfibrinogenemia, beta types

Glutaric acidemia type IIC
Faecioscapulohumeral muscular dystrophy

Factor XI deficiency
Fletcher factor deficiency

(b) Genes on one human chromosome that are associated with disease when mutant

Figure 1-10. This figure shows the relationship between the genetic content of a cell and of one of its chromosomes, the linkage group of human chromosome 4. (Reprinted with permission from Brooker RJ: *Genetics: Analysis and Principles*, 3rd ed. New York: McGraw-Hill, 2008.)

the genetic makeup of one representative of each type of chromosome, the haploid genetic complement. But when considering the specific genetic composition of an individual, we are again thinking concretely. An individual's genotype can be homozygous (*AA* or *aa*) or heterozygous (*Aa*) for different forms, the *A* and *a* alleles, of the "A" gene.

What Is a Gene?

Not long ago, this would have been a fairly easy question to answer. We would have said that a gene is a sequence of nucleotides in a molecule of DNA which, by way of mRNA, codes for the synthesis of a specific protein. But insights from fully sequenced genomes, such as those produced by the Human Genome Project, now show many more subtle and complex informational functions associated with DNA.

One of the first hints at the complexity of the gene concept was the discovery that genes may be split into pieces on the chromosome. The sections that code for protein, the exons, are interspersed with stretches of nucleotides that can be noncoding, the introns. Introns are spliced out of the initial RNA transcript to produce the functional mRNA used in protein synthesis. But the later discovery of alternative splicing complicated even that story. Alternative splicing allows exon and intron modules to be combined in a variety of ways, leading to several different transcripts being translated from the same gene. In fact, the number of different transcripts can be amazingly large. In *Drosophila*, for example, the *Dscam* gene (coding for the *Drosophila* Down syndrome cell adhesion molecule) expresses 38,016 different mRNAs due to alternative splicing.

Other discoveries include overlapping genes, in which one section of nucleotides is transcribed as part of two different genes; genes within genes; and run-ons where transcription continues through one gene into an adjacent gene coding for a totally different protein. These fused transcripts are another way that diversity in proteins can be generated from a comparatively small number of genes.

But perhaps the greatest expansion in complexity of the gene definition comes from discoveries that many more types of RNA play a regulatory role than previously imagined. MicroRNAs are now known to have critical roles in regulating many cellular processes without acting as intermediaries for protein synthesis. Just how important they are, compared to the traditionally recognized RNAs from protein coding genes, is still being debated. Whether the DNA that codes for a microRNA deserves to be called a "gene" is also an unsettled question. But there can be little doubt that detailed information about the genomes of humans and other species will uncover even more complexity.

The Human Genome Project

The genetic makeup of each individual is unique. From that perspective, there is not just one human genome; there are billions. Yet despite genetic variation, there is a surprising degree of similarity in the final structure of our bodies and our physiologies. The great similarity of biochemical events that control normal development is accompanied by extensive genetic diversity within the human gene pool. It yields the common, complex, and often subtle genetic differences that result in the personal individuality upon which a human society is anchored. We recognize and respect each other as equal members of *Homo sapiens*, but modern medicine must be sensitive to the underlying differences among us. Sequencing a representative human genome is a first step. But it means little until the function, or lack of function, is understood for each portion.

The Human Genome Project (HGP) is a multinational effort begun in 1990 to obtain the nucleotide sequence of a complete human genome of approximately 3 billion nucleotides and to identify all the protein coding genes it contains. Technological advances in sequencing methodology enabled the project to be completed in 2003, slightly ahead of schedule. Developing the computer databases to manage and search this massive amount of information has led to a new field of genetics called bioinformatics. Sequencing advancements and bioinformatics are at the foundation of many promising medical applications, including the potential to generate personal genome profiles to assist in tailoring diagnosis to the individual.

As envisioned from the beginning, the HGP had several well-defined goals. The major objectives included:

(1) *Identify* all of the genes coded for in human DNA

(2) *Determine* the sequences of the 3 billion chemical base pairs that make up human DNA

(3) *Store* this information in databases

(4) *Improve* existing tools for data analysis

(5) *Transfer* related technologies to the private sector

(6) *Address* the ethical, legal, and social issues (ELSI) that may arise from this knowledge

Particularly important among these goals for the practice of medicine was making the information derived from the project available to the general public. Several excellent databases that are direct spin-offs of HGP are readily accessible and have great utility in the practice of medicine. Among these are GeneTests, Online Mendelian Inheritance in Man (OMIM), and the HGP website itself. The HGP also included a serious effort to understand and address the legal, ethical, and other social issues associated with this advancement in knowledge. Our presentation of genetic applications in medicine will include discussions of some of these issues.

But understanding the range of normal diversity is also very important. That is a goal of the 1000 Genomes Project. Launched in 2008, this international collaboration will sequence the genomes of approximately 1200 people to provide a database of biomedically relevant variation in DNA. Advances in human population genetics and in comparative genomics provide useful insights into the genetic diversity of our species. It also generates information about single nucleotide polymorphisms (SNPs), structural variations, and copy number variations that can serve as DNA landmarks for mapping genes of biomedical interest.

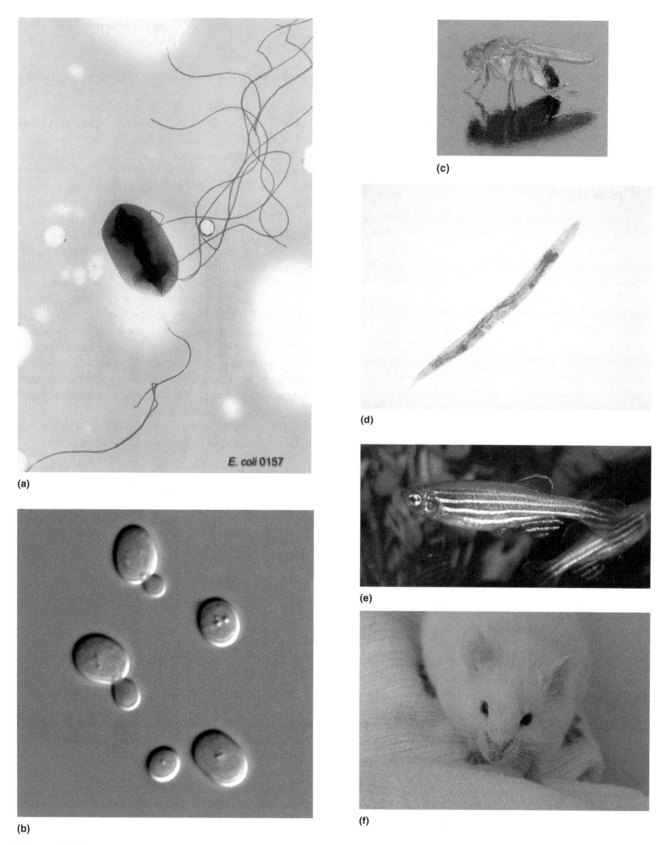

Figure 1-11. Some of the organisms that are used as highly informative models to study gene action and development. (a) *Escherichia coli* is a common bacterium; (b) *Saccharomyces cerevisiae* is a yeast; (c) the fruit fly *Drosophila melanogaster* and (d) *Caenorhabditis elegans*, a nematode, allow sophisticated studies of comparatively simple animal body plans; (e) *Danio rerio*, the zebrafish, and (f) *Mus musculus*, the laboratory mouse, represent more complex vertebrate model systems; (g) *Arabidopsis* was one of the first plant model organisms in genome projects. (a: CDC/Peggy S. Hayes; b: Photograph by Mansur. Released to the public domain, via Wikimedia Commons; c: Photograph by André Karwath. Licenced under CC-BY-SA-2.5, http://creativecommons.org/licenses/by-sa/2.5, via Wikimedia Commons; d: Photograph by Tormikotkas. Licensed under CC-BY-SA-3.0, http://creativecommons.org/licenses/by-sa/3.0, via Wikimedia Commons; e: Photograph by Azul. Released to the public domain, via Wikimedia Commons; f: Steven Berger Photography, licensed under Creative Commons BY-SA 2.0; g: Photo by Peggy Greb, Agricultural Research Service, United States Department of Agriculture.)

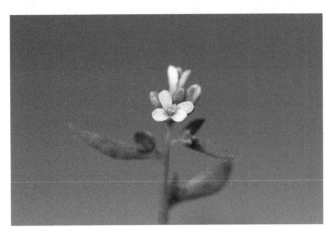

(g)

Figure 1-11. (Continued)

The Importance of Model Organisms

In addition to sequencing human DNA, the HGP also tackled the genomes of several important model organisms, including the human intestinal bacterium *Escherichia coli*, the fruit fly *Drosophila melanogaster*, the laboratory mouse *Mus musculus*, a plant *Arabidopsis thaliana*, and others (Figure 1-11). Earlier in this chapter we explored the shared ancestry reflected in the conservation of DNA makeup and protein sequences over a broad taxonomic spectrum. Information about gene functions in a simple model organism can aid in identifying the functions associated with coding regions of the human genome. Throughout this book, we will draw examples from model organisms to show how insights from a simpler organism can lead us to understand the complex interactions of genes, inducers, environmental variables, and cell structure in defining the roles that genes play in human development and activity.

Part 2: Medical Genetics

The medical application of the principles described earlier is limitless. There is little question that the field of genetics has become the focal point for most of medicine over the past two decades. It is also likely that the focus on genomics (with its translational components of proteomics and metabolomics) will continue to direct medicine for decades to come. The success of the HGP has acted as a force that has propelled genetics out of the laboratory and into the hospitals and clinics. It has put functional tools into the clinician's hands that directly improve the health and treatment of patients. All persons working in the health care disciplines need a working knowledge of basic genetic principles. In addition, they will need a firm understanding of the application of "medical genetics" in their own specialty. Of primary importance, this will include a functional knowledge of how to identify at-risk patients effectively and efficiently in the context of regular clinic flow. They will also need a firm grasp of possible testing methods, referral sources, patient and professional resources, and potential therapies. The role of the practicing physician also requires a continuing education component, keeping current with an appreciation for the rapid pace at which things are changing in the realm of medical genetics.

An introduction to the field of medical genetics should probably begin with a few definitions. The broad category of **Genetics** applies to the scientific study of the principles of heredity and the variation of observable features among organisms. **Human Genetics**, then, would apply to the study of genetics in people. Human genetics today comprises a number of overlapping fields, which go beyond just the practice of medicine. A list of some of the major disciplines in human genetics is provided in Table 1-1. That subset of human genetics that explores the genetic contributions to the etiology, pathogenesis, and natural history of diseases and disorders is referred to as **Medical Genetics**. This is to be distinguished from **Clinical Genetics**, which is the application of Medical Genetics to the diagnosis, prognosis and, in some cases, the treatment of genetic diseases.

With the development of medical genetics as a recognized discipline in medicine, there has been a commensurate appearance of new health care professionals (genetic professionals). **Medical Geneticists** are physicians who provide

Table 1-1.	Disciplines Within the Field of Human Genetics

Medical genetics. The study of the etiology, pathogenesis, and natural history of diseases and disorders that are at least partially genetic in origin

Clinical genetics. The diagnosis, counseling, treatment, and case management of genetic conditions

Behavior genetics. The study of genetic factors in behavioral disorders including psychiatric disorders and disorders of cognition, mood, and affect

Biochemical genetics. The study of biochemical reactions and the disorders (inborn errors of metabolism) of these reactions

Cytogenetics. The study of the structure and function of chromosomes in health and disease

Developmental genetics. The genetics of normal and abnormal development including congenital malformations and teratogens

Forensic genetics. The application of genetic knowledge and technology to medical-legal investigations

Genetic counseling. A patient care discipline that utilizes both the science of genetics and the social sciences (psychology, social work, and so forth) to provide counseling and support for patients and families with genetic conditions

Molecular genetics. The study of DNA and RNA variability; the effects of changes on human health

Pharmacogenetics. The study of genetic influences on drug response and metabolism

Population genetics. The study of genes within populations including frequencies, movement, and trends

Reproductive genetics. The study of the genetic aspects of reproduction including preconceptional health, preimplantation science, prenatal diagnosis, and pregnancy management

typical physician services for patients with genetic conditions. The major types of medical geneticists working today include subspecialists in pediatric, metabolic, perinatal, and adult care. **Genetic Counselors** are allied health professionals that specialize in the science of genetics as it relates to conveying complex information to patients and families as well as providing psychosocial support to persons in crisis. They are an invaluable part of the medical genetics team who help bridge the gap between often overwhelming medical care systems and patients in need of access and information. **Clinical Genetic Laboratories** are managed by doctoral-level scientists with specialized training in biochemical, molecular, and cytogenetic testing. Close communication between the medical geneticist and the genetic counselor is essential for ensuring that the right test is performed and that accurate information is provided to the patient. All of these specialties require specific training in certified training programs with oversight from the primary certifying agency, the American College of Medical Genetics (ACMG). As genetics has evolved as a medical specialty, there has also been an evolution of the medical administration of the field. The development and admission of the ACMG in 1995 as a recognized specialty by the American Medical Association testify to the legitimacy and overall acceptance of these professions within the medical community.

The vast majority of practicing specialists in Medical Genetics work at academic institutions. The scope of practice typically involves consultation in both the outpatient and inpatient settings. Thus health care providers should be familiar with the closest or most readily accessible Medical Genetic service providers in their region. Medical geneticists may also offer services as a member of an interdisciplinary health team that provides integrated and comprehensive services for persons with conditions that require access to multiple specialists. The list of possible interdisciplinary teams that may utilize medical geneticists is extensive. Table 1-2 lists some of the most common such services. Interdisciplinary clinics are especially helpful for persons with complex conditions and their families. They allow the patient to access multiple specialists that they may need to see in one session and allow for direct communication among the specialists about the same patient.

Throughout this book consistent language will be used in reference to specific conditions. In this book—as in a good clinical practice—"person first" language will be used. It is better to refer to "a person with diabetes" than "the diabetic." We refer to a child as having dysmorphic features, not as a funny looking kid (FLK). As society has changed, so has the application of medical terminology. A better understanding and familiarity of rare and often sensational conditions has led to a change in assigned terms—for the better. For instance *circa* 1912, the accepted classification of mental retardation included the categories of moron, imbecile, and idiot, which roughly correlate with the current groupings of mild, moderate-severe, and profound, respectively. Another more recent example would be that of Angelman syndrome (Figure 1-12).

Table 1-2.	Common Interdisciplinary Teams That May Incorporate Medical Genetics
Cancer genetics	
Connective tissue disorders	
Craniofacial	
Cystic fibrosis	
Down syndrome	
Fetal alcohol syndrome	
Gender disorders	
Hemoglobinopathies	
Metabolic disorders	
Neurofibromatosis	
Neurogenetics	
Neuromuscular (including muscular dystrophies)	
Neurosensory (hereditary hearing and vision problems)	
Orofacial clefting (cleft lip/cleft palate)	

Angelman syndrome is a recognizable genetic syndrome associated with a characteristic facial appearance, cognitive impairments, seizures, and a spastic gait with jerky arm movements said to resemble the movements of a marionette. Dr. Angelman originally described the condition in 1965 as a report of three "puppet children." Because these individuals often have episodes of inappropriate laughter, they were also described as being "happy." Subsequently, as late as the mid 1980s, this condition was referred to as the "Happy Puppet syndrome." This type of designation, not surprisingly, was concerning to many families. Acknowledging this, the medical genetics community has now made a deliberate change in the nomenclature to the eponym "Angelman syndrome." The power of language and the specific application of medical terms and their effects on the patients and their families cannot be over-stated.

It is important for all health care providers to understand the context and rationale for multiple terms. There are multiple ways to designate a person receiving medical services. In some settings, terms such as consumer or customer or client may be used. All of these terms convey specific aspects of the provider-patient relationship that may be appropriate. In this book, the term of choice will be "patient." It is also very important to be aware of the specific connotations of discussing a medical condition that a patient may have. While there are some differences in how people may apply certain terms, they will be used consistently in this text. **Disease** refers to a condition that causes discomfort or dysfunction for a person (in contrast to injury, which is typically immediate and acquired). A **disorder** is a condition in which there is a disturbance of normal functioning. Equally important, the health care provider needs to understand the potential impact that the use of such terms may have on their patients. Clearly the context is crucial in the

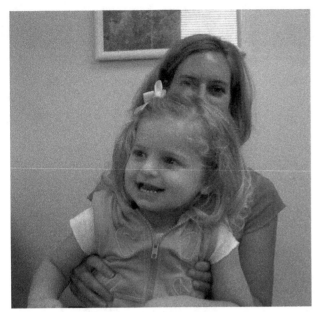

(a)

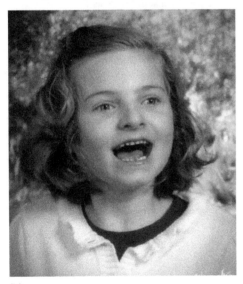

(b)

Figure 1-12. Girl with Angelman syndrome. (a) 3 years old. (b) 7 years old.

Table 1-3.	Timeline of Major Technological Events in Genetics
1869	Extraction of DNA
1882	Chromosomes identified
1913	First genetic "map"
1927	Mutagenic effects of x-rays
1934	X-ray crystallography to illuminate the structure of proteins
1941	"One gene-one enzyme" hypothesis
1944	Deoxyribonucleic acid (DNA) identified as the compound responsible for heredity
1950	DNA bases (AGTC) analyzed
1953	Watson and Crick: The double helix
1956	DNA polymerase isolated
1960	messenger RNA (mRNA) discovered
1961	First nucleotide "triplet" identified
1967	Somatic cell hybridization
1970	Site-specific restriction enzyme
1970	Reverse transcriptase
1972	First recombinant DNA molecule
1973	Cloning of DNA molecules into different cells
1977	DNA sequencing
1978	Restriction fragment length polymorphisms (RFLPs)
1985	Polymerase chain reaction (PCR)
1986	Automated DNA sequencer
1987	Fluorescent in situ hybridization (FISH)
1991	Expressed sequence tags (ESTs)
1992	Comparative genomic hybridization (CGH)
1998	Denaturing high-performance liquid chromatography (DHPLC)
2004	Copy number variants/changes (CNVs/CNCs)
2007	New-generation sequencing
Full Genomes Sequenced	
1995	*Haemophilus influenzae Rd*
1996	*Methanococcus jannaschii and yeast*
1998	Worm
1999	Fruit fly
2000	Human
2002	Mouse
2004	Rat
2005	Chimpanzee
2006	Honeybee
2007	Horse
2009	Cow
2009	Draft completions of domestic pig and Neanderthal genomes
2013	More than 1000 sequenced prokaryotic genomes

interpretation. For instance, much debate exists about how to describe deafness appropriately. Does a person with a hearing loss have a disorder, or do they simply have a different means of communication (language)?

Another point that needs to be emphasized is the proper way to denote a condition that is associated with a person's name. Most commonly, syndromes may bear the name of the person with a strong association with the condition, such as the person who first described the condition or who published the first comprehensive description. Such eponyms are typically associated with some of the most well-known common syndromes. More recently, advances in genetic testing are now identifying conditions that do not have an associated name, but rather are described by the actual genetic abnormality (discussed further in Chapter 5) and the specific genetic nomenclature. For conditions that are associated with a particular name, it is important to note that an apostrophe is not used in the designation. For example, it is Down syndrome, not Down's syndrome. Dr. Langdon Down neither had the condition nor did he "own" it.

What is truly amazing about the application of genetic technology in clinical medicine is the rapidity with which it has occurred. Almost all of the incorporation of genetics into medicine has occurred within a single generation. Only a few currently active practicing geneticists were already training or practicing before the human chromosome count was firmly established at 46 in 1956. Tables 1-3 and 1-4 provide timelines for selected advances in medical genetics. Table 1-3 lists major technological advances, while Table 1-4 highlights clinical milestones. In looking over these, one can begin to appreciate the relative "newness" of the field. Also, the ever-accelerating pace at which things have progressed should be noted. This, in fact, presents us with a somewhat daunting task in writing this textbook. How much of its information will be outdated by the time of publication? Our intention, therefore, will be to establish a firm foundation in concepts and in the ways to think about the role of genes in human development and disease. The specific facts that build upon that foundation will continue to grow.

Finally, it is important to be alert to recurring themes that are woven throughout the book. These themes are the essence of the application of genetic principles and technology in the practice of medicine. References to these principles include:

- Genotype—phenotype correlation(s): the need to correlate clinical observations with information obtained by genetic laboratory techniques
  - What is a phenotype?
  - Levels of describing a phenotype
  - Defining endophenotypes as a critical strategy for therapy
- Pathogenesis: how do changes in genes translate into human medical conditions?
- Variability and expanded phenotypes
- Genetic/etiologic heterogeneity

Table 1-4.	Timeline of Selected Milestones in Modern Medical Genetics
1953	Structure of DNA double helix elucidated
1956	Human chromosome count finally established at 46
1957	Victor McKusick establishes medical genetics clinic and training program at Johns Hopkins
1959	Association of Down syndrome and trisomy 21 reported
1959	Guthrie test (bacterial inhibition by phenylalanine) as harbinger of newborn screening
1960	Discovery of the Philadelphia chromosome as a marker of acute myelogenous leukemia
1962	David Smith coins term "dysmorphology" in the study of human malformations
1966	Victor McKusick's first edition of *Mendelian Inheritance in Man* (*MIM*) published
1966	DNA discovered in mitochondria
1969	First single gene isolated
1970	David Smith's first edition of *Recognizable Patterns of Human Malformations* published
1975	Maternal serum testing for prenatal screening begins
1978	Insulin becomes first biopharmaceutical produced by genetic engineering
1981	Prader-Willi syndrome is first recognized microdeletion syndrome
1987	MIM goes online as "Online Mendelian Inheritance in Man (OMIM)"
1990	HGP begins
1990	First gene therapy trial
1997	Detection of fetal DNA in maternal blood
2002	HGP completed 3 years ahead of schedule
2004	Human genome estimates of functioning genes reduced to ~22,000
2007	Genetic Information Nondiscrimination Act (GINA) successfully legislated
2008	Death of Victor McKusick "Father of Medical Genetics"
2009	Jack Szostak wins Nobel Prize in Medicine for work on telomeres/telomerases

Part 3: Clinical Correlation

Each chapter in this book will have a clinical correlation section to complement the basic science and medical genetic information. This first chapter stands out as somewhat unique. In later chapters, the clinical correlations will present specific conditions that assimilate the principles described in the preceding two sections. Given the introductory nature of this first chapter, however, a specific condition does not readily come

to mind as an example that integrates its information. Still, this does not mean that there is not a clinical corollary to the concept of genetic unity and diversity. The concept of personalized medicine will be the correlation provided.

At first glance, personalized medicine might not seem the most logical topic for a clinical correlation. But, in fact, nothing ties together the concept of "unity and diversity" as well as the practice of personalized medicine does. In traditional medical approaches, unity is found within diagnostic categories. At the core of most related medical conditions is a shared physiological and genetic basis. Still, from the inception of medical interventions, it has been readily appreciated that there is great diversity in clinical responses even within an apparently homogeneous diagnostic group. Simply put, patients with exactly the same condition, with exactly the same cause can have a multitude of responses to the same intervention. People differ in how (if at all) they respond to a given treatment, what is the most effective dose, what side effects are experienced, and possible adverse interactions.

Personalized Medicine: Personalized Health Care, Personalized Health Management

A major current movement in health care is the concept of tailoring therapy to the patient based upon patient-specific information. This type of customized medical practice is referred to as personalized medicine. Personalized medicine may be defined as health care targeted to the inherent biology and physiology of an individual leading to improvements in their medical care. The intended goal is that new molecular diagnostic tools will enhance patient care at several different levels. Currently, it is the common medical practice to follow to some degree a trial-and-error process for finding the right treatment and the right pharmaceutical dosage for each patient. By and large, most established dosage recommendations are adjusted based upon a limited number of variables such as size, age, and occasionally gender. In reality, many more variables are at play in differing responses, not the least of which are genetic factors. In theory, personalized medicine should help in arriving at a correct diagnosis in a shorter period of time. It should enable the provider to prescribe the right medication for an individual with less trial-and-error in the decision making process.

Most importantly, the hope is that these tools will prevent, delay, or reduce morbidity and mortality. Depending upon the particular features of a given medical condition, prevention may occur at many different levels. Primary prevention refers to the actual reduction of disease incidence. Secondary prevention involves the earlier detection (potentially presymptomatic) and intervention. Tertiary prevention utilizes personalized treatments based upon individually identified parameters. In this regard, subtyping conditions into "endophenotypes" based upon any number of genetic or other parameters should allow for the development of better, more specific therapies. Finally, some would define yet another level—quaternary prevention—as strategies that do not necessarily affect the actual medical aspects of the condition, but that somehow improve the quality of life for the individual. For instance information is typically viewed as being empowering for patients. Increased information that does not necessarily affect disease may reduce psychosocial stressors.

Personalized genomics is a subset of this practice. It has been defined as specific genetic testing that identifies individual risk profiles for a specific medical condition and/or treatment option. It also involves modifying treatment and surveillance based on genotype. Personalized genomic strategies are already being applied in a variety of clinical settings. There are many possible venues in which genetic information can be used to direct medical interventions (Table 1-5). A few examples include:

1. *Cancer therapeutics.* Personalized genomics is probably best established in the realm of oncology. Genetic information, such as cytogenetic findings, has been used for decades to stratify patients into the best predicted treatment option(s). Recent advances have identified a number of single gene changes that help direct cancer treatments. In addition, targeted therapies are available in which the use of the medication is designed to target

Table 1-5.	Applications of Genomics in Personalized Medicine

Targeted cancer therapy
- HER2/neu and trastuzumab (Herceptin) therapy
- Chronic myelogenous leukemia and tyrosine kinase inhibitors
- Neurofibromatosis and *ras* inhibitors

Pharmacotherapy
- Warfarin and CYP2C9/VKORC1
- Proton pump therapy and CYP2D6, CYP2C19, CYP2CP
- Clozapine and serotonin neurotransmitter receptor
- ACE inhibitors and ACE polymorphisms
- HIV mutation detection and drug resistance
- Bucindolol and adrenergic receptors polymorphisms

Genetic susceptibility
- Cancer susceptibility genes (clinical testing available)
  - BRCA1/BRCA2 (breast/ovarian cancer)
  - APC (Familial adenomatous polyposis)
  - p53 (Li-Fraumeni syndrome)
  - MLH1, MSH2, MSH6, PMS2 (hereditary nonpolyposis colorectal cancer)
  - PTEN (Cowden disease)
- Altered susceptibility to other conditions
  - ApoE (Alzheimer, outcome in head trauma)
  - DRD (complex decision making, smoking cessation, delinquency)
  - TPH2 (affective disorder spectrum)
  - CCR5 receptor (HIV infections)
  - Type 1 diabetes (at least 11 genes including HLA-DR)
  - Type 2 diabetes (multiple genes including HNF4A)

Diseases for which clinically significant SNP associations have been identified
- Age-related macular degeneration
- Type 2 diabetes
- Prostate cancer
- Asthma
- Cardiovascular disease
- Crohn disease
- Alzheimer disease
- Amyotrophic lateral sclerosis
- Progressive supranuclear palsy
- HIV/AIDS

Genes

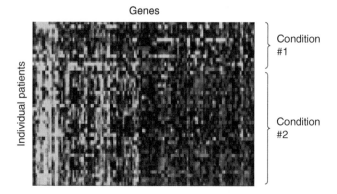

Individual patients

Condition #1

Condition #2

Figure 1-13. Tools are being developed to help clinicians predict the patient's prognosis, as in this example of breast cancer outcomes based on the primary tumor's gene expression profile.

known pathophysiological processes in the disease. Individual testing is typically needed to identify if a specific process is at work in that individual (Figure 1-13).

2. *Pharmacogenetics.* There are many variables in the use of pharmaceuticals among people. Individual differences exist in uptake, metabolism, clearance, and response. At the present time over 30 gene variations that can affect the way individuals respond to different drugs are known. Understanding these genetic variations can help determine the best drug and optimal dosing for individual patients.

3. *Candidate genes for disease susceptibility.* Many human medical conditions occur as the result of specific individual genetic differences (polymorphisms) that invoke a specific

susceptibility to that condition. Often interactions with the right environmental trigger(s) can elicit the onset of the disorder.

4. *Single nucleotide polymorphisms (SNPs).* Minor variations in short DNA sequences have been linked to the occurrence of particular diseases. Numerous SNPs have been reported to associate with an increased risk of common diseases. SNPs may be identified rapidly and in large numbers using microchip technology. These tests typically scan 500,000 to 1,000,000 SNPs, although the clinical significance is known for only a small percentage. For those in which the significance is known, physicians can create a disease risk profile for individual patients.

Personalized genomics is ushering in a new role for the patient and blurring the lines of the traditional doctor to patient relationship. For instance, the first commercially available SNP chips for disease susceptibility predictions were introduced in 2007 with direct-to-consumer (DTC) marketing. This system of bypassing the health care provider and providing a direct link from the consumer to the genetics laboratory has raised a number of fascinating ethical and practical questions.

Lastly, the question remains as to how close these technologies are to truly helping prevent or ameliorate disease. While the pace of information development may be occurring at an extremely rapid rate, there are competing forces that are appropriately slowing down the introduction of these services in an effort to guarantee consumer safety. In this light, validation and incorporation of new genetic testing products and new bioinformatics in standard clinical practice will take years to decades.

■ Board-Format Practice Questions

1. In reference to a "genome"
   A. the term exclusively refers to DNA that is found in the nucleus.
   B. it is the genetic information needed to code for the development of an individual.
   C. it can be defined in terms of the protein content of an individual's cells.
   D. the genome size and the amount of information coded typically have a 1:1 correlation.
   E. is the small person who lives underground and hoards treasure.

2. The Human Genome Project
   A. gave a best estimate of 100,000 as the total number of functioning human genes.
   B. has identified a much greater diversity of the genetics among different species than expected.
   C. is completed and has identified the sequence of all human genetic conditions.
   D. made a concerted effort to address ethical and social issues associated with the information generated.
   E. in general has kept the information it generated locked up and away from public access.

3. Personalized medicine
   A. is likely to drive up medical costs if implemented.
   B. is a theoretical type of practice that may have future applications in clinical practice.
   C. should have little impact on the diagnostic process.
   D. may be used to direct therapy or identify individual susceptibilities.
   E. should have application in the primary prevention of disorders.

4. Medical Genetics
   A. is a unique field that has relatively little interaction with other aspects of clinical medicine.
   B. is so new that it currently is not an officially recognized specialty.
   C. is the subset of human genetics that explores the genetic contributions to disease.
   D. as a medical practice is largely limited to defining syndromes.
   E. is better understood if catchy terms are applied to specific conditions or syndromes.

chapter 2

Information Flow and Levels of Regulation

CHAPTER SUMMARY

Deoxyribonucleic acid (DNA) is sometimes described as a "blueprint" for development. Although easy to visualize, that view is a damaging oversimplification. A blueprint defines the location of each element in a given structure. In contrast, genetic control of development is much more dynamic. A better description for the role of DNA is as a "recipe for interactions." DNA codes for the assembly of proteins by way of a ribonucleic acid (RNA) intermediate, the messenger RNA (mRNA). But it is the interactions among the resulting proteins, other RNAs like microRNAs, and their feedback influences on the genome that will determine how cells, tissues, organs, and the body as a whole will take on its form and function.

As the ultimate information resource for biological processes, DNA is essential. But in many ways it is the simplest part of the development puzzle. In 1953, Watson and Crick proposed a model for the structure of DNA that has been confirmed by experiments to test predictions about processes like DNA replication during cell division. But knowing the structure of DNA does not explain how it works. Sequencing the human genome was also not the final answer. Instead, knowing the genome's DNA structure leads to a higher level of questions. How is DNA organized into genes that control the activities of a cell to create individual phenotypes? How do genes influence each other? How do proteins interact with each other to form networks of biochemical change? How do functional pathways and feedback loops influence the organism at a level beyond the simple turning-on of a gene? Answering questions like these is the focus of new fields like genomics, bioinformatics, proteomics, and metabolomics. Furthermore, genes do not work in isolation from their cellular and developmental environment. What roles do environmental variables like temperature play in forming a trait?

Building from that perspective, we can think of our development as the product of a molecular storm. Storms may be influenced by rules, but the rules are often complex and random events can be influential. Rather than genes providing a simple blueprint, the unfolding of each step in development is actually the result of hundreds, if not thousands, of different molecular interactions. This perspective is introduced here but will be explored in detail in later chapters. DNA is only the beginning.

Part 1: Background and Systems Integration

From DNA to Protein: the Central Dogma of Molecular Biology

A dictionary definition of "dogma" is that it is information presented as an established opinion or an authoritative view, but without significant grounds of support. In that sense, the Central Dogma of Molecular Biology is famously misnamed. The flow of information it describes is extensively supported by experimental evidence. Still, it compactly summarizes the unifying theme of molecular genetics: DNA $\leftrightarrow$ RNA $\rightarrow$ polypeptide (Figure 2-1). The nucleotides that make up a region of DNA are transcribed into a complementary strand of RNA that is then translated into a strand of amino acids, a polypeptide. A large polypeptide is called a protein.

One portion of this information flow is reversible in special circumstances. Retroviruses that utilize RNA as their

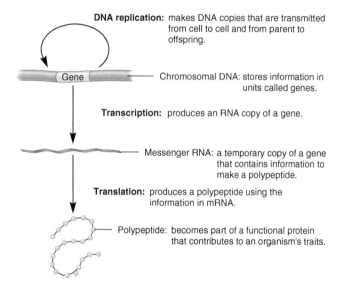

DNA replication: makes DNA copies that are transmitted from cell to cell and from parent to offspring.

Gene

Chromosomal DNA: stores information in units called genes.

Transcription: produces an RNA copy of a gene.

Messenger RNA: a temporary copy of a gene that contains information to make a polypeptide.

Translation: produces a polypeptide using the information in mRNA.

Polypeptide: becomes part of a functional protein that contributes to an organism's traits.

Figure 2-1. The Central Dogma is a unifying theme of molecular biology. (Reprinted with permission from Brooker RJ: *Genetics: Analysis & Principles*, 3rd ed. New York: McGraw-Hill, 2008.)

genetic material use **reverse transcriptase** to create a DNA copy that can integrate into the host's genome so it is transmitted to daughter cells during cell division. The other step, translation of the RNA sequence into protein, is not reversible. This provides a molecular argument against the early evolutionary hypothesis by Jean-Baptiste Lamarck that traits acquired during an organism's lifetime, such as modifications through use or lack of use, can become heritable. The "inheritance of acquired characters" was a powerful idea that competed with later Mendelian genetic models and was even promoted by Trofim Lysenko, with strong political support, to the serious detriment of Russian agriculture as late as the 1960s.

But biology is complex and can sometimes hide surprises. We know that the biochemical process of protein synthesis on ribosomes is not reversible, so altering a protein or other body part does not change the heritable DNA. Acquired traits cannot be passed to offspring that way. But recent advances in our understanding of the biochemistry of DNA suggest that there might be important exceptions to this rule. Some regulatory mechanisms may leave an imprint on chromosomal DNA that can alter its later activity. In such a case some acquired conditions can influence development in later generations, an idea that is being explored further.

The outline of the Central Dogma came about by recognizing that the genome in the nucleus is physically separated from the site of protein synthesis on ribosomes in the cytoplasm. There must be some intermediary molecule that Francis Crick labeled a "messenger," and mRNA was soon discovered. But the existence of an intermediary like mRNA has other far-reaching implications. In cells with a membrane barrier between DNA and the site of protein synthesis, there are opportunities for several levels of regulation that dramatically increase the potential coding power and flexibility of the genome.

Importance of Having a Nuclear Membrane

Prokaryotes like bacteria differ from eukaryotes (animals, plants, fungi, and most single-cell organisms) in several ways (Figure 2-2). But their names indicate one of the most important differences. The term "prokaryote" literally means "before a nucleus," and "eukaryote" means "true nucleus." In prokaryotes, the DNA and other cell components are in the same cellular space, so an mRNA molecule might still be forming when its first part begins binding with ribosomes to start protein synthesis. The connection between transcription and translation is immediate. Eukaryotic cells, on the other hand, have a double membrane separating the chromosomes from other parts of the cell. This creates two functional domains, the nuclear and the cytoplasmic. Eukaryotes also have an array of other important membranous organelles that will be a focus of our later discussions. Among these, mitochondria even have their own DNA. But the nuclear envelope offers a key element in the genetic regulation of biochemical expression. By physically separating the process of transcription from translation, eukaryotic cells are able to modify the initial RNA transcript in various ways before the mature mRNA molecules are transported out of the nucleus. This simple separation of functions thus allows a potentially large expansion of the possible polypeptides that can be produced by each original gene in eukaryotes. It helps explain how the 100,000 or more proteins expressed in a human can be produced by a surprisingly smaller number of genes.

Opportunities for Regulation

The formation of a protein is ultimately encoded in the sequence of nucleotides in a molecule of DNA. But the steps between these points allow many opportunities to influence the outcome (Figure 2-3). By "turning-on" a gene, we simply mean that enzymes and regulatory proteins are activated to synthesize a molecule of RNA using one of the two DNA complementary strands as a template. This initial RNA molecule is then modified in several ways to become a functional mRNA. Certain sequences, **introns**, are spliced out of the initial transcript leaving behind the coding sequences, **exons**, in the mature mRNA. But alternative splicing of introns can result in several slightly different versions of mRNA, so one gene can yield several related products, depending on the cell type or developmental stage. The mRNA is then exported through pores in the nuclear membrane with protein complexes that control the traffic of this and other large molecules between the nuclear and the cytoplasmic domains.

In the cytoplasm, the mRNA binds with ribosome subunits to initiate protein synthesis. Competition among mRNAs, variation in RNA longevity, and temporary inactivation or silencing by microRNAs or other agents can influence how quickly and for how long each type of mRNA will function. But influences on the gene product can occur even after translation. The polypeptide produced at the ribosome

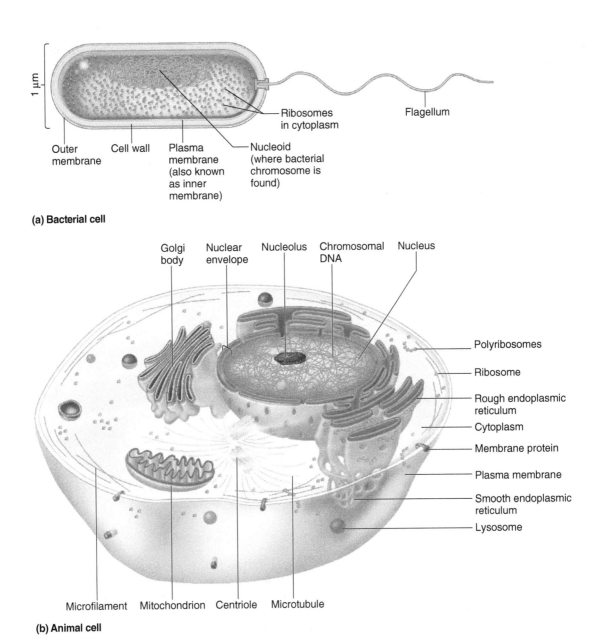

(a) **Bacterial cell**

(b) **Animal cell**

Figure 2-2. The eukaryotic cell has many membranous organelles that influence the way genetic-coded information is processed and expressed. The prokaryotic cell lacks membrane-bound organelles. (Reprinted with permission from Brooker RJ: *Genetics: Analysis & Principles*, 3rd ed. New York: McGraw-Hill, 2008.)

may be active immediately as a structural protein or enzyme. But in many cases a protein is initially inactive until it is activated by some external inducer molecule or it binds with other polypeptides to form a higher-order complex. One example is an inactive proteolytic enzyme, pepsinogen, that is activated into pepsin by hydrochloric acid in the stomach so it does not prematurely digest the proteins in the cell that made it. Thus, there are many opportunities for regulation or intervention in the events between gene and protein. The information flow from a gene to a final phenotype is a network of interactions.

The genetic codes of prokaryotes and eukaryotes are fundamentally similar, and many of the biochemical processes involved in DNA replication and genetic control have parallels that make prokaryotes excellent models with which to

study more complex eukaryotic mechanisms. Much of what we know about DNA replication, transcription, and translation comes from these simpler systems. In the next sections we will outline some of the key events in each process as seen in prokaryotes and point out some ways in which eukaryotes like humans may differ.

DNA Replication

In Chapter 1, we introduced DNA as a double-stranded molecule, a polymer composed of nucleotide subunits. Several characteristics of this helical molecule are important to keep in mind when exploring its replication (Figure 2-4). Each nucleotide carries one of the four nitrogenous bases: adenine

**REGULATION OF
GENE EXPRESSION**

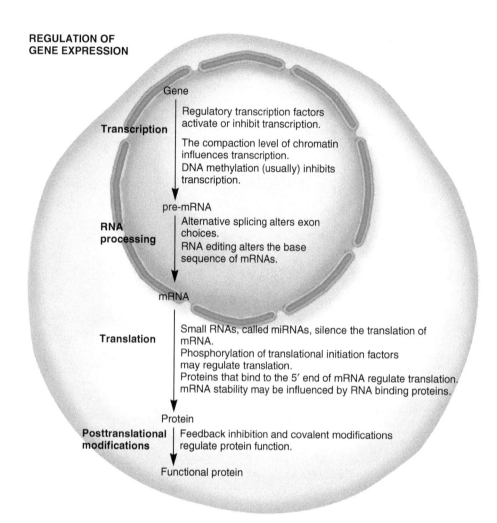

Gene

Transcription

Regulatory transcription factors
activate or inhibit transcription.

The compaction level of chromatin
influences transcription.
DNA methylation (usually) inhibits
transcription.

pre-mRNA

**RNA
processing**

Alternative splicing alters exon
choices.
RNA editing alters the base
sequence of mRNAs.

mRNA

Translation

Small RNAs, called miRNAs, silence the translation of
mRNA.
Phosphorylation of translational initiation factors
may regulate translation.
Proteins that bind to the 5′ end of mRNA regulate translation.
mRNA stability may be influenced by RNA binding proteins.

Protein

**Posttranslational
modifications**

Feedback inhibition and covalent modifications
regulate protein function.

Functional protein

Figure 2-3. The regulation of gene
expression involves determining which
genes are transcribed as well as the
various ways the initial transcripts
are processed. Regulation also takes
place during translation and modifications that can occur in the protein
products. (Reprinted with permission from
Brooker RJ: *Genetics: Analysis & Principles*, 3rd
ed. New York: McGraw-Hill, 2008.)

(A) and guanine (G) are purines, and thymine (T) and cytosine (C) are pyrimidines. Nucleotides have an important directional asymmetry based upon the way subunit components attach to the 5-carbon sugar, deoxyribose. The nitrogenous base is attached to the 1′ carbon, a phosphoric acid group is attached to the 5′ carbon, and there is a hydroxyl (-OH) group on the 3′ carbon. **DNA polymerases** are the enzymes that link nucleotides together to form a single strand. They are only able to add a new nucleotide to a preexisting 3′ OH sugar group. They catalyze the formation of a covalent bond between the 3′ carbon of an existing nucleotide and the phosphoric acid group attached to the 5′ carbon of the new nucleotide, creating a sugar-phosphate backbone with bases at regular intervals. In such a strand, the "earliest" carbon is the 5′ carbon of the first nucleotide, and the newest position is the 3′ carbon of the last nucleotide. In other words, a strand of DNA grows in the 5′ to 3′ direction.

Another key factor is the way hydrogen bonds are formed between nucleotide bases. Adenine only binds to thymine, using two hydrogen bonds; and cytosine only binds to guanine, using three hydrogen bonds. For that reason, the proportion of A is the same as T in double-stranded DNA, and G is the same as C. This relationship, known as Chargaff's rule, can be presented in several different ways, such as A = T and G = C, or A + G = T + C (indicating there is one purine for

each pyrimidine). In the double-stranded DNA molecule, the sugar-phosphate backbones of the complementary strands are antiparallel. One is oriented 5′ to 3′ and the opposite strand is oriented 3′ to 5′. These orientations are important both to the process of replication and to the mechanism for identifying and transcribing genes in the proper sequence during development.

The DNA helix is not a uniform spiral. It has a major and a minor groove. In the major groove, the DNA bases are in contact with water, and proteins that regulate gene action can bind there. To replicate a double-stranded molecule, it is first necessary to separate it into two single-strands to serve as templates for new synthesis (Figure 2-5). But DNA is an alpha-helix. If you have ever tried to pull apart the individual strands of a twisted rope, you will realize that separating the twisted strands generates supercoiling of the remaining part. The occurrence of supercoiling and the fact that strands grow at only the 3′ end of the antiparallel single-strand templates means that the replication of DNA has special challenges. Some of the main enzymes responsible for replication are shown in (Figure 2-6), which diagrams the events at one **replication fork**. Of special note is the fact that once the hydrogen bonds have been broken by DNA helicase and the single strands are stably separated by single-strand binding proteins to form two complementary

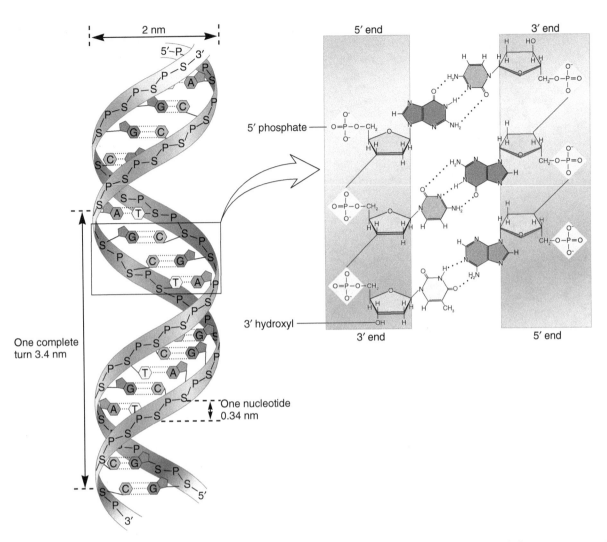

Figure 2-4. The DNA double helix is composed of two antiparallel nucleotide strands oriented in opposite 3′-5′ directions to each other. There are about 10 base pairs in each 360° turn of the alpha helix. (Reprinted with permission from Brooker RJ: *Genetics: Analysis & Principles*, 3rd ed. New York: McGraw-Hill, 2008.)

templates, a short RNA sequence, a **primer**, is laid down by primase. DNA polymerase III (Figure 2-7) can use the 3′-OH position of an RNA nucleotide as a point for attaching the first DNA nucleotide. Replication at this fork occurs in opposite directions on the two template strands.

On the **leading strand**, where the template is oriented with the 5′ end nearest the replication fork, synthesis of a new complementary strand can be continuous because it adds nucleotides at the 3′ end. But on the **lagging strand**, synthesis occurs in discontinuous bursts as new template is opened by the DNA helicase (Figure 2-8) with creation of periodic RNA primer sequences. This results in short sequences, **Okazaki fragments**, of about 1000 to 2000 nucleotides long in bacteria and about 100 to 200 nucleotides long in eukaryotes. To complete synthesis on the lagging strand, therefore, the RNA primers must be removed, DNA nucleotides must replace them, and the final covalent bond must be formed between adjacent fragments. In bacteria, DNA polymerase I removes the primers and inserts DNA nucleotides. DNA ligase catalyzes the final covalent bond.

Some of the enzymes involved in replication are part of a larger complex (Figure 2-9). DNA helicase and primase are bound together as a primosome which separates the parental strands and creates RNA primers spaced along the lagging strand. Linking the proteins helps coordinate their functions more efficiently. The primosome, in turn, is associated with two molecules of DNA polymerase III, one for the leading and one for the lagging strand. This complex is the **replisome**. When the polymerase on the lagging strand completes an Okazaki fragment, it is released from the template and jumps to the next nearest RNA primer to begin again. Although highly accurate, there is some error in all of these processes, and indeed error-prone enzymes are the source of enhanced mutation associated with certain genetic diseases. But many of the errors are detected and corrected during and soon after replication. Repair systems will be discussed in Chapter 7.

The understanding of replication discussed so far comes from studies in simple prokaryotes. Although the biochemistry of eukaryotic DNA replication is not as well understood,

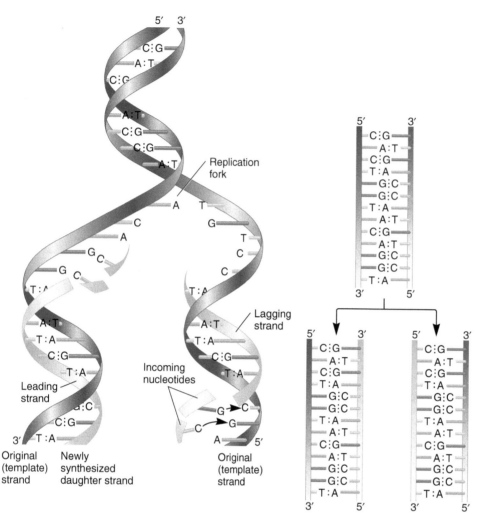

Figure 2-5. The replication of DNA is semi-conservative, or "half saved." Each of the two strands of the original DNA molecule serves as a single-strand template for the synthesis of a new complementary strand. Thus, in the next generation, half of the DNA double helix is directly from the original and half is new. (Reprinted with permission from Brooker RJ: *Genetics: Analysis & Principles*, 3rd ed. New York: McGraw-Hill, 2008.)

(a) The mechanism of DNA replication

(b) The products of replication

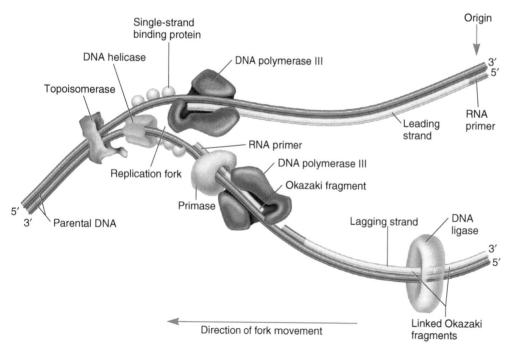

Figure 2-6. DNA replication involves many proteins. DNA helicase unwinds the double-stranded molecule; topoisomerase relaxes the supercoiling that is generated by this unwinding; single-strand binding proteins keep the complementary strands from reassociating with each other; primase forms a short RNA sequence on which DNA polymerase III can attach new DNA nucleotides; and DNA ligase links together the short DNA fragments, the Okazaki fragments, that are formed by replication on the strands in which the 3' end is nearest the replication fork. (Reprinted with permission from Brooker RJ: *Genetics: Analysis & Principles*, 3rd ed. New York: McGraw-Hill, 2008.)

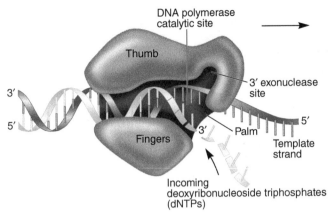

(a) Schematic side view of DNA polymerase III

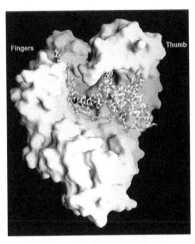

(b) Molecular model for DNA polymerase bound to DNA

Figure 2-7. Diagram of the events that occur when DNA polymerase III moves along the template toward its 5′ end, adding nucleotides to the 3′ end of the new strand. (Reprinted with permission from Ying Li et al: Crystal structures of open and closed forms of binary and ternary complexes of the large fragment of *Thermus aquaticus* DNA polymerase I: structural basis for nucleotide incorporation. *Embo J.* 1998; 17:24, 7514-7525.)

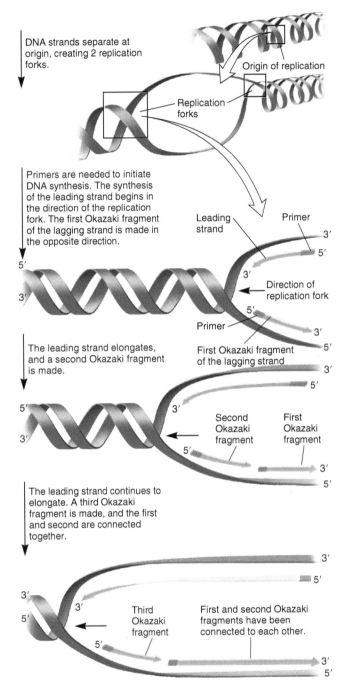

Figure 2-8. Events at a replication fork during DNA synthesis. (Reprinted with permission from Brooker RJ: *Genetics: Analysis & Principles*, 3rd ed. New York: McGraw-Hill, 2008.)

there are many similarities with that in prokaryotes. A comparable array of enzymes is involved, but the process is more complex. One obvious difference comes from the vastly larger size of the eukaryotic genome. In bacteria, there is a single origin with replication proceeding bidirectionally along two forks that eventually meet around the circular bacterial chromosome. Eukaryotic chromosomes are much longer DNA strands and are linear. Multiple origins of replication are required for the process to occur rapidly (Figure 2-10). Like prokaryotic origins of replication, those identified so far in eukaryotes have a high proportion of A and T bases. With two, rather than three, hydrogen bonds in an A-T pair, enzymes can separate these regions into single-strand templates more easily.

In eukaryotes a **prereplication complex** of at least 14 proteins is required to begin replication at an origin site. In addition, eukaryotes have many different DNA polymerases;

mammals have over a dozen. Some of these appear to function in error correction and in repairing various kinds of DNA damage. A final major difference between circular bacterial versus linear eukaryotic strands is the need to handle replication at the ends of a chromosome. Since DNA polymerase must have a preexisting 3′-OH nucleotide to which to attach the first DNA nucleotide, it cannot replicate the initial 3′ end of the chromosome since there is no place for a primer to be synthesized for it. Even if a primer is placed at the tip, the

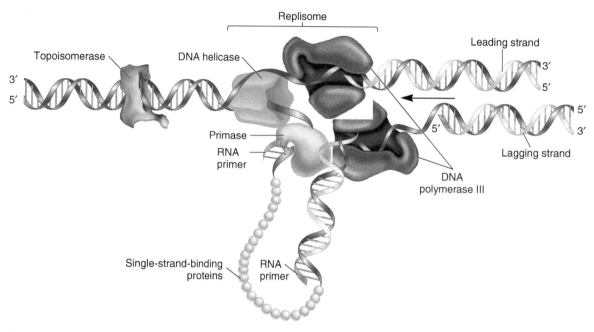

Figure 2-9. During DNA replication, the helicase and primase form a primosome, which associates with two molecules of DNA polymerase III. One of these synthesizes a new strand continuously on the leading strand, but the other synthesizes new fragments in discontinuous bursts on the lagging strand. The primosome plus the two polymerases makeup the replisome. (Reprinted with permission from Brooker RJ: *Genetics: Analysis & Principles,* 3rd ed. New York: McGraw-Hill, 2008.)

DNA polymerase cannot replace the most distal RNA nucleotides with DNA nucleotides without an earlier 3′-OH to link with. To keep the coding region of DNA from becoming shorter at each replication cycle, eukaryotic chromosomes have tandemly-repeated sequences (TTAGGG in humans repeated 250 to 1,500 times) in a region called a **telomere** at each end (Figure 2-11). This extra DNA provides a site for primer formation and avoids chromosome shortening into the information-coding DNA.

Manipulation of DNA Replication: the Polymerase Chain Reaction

Many techniques of molecular biology depend on having pure samples of a specific piece of DNA. This is now routinely accomplished by a manipulation of the process of DNA replication, the polymerase chain reaction (PCR) (Figure 2-12). As we have just seen, replication requires a single-stranded DNA template, primers to provide the 3′-OH group to which a new nucleotide can

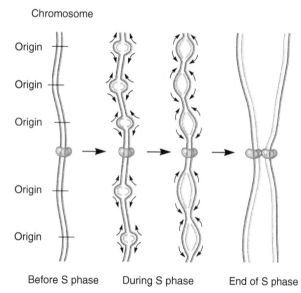

(a) DNA replication from multiple origins of replication

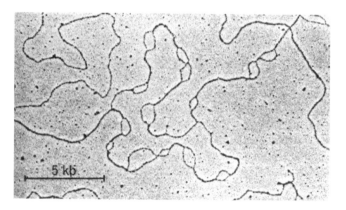

(b) A micrograph of a replicating eukaryotic chromosome

Figure 2-10. The large eukaryotic genome requires multiple replication forks that originate during the S phase of interphase prior to mitosis or meiosis. (Reprinted with permission from Brooker RJ: *Genetics: Analysis & Principles,* 3rd ed. New York: McGraw-Hill, 2008.)

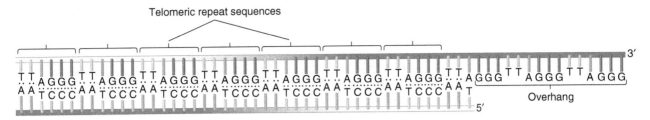

Figure 2-11. Telomeres at each end of a eukaryotic chromosome are made up of tandemly duplicated sequences and a short overhang. (Reprinted with permission from Brooker RJ: *Genetics: Analysis & Principles*, 3rd ed. New York: McGraw-Hill, 2008.)

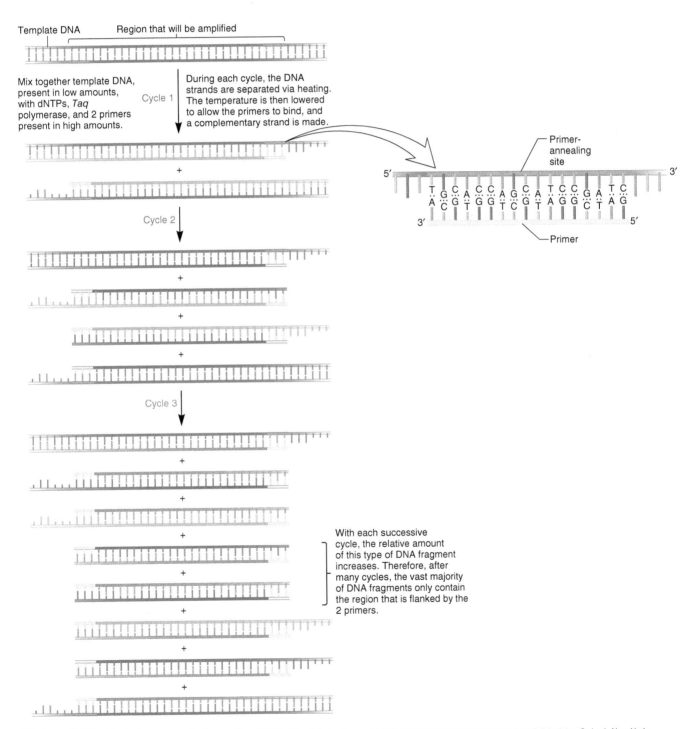

Figure 2-12. The polymerase chain reaction (PCR). (Reprinted with permission from Brooker RJ: *Genetics: Analysis & Principles*, 3rd ed. New York: McGraw-Hill, 2008.)

attach, DNA polymerase, and the four nucleotide triphosphates. The primers are commercially-prepared nucleotide sequences, or **oligonucleotides**, typically about 18 to 22 bases long that flank the region to be amplified. Primers are easily made to order for researchers interested in any particular region of the genome. During PCR, these components in an appropriately buffered solution are manipulated by repeated cycles of heating and cooling to amplify the targeted DNA region.

A small amount of genomic DNA is first heated to 94°C-95°C to separate the double helix into single strands. The reaction is then cooled to a temperature between 52°C and 58°C or slightly higher, which has been predetermined as optimal for hybridizing the two primers to the single-strand templates. After 30 seconds to a minute, temperature is increased to 72°C at which a heat-resistant DNA polymerase from *Thermus aquaticus* (*Taq* polymerase, isolated from a bacterium adapted to living in hot springs) extends the new strand for as much as 1000 bases or so. Temperature is then cooled. This heating and cooling cycle can be repeated, often 25 to 35 times, yielding a large number of copies of the targeted DNA sample. The use of heat-adapted *Taq* polymerase means that the enzyme is not destroyed each time the reaction is heated to 94°C-95°C to melt the DNA.

Transcription and RNA Processing

Transcription is the process of synthesizing a single-stranded RNA molecule from an active gene, literally "transcribing" a copy of the genetic message. The molecular signals that actually initiate the process will be part of our discussion of development and pattern formation in Chapter 3. Here we will focus upon the events that yield the initial RNA transcript and will introduce some of the processes that modify this transcript into one or more functionally-related mature mRNA molecules.

Transcription (Figure 2-13) can be divided conveniently into three phases: initiation of transcription, elongation of the RNA transcript, and termination. Recognition of the beginning of a gene involves the action of **transcription factors**, which are DNA-binding proteins that assist **RNA polymerase** to bind to a **promoter**, a specific sequence of nucleotides upstream from the beginning of the gene's coding region (Figure 2-14). Other transcription factors can bind short nucleotide sequences near the promoter and either enhance or inhibit the rate of transcription. RNA polymerase begins synthesizing an RNA strand starting at the promoter, so each transcript has a stretch of nucleotides before coming to the ones that are eventually translated into the polypeptide.

The transcription factors and RNA polymerase bind to the DNA double helix and must open it to expose the single-strand that will serve as the template for RNA synthesis. In bacteria, the RNA polymerase core enzyme is composed of five subunits, and a sixth protein, the sigma factor (σ, (Figure 2-15), completes the RNA polymerase **holoenzyme** and assists it to recognize the promoter sequence. Synthesis

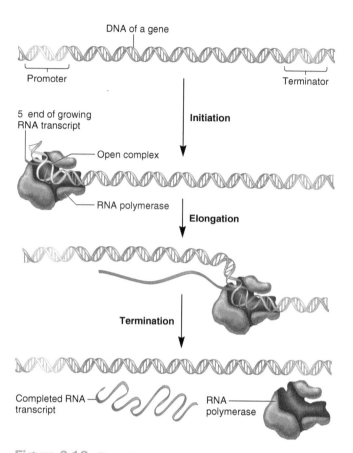

Figure 2-13. Transcription has three stages: initiation, elongation of the RNA transcript, and termination. (Reprinted with permission from Brooker RJ: *Genetics: Analysis & Principles*, 3rd ed. New York: McGraw-Hill, 2008.)

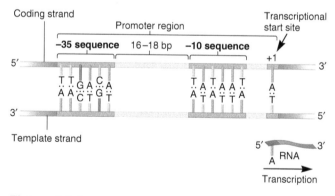

Figure 2-14. The bacterial promoter region, identified by the consensus −35 and −10 sequences shown. The 5′-TATAAT-3′ sequence is sometimes called the Pribnow box. (Reprinted with permission from Brooker RJ: *Genetics: Analysis & Principles*, 3rd ed. New York: McGraw-Hill, 2008.)

occurs as RNA polymerase moves along the template strand and catalyzes the insertion of an RNA nucleotide complementary to the template DNA sequence (Figure 2-16). A pairing similar to that in replication occurs, except that uracil (U) is attached in place of thymine, so when the template presents an

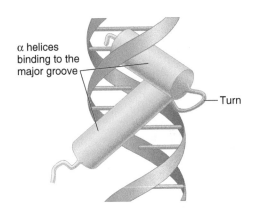

Figure 2-15. The σ factor illustrates how proteins that facilitate transcription interact with the DNA double helix. DNA has a major and a minor groove. The σ factor protein is composed of two α-helices connected by a turn, called a helix-turn-helix motif. The amino acids in the α-helices bond with nucleotide bases in the major groove. (Reprinted with permission from Brooker RJ: *Genetics: Analysis & Principles*, 3rd ed. New York: McGraw-Hill, 2008.)

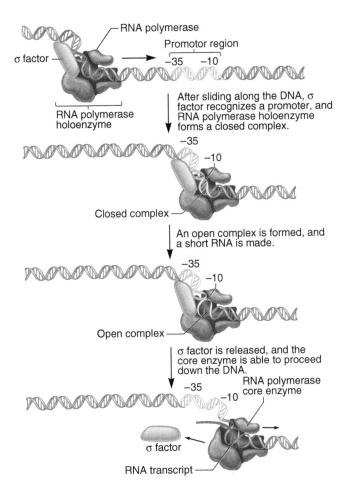

Figure 2-16. The initiation of bacterial transcription. The σ factor helps RNA polymerase recognize the promoter region, and the open complex makes one DNA strand available as a template for RNA synthesis. (Reprinted with permission from Brooker RJ: *Genetics: Analysis & Principles*, 3rd ed. New York: McGraw-Hill, 2008.)

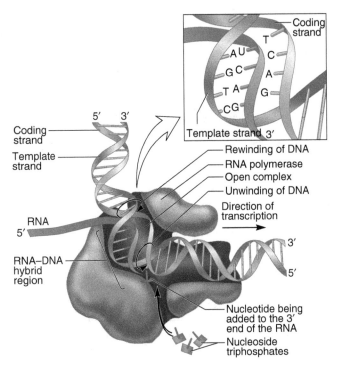

Figure 2-17. Key events in the synthesis of an RNA transcript. (Reprinted with permission from Brooker RJ: *Genetics: Analysis & Principles*, 3rd ed. New York: McGraw-Hill, 2008.)

A, the RNA transcript will add a U to the 3′ end of the growing chain (Figure 2-17).

Special cases are known like overlapping genes that share the use of portions of the same DNA sequence and nested genes that use different parts of the same sequence in separate transcription cycles. But typically, transcription can be thought of as using only one of the two strands as a template. The template strand is defined by the nucleotide sequence of the promoter and regulatory gene regions. Along an extended stretch of DNA, one strand may be the template for gene #1 and be transcribed let us say to the right, and further along the other strand might be the template for gene #2 and be transcribed to the left. The key is the 5′ to 3′ nucleotide sequences of the transcription signals.

Nucleotides are added to the RNA transcript at the 3′-OH end, just as in DNA replication. The template strand is, therefore, being read in the 3′ to 5′ direction, since the RNA is antiparallel to the DNA template and is growing at the 3′ end. One consequence of this is that the unused complementary DNA strand, often called the **coding strand** or **sense strand**, has the same nucleotide sequence as the RNA being formed, except that RNA has uracil (U) wherever the DNA had thymine (T). For that reason, publications often present a gene by showing the nucleotide sequence of the sense strand rather than the template strand that is actually being used, making it easy to convert the information into a form in which amino acid content can be determined mentally.

The overview we have presented of transcription in prokaryotes has direct parallels in eukaryotes, although there is

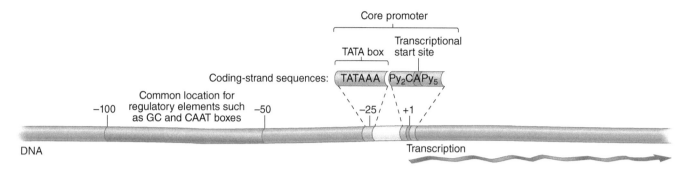

Figure 2-18. Representative elements of the promoter for structural genes in eukaryotes, which are typically more complex and variable than in prokaryotes. For structural genes recognized by the eukaryotic RNA polymerase II, there are sites at which regulatory elements bind, a TATA box, and a start site for transcription. The start site is typically an adenine with a cytosine and two pyrimidines before it and five after it. The promoters for other RNA polymerase differ from this pattern. (Reprinted with permission from Brooker RJ: *Genetics: Analysis & Principles*, 3rd ed. New York: McGraw-Hill, 2008.)

greater variation among promoter sequences and a larger role for a range of regulatory elements. Transcription begins when RNA polymerase II, general transcription factors, and a mediator bind to a promoter sequence (Figure 2-18). With typically 12 subunits in RNA polymerase II, 5 general transcription factors, and a mediator with multiple subunits, this is a complex in every sense of the word (Figure 2-19). Another complication in eukaryotes is that the chromosome has its DNA wrapped around histone protein complexes, the **nucleosomes**. The chromatin must be remodeled to remove the nucleosomes before transcription can proceed. Chromatin remodeling and related issues will be discussed when we explore chromosome structure in more depth in Chapter 5.

RNA Processing in the Nucleus

Ribonucleic acid is processed in various ways before the final molecule is ready for use by the cell. For example, in some cases, a long transcript is cleaved into smaller pieces, such as in the production of **ribosomal RNA** (rRNA) or **transfer RNA** (tRNA) molecules created from a region of a chromosome where their structures are tandemly repeated many times.

As mentioned earlier, the coding portion of a typical eukaryotic gene is interrupted by intervening sequences that occur between those that will eventually define the content of an mRNA. The initial RNA transcript, sometimes called **heterogeneous nuclear RNA** (hnRNA) is processed to cleave out the non-coding intervening sequences, the **introns**, leaving behind the coding part of the mRNA molecule, the exons. Introns are removed by a spliceosome, composed of subunits called snRNPs, **small nuclear ribonucleoproteins**. These RNA plus protein complexes bind splice sites at the edges of an intron, cut the DNA, attach the adjacent exons, and remove the intron in the form of a lariat (Figure 2-20). Different cell types may not splice the introns in exactly the same way, causing **alternative splicing** that can yield slightly modified versions of the protein in different tissues.

The ends of the mRNA are also modified in the nucleus by adding a cap of 7-methylguanosine to the 5′ end (Figure 2-21)

and a string of adenine nucleotides as a **poly-A tail** to the 3′ end. The 5′ cap is recognized by cap-binding proteins that may be required for proper export of the mRNA from the nucleus, and the cap is recognized by initiation factors to begin translation at the ribosome. The poly-A tail is important for mRNA stability.

Translation

Genetic information is translated from one molecular language to another, from nucleotides in DNA/RNA to amino acids in polypeptides, at the ribosomes in the cytoplasm. Like the process of transcription, translation can be viewed as a sequence of stages: initiation, elongation, and termination. The mRNA can be translated many times until it eventually breaks down and its nucleotides are recycled. The translator is a population of RNA molecules called transfer RNA (tRNA) that each carry one of the 20 naturally-occurring amino acids and cause their code-appropriate insertion into a growing polypeptide. The translation dictionary is the **Genetic Code**.

The 20 naturally-occurring amino acids have in common an amino (NH_2) group attached to a carbon and then to a carboxyl (O=C-OH) group (Figure 2-22). The group attached to the middle carbon of this nitrogen-carbon-carbon backbone affects the molecular behavior of its part of the polypeptide. During translation, amino acids are linked together by adding the next one to the carboxyl-end of the chain. Thus, polypeptides have an important asymmetry. The "earliest" amino acid in a growing chain has a free amino group (thus, the N-terminal), and the newest amino acid has a free carboxyl group (the C-terminal). The groups attached to the central carbons influence the 3-dimensional polypeptide shape and thus its function. For example, some side chains make the amino acid non-polar so they are less likely to intermix with water. They are hydrophobic, or "water fearing." Regions of a polypeptide with non-polar amino acids tend to coil toward the inner part of the folded chain, away from water. Polar amino acids, on the other hand, readily interact with polar water molecules. They are hydrophilic, or "water loving," and fold toward the outside in contact with the aquatic cytoplasm or intercellular fluid.

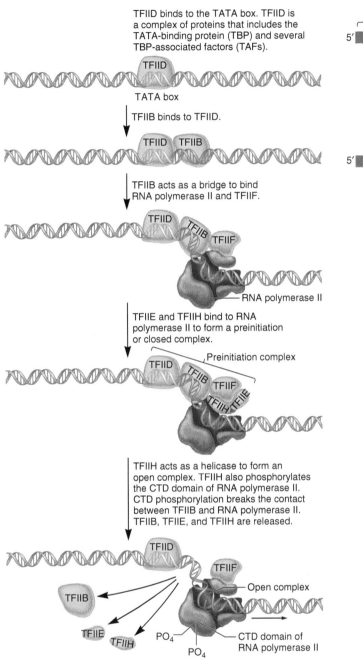

Figure 2-19. The events that occur in producing the open complex for transcription in eukaryotes. (Reprinted with permission from Brooker RJ: *Genetics: Analysis & Principles*, 3rd ed. New York: McGraw-Hill, 2008.)

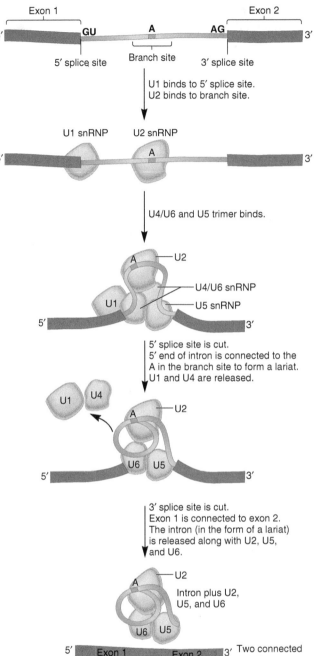

Figure 2-20. Removal of an intron by a spliceosome during RNA processing in the nucleus. (Reprinted with permission from Brooker RJ: *Genetics: Analysis & Principles*, 3rd ed. New York: McGraw-Hill, 2008.)

The information in the nucleotide sequence of mRNA is colinear with the order of amino acids in a polypeptide. In other words, there is a direct linear correspondence between the two molecular languages without gaps. During translation, nucleotides are read three at a time from a starting point near the 5′ end of the mRNA molecule. Such a triplet is called a **codon**. Each triplet is unambiguously associated with a specific amino acid carried by its corresponding tRNA molecule (Figure 2-23) to which it is attached by a covalent bond at the 3′ end. The appropriate amino acid

is covalently attached to the correct tRNA molecule by an aminoacyl-tRNA synthetase (Figure 2-24). Each type of tRNA molecule also has a loop with three nucleotides forming the **anticodon**, which is complementary, and antiparallel, to the three nucleotides of the mRNA codon. In that way, the codon binds the complementary anticodon of a specific tRNA carrying its specified amino acid (Figure 2-25). In effect, the tRNA molecules are the translators at a ribosome. By keeping track of the A with T (or U) and G with C complementary pairing of DNA and RNA nucleotides and the

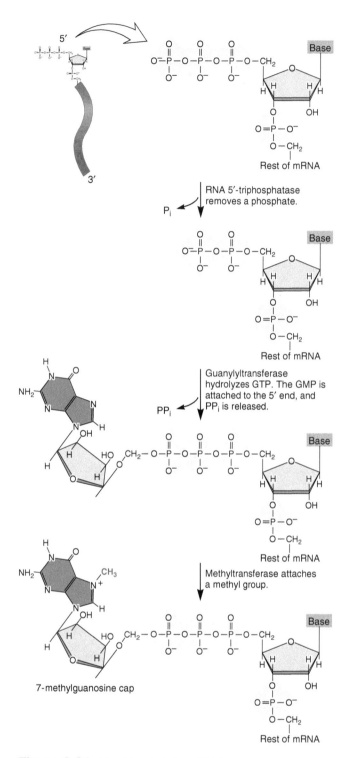

RNA 5′-triphosphatase removes a phosphate.

Guanylyltransferase hydrolyzes GTP. The GMP is attached to the 5′ end, and PP$_i$ is released.

Methyltransferase attaches a methyl group.

7-methylguanosine cap

Figure 2-21. The 5′ end of the mRNA is capped with 7-methylguanosine. (Reprinted with permission from Brooker RJ: *Genetics: Analysis & Principles*, 3rd ed. New York: McGraw-Hill, 2008.)

antiparallel 5′-3′ orientation of each nucleotide strand, one can trace the colinear alignment of genetic information from the double helix to its resultant polypeptide. For example, the 3′ end of the DNA template strand corresponds to the 5′ end of the mRNA, which in turn corresponds with the N-terminal end of the polypeptide. Catalytic RNAs that are part of the

ribosome structure link sequential amino acids into the growing polypeptide chain.

There are only four different nucleotides to account for 20 different amino acids in living cells. For that reason, a triplet code is the simplest possible translation vocabulary. If it were just a two-letter code, for example, there would be only 4^2 different combinations of the four nucleotides, yielding only 16 unique two-letter codons. In a three-letter code, there are $4^3 = 64$ different codons. At that level, however, there clearly must be some redundancy, called **degeneracy**, of the code, since there are more possible triplets than amino acids (Figure 2-26). Of the 64 possible triplets, three (UAA, UAG, and UGA) do not bind a tRNA molecule. Instead they are involved in terminating protein synthesis. There are, therefore, 61 **sense codons**, meaning that 61 triplets bind a tRNA anticodon and result in the addition of an amino acid during translation. Although it has a functional role in the process, the triplet AUG binds a Met-tRNA molecule and is, therefore, one of the sense codons.

In some cases six codons yield the same amino acid (such as leucine or serine). In other cases, four (proline and alanine), two (histidine and glutamine), or only one (methionine) possible codon is found. An examination of the codons within the same amino acid group reveals that it is the third nucleotide, the one in the 3′ position of the mRNA triplet, that primarily accounts for degeneracy of the Genetic Code. This is called the **wobble position** and is explained in part by the tolerance of some mismatched pairing in that position and the incorporation of modified bases into tRNA anticodon (Figure 2-27) that pair differently than the normal four bases. One consequence is that a cell does not need to produce 61 different types of tRNA to accommodate all of the sense codons, although new information about tRNA diversity in humans suggests it may be more extensive than previously thought.

The Genetic Code is almost universal. Few differences among organisms have been found. Among these, however, are differences in the code used in mammalian mitochondria, a cell organelle with its own DNA. For example, the triplet AUA usually codes for isoleucine, but it codes for methionine in mammalian mitochondria, and UGA codes for tryptophan rather than being a stop codon. But in general the near-universality of the Genetic Code is evidence for the continuity of life and is a boon for the use of model organisms to decipher its puzzles.

A key to understanding the process of protein synthesis rests in the ribosome and its active regions. Ribosomes are complexes with a small and a large subunit, each containing one or more types of ribosomal RNA (rRNA) and a large number of proteins (Figure 2-28). Most of the mass and important catalytic activity is associated with the RNA component. There is only one kind of ribosome in bacterial cells, but in eukaryotes, the structure of the main ribosomes, those found in the cytoplasm, differs from those found in the mitochondria (and in the chloroplasts of plant cells). The sizes of the rRNA and the subunits are described in terms of their rate of sedimentation under centrifugation. Svedberg units (S) are

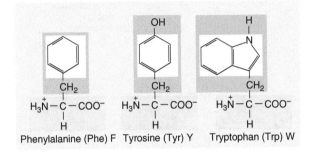

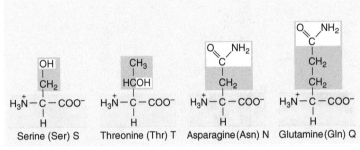

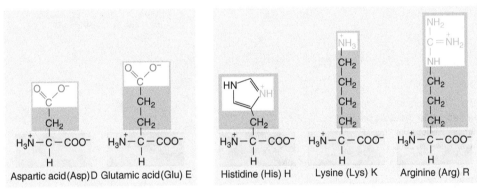

(a) Nonpolar, aliphatic amino acids

(b) Nonpolar, aromatic amino acids

(c) Polar, neutral amino acids

(d) Polar, acidic amino acids

(e) Polar, basic amino acids

Figure 2-22. Proteins contain 20 different amino acids that have chemical characteristics that contribute to protein structure.
(Reprinted with permission from Brooker RJ: *Genetics: Analysis & Principles*, 3rd ed. New York: McGraw-Hill, 2008.)

named after the inventor of the ultracentrifuge. The cytoplasmic ribosomes in a eukaryote have a 40S small subunit composed of an 18S rRNA and 33 proteins plus a 60S large subunit composed of 5S, 5.8S, and 28S rRNAs with 49 proteins. These two subunits are assembled at initiation to produce an 80S ribosome (Svedberg units are not simply additive) with several active sites. Bacterial ribosomes have a 30S small subunit and 50S large subunit.

An overview of events in protein synthesis is shown in Figure 2-29. The initiation of translation requires the assembly of a ribosome from its two subunits and binding with a molecule of mRNA and the initiator tRNA. Elongation of the polypeptide occurs when a triplet is drawn into the aminoacyl site (A site) of the ribosome and the amino acid it carries is covalently linked to the polypeptide carried by the tRNA in the peptidyl site (P site). The tRNA at the P site is released from the ribosome through the exit site (E site), and the ribosome brings the remaining tRNA into the P site by moving along the mRNA. This draws a new triplet into the A site. The process is repeated a few hundred times or more for an average size protein.

Termination occurs when a **stop codon** is brought into the A site. There the stop codon binds with a protein that acts as a release factor. Each type of tRNA molecule is recharged with its appropriate amino acid, and all components are reused until they break down.

With that overview of the process, we will now look at the events of initiation, elongation, and termination of protein synthesis in more detail. As before, these events will be described first for bacterial protein synthesis where they are perhaps best understood, and key features of eukaryotic protein synthesis will then be described.

The bacterial initiation complex (Figure 2-30) involves the small ribosomal subunit, the mRNA, three protein **initiation factors**, and the initiator tRNA that we will denote as fMet tRNA or tRNA^{fMet} (you may encounter different

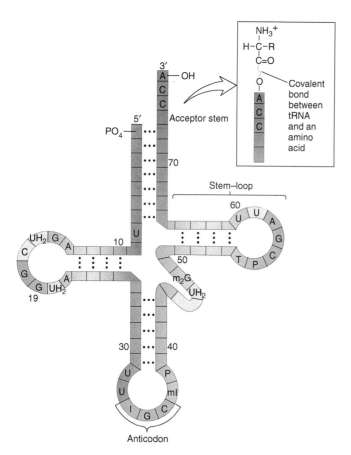

Figure 2-23. A schematic diagram of a tRNA molecule, showing the acceptor stem that binds an amino acid and the anticodon that binds a codon on mRNA. (Reprinted with permission from Brooker RJ: *Genetics: Analysis & Principles*, 3rd ed. New York: McGraw-Hill, 2008.)

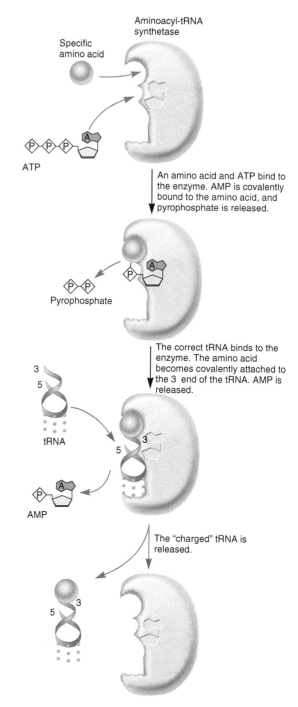

Figure 2-24. Aminoacyl-tRNA synthetase "charges" a tRNA molecule by catalyzing the attachment of the correct amino acid. (Reprinted with permission from Brooker RJ: *Genetics: Analysis & Principles*, 3rd ed. New York: McGraw-Hill, 2008.)

abbreviations in other references). This tRNA is a special form that carries a methionine amino acid covalently bound to a formyl-group that effectively blocks the amino end from forming bonds with another amino acid. It is only used at initiation and helps insure the unidirectional growth of the polypeptide at the C-terminal.

Bacterial mRNA contains a 9-nucleotide-long **ribosomal binding site** called the **Shine-Dalgarno sequence**. This facilitates binding of the mRNA to the small 30S ribosomal subunit, because it is complementary to a sequence of nucleotides in the rRNA molecule present there. Again we see that complementary base pairing is found throughout these processes. One of the initiation factors assists the binding of tRNA[fMet] to the start codon, which is usually AUG. After translation has been completed, the formyl group or the complete fMet may be removed from the protein, so methionine is not the first amino acid of every protein. Finally, initiation phases into elongation of the polypeptide when the large 50S ribosome subunit is attached to complete the protein synthesis workbench with its active A, P, and E sites.

Elongation begins when a charged tRNA, i.e., a tRNA molecule carrying its specified amino acid, binds to an mRNA codon at the A site of the ribosome (Figure 2-31). Accuracy of the codon-anticodon pairing is assisted by the **decoding**

function associated with the 16S rRNA in the small subunit. If mispairing occurs, elongation is halted until the mispaired tRNA leaves the A site. An uncorrected error in elongation occurs only about once per 10,000 amino acids. This level of accuracy is especially impressive when we note that elongation of a polypeptide chain occurs at a rate of approximately 15 to 18 amino acids per second in bacteria and about 6 per second in eukaryotes.

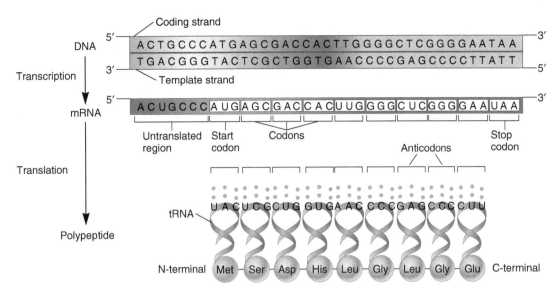

Figure 2-25. An overview of the relationships between the coding and template DNA strands, the mRNA, the tRNAs, and the polypeptide. (Reprinted with permission from Brooker RJ: *Genetics: Analysis & Principles*, 3rd ed. New York: McGraw-Hill, 2008.)

Second base

		U		C		A		G	
First base	**U**	U U U / U U C	Phenylalanine (Phe)	U C U / U C C	Serine (Ser)	U A U / U A C	Tyrosine (Tyr)	U G U / U G C	Cysteine (Cys)
		U U A / U U G	Leucine (Leu)	U C A / U C G		U A A / U A G	Stop codon / Stop codon	U G A / U G G	Stop codon / Tryptophan (Trp)
	C	C U U / C U C	Leucine (Leu)	C C U / C C C	Proline (Pro)	C A U / C A C	Histidine (His)	C G U / C G C	Arginine (Arg)
		C U A / C U G		C C A / C C G		C A A / C A G	Glutamine (Gln)	C G A / C G G	
	A	A U U / A U C / A U A	Isoleucine (Ile)	A C U / A C C	Threonine (Thr)	A A U / A A C	Asparagine (Asn)	A G U / A G C	Serine (Ser)
		A U G	Methionine (Met); start codon	A C A / A C G		A A A / A A G	Lysine (Lys)	A G A / A G G	Arginine (Arg)
	G	G U U / G U C	Valine (Val)	G C U / G C C	Alanine (Ala)	G A U / G A C	Aspartic acid (Asp)	G G U / G G C	Glycine (Gly)
		G U A / G U G		G C A / G C G		G A A / G A G	Glutamic acid (Glu)	G G A / G G G	

(Third base column: U, C, A, G for each row group)

Figure 2-26. The Genetic Code. (Reprinted with permission from Brooker RJ: *Genetics: Analysis & Principles*, 3rd ed. New York: McGraw-Hill, 2008.)

Figure 2-27. The wobble position is the third base of the 5′ to 3′ codon, which corresponds to the first base of the antiparallel anticodon. The tRNA can carry modified bases in addition to the normal A, U, G, and C. Examples are inosine (I), 5-methyl-2-thiouridine (xm⁵s²U), 5-methyl-2′-O-methyluridine (xm⁵Um), 2′-O-methyluridine (Um), 5-methyluridine; (xm⁵U), 5-hydroxyuridine (xo⁵U), and lysidine (k²C). The bases in parentheses are not well-recognized by tRNA. (Reprinted with permission from Brooker RJ: *Genetics: Analysis & Principles*, 3rd ed. New York: McGraw-Hill, 2008.)

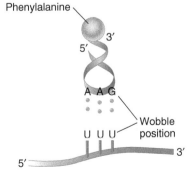

(a) Location of wobble position

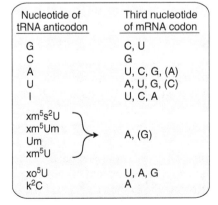

(b) Revised wobble rules

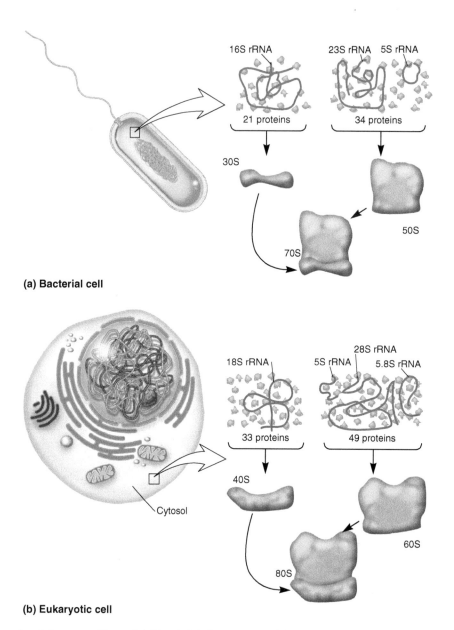

Figure 2-28. RNA and protein compositions of: (a) bacterial ribosomes; and (b) eukaryotic ribosomes. (Reprinted with permission from Brooker RJ: *Genetics: Analysis & Principles*, 3rd ed. New York: McGraw-Hill, 2008.)

Next, the peptide attached to the tRNA in the P site is transferred to the tRNA at the A site, and a covalent peptide bond is formed with the new amino acid. This peptidyl transfer is catalyzed by a component of the 50S subunit called **pepti-dyltransferase**, composed of rRNA and several proteins. It is actually the 23S rRNA that catalyzes the dehydration reaction to synthesize the peptide bond, an example of the enzymatic capability of RNA. The ribosome then translocates three nucleotides in the 3′ direction. This does two things. It moves the two tRNA molecules into the E and P sites, respectively, and it brings a new codon into the now-empty A site. The uncharged tRNA in the E site is released from the ribosome, and a new charged tRNA binds the codon in the A site. This process is repeated until one of the stop codons enters the A site.

In most organisms, the stop codons are UAA, UAG, and UGA. Instead of binding with a tRNA, they bind with proteins called **release factors** (Figure 2-32). The bond between the complete polypeptide attached to the tRNA in the P site is broken (hydrolyzed). The polypeptide and uncharged tRNA are released from the ribosome, then the ribosome disassembles into its subunits and a free mRNA. Components are reused until they degrade.

The translation process in eukaryotes parallels the bacterial events outlined here, but with some not-unexpected added complexity. Some translational proteins are conserved (i.e., found in both systems), but there are additional initiation factors in eukaryotes and only one release factor, compared to the three present in bacteria. Furthermore, eukaryotic mRNA

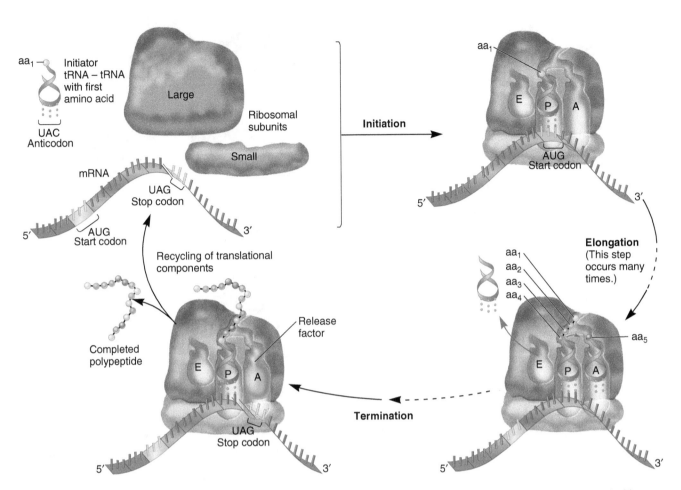

Figure 2-29. Summary of protein translation in bacteria: initiation, elongation, and termination. These stages are presented in more detail in Figures 2.31 to 2.33. (Reprinted with permission from Brooker RJ: *Genetics: Analysis & Principles*, 3rd ed. New York: McGraw-Hill, 2008.)

does not have a Shine-Dalgarno sequence. Instead, several initiation factors bind to the mRNA, one of which (cap-binding protein I, CBPI) recognizes the 5′ cap of 7-methylguanosine added in the nucleus during mRNA processing. These initiation factors also unwind any secondary folding that might be present in the mRNA and assists binding to the ribosome's 40S small subunit. Typically, translation uses the first AUG triplet in the 3′ direction as the start codon, although the sequence of flanking nucleotides plays an important role in scanning by the ribosome. One of the initiation factors helps to complete ribosome assembly by the addition of the 60S large subunit.

Factors Affecting Protein Shape and Function

The amino acid sequence of the gene product determines its function. But the relationship is not a straightforward one. The amino acid side chains have their own individual chemical characteristics. Individual amino acids or subregions of the polypeptide can also react with each other and with different domains in the cell, such as the aquatic cytosol or the non-polar membrane lipid bilayer. In addition, binding with other polypeptides or cofactors can influence shape and

function. For simplicity, it is helpful to begin by recognizing four general levels at which protein structure can be described (Figure 2-33).

The primary (1°) level of protein structure is the amino acid sequence. This is presented in the literature by listing the amino acid abbreviations or their one-letter codes (Figure 2-22) in sequential order from the N-terminal to the C-terminal. The secondary (2°) level derives from the way hydrogen bonds can create repeating shapes within some localized portions of a protein. There are two forms of secondary structure. The α-helix is a right-handed coil of the nitrogen-carbon-carbon backbone, and the β-pleated sheet is formed between parallel regions. Both are stabilized by hydrogen bonds between amino- and carboxyl-groups of different amino acids. When protein shape is denatured by heat or increased acidity, it is often these comparatively weak hydrogen bonds that are broken, causing the protein to fall into a random coil.

As it is synthesized, the polypeptide folds into a tertiary (3°) structure in which the three-dimensional shape determines many of its functional characteristics in the cell. Often other proteins, called **chaperones**, help produce the proper shape. Some proteins are long and fibrous, such as collagen and elastin that affect the strength and flexibility of connective tissue or actin that participates in cell movement.

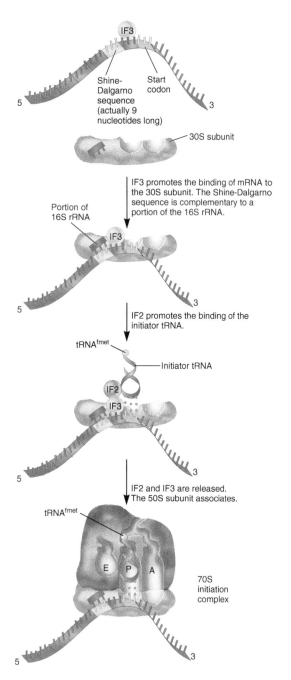

Figure 2-30. Bacterial translation: initiation. In addition to the 30S ribosome subunit, the mRNA with the 9 nucleotide long Shine-Dalgarno recognition sequence and AUG start codon, three initiation factors (IF) are required. The initiator tRNA carries the modified formyl-Methionine (f-Met) amino acid, and the initiation complex is complete when the 50S ribosome subunit becomes attached. (Reprinted with permission from Brooker RJ: *Genetics: Analysis & Principles*, 3rd ed. New York: McGraw-Hill, 2008.)

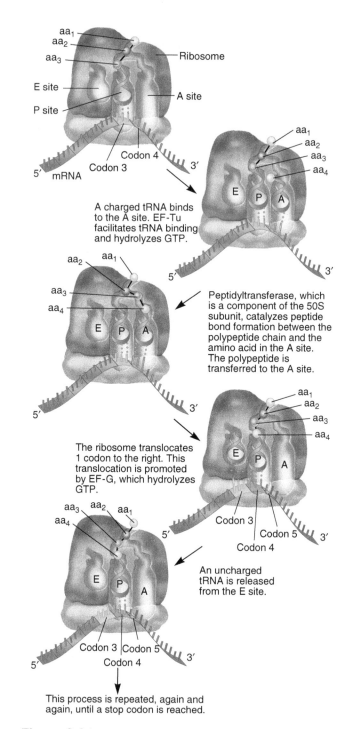

Figure 2-31. Bacterial translation: elongation. Catalytic activities and binding sites are associated with the large ribosome subunit, and elongation factors (EF) promotes tRNA binding and translocation. (Reprinted with permission from Brooker RJ: *Genetics: Analysis & Principles*, 3rd ed. New York: McGraw-Hill, 2008.)

Most proteins, however, are globular with one or more active sites that allow proteins to carry out a broad array of functions. Perhaps the most familiar class of globular proteins is enzymes that catalyze the biochemical events of metabolism. Globular proteins also include membrane receptors, ion channels, cell signaling molecules, protein hormones, and many other critical elements of a cell and its products.

Many proteins are also found to have an additional level of structural complexity, the quaternary (4°) level, in which two or more polypeptides are linked together to form a complex. These polypeptides are often produced by different genes, so several genes yield one active product. Hemoglobin, microtubules, microfilaments, connective tissue proteins, and many of the enzymatic complexes we described in DNA replication,

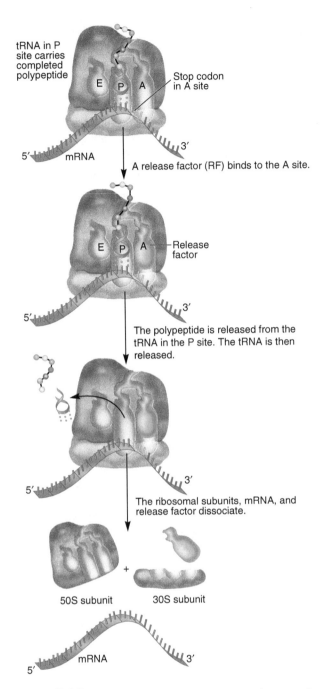

tRNA in P site carries completed polypeptide

E P A

Stop codon in A site

5' mRNA 3'

A release factor (RF) binds to the A site.

E P A

Release factor

5' 3'

The polypeptide is released from the tRNA in the P site. The tRNA is then released.

5' 3'

The ribosomal subunits, mRNA, and release factor dissociate.

50S subunit   +   30S subunit

mRNA 3'
5'

Figure 2-32. Bacterial translation: termination. A stop codon is recognized by release factors (RF) that promote termination and the dissociation of components. (Reprinted with permission from Brooker RJ: *Genetics: Analysis & Principles*, 3rd ed. New York: McGraw-Hill, 2008.)

transcription, and translation must be understood at this level. A change in any one of the component proteins can affect the function of the complex, so several different genetic mutations can have related consequences for the cell. Indeed, the way **multimeric proteins** are assembled can affect their function and be abnormal, even if each of the component subunits is normal.

Protein shape is not rigid. In fact, many proteins must be flexible in order to carry out their metabolic role. The motor molecule dynein "walks" up an adjacent tubule to cause movement of cilia and flagella. Movement of the end of myosin molecules

in muscle cells is essential to contraction. Temporary shape changes can also have a regulatory influence. **Allosteric proteins** are those that go through reversible changes in shape by binding with another molecule.

Allosteric interactions with an activator or inhibitor molecule play important regulatory roles in biochemical pathways and in processes like facilitating or inhibiting the binding of RNA polymerase to initiate transcription in eukaryotes. We will explore this last example in more detail in Chapter 3.

From the genetic point of view, it is easy to understand the impact a mutation can have by causing an amino acid substitution. But there is a range of severity among mutations. Not all amino acid changes will alter a protein in a major way, and some amino acid substitutions are biochemically equivalent. Many **point mutations** cause the substitution of one amino acid with another that differs in chemical properties and affects protein shape in a major way. Thus, the consequences of a mutation can range from being phenotypically neutral, to being conditional on the biochemical environment, to being severe or even fatal.

Posttranslational Modification and Protein Sorting

We have seen that the process of information flow from DNA to phenotype has many points at which regulatory events can operate. In the previous section, some examples of regulation at the protein level were described. But we can formalize this idea by introducing the concept of **posttranslational modification**. Protein structure can be changed after translation in several ways. For example, a few amino acids can be removed from an end of the polypeptide, and that can change the protein's activity. Some proteolytic enzymes of the digestive tract, such as trypsin, are initially synthesized and secreted in an inactive form (e.g. trypsinogen in this case) so they do not damage the cells that make them. They are then activated when they reach their working location. Similarly, the inactive fibrinogen is activated into the fibrin monomer of a blood clot by platelet breakdown or other activating signal.

Several small polypeptides can be produced from a larger one by cleavage. An example is pituitary hormones. Depending on how it is cleaved, propriomelanocortin (POMC) yields a total of five different hormones, including ACTH and β-endorphin. Posttranslational modifications can also include adding chemical groups, such as methyl groups (methylation), phosphate groups (phosphorylation), and carbohydrates (glycosylation). Phosphorylation, for example, is dependent on a class of enzymes called kinases and can either activate or inactivate a protein. In Chapter 5 we will see how cyclin-dependent kinases (CDKs) are involved in regulating the cell division cycle by phosphorylating proteins like those required for DNA replication and for chromosome condensation.

A related idea is directed transportation or sorting of proteins within the cell. Many protein sequences include signals that will sort proteins to particular targets, such as a specific membrane-bounded organelle (Figure 2-34), since each protein typically works in a restricted area of the cell.

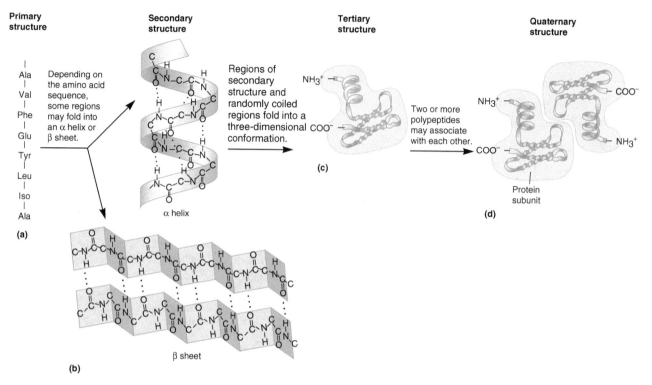

Figure 2-33. Levels of protein structure. (Reprinted with permission from Brooker RJ: *Genetics: Analysis & Principles*, 3rd ed. New York: McGraw-Hill, 2008.)

Proteins involved in ATP synthesis but encoded in the nuclear genome, for example, must be sorted to the mitochondria. Sometimes the polypeptide includes a sequence that is recognized by an RNA-protein complex called the signal recognition particle (SRP) that temporarily halts translation until the ribosome has been bound to the membrane of the endoplasmic reticulum (ER). The polypeptide is then synthesized into the inner lumen of the ER. **Sorting signals** are short amino acid sequences that are recognized by specific ultrastructural elements. The SRP signal is a group of about 20 primarily nonpolar amino acids near the amino terminal, while the mitochondrial-sorting signal is a short sequence that includes positively charged amino acids that fold into an alpha helix with the positive charges on the outside. Clearly, the flow of information in a cell is much broader and more dynamic than expressed by the Central Dogma, DNA ↔ RNA → polypeptide.

Pleiotropy

In contrast to the Central Dogma, the flow of genetic information is often not linear. The gene and phenotype do not always show a one-to-one relationship. Pathways branch and merge. Sometimes one mutation can have several apparently unrelated phenotypic effects, a phenomenon called **pleiotropy**. Sickle cell anemia is a classic example (Figure 2-35).

Hemoglobin is a multimeric protein composed of two α-globin and two β-globin polypeptides. The change from glutamic acid to valine at position 6 of β-globin causes the hemoglobin to crystallize in low oxygen conditions, such as during strenuous exercise or at high altitude. Deformed and rigid

RBCs block capillaries and cause heart attacks and strokes. They also rupture and cause anemia that places high demands on RBC forming tissues in bone marrow, which can alter bone size and shape. Thus, one amino acid substitution has a range of superficially unrelated phenotypic consequences.

Understanding pleiotropic expression can uncover the central event of a genetic change. For example, what can small ears and kidney problems in a mouse have in common? First, let us consider the ear phenotype. What can account for having small ears? One possibility is a defect in cartilage production. If cartilage formation is retarded, what other body structures might be similarly affected through their cartilage? The nose and the cartilage disks between vertebrae are candidates. It might be hard to tell if a mouse's nose is shorter than usual. But the vertebral disks can certainly have a noticeable effect on body length. Having normal-sized organs in a shortened abdomen can cramp structures like the ureters, leading to back pressure of urine into the kidneys and eventually to tissue damage. Atrophy of the kidney, or hydronephrosis, is therefore a functional consequence of the same genetic defect that caused the ears to be small.

The opposite defect, abnormal proliferation of cartilage cells or their precursors in rats, was one of the first examples of pleiotropy studied in detail. Excess cartilage narrows the lumen of the trachea and causes ribs to be larger. For that reason, breathing is inhibited and there is chronic oxygen deficiency. Hemoglobin levels increase to compensate and the blood thickens. Higher resistance to pulmonary circulation contributes to hypertrophy of the right ventricle. The affected rats cannot suckle or sneeze. Death occurs soon after birth.

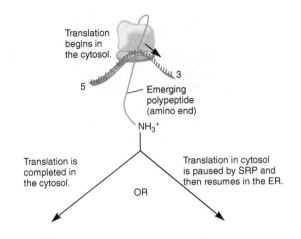

Translation begins in the cytosol.

Emerging polypeptide (amino end)

NH_3^+

5

3

Translation is completed in the cytosol.

OR

Translation in cytosol is paused by SRP and then resumes in the ER.

Figure 2-34. One means of regulation involves sorting of the protein into various cell regions. Posttranslational sorting occurs with proteins synthesized in the cytosol. They either remain in the cytosol or are sorted to the mitochondria, chloroplasts, peroxisomes, or nucleus. Cotranslational sorting involves the signal recognition particle (SRP) detecting a short amino acid sequence near the amino terminal. These proteins are sorted first to the endoplasmic reticulum and then to the Golgi complex, lysosomes, secretory vesicles, or the plasma membrane. Note that the diagram represents snapshot points in translation, not three ribosomes translating an mRNA at the same time. (Reprinted with permission from Brooker RJ: *Genetics: Analysis & Principles*, 3rd ed. New York: McGraw-Hill, 2008.)

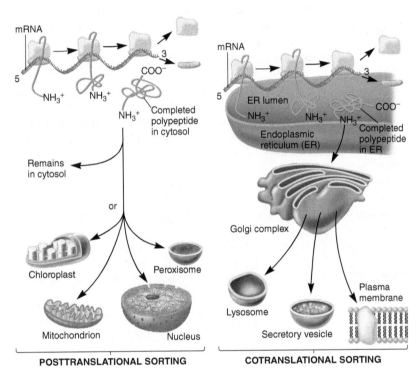

mRNA

5

3

NH_3^+ NH_3^+

NH_3^+

COO^-

Completed polypeptide in cytosol

Remains in cytosol

or

Chloroplast

Peroxisome

Mitochondrion

Nucleus

mRNA

5

3

ER lumen

NH_3^+ NH_3^+ NH_3^+

COO^-

Completed polypeptide in ER

Endoplasmic reticulum (ER)

Golgi complex

Lysosome

Secretory vesicle

Plasma membrane

POSTTRANSLATIONAL SORTING

COTRANSLATIONAL SORTING

NORMAL: NH_2 – VALINE – HISTIDINE – LEUCINE – THREONINE – PROLINE – GLUTAMIC ACID – GLUTAMIC ACID...

SICKLE CELL: NH_2 – VALINE – HISTIDINE – LEUCINE – THREONINE – PROLINE – VALINE – GLUTAMIC ACID...

(a) A comparison of the amino acid sequence between normal β-globin and sickle-cell β-globin

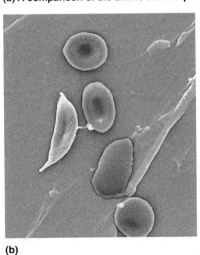

(b)

Figure 2-35. (a) A comparison of the amino acid sequence between normal beta-globin and sickle cell beta-globin. (b) Abnormally shaped (sickled) red blood cells in sickle cell anemia. (a: Reprinted with permission from Brooker RJ: *Genetics: Analysis & Principles*, 3rd ed. New York: McGraw-Hill, 2008. b: CDC/Sickle Cell Foundation of Georgia: Jackie George, Beverly Sinclair.)

This range of phenotypes, including death, can be traced to the action of a single gene.

In this example, death is a phenotype. In fact, recessive lethal mutations are the largest class of gene mutations. When a recessive lethal mutation also has developmental effects that can be detected in heterozygotes, they are showing pleiotropic expression. An example is the creeper mutation in chickens. The heterozygote displays skeletal defects of the legs, but the homozygote dies in early development. Thus, in this pleiotropic mutation, the leg malformation is dominant and lethality is recessive. In fact, given enough information about their developmental influences, most if not all genes are probably pleiotropic at some level.

Genotype × Environment Interactions

It would be a mistake to limit one's evaluation of genetic influences to their direct products: the RNA and proteins. Since temperature can affect the rate of chemical reactions, it is hardly surprising that environmental conditions can affect the phenotype produced by a gene. Genotype × environment interactions are situations in which the genetic effects on a phenotype differ due to environmental factors like nutrition, climate, or presence of a specific chemical or drug. The field of medicine called pharmacogenetics is devoted to identifying situations in which a person's genetically defined physiology puts them at risk for serious reactions to properly prescribed treatments.

An environmental factor can even have genetic consequences one or two generations later. An example is dietary intake by a mother and its potential influence on body weight of grandchildren. In a female fetus, primary oocytes are already present in developing ovaries by week 10 after conception. Meiosis, the cell division leading to gamete formation, begins in these primary oocytes but is temporarily arrested at an early stage until it is stimulated to continue years later after puberty. This timing has many important implications and will be discussed in more detail in Chapter 3. Here, the main point is that the cellular events in early development essentially collapse the physiological separation between a grandmother and a grandchild. Genetic and environmental factors affecting a pregnant female can influence the developing oocytes in the fetal ovaries of her daughter in utero.

Biochemical Pathways

As we have seen, genes do not produce their phenotypes in isolation. Proteins influence development by participating in networks of synthesis and degradation. An early insight into the role of genes was formalized in the "one gene, one enzyme" hypothesis by George Beadle and Edward Tatum in 1941, one of the first major insights establishing the field of molecular biology. But it soon became clear that this was an over-simplification, because some proteins, such as hemoglobin, are formed by combining two or more different polypeptides into one functional unit and, of course, not all proteins are enzymes. So the hypothesis was revised as "one gene, one polypeptide." Current advances, like identifying numerous proteins produced from the same gene by alternative splicing and other processes will continue to refine our appreciation of

the complexity of gene effects. But historically this idea was useful in guiding early studies of the role that genes play in determining phenotypes.

Even in its earliest formulation, the role of a gene was understood as controlling sequential steps in a metabolic pathway. By following the inheritance patterns of a rare metabolic disorder, alkaptonuria, Archibald Garrod pioneered the study of inherited diseases of metabolism in 1902. A mutation in homogentisic acid oxidase causes a build up of homogentisic acid, which oxidizes to a black color in urine. Its easy detection in diapers made it the first human metabolic disease clearly associated with a genetic mutation. Expanding the work to include metabolic studies of related compounds, Garrod developed an appreciation of genetic network relationships. A classic example is the metabolism of phenylalanine derived from dietary protein (Figure 2-36).

Phenylketonuria (PKU) is due to a mutation affecting the activity of the enzyme phenylalanine hydroxylase blocking the conversion of phenylalanine to tyrosine. Such an enzymatic defect can potentially affect a phenotype in two ways: it can reduce the available pool of the product of the

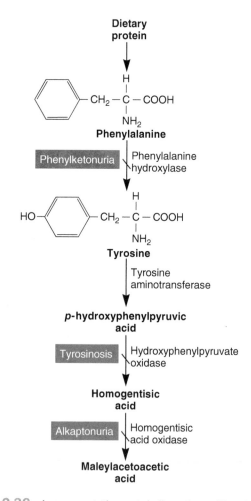

Figure 2-36. A representative metabolic pathway. Phenylalanine from the diet is broken down through tyrosine to maleylacetoacetic acid. Mutations at several points in the process lead to well-known human genetic diseases. (Reprinted with permission from Brooker RJ: *Genetics: Analysis & Principles,* 3rd ed. New York: McGraw-Hill, 2008.)

reaction and it can cause excess build up of the precursor acted upon by the normal enzyme. In this case, a build up of phenylpyruvic acid via phenylalanine interferes with normal neurological development leading to cognitive impairment.

Now imagine a much larger database of protein relationships. Specialties like proteomics combine advanced computational tools with rapidly growing knowledge about the genome and biochemical makeup of humans and model organisms. The technical challenges of analyzing such immense data collections should not be underestimated. It is spurring rapid progress in another fairly new field, bioinformatics. In contrast to the simple relationships seen in the pathway for phenylalanine metabolism, a more current view looks like the protein-interaction map shown in (Figure 2-37).

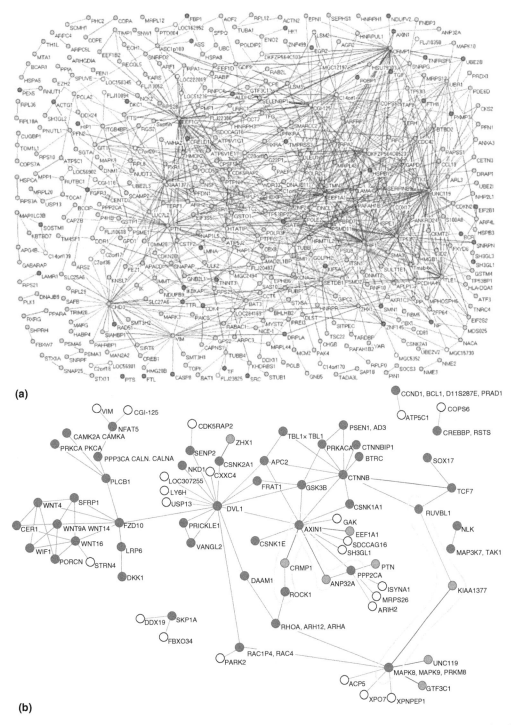

Figure 2-37. (a) Diagram showing 911 high confidence (HC) interactions involving 401 proteins for disease proteins (orange), proteins with gene ontology (GO) annotation (light blue), and proteins without GO and disease annotation (yellow). Interactions that connect the nodes are color-coded to denote confidence scores: green for 3, blue for 4, red for 5, and purple for 6 (b) Proteins linked to one specific role, the Wnt signaling pathway. (From Stelzl et al., 2005, Cell 122: 957-968).

One theme of this chapter, and indeed of the whole book, is the way model organisms can help us understand the human genome and its role in physiology, development, and disease. The molecular interactions and mutation effects in model organisms like *Drosophila* are very similar to events in human development and our genetic diseases. For that reason, the proteins identified in model organisms suggest prime targets for developing potential drugs and new medical therapies. In a sense, then, the flow of genetic information extends beyond the organism and into medical applications.

Part 2: Medical Genetics

A question often asked in the medical school classroom is, "Why do I need to know (or review) this basic science material? I want to train to be a doctor." A corollary question would be, "Why should the medical student know the basic mechanics of information flow at the molecular level as described in this chapter?" The answer lies in the progression of the understanding of the basis of human disease in terms of appreciating systems, and how they relate to the structure and function of an organism. In general this progression can be tied to periods of time in the advancement of medical knowledge that correspond to its "Golden Ages." The history of acquiring medical knowledge parallels the "hot" subject of an era. In periods gone by, advances in medical information have reflected the discipline yielding the "cutting edge" of the day. Previous periods of emphasis have occurred in anatomy, physiology, and microbiology. The last 20 years have clearly ushered in the era of genetics. Most recently, the role of genetics in medicine has evolved into the further refined disciplines of genomics, leading to proteomics and eventually metabolomics discussed in later chapters.

One of the greatest challenges for the student in assimilating the ever increasing knowledge base in genetics is how to organize the material in some sort of functional construct. What is needed is a way to group the information into tangibly related categories without losing important detail in the process. This can be seen in the realm of clinical classification with the two major types of diagnosticians: the "lumpers" and the "splitters." As with any dichotomy in science the best answer probably lies somewhere between the extremes.

The discipline of **dysmorphology** involves identifying specific physical features in a patient and then trying to group the findings into a recognizable pattern (Chapter 3). As dysmorphology emerged as its own discipline in the 1970s, painstaking emphasis was placed on identifying specific, often subtle, developmental features that could be identified in an individual. The patterns of these features were then grouped into diagnoses that were designated as syndromes or associations or sequences. A collection of these conditions was assembled into the seminal book on dysmorphology by the father of the field, Dr. David Smith (*Recognizable Patterns of Human Malformations*). As many such conditions have been described, there are now observations of persons with similar, but not identical, features. The diagnostic key then is to determine critical features that at a minimum should be present to make a diagnosis.

For most of the more common conditions, specific diagnostic criteria have been determined by expert panels. Those patients that have many of the features of a particular condition, but not enough to meet criteria, represent a diagnostic dilemma. Should their condition be classified as a milder expression of the primary disorder or an unrelated but similar condition? Advances in molecular diagnostics have shown that the correct answer can be either. These diagnostics have also demonstrated that there can be a tremendous range of variability in expression from changes in the same gene, such that two clinically very different conditions may be linked by a common gene, i.e., be allelic disorders. Thus, the best approach appears to be the use of strong clinical characterization supported by molecular confirmation.

As these types of correlations emerge, apparently unrelated conditions may be grouped by any number of differing parameters. Depending on the reasons that necessitate grouping (or simply by personal preference), they may be grouped by clinical, biochemical, physiological, or molecular characteristics. At one end of the spectrum, diseases may be classified by how the condition actually affects the patient. In this way of thinking, diseases are linked by the total spectrum of the disease and the *clinical presentation* of the condition (Table 2-1). A particularly attractive way to pull apparently disparate scenarios together is by *pathogenesis*, i.e., the underlying mechanism of the disease. Thus, in light of the discussions in the first section of this chapter, specific conditions may be linked by identifying the point in the flow of information at which normal function is disrupted.

As these mechanisms have been discovered, the answers have not always been intuitive. For example, Hutchinson-Gilford syndrome is a premature aging condition. Patients with this condition usually start showing problems by 2 years of age. They have marked decrease in linear growth, hair

Table 2-1.	Common Medical Presentations of Genetic Changes (Phenotype from Genotype)

Acquired/degenerative condition

Adverse reproductive outcomes
• Infertility
• Prenatal lethal condition
• Spontaneous miscarriage

Congenital anomaly

Endocrinopathy

Genetic susceptibility to an environmental agent

Inborn error of metabolism

Neoplasia/tumor formation

Neuromuscular dysfunction

Specific organ dysfunction

growth, and decreased subcutaneous fat. Features of premature aging include atherosclerosis, presbycusis (hearing loss associated with aging) and arthritic changes as early as 4-5 years old. This condition has now been shown to be due to abnormalities of the LMNA gene, which codes for a protein called lamin A, one major component of the nuclear membrane. Molecular tools were needed to make this association, as no clinician would have ever deduced on their own that the clinical features of premature aging would be caused by a gene that codes for a protein in the nuclear membrane. Other examples of clinical disorders associated with disruption of a specific component of information flow are given in Table 2-2.

Alternatively, genetic "families" may be defined based on the *common gene / locus* involved. Thus a spectrum may

be defined as a range of conditions that represent different levels of severity in the disruption of that particular gene's function. Type II collagen is a structural connective tissue protein that lends strength to tissues, such as bones and cartilage. Abnormalities in type II collagen lead to problems with the bones, joints, eyes, and other tissues. Molecular studies have now demonstrated that several clinically described conditions share in common mutations in type II collagen. These conditions range from skeletal disorders that are so severe that the child dies shortly after birth to less severe conditions like the early onset of osteoarthritis (Table 2-3).

Similarly, conditions may be linked by a common *signaling pathway* with similar expression resulting from the involvement of different genes that share a common input into the

Table 2-2.	Processes in Information Flow and Corresponding Disorders		
Process	**Category**	**Example of Disorders**	**Description**
Transport across nuclear membranes	Laminopathies	Hutchinson-Gilford progeria	Premature aging syndrome
DNA replication	Suppression of DNA replication	Bloom syndrome	Short stature, microcephaly, facial telangiectasias, predisposition to cancer
DNA repair	Mismatch repair genes	Hereditary non-polypotic colorectal cancer	Familial colorectal and other tumors
Transcription	Chromatin remodeling disorders	CHARGE syndrome	Multiple structural congenital anomalies
RNA processing	RNA editing in the pancreas	Diabetes mellitus	Carbohydrate intolerance
Translation	Poly A variants	Cystic fibrosis	Disordered chloride transport in exocrine glands leads to pulmonary and pancreatic insufficiency
Posttranslational modification	Congenital disorders of protein glycosylation	CDG1a (phosphomannomutase 2 deficiency)	Multi-system failure including nervous, ocular, skeletal, clotting, or immune systems
Protein shape and function	Hemoglobinopathies	Sickle cell anemia	Abnormal hemoglobin leads to misshaped red blood cells with secondary vascular occlusion
Enzymatic	Inborn errors of metabolism	Phenylketonuria	Impaired conversion of phenylalanine to tyrosine interferes with brain myelin formation
Multimeric protein Assembly	Type I collagen	Osteogenesis imperfect	Abnormal collagen folding produces 'brittle bones'
Epigenesis	Imprinting	Beckwith Wiedemann syndrome	Overgrowth, hyperinsuliema, omphalocoele

Table 2-3.	Examples of "Genetic Families"		
Gene Family	**Gene**	**Abnormal Example of Disorders**	**Description**
Type II Collagenopathies	COL2A	Achondrogenesis (some types)	Lethal neonatal dwarfism
		Kniest dysplasia	Skeletal dysplasia with short stature, flat facies, joints, cleft palate, major ocular changes
		Spondyloepiphyseal dysplasia congenital	Similar to Kniest but milder
		Stickler syndrome	Hereditary arthro-ophtalmopathy
		Premature osteoarthritis	Onset in third decade
GLI-Kruppel Family Member 3	GLI3	Pallister-Hall syndrome	Hamartoma in the hypothalamus, postaxial polydactyly, imperforate anus, malformations of many other systems
		Greig Cephalosyndactyly	Macrocephaly, frontal bossing, pre- and postaxial polydactyly
		Postaxial polydactyly type A	Extra digits on the postaxial (outside) part of the hands/feet
		Preaxial polydactyly type IV	Extra digits on the preaxial (inside) part of the hands/feet

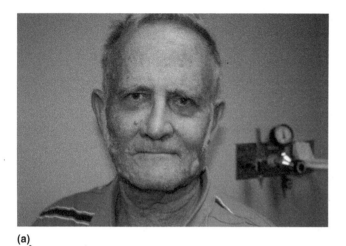

(a)

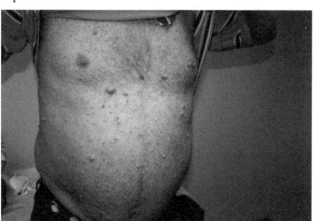

(b)

Figure 2-38. (a) Adult male with neurofibromatosis. (b) Note the multiple cutaneous tumors (neurofibromas).

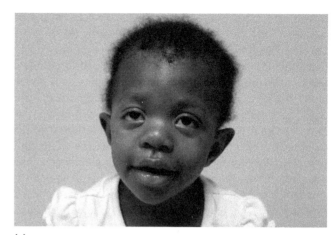

(a)

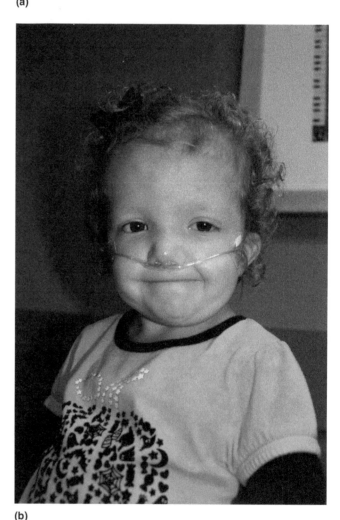

(b)

Figure 2-39. Two patients with Noonan syndrome. (a) Known mutation in SOS1 gene, and (b) Known mutation in KRAS gene.

same system of transmission of molecular information. Neurofibromatosis is a neurocutaneous condition characterized by pigmentary changes in the skin (café au lait spots and abnormal freckling), tumors of the nerves, and various skeletal problems (Figure 2-38). Noonan syndrome is a multiple anomaly syndrome characterized by short stature, characteristic facies, pulmonic stenosis, and skeletal changes (Figure 2-39). Clinical geneticists familiar with both conditions on occasion had noted patients who had the typical changes of neurofibromatosis and some of the features of Noonan syndrome (typical facies and pulmonic stenosis). These conditions were then ascribed names such as Watson syndrome and Noonan-neurofibromatosis. Molecular studies eventually showed that these conditions were actually allelic to neurofibromatosis (neufibromin gene on chromosome 17). Recent molecular studies have now demonstrated that the link between these two conditions is that both conditions are due to mutations in genes that contribute to a common signaling pathway—the RAS/MAPK system (Table 2-4). Most importantly, beyond its role in diagnosis, this type of understanding will have significant implications for potential therapies. For more detailed discussion on pathogenesis and categorizing conditions see Chapter 16.

Table 2-4.	Examples of Disorders Linked By a Common Signaling Pathway	
Signaling Pathway	**Example of Disorders**	**Description**
RAS/MAPK	Neurofibromatosis	Pigmented macules on the skin, neurofibromas, bony lesions
	Noonan syndrome	Short stature, characteristic facies, pulmonic stenosis, chest wall changes, bleeding problems
	Costello syndrome	Macrocephaly, 'coarse' facial appearance, mucosal papillomas. Ectodermal, skeletal and cardiac changes
	Cardiofacialcutaneous (CFC)	Growth and developmental delays, ectodermal changes, cardiac anomalies,
Fibroblast Growth Factors	Crouzon syndrome Apert syndrome Jackson Weiss syndrome Pfeiffer syndrome Muenke syndrome Beare-Stevenson syndrome	All have varying degrees and combinations of craniosynostosis, and digital changes (poly- syn- dactyly)

Part 3: Clinical Correlation

Increasing knowledge of the molecular basis of human medical conditions has identified clinical correlates of the disruption of each part of the information flow outlined in the first section of this chapter. Table 2-2 lists the major processes we have described and gives examples of the types of conditions that may occur when there is interference with that process.

Congenital Disorders of Glycosylation

Glycosylation is one of several known posttranslational modifications of biological chemicals. This process is both intricate and specific. Glycosylation pathways are some of the most complex metabolic processes known. To date there

have been at least eleven glycosylation pathways identified. It plays an important part in the completion of protein production. Two major types of protein glycosylation have been described. N-linked glycosylation involves the link of a glycan to the amide nitrogen of asparagines; O-linked glycosylation involves the attachment to the hydroxy oxygen of serine or threonine.

The first clinical disorder recognized as being due to a problem with protein glycosylation was described in 1980. Since then over 30 such conditions have been reported. These conditions were originally known as "carbohydrate deficient glycoprotein syndromes." Current nomenclature now identifies them as congenital disorders of glycosylation (CDGs). The

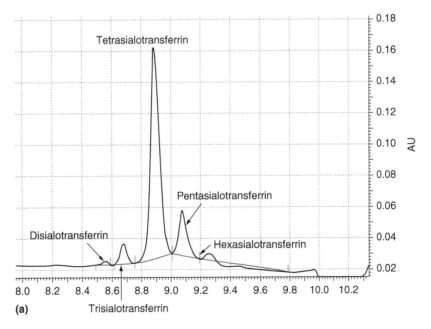

Figure 2-40. Isoelectric focusing of the protein transferrin. (a) Normal pattern. (b) Isoelectric focusing of the protein transferrin from a patient with CDG Ia. Note the increases in disialotransferrin and asialotransferrin in an affected patient and the general shift in the pattern to the left. (Graphs courtesy of Dr. Tim Wood, Greenwood Genetics Center, Greenville, SC.)

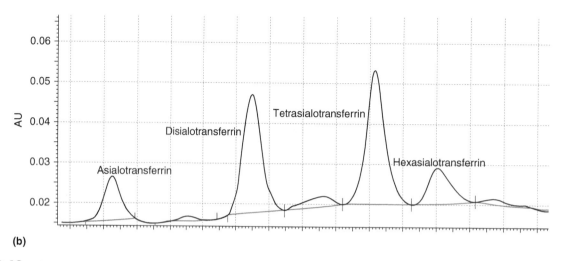

(b)

Figure 2-40. *(Continued)*

clinical spectrum of CDGs is widely variable. Patients may present as extremely ill neonates or as mildly affected adults. They often manifest as multi-system disorders. CDGs should be included in the differential diagnosis of symptoms as varied as problems with the nervous, ocular, skeletal, clotting, or immune systems. They may present with nonspecific features such as growth abnormalities or low muscle tone. CDGs should be considered in almost any patient with otherwise unexplained multi-system problems. Fortunately, a simple and relatively inexpensive screening test is available as a first-tier evaluation. This test, called "transferrin isoelectric focusing," looks at the migration of the protein transferrin on an electrophoretic gel. In the case of abnormal glycosylation, the protein will migrate on the gel in a pattern different from normal (Figure 2-40).

Congenital disorder of glycosylation type 1a (CDG 1a) has also been called Jaeken syndrome. It is the most common form of CDG and was the first to be reported. It is known to be due to a deficiency of the enzyme phosphomannomutase 2. This deficiency results in glycoproteins with decreased levels of sialic acid. Patients with CDG 1a typically present with neurologic symptoms including cognitive deficits, central (supranuclear) hypotonia, decreased stretch reflexes, and truncal ataxia. Other features that may be present include cardiomyopathy, enlarged fibrotic liver, and problems with the kidneys. Endocrine, immune, and clotting abnormalities may also be involved. There may be a number of important clues seen on physical exam that may alert the clinician to the possible diagnosis. Such features include dysmorphic facial features (Figure 2-41), inverted nipples, abnormal distribution of subcutaneous fat, and an "orange peel" appearance to areas of the skin.

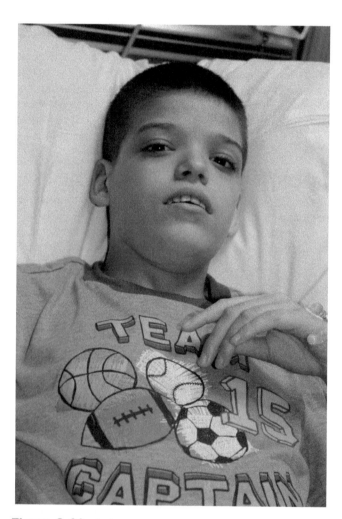

Figure 2-41. Patient with a congenital disorder of glycosylation (CDG). This patient has CDG type 1a (Jaeken syndrome) due to phosphomannomutase-2 enzyme deficiency.

■ Board-Format Practice Questions

1. Different types of RNA can play a role in which of the following processes:
   A. DNA replication.
   B. Enzymatic/catalytic functions.
   C. Secondary messengers for cell membrane receptors.
   D. Endocytosis.
   E. Synaptic communication.

2. Which is the best example of pleiotropy?
   A. One patient with neurofibromatosis has only a few hyperpigmented spots. A second (unrelated) patient has multiple tumors including spinal tumors that cause extreme pain.
   B. A patient who carries a mutation inherited from a parent who is affected with a medical condition due to the mutation shows no expression of the condition themselves.
   C. A mutation in the SOS1 gene produces Noonan syndrome. Patients with Noonan syndrome have short stature, heart malformations, dysmorphic facies, and learning difficulties.
   D. A mutation in one part of gene produces one clinical problem. A mutation in another part of the gene produces a completely different problem.
   E. A specific gene change causes no clinical problem.

3. It is estimated that humans only have 22,000 functioning genes. Much simpler organisms have many more functioning genes. A major reason that the more complex human development can occur with fewer genes is:
   A. the presence of multiple pseudogenes per each copy of a 'real' gene.
   B. posttranslational modification of produced proteins.
   C. gene amplification.
   D. single splicing options.
   E. epimerases.

4. Mutations in a gene known as PTEN can produce many different clinical conditions. These would include Cowden disease (a familial cancer syndrome), autism with macrocephaly, and Bannayan-Riley-Ruvalcaba syndrome (a multiple anomaly syndrome with mental retardation and dysmorphic features). These conditions could be grouped together as:
   A. pleiotropic conditions.
   B. genetically linked conditions.
   C. co-dominant conditions.
   D. a genetic family.
   E. contiguous gene disorders.

chapter 3

The Organization of Development

CHAPTER SUMMARY

A conclusion one could draw from the first two chapters is that the role of genes in determining phenotypes is complex and dynamic. That is true. It is an important insight that should be kept in mind when evaluating a genetic question. But, by the same token, complexity does not necessarily mean that rules and order are weak. In this chapter we will explore some of these rules, specifically the question of how gene regulation activates a particular gene in the appropriate developmental context and how molecular signals carry out large-scale patterning to organize the structure of the body in early development.

To a degree that still impresses most biologists, there is extensive similarity, or homology, in the genes that control development in humans and in model organisms like fruit flies, nematodes, and zebrafish. These homologies underlie the unity of life. The insights the field has gained from model organisms will help tell the story of genetic control of development in humans.

Part 1: Background and Systems Integration

Overview of Timing and the Processes at Work

The nuclear control of development does not actually begin when the genes of an egg and a sperm fuse at fertilization. The earliest stages of embryonic development are actually controlled by the mother's genome. Molecular signals like inducers and mRNA coded by the maternal genome are stored in the cytoplasm during egg formation. Very few genes in the new individual are transcribed at first. Genetic influences at this early stage are called **maternal effects**. Details vary among organisms, but basically the fertilized egg nucleus divides several times to become a ball of cells, the **morula**. The cells then form a fluid-filled ball, the **blastula** or in mammals the **blastocyst**, in which cells are set off to one side. The internal space keeps cells that will become ectoderm and endoderm from interacting prematurely and provides a space for cell movement. In humans the embryo forms the morula as it travels along the fallopian tube, and by 41/2 to 5 days it has formed into a blastocyst and enters the uterine cavity. This blastocyst implants into the uterine wall about 6 days after fertilization.

It is at this blastula stage that the embryo's own genes first become active and take over control of development. One process that may trigger this transition is the demethylation of various promoters that then bind with transcription factors to initiate transcription. At that point there can be cytoplasmic differences among the blastula cells, **blastomeres**, due to process like the partitioning of inducers and RNA molecules in the original egg cytoplasm. The resulting transcriptional cascades in different parts of the blastula ultimately contribute to the patterned organization of tissues, organs, and organ systems of the fetus and adult.

The process of early development can be conveniently described in terms of three types of processes: cellular differentiation, pattern formation, and morphogenesis. They are not mutually exclusive. **Cellular differentiation** is the gradual specialization of cells. Cell specialization is determined by the specific array of genes that are active in the cell lineage as it forms, and it can be described in terms of the cell's biochemical profile, thus its molecular structure and function. **Pattern formation** is the establishment of spatial organization of differentiated cells. It is the series of processes like cell signaling and gradient formation that establishes the spatial addresses of cells and tissues with respect to each other. Patterned interactions form the basis for succeeding phases of developmental specialization and the temporal changes in spatial arrangement that occur as the embryo forms. **Morphogenesis** is literally the "origin of form." The sculpting of form involves the movement of cells and sheets of cells as well as events like programmed cell death, **apoptosis**. Our focus will be on the way the genome controls these processes during early development. In humans most of this occurs during the first trimester of development, because, except for the brain, the main thing the embryo does after the first trimester is simply grow larger.

Control of Gene Action–Models From Bacteria

The organization of gene action in bacteria is different from that in eukaryotes in many ways. But insights gained from studies of bacterial gene regulation help us better understand the more complex and flexible eukaryotic processes. For this discussion we will define **structural gene** as a gene that codes for the synthesis of a polypeptide (although we will not argue if someone wants to include the genes for RNAs like the tRNAs and rRNAs in the mix). Other genetic sequences have a regulatory role, such as serving as binding sites for transcription factors and polymerase. Indeed, the wide array of functions that are being discovered for regions of the genome make it increasingly difficult to define what we really mean by "a gene." An important characteristic of bacteria is that several genes needed at the same time to carry out a particular activity can be linked under the control of a single set of regulatory genes, a genetic organization called an **operon**. In eukaryotes, each structural gene has its own individual regulatory gene control system. Bacterial operons give us ideas about the regulatory strategies the more complex eukaryotic cell might employ. Our discussion of operons will, however, be relatively brief and will not cover the full range of specific examples that are now well understood. But it is a convenient way of introducing some useful terminology.

Gene action, or turning genes "on" and "off," is simply another way of describing the regulation of transcription. Typically this involves **transcription factors**, which are regulatory proteins with at least two active sites. One active site binds to DNA and the other binds to a small effector molecule that can change the conformation of the regulatory protein and, thus, its DNA binding domain. Some regulatory proteins are **repressors** that inhibit transcription when they bind to DNA. Others are **activators** that increase the rate at which transcription occurs. Representative molecular interactions are shown in Figure 3-1 for inducible genes and repressible genes. We can see how this works by looking at the relatively simple regulation of bacterial operons.

When you think about how a process can be controlled, there are two obvious alternatives. It can be "off" because it is not needed except under specific conditions. When needed, a molecular signal turns it "on." It is **inducible**. Or it can be "on" because its product is needed continuously, but it is turned "off" when its product has reached a required level. It is **repressible**. It is wasteful of precious energetic resources to continue to produce even a necessary product when there is a sufficient supply. During development, probably most genes operate inducibly. They are turned on when their coded enzyme or structural protein is needed by the cell in which they will work. Both approaches are dynamic, in the sense that they are reversible as the need changes.

One of the first bacterial operons to be studied in detail was the inducible lactose, or *lac*, operon (Figure 3-2). There are three structural genes, *lacZ*, *lacY*, and *lacA*. Several regulatory gene functions are also involved. In this example (Figure 3-3), a regulatory gene, *lacI*, codes for a repressor protein. By binding to the Operator site (*lacO*), the repressor protein physically blocks binding or transcription by RNA polymerase. If the Operator gene site is not blocked, the Promoter gene (*lacP*) can bind with RNA polymerase. Transcription continues until a termination signal is reached. The resulting mRNA is a transcript of several tandem structural genes. For each coding region, it has individual start (AUG) and stop (UAA, UAG, or UGA) codons. The term cistron is sometimes used by geneticists to describe a gene. The word comes from a test for allelism. The mRNA transcript in bacteria is, therefore, polycistronic, in that each transcript carries the information of several functionally-related genes.

Since a regulatory gene makes a repressor molecule that is diffusible throughout the cell, its regulatory action is at a distance from the regulatory gene itself. It is said to be trans-acting, literally "acting across." The Operator, on the other hand, regulates transcription of the structural genes to which it is directly attached. It is said to be cis-acting.

The *lac* operon is inducible, because the *lacI* regulatory gene codes for an active repressor protein. This has DNA binding sites that attach to the operator and inhibit RNA polymerase. Transcription of the operon is, therefore, at a very low level (essentially "off") until something induces it to begin working. In this case, the inducer is the sugar allolactose, a derivative of lactose, the carbon and energy source that proteins coded by the lac operon process for the bacterial cell. It is not the preferred sugar resource, so the operon is off until its preferred source, glucose, has been depleted.

In contrast, a repressible operon controls a pathway that is needed continuously by the cell. The tryptophan, or *trp*, operon is a good example (Figure 3-4). It codes for enzymes that catalyze the production of tryptophan, an amino acid. The essence of the process is that when tryptophan levels are low, the operon is transcribed normally. But when tryptophan levels are high, the tryptophan participates in a feedback reaction to inhibit transcription temporarily. It is a waste of energetic resources to continue producing it. When sufficient product is present, the operon is repressed. Feedback inhibition is an important element in many regulatory pathways. An example of such a mechanism is illustrated in Figure 3-5. When the concentration of an end product of a biochemical pathway is high, it can bind with an inhibitor site on an earlier enzyme to inactivate it temporarily.

Control of Gene Action in Eukaryotes

Eukaryotes have a much more complex cell structure than that found in prokaryotes. Most are multicellular with a range of cell types reflecting the division of labor for specialized structures and functions. This requires a higher degree of flexibility in genetic regulation to allow gene products to be produced

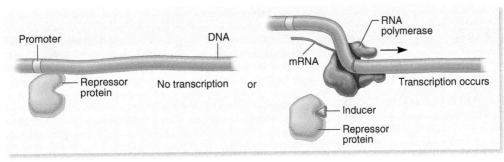

(a) Repressor protein, inducer molecule, inducible gene

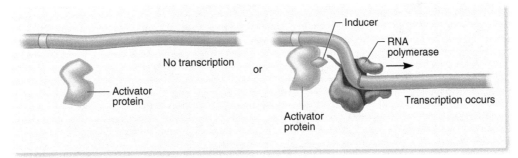

(b) Activator protein, inducer molecule, inducible gene

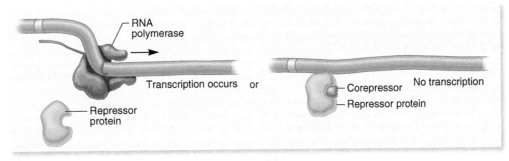

(c) Repressor protein, corepressor molecule, repressible gene

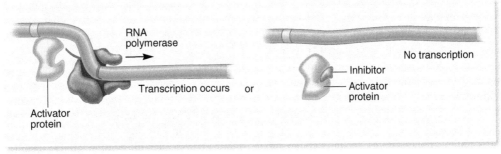

(d) Activator protein, inhibitor molecule, repressible gene

Figure 3-1. Regulatory proteins for inducible and repressible genes. An active repressor protein will inhibit transcription, but binding with an inducer will alter its structure so it cannot bind to DNA. An active activator protein bound to an inducer will promote transcription, but binding to an inhibitor will shut transcription down. In these examples, the regulatory protein has two binding sites. One region can bind to DNA, and the other can bind to a small effector molecule (inducer, corepressor, or inhibitor). (Reprinted with permission from Brooker RJ: *Genetics: Analysis & Principles*, 3rd ed. New York: McGraw-Hill, 2008.)

in the various combinations needed by different cell types. In eukaryotes, transcription factors regulate the binding of the transcription complex to the core promoter, and they initiate the elongation phase of RNA transcription. There are three classes of transcription in eukaryotes characterized by their

promoters, and different RNA polymerases transcribe each one. **RNA polymerase I** transcribes rRNA in the nucleolus region of the nucleus. **RNA polymerase II** transcribes mRNA throughout the genome. **RNA polymerase III** transcribes tRNA and some other types of small RNA.

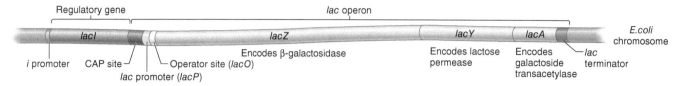

(a) Organization of DNA sequences in the *lac* region of the *E.coli* chromosome

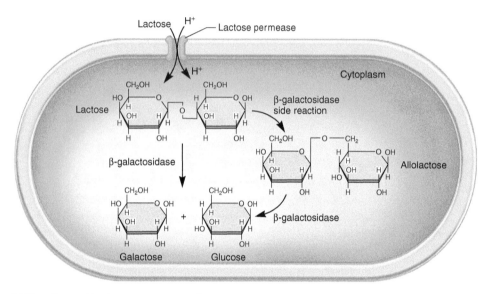

(b) Functions of lactose permease and β-galactosidase

Figure 3-2. Organization and function of the bacterial lactose (*lac*) operon. (Reprinted with permission from Brooker RJ: *Genetics: Analysis & Principles*, 3rd ed. New York: McGraw-Hill, 2008.)

General transcription factors are needed to bind RNA polymerase to DNA at any type of promoter region. Some promoters have short upstream sequences (i.e., a string of nucleotides located before the beginning of a coding sequence) that bind **upstream factors** that increase the efficiency of transcription initiation. Inducible or regulatory transcription factors have a regulatory role and are produced at specific times in each cell type. They bind at short DNA sequences called **response elements** and affect the patterns of transcription sequentially through development. Not surprisingly, transcription factors make up a large family of genes. About 10% of the proteins coded for in the human genome have DNA binding domains, so most of these are likely to be transcription factors. This makes them perhaps the largest family of proteins coded by the human genome.

Regulatory transcription factors can either activate or repress transcription (Figure 3-6). Indeed, transcription in eukaryotes has many possible influences. In addition to activator and repressor proteins that might themselves be affected by binding with small regulatory molecules, transcription can be inhibited by methylation. The degree of DNA compaction, i.e., its looping, supercoiling, and bonding with nucleosomes, is also an important variable in the process. At this point, however, we will focus on the role of transcription factors. DNA structure will be discussed further in Chapter 4.

Since the mechanisms of transcriptional regulation are so central to the expression of genetic information, it should be no surprise that structural similarities can be seen in families of transcription proteins from even distantly-related organisms. Proteins have **domains** with specific functions. One transcription factor domain has characteristics that enable it to bind with DNA, while one or more other domains might bind with small effector molecules or other proteins. In Figure 3-7, several common domain structures, or motifs, are shown. Many transcription factors have regions of α-helix coiling. The width of the α-helix fits well into the major groove in DNA. The helix-turn-helix and the helix-loop-helix structures can form hydrogen bonds with nucleotides in the major groove, thus allowing each transcription factor to bind to a specific DNA region. In a similar way, a zinc finger and a leucine zipper bind specific nucleotides in the DNA major groove. The helix-loop-helix and the leucine zipper often cause pairs of transcription factors to bond, forming a protein dimer. A **homodimer** is where the two factors are the same; a **heterodimer** is made up of two different transcription factors. This contributes to the wide diversity of regulatory structures that can be produced.

The promoter sequence in eukaryotic genes is, therefore, more complex than the promoter in prokaryotes (Figure 3-8). Regulatory transcription factors that serve as activator proteins will bind with an enhancer sequence to increase the rate

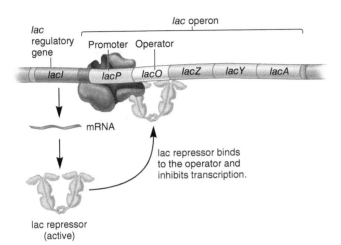

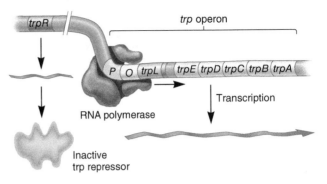

(a) Low tryptophan levels, transcription of the entire *trp* operon occurs

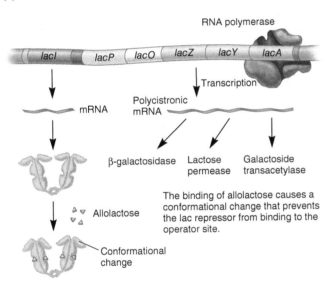

(b) Lactose present

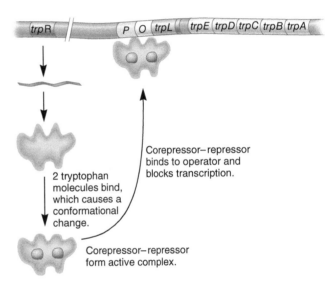

(b) High tryptophan levels, repression occurs

Figure 3-3. The *lac* operon is inducible. The *lac* repressor is synthesized in an active form, so transcription is inhibited until the appropriate inducer, allolactose, enters the cell. When it binds to the repressor protein, a conformational change causes it to release from the DNA and allow RNA polymerase to transcribe the three genes of this operon. (Reprinted with permission from Brooker RJ: *Genetics: Analysis & Principles*, 3rd ed. New York: McGraw-Hill, 2008.)

Figure 3-4. The tryptophan (*trp*) operon is repressible. At high-end product levels, tryptophan binds to the *trp* repressor protein and inhibits further transcription. (Reprinted with permission from Brooker RJ: *Genetics: Analysis & Principles*, 3rd ed. New York: McGraw-Hill, 2008.)

of transcription. This is up regulation. When a repressor protein binds to a silencer sequence, the rate of transcription is down regulated. Enhancer and silencer elements are often found within about 100 bp from the initiation start site, but they can be located much further away and still have a strong effect due to conformational changes in DNA folding.

Instead of binding to the RNA polymerase directly, most regulatory transcription factors work indirectly by influencing other proteins that bind with the polymerase. Two such intermediaries are TFIID and mediator. TFIID is a protein complex that works as a general transcription factor. It binds to a sequence called the TATA box in the core promoter of eukaryotes (Figure 2-18) and then binds with other transcription factors that facilitate binding RNA polymerase II to structural gene promoters. Mediator is also a protein complex that binds with other general transcription factors and with RNA polymerase. Depending on these binding interactions, mediator can either lead to up regulation or down regulation of transcription. Additional information on transcriptional regulation will be introduced in other chapters. An especially important example will be the interaction of steroid hormones with their specific regulatory transcription factor, the steroid receptor.

Cellular Differentiation

From the examples presented here, it is clear that eukaryotes call upon a range of mechanisms to influence the transcription rate of each gene. In some cases, an effector molecule like a hormone can activate a transcription factor (Figure 3-9). In other cases, protein-protein interactions or phosphorylation can turn a gene on. An activator protein might bind at several

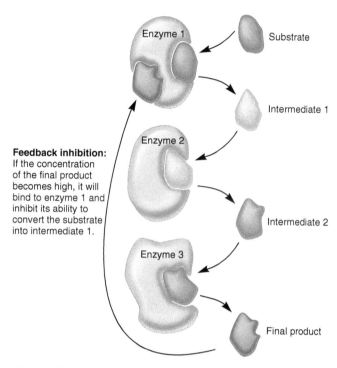

Feedback inhibition:
If the concentration of the final product becomes high, it will bind to enzyme 1 and inhibit its ability to convert the substrate into intermediate 1.

Figure 3-5. An example of feedback inhibition of enzyme activity. (Reprinted with permission from Brooker RJ: *Genetics: Analysis & Principles*, 3rd ed. New York: McGraw-Hill, 2008.)

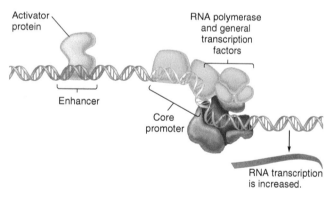

(a) Gene activation

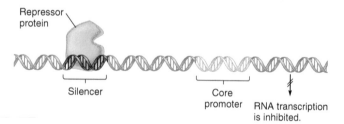

(b) Gene repression

Figure 3-6. Regulatory transcription factors can act by either increasing or decreasing the rate of transcription. (Reprinted with permission from Brooker RJ: *Genetics: Analysis & Principles*, 3rd ed. New York: McGraw-Hill, 2008.)

different genes that have the same response element sequence, and the product of one gene might affect the regulatory signals of other genes. These interactions can cause a cascade of transcriptional activities that is different from one cell type to another. **Cellular differentiation** is essentially the process by which cells become different. That difference is reflected in the profile of proteins that affect its composition and function at any given time during development.

Cell-to-cell communication is a critical component of the cellular differentiation process since many of the signals that determine the appropriate transcriptional responses come from outside the cell. In most cases, the extracellular signal is a molecule that cannot pass through the cell membrane. Instead, it binds to a receptor in the membrane and initiates a chain of events by way of a secondary cascade inside the cell. When an activated membrane receptor initiates a response pathway inside the cell, the process is called **signal transduction**. The signal is literally transduced or "carried across" the membrane. A molecule that is produced intracellularly in response to signal transduction is called a **second messenger**. Thus, in order to respond, the target cell must be preprogrammed to detect the presence of the extracellular signal.

First, a signaling molecule binds to a specific protein receptor on the outer membrane. Either directly through protein kinase activity associated with the receptor or indirectly through a G protein, it activates a target protein in the cytosol. A **protein kinase** is an enzyme that affects activity by adding a phosphate group to an amino acid of another protein. **G proteins** have the ability to bind guanine nucleotides. The inactive form is a trimer bound to guanine diphosphate (GDP). The active receptor replaces this with guanine triphosphate (GTP), which then causes the G protein to dissociate into a monomer carrying GTP or a dimer. One of these acts upon a target protein that causes production of a second messenger.

An example of this chain of events is the cAMP response element-binding (CREB) protein (Figure 3-10). Cyclic-AMP (**cAMP**) plays the role of an intracellular messenger in many pathways. In this case, an activated membrane receptor activates adenylate cyclase (also denoted, adenylyl cyclase) that catalyzes the production of cAMP from ATP. The cAMP second messenger then activates protein kinase A, which phosphorylates the CREB protein in the nucleus to form a dimer. This dimer is an active regulatory transcription factor that initiates transcription at genes that have a cAMP response element (CRE) upstream of the core promoter of a target gene.

These events are, of course, also accompanied by cell division. The control of cell division rate shares many of the general mechanisms described here. But we will focus upon that important process separately in Chapter 4. By cascades of molecular interaction within both the cytosol and nucleus and through signal transduction in response to extracellular signals, transcription of genes in a cell lineage ultimately leads to the formation of each of the differentiated cell types of the adult body.

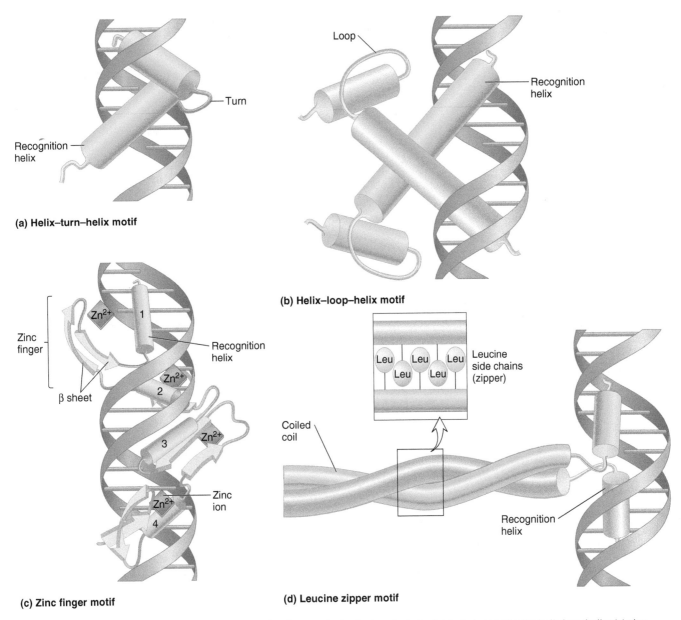

Figure 3-7. Some of the common structural motifs of transcription factors include: (a) helix-turn-helix; (b) helix-loop-helix; (c) zinc finger; and (d) leucine zipper. (Reprinted with permission from Brooker RJ: *Genetics: Analysis & Principles*, 3rd ed. New York: McGraw-Hill, 2008.)

Pleuripotency and Developmental Plasticity

The ability of a cell to differentiate into various cell types is unlimited in the fertilized egg and early cells, such as those in the morula of the human embryo. At this point, cell fates are unrestricted, since all cell types of the developing body plan must trace their lineage from them as the embryo grows. The nuclei are said to be **totipotent**, i.e., "totally potent, or totally competent" in developmental opportunity. If the embryo is divided into two or more separate groups of cells at this stage, as in monozygotic (identical) twins, each subgroup of cells has the capacity to yield all cell types in the adult body. But developmental plasticity is gradually lost as the individual develops (Figure 3-11). Many nonmammalian organisms lose

totipotency earlier than in mammals, and plants tend to retain it much longer. In the blastocyst stage of human development, when the individual's own genome begins to control cellular differentiation, the embryonic stem cells have become **pluripotent**. Each is capable of differentiating into many different cell types, but not into all of them.

Totipotency and pluripotency are significant for several reasons. If one or a few cells die in early development or are removed from the embryo, their developmental role can be taken over by the remaining cells. Cells removed from an embryo at this time are totipotent or pluripotent stem cells that can divide in cell culture and potentially differentiate into a range of specialized cell types for therapeutic applications. But as embryonic development continues, cells lose even more plasticity. In the adult there are still some stems

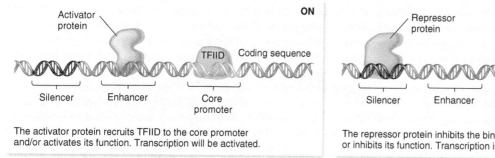

(a) Regulatory transcription factors and TFIID

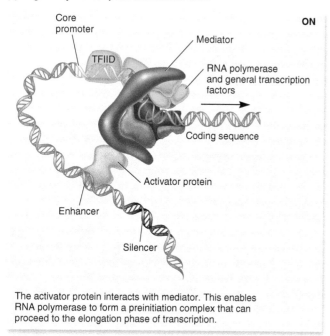

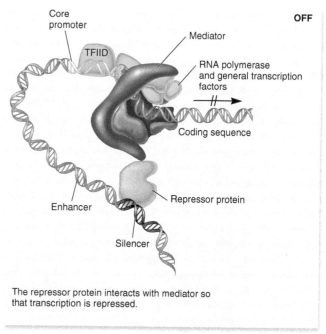

(b) Regulatory transcription factors and mediator

Figure 3-8. Examples of how a regulatory transcription factor influences transcription. (Reprinted with permission from Brooker RJ: *Genetics: Analysis & Principles*, 3rd ed. New York: McGraw-Hill, 2008.)

cells that retain the ability to differentiate into a limited range of types. Hematopoietic stem cells in the bone marrow, for example, are multipotent. But many cell types become fully restricted. Unipotent stem cells are only capable of replacing cells of the same type.

Not all organisms share the same limitations of plasticity. In some the cell fate is determined very early. If a few cells in the *Drosophila* blastoderm are destroyed with a hot needle, a corresponding part of the adult body is missing. The cell lineage in the nematode, *Caenorhabditis elegans*, has now been mapped in such detail that the steps of cellular differentiation are known for every cell in the body (Figure 3-12). As mentioned earlier, plants are at the other end of the spectrum. Their cells seem to retain a greater degree of plasticity longer than do most animal cells. Plant cells also have a greater potential to revert from a specialized type into a totipotent one, but this potential can also be generated in mammals as seen for example in cloning an animal like Dolly, the sheep.

Pattern Formation

It is not enough that cells have the capacity to specialize into the range of cell types found in the body. They must do so in the correct place, relative to other cell types. Pattern formation is the result of processes that specify the spatial "address" of cells and determine the pathway toward specialization that they will follow. We will illustrate this concept by exploring how the diffusion gradient of an effector molecule, a **morphogen**, can signal positional information within a developmental field (Figure 3-13). Positional information can also be signaled by direct cell-to-cell or cell-to-extracellular matrix contact by means of cell adhesion molecules and other signaling mechanisms.

A morphogen is a small diffusible molecule whose concentration can be detected by cells within a limited region of tissue, the developmental field. If the diffusible morphogen is synthesized in one region, sometimes called the source, its concentration declines as a function of distance from the source. Such a concentration gradient can become stable over

Figure 3-9. The activity of regulatory transcription factors can be influenced by binding to small effector molecules, such as certain types of hormones, or by protein-protein interactions or phosphorylation. (Reprinted with permission from Brooker RJ: *Genetics: Analysis & Principles*, 3rd ed. New York: McGraw-Hill, 2008.)

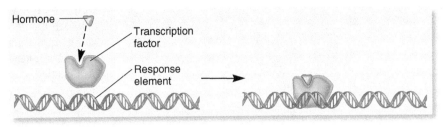

(a) Binding of a small effector molecule such as a hormone

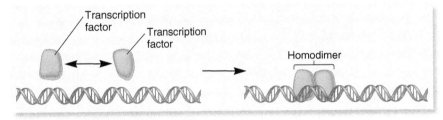

(b) Protein-protein interaction

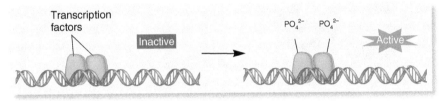

(c) Covalent modification such as phosphorylation

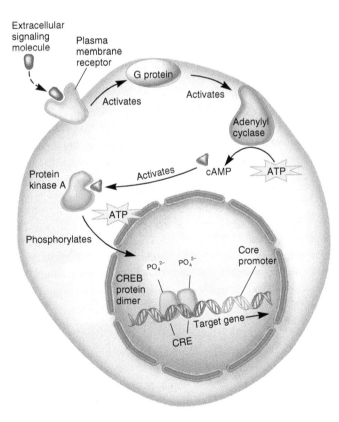

Figure 3-10. Signal transduction is illustrated by the sequence of events involving the CREB protein. (Reprinted with permission from Brooker RJ: *Genetics: Analysis & Principles*, 3rd ed. New York: McGraw-Hill, 2008.)

a small distance if the morphogen is inactivated or destroyed at another point, the sink. Concentration of the morphogen along the gradient communicates a cell's relative position within the field. In one well-studied example, the anterior-posterior body axis of *Drosophila* is established by diffusible proteins, such as bicoid, produced by maternal mRNAs deposited in the developing oocyte (Figure 3-14).

Morphogenesis

In addition to positional information signaling the events of differentiation, it can also specify the pattern of cell death that helps shape the body. Body form is also determined by the movement of cells and sheets of cells that define positional and signaling interactions. **Morphogenesis** is the process of shaping body form.

The earliest morphogenetic event in the embryo is **gastrulation**, in which a portion of the outer layer of the hollow blastocyst folds inward to produce a two-layer embryo with an outer **ectoderm** and inner **endoderm**. At about the same time, out pockets of tissue from this inner layer become a middle layer, the **mesoderm**. All tissues of the adult derive from one or other of these three layers (Table 3-1).

The next critical morphogenetic event in mammals is neurulation in which a fold occurs in the ectoderm. This defines the dorsal midline and produces the dorsal hollow neural tube, the first step in organogenesis. Many later developmental events are organized around this axis. The establishment of body axes at an early stage of embryonic development is the

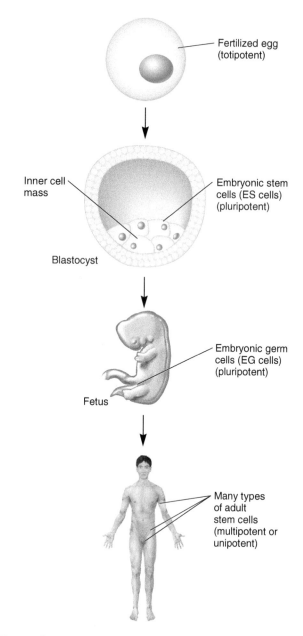

Fertilized egg
(totipotent)

Inner cell
mass

Embryonic stem
cells (ES cells)
(pluripotent)

Blastocyst

Embryonic germ
cells (EG cells)
(pluripotent)

Fetus

Many types
of adult
stem cells
(multipotent or
unipotent)

Figure 3-11. The ability of stem cells to differentiate into other cell types is gradually restricted during development. (Reprinted with permission from Brooker RJ: *Genetics: Analysis & Principles*, 3rd ed. New York: McGraw-Hill, 2008.)

foundation of embryonic organization. The genes responsible for such fundamental steps are surprisingly well conserved across a wide taxonomic spectrum. But like many key genetic mechanisms, they were first discovered in *Drosophila*.

The Organization of Embryonic Development

The organization of embryonic development in *Drosophila* involves two sets of genes. **Segmentation genes** divide the body into a series of similar segments, and the **homeotic genes** define the way in which each of these segments will develop.

Homeotic mutations in *Drosophila* have strange phenotypes in which the normal specification of one body part is altered into that of another, such as legs growing in the normal position of antennae (Figure 3-15).

Studies of the genetic makeup of homeotic genes led to the discovery of a regulatory sequence, the **homeobox**, which has now been identified in many genes that establish key aspects of body organization in animals as structurally diverse as mammals, insects, nematodes, and the simplest animals, sponges. Indeed the same homeobox is even found in many genes that regulate plant development.

Homeotic genes code for proteins that act as DNA transcription factors (Figure 3-16). In each of them, the homeobox is a conserved 180 bp consensus sequence that codes for a 60 amino acid region called the **homeodomain** (remember that each DNA triplet corresponds to 1 amino acid). The homeodomain contains α helices that bind in the major groove of DNA at sites within transcription enhancer elements. A transcriptional activation domain in the homeotic protein then increases the rate of transcription in the genes it regulates. This can lead to a cascade of further transcriptional activation in cell signaling pathways that causes each segment to take on its prescribed morphological characteristics.

The homeotic genes that control segment specialization in *Drosophila* are arranged in two clusters on the third chromosome (Figure 3-17). The *antennapedia* complex includes genes that control the fate of segments in the head and anterior thorax. The *bithorax* complex controls segment specification in the posterior thorax and abdomen. The anterior to posterior order of the genes in each complex almost perfectly parallels the order of body segments that they control.

In other organisms, the homeotic gene clusters are called ***Hox* complexes**, a contraction of "homeobox." The general organization of these clusters is largely conserved among organisms, but vertebrates have an increased number of *Hox* complexes. All invertebrates have one *Hox* complex, as described in *Drosophila*. But vertebrates have at least four copies that may be located on different chromosomes. One hypothesis is that this increase in *Hox* gene number allows the creation of greater complexity in cell types. Some genes within these duplicates have lost their ability to function and new homeotic genes are present. In mice, there are four *Hox* clusters (Figure 3-18). As originally seen in *Drosophila*, there is a correlation between the genetic order of the adjacent *Hox* genes and the anatomical region within which each one acts (Figure 3-19).

Our discussion of developmental organization has focused on events defining body structure along the anterior-posterior and the dorsal-ventral axes. But there is another important dimension, laterality. We are essentially symmetrical, in organization if not in actual appearance. Yet, some internal organs are not. The heart, stomach, and liver do not develop symmetrically on the midline. Laterality in such structures is determined very early in development, and errors in signaling can lead to laterality defects like mirror image arrangement. In animals with less plasticity in developmental programming, early changes in cell lineage can yield distinct bilateral differences

Figure 3-12. A brief summary of the cell lineage of the nematode, *caenorhabditis elegans*, which has now been mapped for each cell of its body.

(Reprinted with permission from Brooker RJ: *Genetics: Analysis & Principles*, 3rd ed. New York: McGraw-Hill, 2008.)

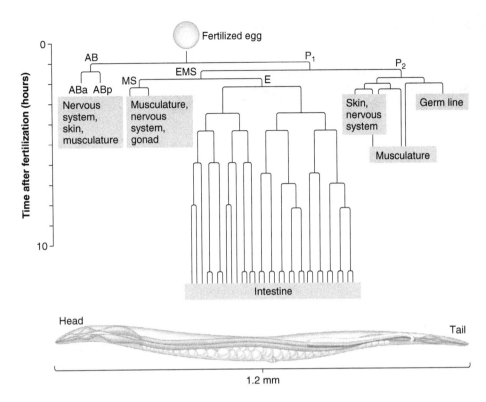

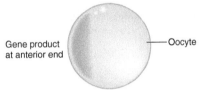

(a) Asymmetric distribution of morphogens in an oocyte

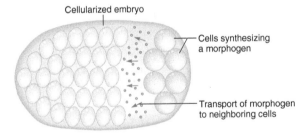

(b) Asymmetric synthesis and extracellular distribution of a morphogen in an embryo

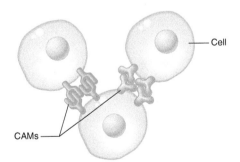

(c) Cell-to-cell contact conveys positional information

Figure 3-13. Three different mechanisms by which positional information can be communicated within a cell population.

(Reprinted with permission from Brooker RJ: *Genetics: Analysis & Principles*, 3rd ed. New York: McGraw-Hill, 2008.)

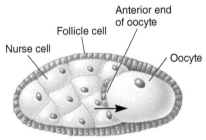

(a) Transport of maternal effect gene products into the oocyte

(b) In situ hybridization of *bicoid* mRNA

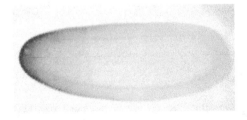

(c) Immunostaining of Bicoid protein

Figure 3-14. Immunostaining of *bicoid* mRNA and protein illustrates a morphogen gradient in the early *Drosophila* egg. The *bicoid* mRNA is trapped near the anterior end of the developing oocyte.

(b, c: Christiane Nüsslein-Volhard, *Development*, Supplement 1, 1991. © The Company of Biologists Limited.)

Table 3-1.	Derivatives of the Three Embryonic Layers
Layer	Representative derivatives
Ectoderm	Epidermis and its derivatives, including hair, nails Brain, spinal cord, and nerves Schwann cells Adrenal medulla
Mesoderm	Circulatory system, heart, vessels, and blood Dermis Skeleton Muscles Kidney Gonads Outer covering of internal organs Lining of thoracic and abdominal cavities
Endoderm	Lining of digestive tract Lining of respiratory tract Pancreas Liver Pharynx

like the two-colored lobster in Figure 3-20. In *Drosophila*, bilateral mosaics called gynandromorphs, in which one half of the body is female and the other half is male, are used as experimental tools to study a variety of developmental mechanisms.

Thus, a study of simple developmental systems in prokaryotes and invertebrates can give us an insight into the mechanisms that regulate the developmental events in more complex animals like ourselves. Genetic changes operating at each of the levels we have discussed here have parallels in medically important conditions.

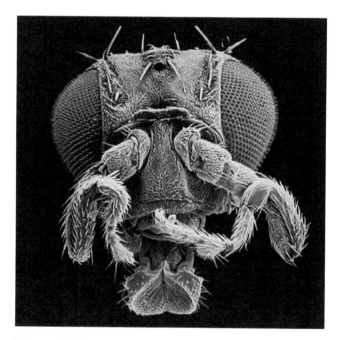

Figure 3-15. The *antennapedia* mutation is a homeotic mutation that changes the fate of cells in a segment that would normally yield an antenna. Instead, a leg forms. (© F.R. Turner, Indiana University/Visuals Unlimited.)

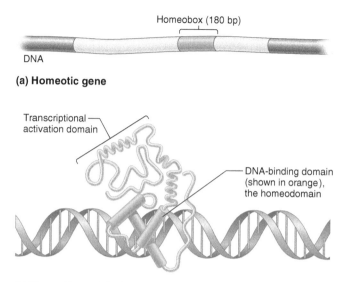

(a) Homeotic gene

(b) Homeotic protein bound to DNA

Figure 3-16. A homeotic gene, shown in tan and orange, contains a 180-bp homeobox, which codes for a DNA-binding protein region called the homeodomain. This binds at an enhancer genetic regulatory element and activates transcription. (Reprinted with permission from Brooker RJ: *Genetics: Analysis & Principles*, 3rd ed. New York: McGraw-Hill, 2008.)

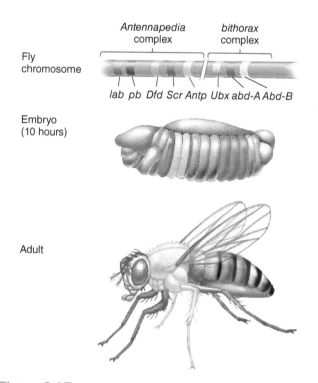

Figure 3-17. The direct correspondence between the order of homeotic genes of two complexes, the *antennapedia* complex and the *bithorax* complex, and the body regions in which they are expressed. (Reprinted with permission from Brooker RJ: *Genetics: Analysis & Principles*, 3rd ed. New York: McGraw-Hill, 2008.)

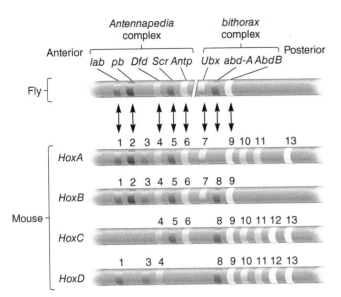

Figure 3-18. The organization of homeotic genes is highly conserved among taxonomically diverse animals. As a representative mammal, for example, mice have four homeobox (*Hox*) gene clusters that correspond with genes in *Drosophila*. (Reprinted with permission from Brooker RJ: *Genetics: Analysis & Principles*, 3rd ed. New York: McGraw-Hill, 2008.)

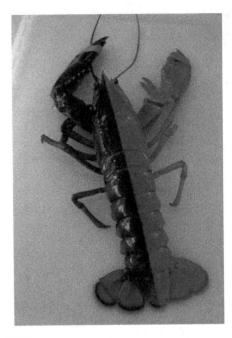

Figure 3-20. A rare laterality in color in a lobster caught by a Digby County, Nova Scotia, fisherman. (© Tina Comeau/Yarmouth Vanguard, Reprinted with permission from "Just how rare is a two-coloured lobster?" *The Vanguard*. Published on January 11, 2008. http://www.novanews-now.com.)

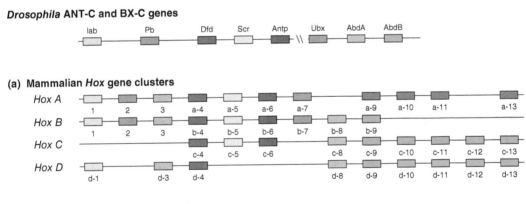

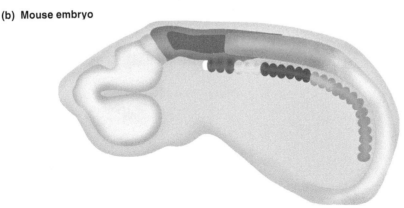

Figure 3-19. The correspondence between *Hox* gene arrangement and the body segments in which they are expressed in mice. (Reprinted with permission from Hartwell LH, et al: *Genetics: From Genes to Genomes*. 3rd ed. New York: McGraw-Hill, 2008.)

From a single fertilized egg, the development of the complex organism that will become a human being seems nothing less than miraculous. Understanding the process does not lessen the awe. The process of development is a series of steps that begins with the organization (set up) of the embryo, followed by progressive refinement of cells into specialized functions, leading to the organization of differentiated cells into tissues, and finally the formation of discrete anatomic structures.

As discussed earlier, this developmental cascade is under precise regulation by a series of programmed genetic "switches" that are intensely integrated. In the coordination of development, order and timing are crucial. At any given step in the process of development, something can go wrong. Structural congenital anomalies, or "birth defects," are then the result of alterations in these normal developmental processes. Depending on the timing and the process involved, different types of anomalies may occur. Table 3-2 lists examples of disorders of embryonic organization with the corresponding levels of embryonic developmental control.

General Principles of Embryology

Before we proceed with a discussion of congenital anomalies, a brief review of embryology is in order. It is beyond the scope of this text to review human embryology fully. However, a solid understanding of human embryology is critical to interpret congenital anomalies correctly.

Table 3-2.	Examples of Disorders of Embryonic Organization at Various Levels	
Level of Organization	**Type**	**Disorder**
Trilaminar embryo	Ectoderm	Ectodermal dysplasias
Anterior:posterior	Neural tube	Caudal regression
Sidedness	Disorders of laterality	Kartagener syndrome Ivemark syndrome
Ventral:dorsal	Front:back	
Segments	Branchial arches (1st/2nd) (3rd/4th)	Treacher Collins syndrome DiGeorge syndrome
Developmental fields	Midline	Opitz syndrome
Organ	Heart	Congenital heart malformations
Tissue	Connective tissue	Connective tissue disorders

Developmental periods

One of the best ways to conceptualize development is to organize it by developmental periods. As the organism develops, each period is characterized by the pattern of which critical structures and processes are emerging. The key point here is timing. Timing is critical both from the standpoint of which structure is developing when, and from knowledge about which processes are dependent on each other in a developmental sequence.

In a very real sense, the organization of a human embryo begins even before conception. Recent studies have demonstrated the central role of preconceptional influences on human development. In fact it probably begins during the middle part of the mother's gestation! Beginning in the third fetal month, the oogonia begin to differentiate into oocytes. Oocyte formation in the female fetus requires organization of the cell that includes establishing polarity, intracellular sub-compartmentalization, and chemical gradients. Defects in these processes may have downstream effects on the development of the offspring from this individual. In the mature (adult) female, external (prepregnancy) influences can still affect fetal development presumably by their effects on the oocyte milieu. For example, abundant research has shown that the maternal use of relatively high doses of folic acid can significantly reduce the occurrence and recurrence of neural tube defects. The maximum effect can be achieved if the folate supplementation is started 2-3 months prior to conception, presumably due to changes in the oocyte prior to conception.

The process of *in utero* development can be divided into major time periods typically marked from the time of conception. It is important to note that an alternative designation can be used that defines the periods of development in relationship to the last menstrual period (LMP). By this designation, pregnancies are dated in weeks beginning from the first day of the woman's LMP. On average, ovulation occurs on day 14 of the menstrual cycle, and conception occurs about 2 weeks after her LMP. Thus a woman's "obstetrical date" of 6 weeks would be 2 weeks after her first missed period. This definition is preferentially used in perinatal assessments such as prenatal ultrasounds. This is in contrast to the embryologic date (the age of the embryo). The obstetric date is about 2 weeks longer than the embryologic date. For the purposes of identifying critical periods for the occurrence of congenital anomalies, the embryologic date is used. The clinically important time periods of *in utero* development can be defined as:

- Early pregnancy (first 3 weeks)
- First trimester (3-11 weeks)
- Second trimester (12-25 weeks)
- Third trimester (26-40 weeks)

Embryonic development essentially refers to the time of organ formation. For practical purposes this corresponds to the first trimester. All major structural features of the individual are in place by the end of the 11th week, with one major exception. Macroscopic structural changes can still be seen in the central nervous system until about the middle of pregnancy. The last major structural development that can be seen in developing humans is the corpus callosum of the brain. The completion of its development is seen at about 21 weeks.

The response of the embryo or fetus to various deleterious factors differs by the embryologic period. In brief, major insults in the first 3 weeks of pregnancy result in pregnancy loss. Problems during the first trimester result in malformations (discussed further later). Insults in the second and trimester tend to disrupt growth and organization more at the cellular level.

Key factors in normal morphogenesis

Conceptually, most congenital anomalies can be understood as the disruption of specific normal processes in development. Some of the key processes to be considered are:

1. *Cell growth rate* as a "force" in human development. Many observable physical features can be explained by differences in cell growth rate. For instance, things like fingerprint patterns are the results of relative growth rates of the cells of the finger tip pads. Higher elevated pads (associated with increased cell growth) will result in whorl patterns, whereas lower elevated pads tend to produce arch patterns. The so-called "embryopathic face" is a set of common facial features, such as underdevelopment of the midface, flattened nasal bridge, thin upper lip, and smoothened philtrum. These features can be caused by many factors (including teratogens) that work by the common mechanism of reducing the overall rate of cellular growth.

2. *Cell migration.* In the normal process of embryonic development, many specialized cells need to migrate from their place of origin to their definitive position in the body. Migrational defects occur when the movement of cells from one place to the next is interrupted.

3. *Cell-cell interactions.* Throughout development, specialized cells are being defined. Among cell types, there is a need for interactions between these groups. In the normal process of development and organization, interactions among cells, such as induction, adhesion, and destruction, are critical. Interference with these interactions may produce areas of dysplasia. It is also important to note that most of these processes are normal events during embryogenesis. At the conclusion of embryonic development, they should be rendered inactive. Reactivation of some of these processes plays a central role in the ontogeny of cancer.

4. *Selected cell death.* Certain cells are developmentally preprogrammed for **apoptosis** (cessation of function). Eliminating these cells is just as crucial for normal development as the generation of cells in the first place. For example, failure of the (normal) programmed cell death for those cells between developing fingers will result in syndactyly (fusion of the digits).

5. *Growth factors/hormones.* Cell growth and migration are directly influenced by a variety of hormones and growth factors. These substances are typically produced elsewhere and are then transported to the target site to direct those cells in further development. Many of these factors exert their influence under a narrowly-defined set of chemical concentrations established by interactive gradients.

Congenital Anomalies

The term **congenital anomaly** literally means "something not right at birth." In the broadest sense, any abnormality present at birth and its resulting phenotype could be classified as a "birth defect." This could be an abnormality of structure, function, or body metabolism (i.e., an inborn error of body chemistry) present at birth that results in physical or mental disability, or is fatal. Taken to the extreme any mutation present at conception and its resulting phenotype could be classified as a congenital anomaly. For instance, a seminar was held several years ago entitled "Breast Cancer and Other Birth Defects." Their reference was to heritable abnormalities of certain "cancer genes" that give a genetic predisposition to breast cancer. For the purposes of this chapter, however, we will limit our discussions to structural congenital anomalies.

Epidemiology

Overall, 4 million babies are born each year in the United States. Approximately 150,000 of these are born with a congenital anomaly. Roughly half of these are detectable as part of the child's first physical examination shortly after birth. The other half may be hidden from view and not readily detected initially.

The overall incidence of a major congenital anomaly is around 4% of all live born infants. This represents a baseline or "population" incidence. It represents the lowest relative risk that exists for a given pregnancy—a number from which no couple is exempt. Few couples approach a pregnancy with the expectation of a child with a birth defect. Yet, this baseline number means that 1 in 25 couples are expected to experience the birth of a child with a medically significant problem. Obviously, other factors such as family history, medical conditions, environmental factors, ethnicity, and genetic factors can modify, i.e., increase, these risks. Interestingly, there are no well-identified factors that can actually lower this 4% risk.

If the actual number of congenital anomalies per live birth is calculated, it is more than double (9%) the rate of newborns with an anomaly. The reason for this, of course, is that some children have more than one anomaly. In fact the presence of one congenital anomaly carries a 50% chance that there is a second significant anomaly present. This is critically important in the evaluation of a child with a congenital anomaly. Once a structural congenital anomaly is identified, it is imperative that a search for potentially associated anomalies be implemented. Table 3-3 lists the most commonly found congenital anomalies and the incidence of these at birth.

Table 3-3.	Most Common Structural Congenital Anomalies	
Anomaly	**Incidence (per 10,000 births)**	
Congenital heart defects	200
Hypospadius	35
Polydactyly/syndactyly	25
Club foot	21
Hip dislocation	20
Orofacial clefts	18
Pyloric stenosis	15
Spina bifida/anencephaly	10
Hydrocephalus without spina bifida	8
Limb reductions	6
Omphalocoele	5
Cystic kidney disease	4
Diaphragmatic hernia	3
Gastroschisis	1

Trends

Because of the enormous impact of these conditions, most state health departments have some sort of birth defects registry in place. These registries vary from state to state in their scope and policies. The common link is the goal to track the number and types of congenital anomalies occurring in that state for any given year. These projects have been ongoing for decades now. In addition, several federal initiatives have been implemented to coordinate and compare data collection efforts across states in the United States and worldwide. As might be expected, there are distinct regional variances. But, in general, the information obtained is fairly consistent and identifies several common themes and trends.

The overall birth defect rates have been surprisingly consistent over the past several decades. A few changing trends have been identified. Neural tube defects (excluding anencephaly) have steadily decreased. Notably, this decline seems to have started before the advent of folate supplementation or fortification. The occurrence of congenital heart malformations has been steadily increasing over the past several years for reasons still unknown. Other anomalies showing an increasing incidence include obstructive uropathies and certain neurodevelopmental disorders.

Consistently higher birth defect rates are reported in the southern United States and parts of the Midwest as compared to other parts of the United States. It is likely that these differences are not related to an actual increase in congenital anomalies in these regions, but rather are a function of the tracking systems in place. There is a direct correlation in which the states that have a "better" tracking system have a higher reported incidence of birth defects; i.e., a correlation of higher numbers with better reporting.

Congenital anomalies affect people of all racial and ethnic groups. While certain specific genetic conditions clearly do occur with a higher frequency in certain ethnic groups, in general these differences are relatively small for congenital anomalies. The birth defect rates are mildly increased in African Americans and Hispanics in the United States, as compared to Caucasians. Potentially this may be related to socioeconomic factors, although there is some suggestion that this may not be the sole answer.

Impact

The medical and fiscal impact of congenital anomalies is staggering. This is due in part to the sheer number of these conditions as well as the magnitude of their effects. Persons with congenital anomalies are affected in their medical care and can suffer serious health, emotional, and social burdens. The burdens affect not only the child, but also that child's family and society as a whole. In one study, the estimated lifetime expense associated with 12 selected, isolated birth defects was calculated to be more than $8 billion, ranging from $140,000 to $700,000 per child.

One of the most notable impacts of birth defects is their effect on longevity. Consistently, birth defects and prematurity are fairly well tied as the two leading causes of death among infants in the United States. Birth defects account for an estimated 20% of infant deaths per year, which translates to 6,500 deaths annually. Infants with major congenital anomalies have a six-fold higher incidence rate of infant deaths when compared to those without congenital anomalies. Forty-five percent of all deaths in the neonatal intensive care units are due to congenital anomalies. For African Americans, they represent the second most common cause, with preterm labor or low-birth-weight infants being the most common cause of infant mortality. They are also the second leading cause in Native Americans and Alaskan natives.

Birth defects account for a similar proportion of total deaths for children aged 1 to 14. They account for approximately 15.5% of deaths among children 1 to 4 years old; 8% in the 5- to 9-year-old age group; and 6% in the 10- to 14-year-old category. In fact, among children aged 1 to 14, one study estimated that birth defects could account for 21.5% of total deaths.

Types of Congenital Anomalies

Individual congenital anomalies can be classified according to the pathogenetic mechanism responsible for their occurrence. In general four distinct mechanisms have been purported: malformations, deformations, disruptions, and dysplasias. Clinical geneticists are meticulous about the use of these terms in the classification of congenital anomalies. The student should be cautious when reviewing the medical literature in this regards. Outside of the discipline of clinical genetics the terms may be applied more loosely.

A **malformation**, as the term would imply, is a congenital anomaly in which the tissue is malformed, i.e., it did not

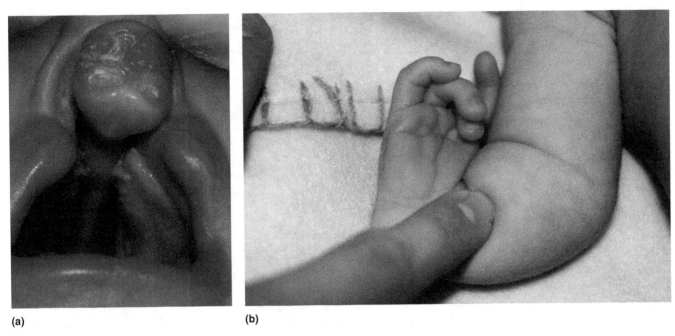

(a)   (b)

Figure 3-21. Two examples of major malformations. (a) Bilateral cleft lip and palate. (b) Agenesis (absence) of the radius.

form correctly from the start. As noted in our earlier discussions, the vast majority of malformations occur in the first trimester of pregnancy given the timing of normal embryogenesis. A distinction is made between major and minor malformations. **Major malformations** are defined as those that have significant clinical implications and are not found in the general (normal) population (Figure 3-21). In contrast, **minor malformations** do not produce clinically significant problems and may occur in a small number of "normal" individuals (Figure 3-22). Current estimates suggest that 15% of newborns will have a single minor anomaly (not including dermatoglyphic changes) when carefully assessed by a trained dysmorphologist. In addition about 1% of all newborns will have two or more minor anomalies. Although minor malformations are not of major clinical import, they are very important in the assessment of persons with congenital anomalies as clues to more serious problems and the recognition of malformation syndromes. As the number of detected minor malformations goes up, the chance of having a major malformation likewise increases. As such, it is recommended that any individual with three or more minor malformations have a formal assessment looking for major malformations. It is also important to note that minor malformations may present as a familial trait. In this context, it is important to define whether this represents a normal familial variant or is an indicator of a heritable disorder. From a mechanistic standpoint, malformations can result from the lack of development (**agenesis**) or underdevelopment (**hypogenesis**) of a given structure. There may also be abnormal migration of cells (**heterotopia**) or whole organs (**ectopia**). Finally there may be incomplete closure or separation.

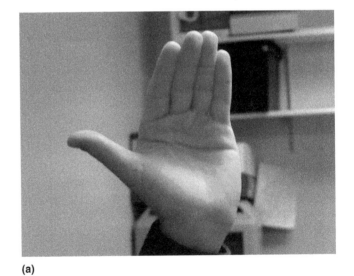

(a)

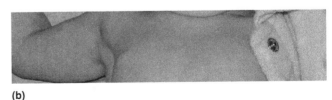

(b)

Figure 3-22. Two examples of minor malformations. (a) A single transverse palmar crease. Most individuals have two creases in the palms. About 2% of the general population has a single crease. In contrast, over 90% of patients with Down syndrome have a single crease. (b) Widely spaced nipples. Note that the nipple is laterally placed almost to the axilla.

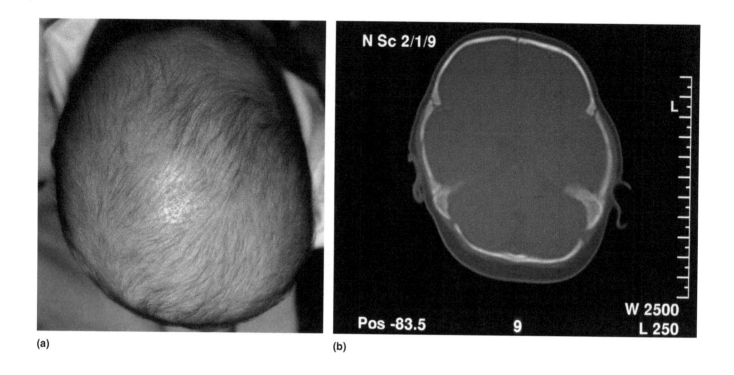

(a)   (b)

Figure 3-23. Deformational plagiocephaly. (a) Note the asymmetry of the cranium with a deformational change in the shape to a rhomboid configuration. (b) Corresponding CT scan of the head. Note the asymmetry of the position of the ears.

Deformations represent another mechanism that causes congenital anomalies (Figure 3-23). Deformational changes are the results of mechanical forces applied to otherwise normally developing structures. In the case of a deformation, the magnitude and the direction of the applied force can often be deduced from careful inspection of the changes coupled with knowledge of normal perinatal anatomy and physiology (Figure 3-24). The mechanical forces that lead to deformations can arise from a variety of sources. In general they are factors that somehow constrain or apply a force to the fetus. Deformations can be of maternal or fetal origin. Maternal factors that may cause deformational anomalies include a small mother, a small uterus, uterine malformations (bicornuate uterus, septate uterus, and so forth), primigravid pregnancy, or oligohydramnios. Fetal factors would include multiple gestation, a large fetus, other fetal anomalies, fetal hypo-mobility, or oligohydramnios. (Note that oligohydramnios appears on both lists as it may occur due to maternal factors such as amniotic leakage or fetal factors such as oliguria.) Table 3-4 lists some of the commonly found deformations.

Normally developing tissue may be subjected to insults that result in actual loss of cells and/or tissue. The resultant anomalies are due to the effects of the missing cells. This type of anomaly is referred to as a **disruption** (Figure 3-25). A variety of insults may occur during pregnancies that result in a disruption. The most common mechanism is some sort of vascular accident (hemorrhage, occlusion, ischemia, or constriction). Other mechanisms include radiation or infection. Table 3-5 lists some of the commonly found disruptions.

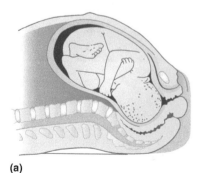

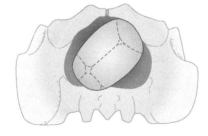

(a)   (b)

Figure 3-24. Schematic demonstrating how deformational plagiocephaly may be induced by early descent into the pelvis. (a) Infant engaged in pelvis. (b) Contralateral pressure on the skull from opposite sides of the pelvic rim. (Redrawn from Bruneteau RJ, Mulliken JB: Frontal plagiocephaly: synostotic, compensational, or deformational. *Plast Reconstr Surg.* 1992; 89(1):21-31.)

Table 3-4.	Commonly Noted Deformations
Torticollis-plagiocephaly	
Scoliosis	
Facial nerve palsies	
Ear anomalies (crumpling, folding, flattening)	
Nose compression/deviation	
Chest protrusion (pectus carinatum) or indentation (pectus excavatum)	
Joint dislocations	
Retromicrognathia (small recessed jaw)	
Overlapping or crowded toes	

Dysplasia (Figure 3-26) literally means "bad form." A dysplasia represents aberrant formation specifically at the level of the organization of cells into tissues (**dyshistogenesis**). As such they tend to occur later in development and somewhat independently of morphogenesis. Morphogenesis is exclusively prenatal in origin, whereas histogenesis continues postnatally in all tissues that have not undergone end differentiation. A unique aspect of congenital anomalies that are dysplastic in nature is that they may predispose to cancer later in life.

Patterns of Congenital Anomalies

As mentioned earlier, congenital anomalies may occur as isolated anomalies, but frequently multiple anomalies occur in the same individual. In fact, if one structural congenital anomaly is present in a patient, there is a 50% chance that that person has one or more additional anomalies (i.e., multiple congenital anomalies). If multiple anomalies are present, then the next step in the evaluation process is to try and identify a specific pattern that ties the multiple findings together.

Three major categories of patterns of multiple anomalies have been defined. **Syndromes** are patterns of congenital anomalies of more than one organ system with a common etiology. Sotos syndrome (Figure 3-27) is characterized by overgrowth, macrocephaly, an advanced bone age, a characteristic facial appearance, and neurodevelopmental and neurobehavioral changes. Over 90% of patients with Sotos syndrome have a mutation in a gene called NSD1. There are hundreds of other well-described syndromes.

Associations refer to the known occurrence of certain anomalies that happen too often to be by chance, but without a defined etiology. Associations often are designated by acronyms that detail the most common features. VACTERL association (Figure 3-28) defines an association of **V**ertebral anomalies, **A**nal atresia (imperforate anus), **C**ardiac malformations, **T**racheal-**E**sophageal fistula, **R**enal anomalies, and **L**imb anomalies. (Earlier reports defined the condition as the VATER association.) Not every patient has every one of the listed anomalies. Again, what is found is the association—these anomalies

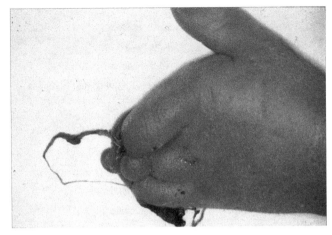

(a)

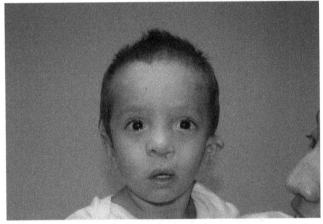

(b)

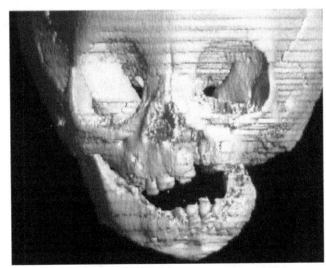

(c)

Figure 3-25. Two examples of disruptions. (a) Terminal reduction of the digits due to constriction from amniotic bands. (b and c) Hemifacial microsomia. Photo and CT scan demonstrating underdevelopment of the left side of the jaw. This anomaly is most commonly due to occlusion of the stapedial artery in the developing fetus.

Table 3-5.	Commonly Noted Disruptions
Cause	**Results**
Radiation	Microcephaly
Infection	Congenital infection syndrome
Toxoplasmosis	
Rubella	
Cytomegalovirus	
Herpes	
Amniotic rupture	Anencephaly
	Facial clefts
	Amputations of limbs/digits
Ischemia	Porencephalic cysts
	Ileal atresia
Vascular occlusion	Hemifacial microsomia
	Gastroschisis

are found together at a frequency too often to be likely by chance. The diagnostic criteria for this condition require that at least three of the highlighted features be present. The key distinction from syndromes is the lack of an identified common etiology.

Because development is so interconnected, an early change can have a "snowball effect" on other components of development. The cascading effect can lead to a reproducible pattern of anomalies. This type of multiple anomaly pattern is referred to as a **sequence**. The Robin sequence (sometimes called the Pierre Robin sequence) is an example of such a pattern (Figure 3-29). It is often errantly referred to as the Robin syndrome. By strict definition, it is not a syndrome, rather it is best designated a sequence. In this condition, there is only one primary anomaly, micrognathia (small jaw). A smaller jaw tends to displace the tongue posteriorly. If this occurs before 9 weeks of gestation (prior to the closure of the lateral palatine ridges), the abnormally displaced tongue physically interferes with the closure of the palate. This results in a cleft palate that is somewhat different in its configuration than the typical

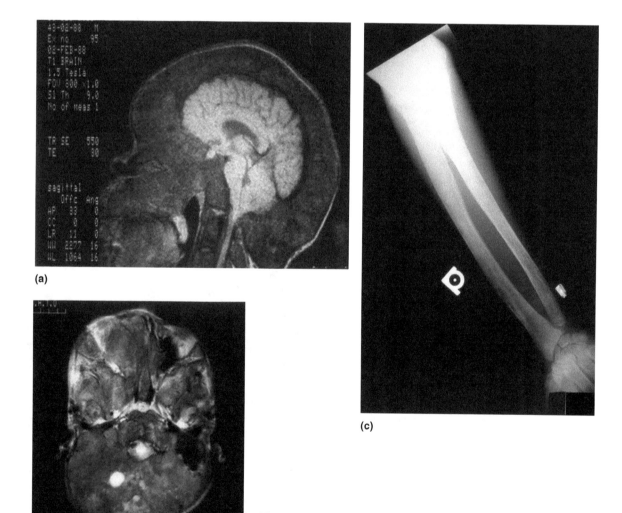

(a)

(b)

(c)

Figure 3-26. Imaging studies of a patient with polyostotic fibrous dysplasia. (a and b) MRI slices of the cranium. Note the markedly abnormal configuration (dysplasia) in the cranial bones. (c) X-rays of the forearms also demonstrating dysplastic changes.

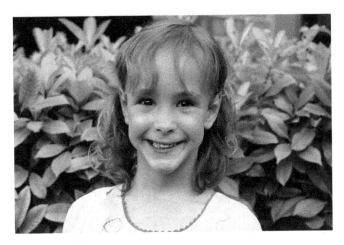

Figure 3-27. Young girl with Sotos syndrome.

Etiology of Congenital Anomalies

When a person is identified as having a congenital anomaly, the first question usually raised is "Why?" For most people there is a strong desire to know the cause (etiology) of the abnormality. In addition, there are often medically important pieces of information that are tied to this answer. Besides simply knowing the cause, identifying an etiology is helpful in defining recurrence risks, prognosis, associated co-morbidities, and even potential targeted therapies. Thus, when a child is born with a congenital anomaly, a consultation with a clinical geneticist is typically requested. The role of the geneticist is to identify the pattern of anomalies and determine the etiology, if at all possible. If an etiology can be determined, then detailed counseling can be provided to the family along the lines noted. The discipline of **dysmorphology** is the art and science of discerning recognizable patterns of congenital anomalies. Some would consider this a separate discipline and request themselves to be called dysmorphologists. We would tend to characterize it as a subdiscipline within clinical genetics. The seminal publication in this arena is *Smith's Recognizable Patterns of Human Malformations* which was originally penned by Dr. David Smith, the man regarded as the father of the discipline of dysmorphology. This book is currently in its 6th edition, ever expanding to include additional syndromes

cleft palate. While the typical cleft is a linear defect, the cleft palate seen in the Robin sequence will have a 'U' or wedge-shaped configuration. Secondary changes are often seen because of malnutrition, the combination of a cleft and a small jaw making feeding quite difficult. The end result is a child with what appears to be a syndrome, but in actuality it has a series of problems cascading from a single early anomaly.

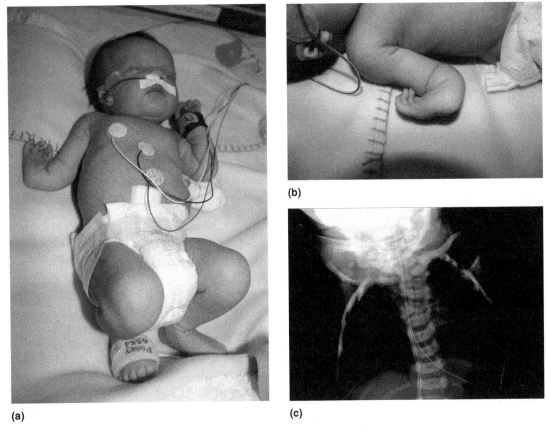

(a)   (b)   (c)

Figure 3-28. Infant with VACTERL (VATER) association. (a) Whole body of infant. (b) Note forearm anomalies due to radial hypogenesis. (c) Multiple anomalies of cervical vertebrae.

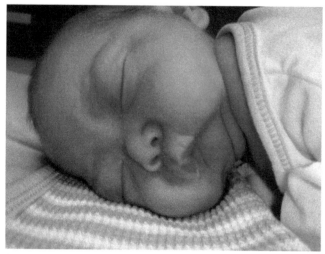

(a)

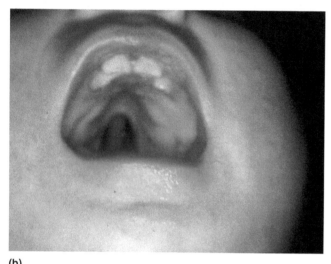

(b)

Figure 3-29. Infant with Robin sequence. (a) Small recessed chin (retromicrognathia). (b) 'U-shaped' cleft palate.

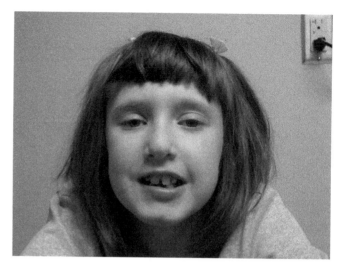

Figure 3-30. Young girl with a known 22q11.2 deletion. She has learning disabilities, cleft palate, congenital heart disease, immune deficiency, and minor facial dysmorphisms. Her phenotype is best characterized as DiGeorge syndrome.

and updates on the molecular genetics of each condition. Several other excellent published collections of syndromes and their descriptions are available.

As one might expect, there are a myriad of causes of congenital anomalies. All known categories of etiologies have been identified in congenital anomalies. Depending upon the particular anomaly, the etiology may be chromosomal, single gene, teratogenic, or multifactorial. More complex genetic changes may also be involved. Traditionally, it has been noted that only about 20% of all congenital anomalies have an identifiable cause. Recent advances in genetic testing are clearly improving this yield. Although we are not aware of any recent study that has been published to quantify and substantiate this, our clinical experience would suggest that currently this diagnostic yield has at least doubled and is on the order of 40% or greater. Clearly further advances will continue to improve the diagnostic yield for congenital anomalies.

In general it is easier to identify the etiology if multiple anomalies are present. Identifying the etiology for single anomalies has historically been quite difficult. But recent advances in diagnostic testing (see Chapter 11) have provided powerful tools that are allowing the identification of the etiology even for isolated (single) anomalies. Some of this can be attributed to the better recognition and understanding of the range of expression of certain conditions. For example, submicroscopic deletions (Chapter 5) on a specific region of chromosome 22, designated as a "22q11.2 deletion" are associated with several patterns of multiple anomalies involving the face/palate, heart, parathyroid glands, thymus, and other organs. When multiple anomalies are seen in conjunction with this deletion, it is often possible to identify an associated recognizable pattern (syndrome) including DiGeorge syndrome (Figure 3-30) and Shprintzen (velo-cardio-facial) syndrome among others. The spectrum of abnormalities seen in conjunction with this deletion is staggering. In fact, the total number of anomalies reported with this deletion is now over 180! The phenotypic range seen with this deletion goes from easily recognizable multiple anomaly syndromes to apparently unaffected individuals. Within this range it is known that some individuals may have only single organ involvement. It is now known that 17% of persons with isolated congenital heart malformations will have a 22q11.2 deletion and 30% of persons with a specific subcategory of heart malformations (conotruncal heart malformations) will have this deletion. Thus, even though the diagnostic yield is nowhere near 100%, these sort of advances have ushered in the era of identifying some causes of congenital anomalies—even at the single organ level.

For much of the rest of this book, we will be discussing two major parameters of human diseases: etiology (the cause) and pathogenesis (the mechanism). In future chapters we will be reviewing in detail etiologies such as single gene disorders, chromosomal abnormalities, gene-environment interactions, and even more complex etiologies such as epigenetic causes. In the context of the discussions in this chapter about congenital anomalies, one specific category of etiology, teratogens, warrants a more detailed discussion here.

Teratogens are environmental agents that can cause birth defects if the mother is exposed to the agent during pregnancy. The maternal exposure is transmitted to the fetus and can invoke congenital anomalies. Early medical thinking had envisioned the "womb" as a highly protective environment that would shield the developing baby from any and all outside influences. Modern understanding recognizes that the maternal-fetal interface is by no means impervious to outside agents. In fact hundreds if not thousands of environmental factors are now known to affect fetal development adversely in the right setting. Some of the major categories of known teratogens include legal and illegal drugs, prescribed medications, herbal and other homeopathic compounds, maternal medical conditions, and environmental/occupational exposures. Table 3-6 lists many of the more common/important human teratogens. The teratogenic potential of any given agent (the likelihood that it could induce a birth defect) is dependent upon a complicated series of interacting

Table 3-7.	Factors That Influence the Potential Teratogenicity of a Particular Agent/Exposure

Timing of the exposure
- Early first trimester—miscarriage
- First trimester—malformations (high degree of sensitivity days 18-60 postconception)
- Second/third trimester—pregnancy viability; brain malformations, organization and maturation; fetal growth
- Perinatal—neonatal adaptation

Ability to cross the placenta
- Molecular size/weight—smaller molecules cross easier
- Charge—highly charged molecules cross less well
- Lipophilic/lipophobic—cell membranes contain large amounts of lipids. Lipophilic compounds cross the placenta better

Characteristics of the exposure
- Dosage
- Duration
- Pattern of exposure

Maternal and/or fetal genetic susceptibility

Mechanism of action
- Vasoconstrictor/vasodilator
- Alters DNA
- Changes rate of cell growth
- Modulates apoptosis

characteristics of the agent and the particular exposures. Table 3-7 lists such factors.

With a better understanding of the importance of teratogenic agents, several major efforts have emerged to identify such agents, report on their characteristics, measure their impact, and establish prevention measures. Large databases available to clinicians and researchers such as TERIS and Reprotox have been established and are constantly being updated. Groups like the Organization of Teratogen Information Specialists (OTIS), the Centers for Disease Control (CDC), the National Institutes for Health (NIH), and the March of Dimes (MOD) have all had major programmatic efforts in understanding and preventing teratogenic birth defects. Herein is by far the most important feature of teratogen-induced birth defects—they are preventable! (For many of the other known causes of congenital anomalies, prevention is simply not possible at this time.) The key to prevention of teratogen-induced congenital anomalies is simple—avoid exposures. This of course is much easier said than done. Some exposures are simply unavoidable. Sometimes the mother's health requires that she take a particular medication. While the drug may have teratogenic potential, it would be more harmful to both mother and child if the mother were not treated.

Likewise, the science may be simple but the implementation extremely difficult. Fetal alcohol syndrome is a recognizable pattern of malformations seen with *in utero* exposure of the fetus to alcohol (ethanol). Fetal alcohol syndrome (FAS) is identified by characteristic facial changes, abnormalities of the growth of the head and body, and neurologic deficits

Table 3-6.	Important Human Teratogens

Substances of abuse
  Legal
    Alcohol (ethanol)
    Cigarettes
  Illegal
    Cocaine
    Marijuana
    Heroin
    LSD
    Benzodiazepines
    Inhalants (toluene)
    Amphetamines

Pharmaceuticals
  Prescription
  Over the counter preparations
  Vitamins
  Herbals
  Hormones

Maternal medical conditions
  Diabetes
  Infections
  Nutrition (folic acid, trace metals)
  Weight
  Health/fitness
  Phenylketonuria
  Lupus
  Hyperthermia

Occupational exposures
  Chemicals (agriculture, lawn care, hair dressing)
  Radiation (X-rays, radiation therapy, industrial)

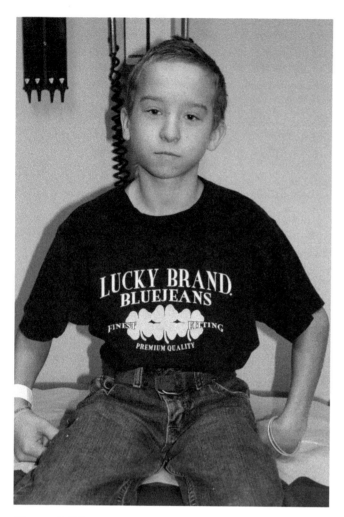

Figure 3-31. Adolescent male with FAS. This child originally presented with short stature of unexplained etiology.

give is that *there should be zero alcohol use at any time for any pregnancy!* As already stated, this is easier said than done. In order to avoid any exposure, a woman must not drink at any point in pregnancy. Since the average gestational age that a woman identifies pregnancy is around 8-9 weeks, it is not enough simply to quit drinking when she recognizes that she is pregnant. Most importantly, health care providers should be aware of this risk and appropriately counsel their patients. As unbelievable as it might seem, there are still practitioners who will advise their pregnant patients to drink a small amount of alcohol during pregnancy to "calm their nerves"! We sincerely hope that you as a conscientious health care provider will instead make the only wise prescription for your patients. No alcohol during pregnancy. None; never.

Evaluation of the Patient With Congenital Anomalies

The approach to the person with a congenital anomaly is largely similar to most other medical assessments. The evaluation revolves around the typical "history and physical" approach. The difference in the evaluation of a person with a congenital disorder is largely a greater emphasis on certain components of the exam and history. Clearly much more attention is paid to the family and prenatal histories. The examination goes beyond a standard physical exam to include quantifying morphologic alterations. Growth patterns—both pre- and postnatal—are emphasized. All of the collected data are then interpreted in light of known embryologic principles. Finally testing is performed if indicated, and counseling is given regarding etiology, recurrence risk, and expected outcomes (Figure 3-32).

(Figure 3-31). Not all children exposed to alcohol in the womb will have FAS. Of those children exposed to "significant" amounts of alcohol *in utero*, 1/3 will have the full expression of FAS, another 1/3 will have neurodevelopmental and neurobehavioral problems without any physical features, and the final 1/3 will have no apparent effects. The reasons for this wide range expression can be attributed to genetic differences in the maternal and the fetal genome as well as environmental modifiers. Collectively, then the full range of problems seen with *in utero* alcohol exposure are best termed **Fetal Alcohol Spectrum Disorders (FASD)**. The magnitude of problems produced by alcohol teratogenesis cannot be understated. FASDs represent the most common preventable cause of mental retardation. As a group they may account for up to 30% of all neurodevelopmental disabilities. The total costs of habilitation for individuals with Fetal Alcohol Syndrome (FAS) have been estimated at over $1 million for a lifetime. Thus it is imperative that all health care providers recognize one simple health care recommendation. The only appropriate advice to

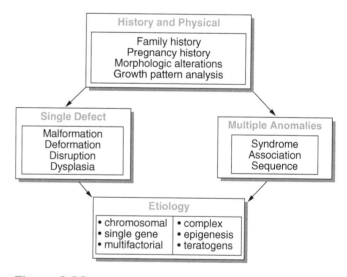

Figure 3-32. A schematic outlining the diagnostic approach to the child with congenital anomalies.

Part 3: Clinical Correlation

The definitions provided above are precise in their meaning and intention. They convey critical information about the nature and feature of a given congenital anomaly. As such, clinical geneticists are meticulous in their use of these terms. Two clinical examples are provided below that highlight the types of information contained in these terms.

1. Potter syndrome as originally described in 1946 was the set of features seen in newborns with renal abnormalities and characteristic facies (hypertelorism, flattened nasal structures, retrognathia, and large, low-set ears lacking in cartilage) (Figure 3-33). Other commonly associated changes include pulmonary hypoplasia and bone and joint abnormalities.

   Subsequently other newborns were reported with identical physical features, but with normal kidneys.

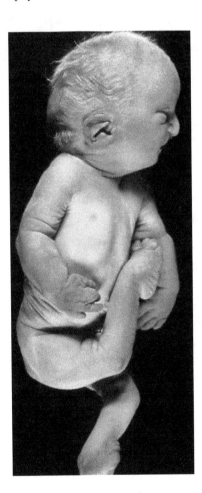

Figure 3-33. A stillborn infant with Potter anomalad. On autopsy, complete absence of the kidneys was noted. In this photograph note the multiple deformational changes of the face and joints.

The physical features in these infants could be attributed to low levels of amniotic fluid (oligohydramnios). The link in this situation is that 80% of amniotic fluid is derived from fetal urine. Thus fetuses with poorly functioning kidneys will have oligohydramnios. In the other group—the newborns with Potter-like features and normal kidneys—there were other causes of the oligohydramnios such as amniotic fluid leakage.

Thus, to apply the terms above accurately, one would say:

- The renal anomalies are *malformations.*
- The facial changes and the bone and joint changes are *deformations.*
- The facial changes and the bone and joint deformations are secondary to oligohydramnios with this pattern, then, best termed the *oligohydramnios sequence.*
- The designation Potter syndrome, then, is actually a misnomer. But, given the historical significance of Dr. Potter's description, many choose to keep this designation and reserve its use for the specific situation of the oligohydramnios sequence when it is caused by bilateral renal agenesis.

2. CHARGE association was originally described in 1979 as a constellation of **C**oloboma of the eyes, **H**eart anomalies, choanal **A**tresia, **R**etarded growth and development, **G**enital anomalies, and **E**ar abnormalities + hearing loss with the acronym designating the key features (Figure 3-34). Most cases identified were sporadic (negative family history). At the time of its description, CHARGE had no known etiology. Much of the literature about CHARGE noted that the features often overlapped with other developmental field defects, especially those known to be due to vascular disruptions. Thus, the designation *CHARGE association* was appropriately given. As molecular diagnostic testing advanced, a small number of patients with CHARGE were found to have 22q11.2 deletions. Scattered patients were identified with various other chromosome imbalances. Then, in 2006, patients were identified with CHARGE association who had identifiable mutations in a gene called CHD7. Further studies have shown that over 2/3 of patients with CHARGE harbor a CHD7 mutation. With this knowledge of the etiology of CHARGE (albeit heterogeneous), the designation has changed. Officially, it is now the *CHARGE syndrome.* This change in terms accurately reflects the change in the knowledge of the basis of this condition. Still, those reviewing the literature may find this shift in terminology confusing.

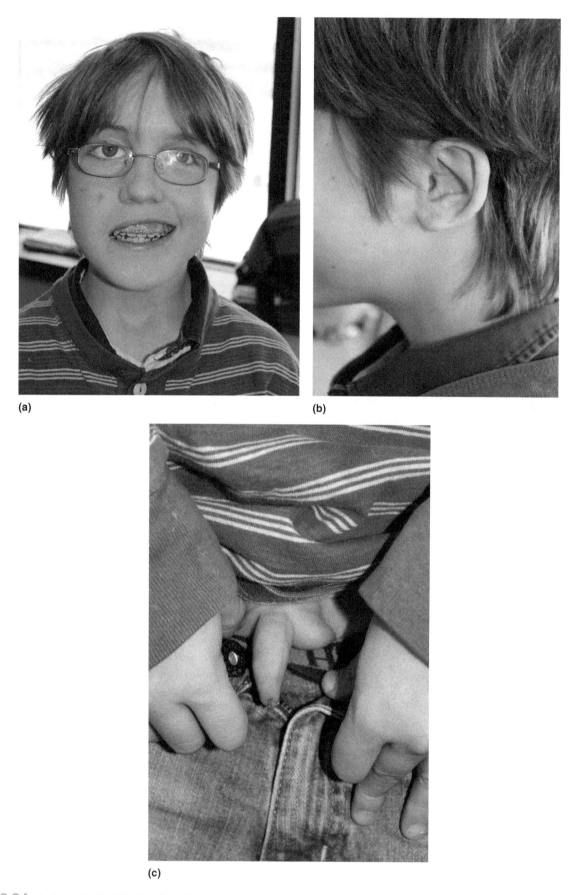

(a)

(b)

(c)

Figure 3-34. (a, b, and c) A child with CHARGE syndrome. This young man has a confirmed CHD7 gene mutation.

■ Board-Format Practice Questions

1. Most people have two major linear creases across the palm of their hands (take a look). Two percent of people in the general population have a single transverse palmar crease (a so-called "simian crease"). This finding is very frequent in patients with Down syndrome. The single transverse palmar crease would be an example of
   A. an association.
   B. a sequence.
   C. a syndrome.
   D. a malformation.
   E. a disruption.

2. Porencephalic cysts are fluid-filled spaces in the brain that are left after the death of brain cells. A porencephalic cyst identified in an infant at 2 hours of age is the result of a
   A. malformation, and must have occurred before 11 weeks of pregnancy.
   B. malformation, but since the organ affected is the brain, must have occurred before 22 weeks of pregnancy.
   C. deformation.
   D. disruption.
   E. transfected DNA sequence.

3. Dysmorphology (the area of clinical genetics concerned with diagnosis and etiology) classifies congenital anatomic malformations according to pathophysiology. This classification includes malformations, deformations, and disruptions. A fourth type exists in which there is abnormal organization of cells into tissues with its morphologic consequences. This would be defined as
   A. dysautonomia.
   B. dysdiadokinesis.
   C. distichiasis.
   D. dysergia.
   E. dysplasia.

4. Birth defects
   A. are uncommon disorders that most practitioners will rarely see.
   B. in general are decreasing in frequency.
   C. are often associated with infant mortality.
   D. are less common in the South as compared to the rest of the United States.
   E. rarely are seen with more than one anomaly per person.

5. Occasionally, an infant is born in which both kidneys are missing because they simply never developed. Since over 75% of amniotic fluid is formed by fetal urine, fetuses with no kidneys produce very little amniotic fluid, a condition called oligohydramnios. If oligohydramnios is present, then there are a variety of changes such as flattening of the face and misshaped joints that occur because the fetus cannot move about freely in the womb. The best description of these anomalies would be
   A. the kidney anomalies are deformations; the face and joint changes are malformations.
   B. the kidney anomalies are malformations; the face and joint changes are deformations.
   C. the kidney anomalies are disruptions; the face and joint changes are malformations.
   D. the kidney anomalies are malformations; the face and joint changes are disruptions.
   E. the kidney anomalies are disruptions; the face and joint changes are deformations.

chapter 4

The Structure and Function of Genes

CHAPTER SUMMARY

When one thinks about the genetic makeup of a human, or indeed any organism, it is natural to focus on the protein-coding genes. After all, that is the part of the genome that controls biochemical activities of cells and the processes of growth and development. But the protein-coding genes whose function is summarized in the "Central Dogma" (DNA ↔ mRNA → polypeptide) account for only about 3% of the DNA in a human cell. The genome also contains a large array of DNA sequences that have other functions (Figure 4-1) or that perhaps have no function at all. Some sequences represent the no-longer functional copies of duplicated genes, pseudogenes, produced at an earlier time in a species' history. In other cases, the regulatory functions of regions like microRNAs have only recently been recognized. Thus, the genome must be understood as a package of informational, historical, and noncoding DNA along with regions that hold secrets that researchers continue to unravel with the tools of molecular biology.

In Chapter 1 we saw that the chromosomes of eukaryotes (Figure 4-2) are made up of DNA complexed with proteins to form a nucleoprotein structure. The DNA molecule in each chromosome is a single, very long double helix. If one took each of the 23 chromosomes in one haploid set of human chromosomes, removed the protein, and stretched the DNA molecules out end-to-end, they would reach about a meter in total length. On average, then, each human chromosome's DNA strand is about 4.3 cm long (100 cm/23 linkage groups) and can be composed of as many as several hundred million nucleotide base pairs. Within this molecule, some genes follow the diploid organization we have assumed to this point, with one copy of each gene per haploid genome. But many genes are actually found in multi-gene families that often have large numbers of copies, and in fact the number of copies can change over time.

The first step is to understand the kinds of sequences present in the genome and their functions, if any, for the cell or their use to researchers, which is not necessarily the same thing. We will then explore how this vast amount of DNA is packed within the tiny confines of a nucleus and how packing can influence the process of gene regulation. This will lead into our discussion of normal and aberrant cytogenetic organization in Chapter 5.

Part 1: Background and Systems Integration

Categories of Sequence Complexity

Sequence complexity refers to the number of times a particular nucleotide sequence is found in the genome. Some are unique in the haploid genome, while other short- or medium-length sequences are repeated dozens, hundreds, or even millions of times. One way to estimate the proportion of the genome at various levels of sequence complexity is to measure the rate of DNA reannealing (Figure 4-3). Genomic DNA is first broken up into short pieces of several hundred base pairs (bp) each. Reaction temperature is then raised so the hydrogen bonds between strands break, yielding single-stranded molecules. In other words, the DNA becomes denatured. You will recognize this as being similar to the first DNA melting step of the PCR technique we described earlier. When the temperature is

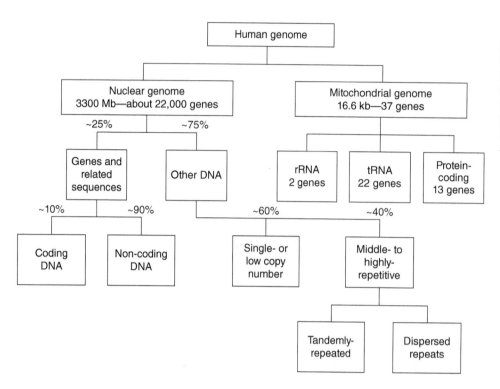

Figure 4-1. Overview of the kinds of DNA sequences found in the human genome (after Stracham and Read, Garland Science, NCBI Bookshelf). For additional details, see Tables 4-1 and 4-2. (Reprinted with permission from Brooker RJ: *Genetics: Analysis & Principles*, 3rd ed. New York: McGraw-Hill, 2008.)

cooled again, complementary strands begin to renature into stable double strands, i.e., they reassociate or **reanneal**.

For repetitive sequences, where there are large numbers of a particular sequence in the genome, it takes less time for two complementary strands to encounter each other and pair than it does for the parts that are present in lower repeat numbers or as single copies in the haploid genome. A C_0t curve plots a metric derived from concentration (C_0) and time (t) *versus* the percentage of DNA that has reannealed. From such experiments, it is estimated that about 60% of the human genome is made up of slowly reannealing DNA, representing largely unique or low-copy sequences. About 30% reanneals at an intermediate rate (middle-repetitive) and 10% is fast-annealing (highly repetitive). The proportion of middle- and highly-repetitive DNA can be even larger in other organisms.

Most protein-coding genes are part of the unique-sequence component. But, it is misleading to think that all of the unique sequence DNA is doing something useful. Similarly, the multiple-copy DNA is not just filler. It can have functions that are critical to the individual, like the tandem repeats that make up the telomeres at the tips of each chromosome (Figure 4-4). In Table 4-1 we summarize some of the roles (or non-roles) played by representative levels of sequence diversity, and we will expand upon some important examples in the next few sections. To avoid confusion, this list will address sequence copies per haploid genome. For example, so-called "unique" or single-copy sequences are of major importance, because they code for many of the key proteins controlling cell structure and function.

But since a diploid carries two copies, it can be confusing to call such unique sequence genes "single-copy" without any qualification.

Anatomy of a Protein-Coding Gene

For the purposes of this chapter, we will tend to take for granted the single-copy genes that code for proteins. But since this chapter focuses on DNA structural components, it might be helpful to review briefly the anatomy of a typical protein-coding gene. The term "**structural gene**" is often used to describe the nucleotide sequence that defines the amino acid composition of a protein. Upstream of the coding region will be a stretch of noncoding DNA that includes regulatory functions, such as the promoter that binds RNA polymerase and the binding sites for various transcription factors (Figure 4-5). Downstream past the end of the coding region is the terminator that ends transcription. While these regulatory sequences are not part of the structural gene per se, they are critical elements in its functional environment.

Coded within the transcribed region are nucleotides that define the ribosome-binding domain, translational start site, the codons corresponding to the polypeptide's amino acid chain, and stop codons that terminate translation. But the gene as it is found on the chromosome has untranslated regions (introns) in addition to the portions (exons) that are part of the mature messenger RNA (mRNA). The dystrophin gene associated with Duchenne muscular dystrophy, for example, has more than 80 exons. Cleaving the introns out of the

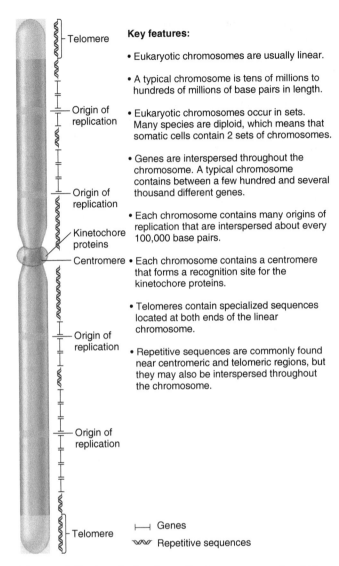

Figure 4-2. A typical eukaryotic chromosome showing some of the genetic structures and activities it can carry. (Reprinted with permission from Brooker RJ: *Genetics: Analysis & Principles*, 3rd ed. New York: McGraw-Hill, 2008.)

2500 kilobase (kb) initial transcript yields a mature mRNA that is only about 14 kb long.

Deciphering the human genome and the genomes of model organisms has clearly demonstrated the range of unusual patterns in what we might call the "molecular geography of functions" in a DNA strand. First, the synthesis of an mRNA transcript always reads the DNA template strand from the 3′ toward the 5′ end (the mRNA strand grows in the antiparallel direction, adding new nucleotides at its growing 3′ end). But the template strand's orientation can differ from one gene to another (Figure 4-6), with some genes reading one of the DNA strands and others being transcribed in the opposite direction using the other strand. The orientation is determined

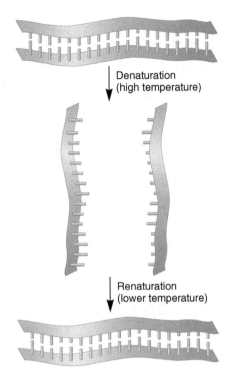

(a) Renaturation of DNA strands

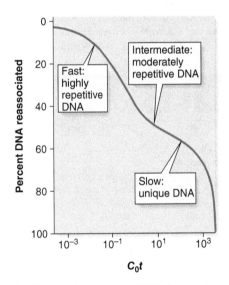

(b) Human chromosomal DNA C_0t curve

Figure 4-3. Detecting levels of sequence complexity by measuring rates of reassociation of melted DNA fragments. (a) The hydrogen bonds between complementary DNA strands are broken at high temperature. When fragmented DNA is denatured by heat, it yields single-stranded DNA fragments that reassociate (renature or **reanneal**) when cooled. (b) Rates of renaturation are measured in a C_0t curve that plots the percentage of DNA that has reannealed against the DNA concentration C_0 times the incubation time, t. (Reprinted with permission from Brooker RJ: *Genetics: Analysis & Principles*, 3rd ed. New York: McGraw-Hill, 2008.)

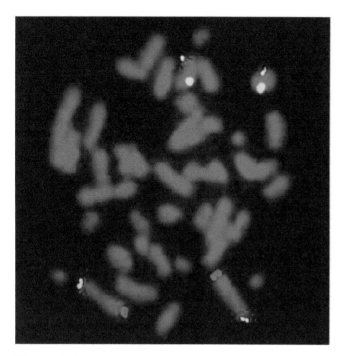

Figure 4-4. An example of a FISH hybridized metaphase spread. Four different probe signals are visible: subtelomeric probes for 2p (green signal), 2q (red signal) are seen. (Reprinted from Wise JL, Crout RJ, McNeil DW, et al: Cryptic subtelomeric rearrangements and X chromosome mosaicism: a study of 565 apparently normal individuals with fluorescent in situ hybridization. PLoS One. 2009 Jun 10;4(6):e5855. doi: 10.1371/journal.pone.0005855.)

Table 4-1.	Categories of Genome Sequence Complexity
Category	**Examples for Eukaryote Genomes**
Known function	
Single-copy sequences	
Protein coding	enzymes, cell signaling membrane receptors, and similar structural proteins
Not protein coding	microRNAs, some regulatory sequences
Multiple-copy sequences	
Protein coding	dispersed gene families, like actin (5-30 copies), keratins (20 + copies), and histones (100-1000 copies)
RNA coding	rRNA genes (nucleolar organizer region) tRNA genes (about 50 sites with about 10-1000 copies per site)
Not coding	telomeres
No known function	
Single-copy sequences	pseudogenes
Multiple-copy sequences	repeated centromeric DNA sequences transposable elements, like LINEs and SINEs Variable Number Tandem Repeats (VNTRS): minisatellites (repeats of about 15-50+bp), microsatellites (repeats of 2-6bp)

by which strand has the proper nucleotide sequence of a promoter.

Furthermore, a strand of DNA is not always the exclusive territory of only one gene. Rare examples are known where genes overlap. Often this involves transcribing the complementary strands in opposite directions, with part of the mRNA transcripts overlapping (using the same portion of the DNA molecule) at one end. But occasionally two genes will transcribe the same strand in different reading frames, as seen for example in the mitochondrial ATPase gene (Figure 4-7). Genes can also be nested as, for example, in the neurofibromatosis type I (*NF1*) gene that has three smaller genes (*OGMP*, *EVI2A*, and *EVI2B*) transcribed within one of its introns (Figure 4-8).

The information flow summarized by the Central Dogma is, therefore, deceptively simple until we look at DNA from the viewpoint of its functional geography. No doubt the picture will become more complex. But, by the same token, seeing the complications that are encoded within DNA gives us the foundation to explain important mechanisms at work in medical conditions. So, from this complexity will ultimately come greater understanding and order.

Varieties of RNA

Early understanding of RNA and its function was mainly focused on the actual transcription and translation of DNA into a protein product. Messenger RNA (mRNA) was recognized as the copy resulting from transcription which then functioned as the template for translation. Ribosomal RNA (rRNA) was appreciated as a major component of the translational machinery, and transfer RNA (tRNA) was known to be the major shuttle vehicle for transporting amino acids to the translational complex. Advances in the understanding of RNA and its various functions has revealed many other "types" of RNA that do not code for a specific product, but that play many important roles in the process of gene expression and regulation. Besides tRNA and rRNA, several more types of **noncoding RNA** have been discovered. It is sometimes confusing that this group of molecules can be referred to by many other names such as non-protein-coding RNA (npcRNA), non-messenger RNA (nmRNA), small non-messenger RNA (snmRNA), and functional RNA (fRNA). The list of noncoding RNAs in humans described thus far totals over 15 types, each with numerous subtypes that have specific regulatory functions in processes such as translation, transcription, posttranscriptional modification, DNA replication, epigenesis, and gene regulation/expression (Table 4-2). The importance of these RNAs cannot be overstated. Not surprisingly, mutations in these RNAs lead to clinical problems. A few are listed later. Much more important is the fact that these molecules have an *ongoing* role of gene regulation and expression beyond embryogenesis—in fact for the life of the individual. This fact, then, gives noncoding RNAs tremendous potential for use in the development of genetic therapies, where the actual DNA code would not have to be changed.

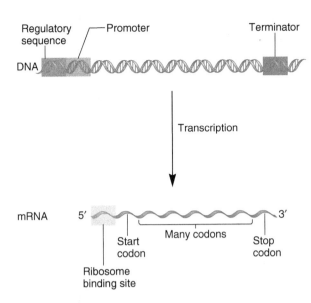

DNA:

• **Regulatory sequences:** site for the binding of regulatory proteins; the role of regulatory proteins is to influence the rate of transcription. Regulatory sequences can be found in a variety of locations.

• **Promoter:** site for RNA polymerase binding; signals the beginning of transcription.

• **Terminator:** signals the end of transcription.

mRNA:

• **Ribosomal binding site:** site for ribosome binding; translation begins near this site in the mRNA. In eukaryotes, the ribosome scans the mRNA for a start codon.

• **Start codon:** specifies the first amino acid in a polypeptide sequence, usually a formylmethionine (in bacteria) or a methionine (in eukaryotes).

• **Codons:** 3-nucleotide sequences within the mRNA that specify particular amino acids. The sequence of codons within mRNA determines the sequence of amino acids within a polypeptide.

• **Stop codon:** specifies the end of polypeptide synthesis.

Figure 4-5. Correspondence between the functional regions of the genome and of the final mRNA product following transcription and RNA processing. (Reprinted with permission from Brooker RJ: *Genetics: Analysis & Principles*, 3rd ed. New York: McGraw-Hill, 2008.)

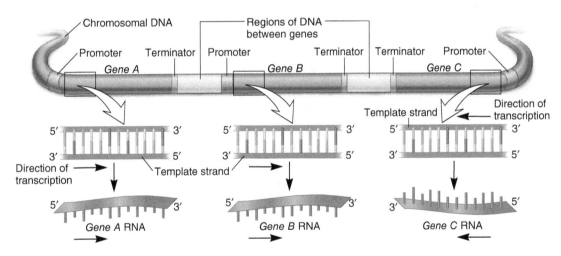

Figure 4-6. Transcription of three different genes, showing that the direction of transcription depends on the placement and orientation of the promoter region. The transcript is synthesized in a 5′ to 3′ direction by reading the template strand from 3′ to 5′. (Reprinted with permission from Brooker RJ: *Genetics: Analysis & Principles*, 3rd ed. New York: McGraw-Hill, 2008.)

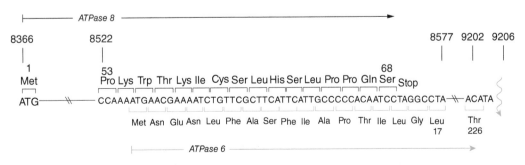

Figure 4-7. Example of overlapping genes.

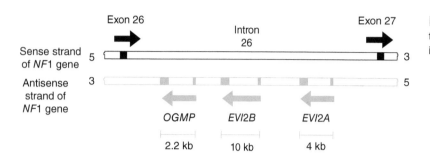

Figure 4-8. Neurofibromatosis type I (*NF1*) with three small genes transcribed from within one of its introns.

MicroRNAs: Single-Copy Sequences That Are Not Protein Coding

MicroRNA (miRNA) is not translated. Instead, it is a recently identified mechanism for gene regulation. MicroRNAs are small RNA molecules that participate in gene regulation by **RNA interference**. Each is about 21 to 23 nucleotides long and is at least partly complementary to one or more mRNA molecules. By binding to an mRNA molecule, miRNA inhibits translation or degrades mRNA and, thus, down-regulates the expression of that gene. MicroRNAs can be produced from a variety of sources. Some are produced from genes, while others are processed from introns, noncoding RNAs, **transposons**, or other sources. The initial, or primary, transcript for a miRNA is a **pri-miRNA** with 5′-cap and poly-A tail that is processed in the nucleus to a 70-nucleotide **pre-miRNA** with a stem-loop structure (Figure 4-9). The pre-miRNA is processed into mature double-stranded miRNA in the cytoplasm by the endonuclease called Dicer. This RNA then associates with protein to form the RNA-induced silencing complex (RISC), and one of the RNA strands is broken down. When the remaining RNA strand of the RISC binds to an mRNA, it can cause the mRNA to degrade or it can block translation.

Functional Multi-Copy Genes

Several proteins in eukaryotic cells are coded for by families of genes that are distributed at dispersed locations among the chromosomes. Examples of dispersed gene families include actin, with 5 to 30 copies in eukaryotes, and the tubulin proteins, with 3 to 15 copies. In some cases, members of a family can diverge, allowing slightly different functions to arise within the group.

Some gene products are needed in large amounts, and having multiple copies is one way to accomplish this. Such genes can sometimes be found in tandemly-duplicated arrays. Histone proteins, for example, are present 100 to 1000 times in duplicated arrays. The tRNAs and rRNAs, in which the final gene product is the RNA itself, are also duplicated tandemly. In humans, there are about 50 chromosomal locations for the different tRNA genes, with from 10 to 100 copies at each. Another example is the rRNA coding structure associated

Table 4-2.	Types of Noncoding RNA
Type	**Specific Processes**
Ribosomal RNA (rRNA)	Recognition site of the translational complex
Transfer RNA (tRNA)	Shuttle of amnio acids to translational complex
MicroRNA (miRNA)	Fine tuning of gene expression
Small interfering RNA (siRNA)	RNA interference (down-regulates gene expression)
7SL RNA (srpRNA)	Part of signal recognition particle (recognizes and delivers protein to endoplasmic reticulum)
Small nuclear RNA (snRNA)	RNA splicing, regulation of transcription factors, maintenance of telomeres
Small nucleolar RNA (sno RNA)	Guide in the process of maturation of rRNA
Ribonuclease P (RNaseP)	RNA molecule with catalytic function on tRNA
Y RNAs	Repressor of Ro ribonucleoprotein particle, required for DNA replication
Telomerase RNA (TERC)	RNA component of telomerease; involved in telomere lengthening
Antisense RNA (aRNA)	Complement of sense strand of messenger RNA. Natural function unclear, (?) protects DNA from infectious agents
Cis-natural antisense transcript (NAT)	Suggested role in imprinting, alternative splicing, Lyonization
Piwi interacting RNA (piRNA)	Inhibition of retrotransposons
Long-noncoding RNAs (>200 nucleotides)	Many aspects of transcription, translation, splicing, and epigenetic processes

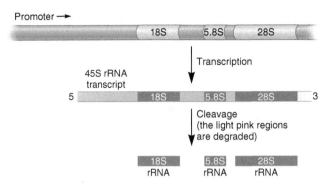

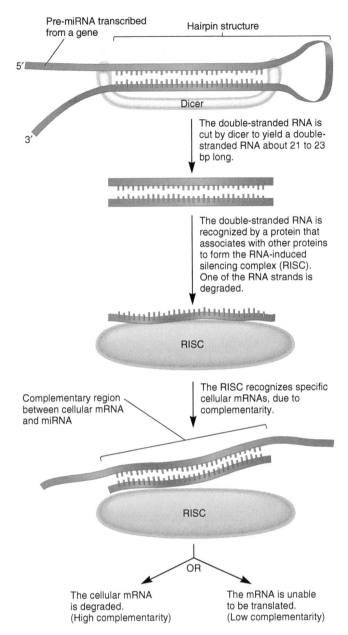

Figure 4-9. The processing of microRNA that is involved in gene regulation by RNA interference. (Reprinted with permission from Brooker RJ: *Genetics: Analysis & Principles*, 3rd ed. New York: McGraw-Hill, 2008.)

Figure 4-10. Tandemly repeated sequences like the one shown here from the nucleolar organizer (NO) region code for three rRNAs needed for ribosome synthesis. This sequence is repeated about 250 times in the human NO region. (Reprinted with permission from Brooker RJ: *Genetics: Analysis & Principles*, 3rd ed. New York: McGraw-Hill, 2008.)

with the nucleolar organizer (NO), which forms a cytologically distinct region, the **nucleolus**, in the nucleus. A human NO region can contain about 250 copies of tandemly arranged rRNA genes (homologous to the "p" arms of the acrocentric chromosomes) to produce the large amount of these RNAs needed to synthesize ribosomes. The processing of one of the repeated units is shown in Figure 4-10.

Pseudogenes

Pseudogenes have sometimes been described as "gene ghosts." Some are duplicated genes that accumulate mutations that make them nonfunctional since selection no longer acts

effectively against mutations in the extra copy. Others may have arisen from the activity of **retrotransposons**, like SINEs and LINEs described later. These transposable elements reverse transcribe, or retrotranspose, from RNA back into DNA that then inserts into a chromosome. In the process, some random mRNA can become involved and yield a pseudogene that generally lacks typical features like a promoter or introns that had already been processed out of the RNA molecule. If such a sequence is inserted into an intron, it may be neutral or it can possibly have an effect due to alternative intron splicing. Other rarer mechanisms have also been documented. But it is also possible that presumed pseudogenes might acquire a new function or be mistakenly classified because of incomplete information about their function. If their promoter is intact, some presumed pseudogenes can be transcribed and may potentially play some role in gene regulation and gene expression.

Repetitive Sequences Having an Uncertain Function

Some repetitive sequences likely affect the biology of the cell, but the mechanism by which they act, if any, is still uncertain. A good example is the repetitive alpha-satellite DNA in the heterochromatic regions around human chromosomal centromeres that makes up about 3% to 4% of the genome. Its repetitive nature makes centromeric DNA very difficult to sequence for comparative genomic studies. In contrast to the conserved sequence similarity found in genes that share a critical function in different organisms, the sequence of centromeric repeats appears to differ extensively from one species to another.

Human alpha-satellite DNA is composed of tandemly repeating units (monomers) of about 171 bp. There are two forms of alpha satellite (Figure 4-11). Higher order repeat arrays (HOR) are chromosome-specific arrays composed of hundreds or thousands of copies per chromosome totaling 3

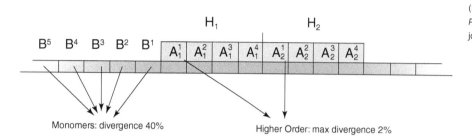

Figure 4-11. Human alpha-satellite DNA showing tandemly repeating units from the centromeric region of a chromosome (Reprinted with permission from Alkan et al: 2007. *PLoS Computational Biology* 3(9): e181. Doi: 10.1371/journal.pcbi.0030181.)

to 5 Mb in size and with only about 2% sequence divergence between the repeat units. The array size varies from one individual to another due to unequal crossing-over during meiosis. This can yield some submicroscopic chromosome length polymorphism. In addition, a second type of alpha-satellite DNA has been found in the areas of transition between the HOR region flanking the centromere and the coding euchromatic portion of the chromosome. Unlike higher order structure, the repeats within this so-called "monomeric" alpha-satellite DNA have a lot of sequence divergence among individuals.

Minisatellites and Microsatellites

The **variable number of tandem repeats (VNTRs)**, or **minisatellites**, form a class of tandemly-repeated sequences that can vary from one location or one individual to another. Each is between about 1 and 5 kb in length with repeated units of about a dozen to perhaps 100 nucleotides. Since they can

readily change in the number of repeated units, minisatellites can be a useful marker to assess chromosome relationships, such as those among geographically separated populations.

As far as genome content is concerned, therefore, lacking a biological function is not the same as lacking a use. Even when they have no particular influence on the biochemistry of cellular processes, VNTRs have a use in applications like forensic DNA fingerprinting. *The Blooding*, by Joseph Wambaugh, for example, is an historical novel recounting the true story of the first murder case solved with the involvement of genetic fingerprinting. The now-familiar process has played a role in an increasingly large number of legal cases. Given the legal profession's awareness of this aspect of genetic diversity in human populations, physicians with knowledge of medical genetics might expect inquiries in this field.

To obtain a DNA fingerprint, total genomic DNA is digested with a **restriction enzyme** that cleaves DNA at specific nucleotide target sequences (Figure 4-12). The population

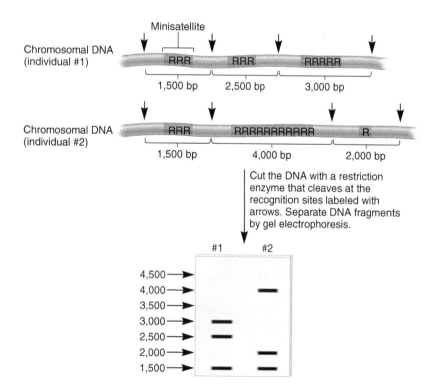

Figure 4-12. DNA fingerprints are produced by digesting chromosomes with a restriction enzyme to yield fragments that differ in the number of tandem repeats, and thus the relative migration rates of the fragments on an electrophoretic gel. (Reprinted with permission from Brooker RJ: *Genetics: Analysis & Principles*, 3rd ed. New York: McGraw-Hill, 2008.)

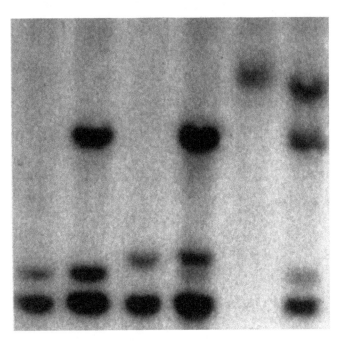

Figure 4-13. An autoradiograph showing DNA fragments which show different migration speeds, interpreted in Figure 4-29.

of fragments is then separated by size with electrophoresis. Once the fragments have been transferred from the electrophoretic gel to a nylon membrane by a process called **Southern blotting**, they can be visualized by hybridizing with a radioactively-tagged **oligonucleotide** probe that complements regions within the minisatellite. The resulting autoradiograph (Figure 4-13) shows the variation in fragment lengths that will occur when the placement of restriction enzyme target sites differs from one individual to another. Similar approaches using fluorescent tags are also in use.

Microsatellites have become an even more widely used category of tandemly repeated sequences. They differ from minisatellites in the length of the repeated unit. Microsatellites are long repeats of two to six nucleotides (often di-, tri-, and tetranucleotide repeats). Changes in microsatellite copy number can have serious medical consequences. In other cases, microsatellites serve as genetic markers that can segregate along with (i.e., cosegregate with) a condition of interest and lead its molecular localization.

Transposable Elements

The study of transposable elements (TEs), sometimes called "jumping genes," was pioneered by Barbara McClintock who received the Nobel Prize for her work in 1983. They are common in most organisms and move by a variety of mechanisms. By transposing from one chromosome location to another, they can insert directly into a gene causing a mutation or diseases, including cancers. Most insertions, however, are into noncoding regions and do not affect development. In the human genome, there are several hundred different transposable element families and subfamilies that together account

for about 44% of the total human genome. But most of these copies are inactive. Only about 0.05% of the more than 4 million annotated TEs in the human genome are still capable of transposition.

Transposons carry out transposition as DNA copies, while **retrotransposons** spread after reverse transcription of an RNA molecule into DNA. These include **short interspersed nuclear elements**, called **SINEs**, that are less than about 500 nucleotides in length. Another type of transposable element in mammals, including humans, is the **long interspersed nuclear elements** (**LINEs**), which have some DNA sequence homology to retroviruses and encode enzymes used in transposition.

The most common human TEs are the retrotransposon *Alu* and the LINE-1 (L1) dispersed repetitive sequences. The complete *Alu* sequence is about 200 nucleotides long, and L1 is 1 to 5 kb in length. *Alu* is present in hundreds of thousands of full and partial copies in the human genome, and L1 is found in 20,000 to 40,000 copies. But most *Alu* and L1 elements are truncated and thus inactive. There is functionally important genetic variation in L1 copies, but only rarely have active L1 copies been documented to transpose and cause disease. Transposition by *Alu* is dependent on the L1-transposition mechanism. Examples of human diseases traced to transposable elements include occurrences of hemophilia A (L1 insertion) and neurofibromatosis type 1 (*Alu* insertion). The genetics and biomedical importance of transposable elements will be explored in more detail in Chapter 12.

Eukaryotic Chromosome Packing in the Nucleus

This introduction to categories of genetic function brings home the point that there is a very large amount of DNA in each cell. The mechanism for packaging this DNA in the nucleus is critical to maintaining its integrity and organization (Figure 4-14). Packaging also influences gene expression. The basic element of chromosome structure is the **nucleosome**, a repeating unit composed of double-stranded DNA wrapped almost twice around a complex of histone proteins (Figure 4-15). This compacts DNA by reducing its length about 7-fold.

The nucleosome's protein core is composed of two molecules of each of four different histone proteins, H2A, H2B, H3, and H4. These contain a large number of lysine and arginine amino acids, making the protein core highly basic. This helps it bind to the negatively-charged phosphate groups in DNA. A short unbound stretch of linker DNA is found between consecutive nucleosomes. A fifth histone, H1, binds to the linker DNA and may help connect adjacent nucleosomes during early chromosome compaction (Figure 4-16), although there are competing models of the resulting 30-nm fiber. This shortens DNA length another 7-fold, to a total of almost 50-fold over the initial DNA molecular length.

In addition to these histone proteins, there is a large non-histone protein component in a chromosome. Non-histone proteins are highly diverse. The largest class is the transcription

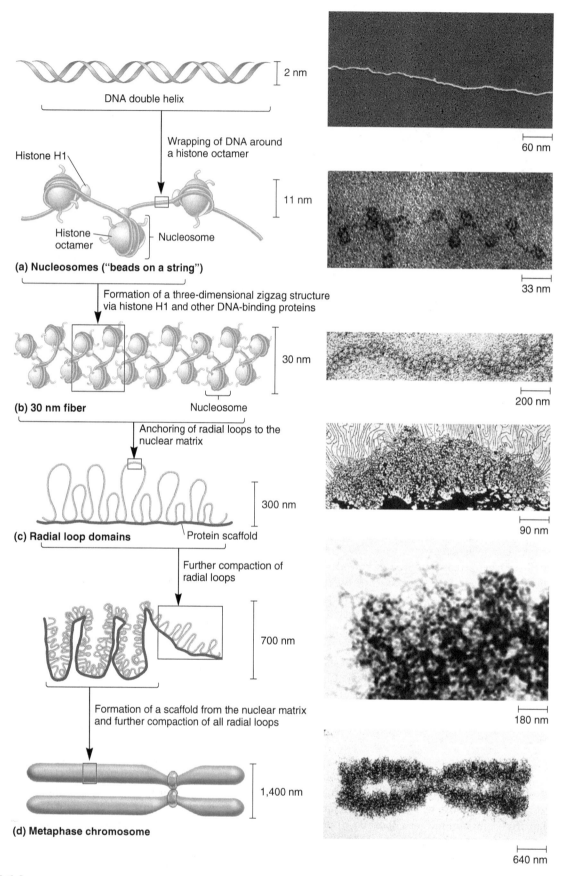

2 nm

DNA double helix

Wrapping of DNA around
a histone octamer

60 nm

Histone H1

Histone
octamer

Nucleosome

11 nm

(a) Nucleosomes ("beads on a string")

33 nm

Formation of a three-dimensional zigzag structure
via histone H1 and other DNA-binding proteins

30 nm

(b) 30 nm fiber

Nucleosome

200 nm

Anchoring of radial loops to the
nuclear matrix

300 nm

(c) Radial loop domains

Protein scaffold

90 nm

Further compaction of
radial loops

700 nm

Formation of a scaffold from the nuclear matrix
and further compaction of all radial loops

180 nm

1,400 nm

(d) Metaphase chromosome

640 nm

Figure 4-14. The hierarchy of DNA packing in a chromosome. (Reprinted with permission from Brooker RJ: *Genetics: Analysis & Principles*, 3rd ed. New York: McGraw-Hill, 2008.)

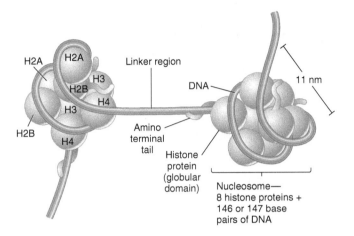

H2A   H2A   Linker region

H3

H2B   DNA   11 nm

H4

H2B   H4   Amino
terminal
tail

Histone
protein
(globular
domain)

Nucleosome—
8 histone proteins +
146 or 147 base
pairs of DNA

(a) Nucleosomes showing core histone proteins

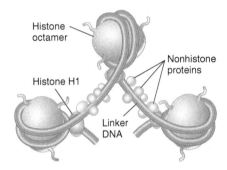

Histone
octamer

Nonhistone
proteins

Histone H1

Linker
DNA

**(b) Nucleosomes showing linker histones
and nonhistone proteins**

Figure 4-15. Nucleosomes are composed of DNA wrapped around the positively-charged histone core. (a) The core of eight proteins includes two each of histone H2A, H2B, H3, and H4. (b) Histone H1 and various non-histone proteins bind to the linker DNA between adjacent nucleosomes. (Reprinted with permission from Brooker RJ: *Genetics: Analysis & Principles*, 3rd ed. New York: McGraw-Hill, 2008.)

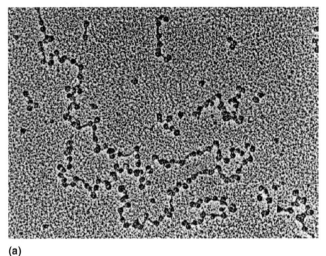

(a)

(b)

Figure 4-16. (a) When H1 histones are not present, the nucleosomes appear like a beaded string. (b) The H1 histones may link together adjacent nucleosomes to yield a first-order level of compaction seen in the 30-nanometer (nm) fibers. (Reprinted with permission from Brooker RJ: *Genetics: Analysis & Principles*, 3rd ed. New York: McGraw-Hill, 2008.)

factors that regulate gene expression. Other examples are the non-histone proteins in the centromeric **kinetochores** that function in chromosome movement during cell division and the structural proteins of the nuclear matrix and supporting scaffold of condensed chromosomes.

At a third level of compaction, the 30-nm fibers are hypothesized to attach as radial loops to filaments of the dynamic network of proteins that make up the **nuclear matrix** (Figure 4-17). These **looped domains** of between 25,000 bp and 200,000 bp in size are anchored to the matrix filaments by other kinds of non-histone proteins. Matrix-attachment regions (MARs) or scaffold-attachment regions (SARs) are dispersed at intervals throughout the genome. This results in a further 200- to 250-fold shortening of the chromosomes to a total of about 10,000-fold above the naked DNA.

Formation of the chromosome scaffold from the nuclear matrix causes additional compaction of the radial looped domains (Figure 4-18). By the end of prophase in nuclear division, all chromosomes are highly condensed, and gene transcription is almost completely halted since transcription factors cannot easily bind the DNA. Each chromosome also has its own characteristic patterns of regional compaction that can be seen by pretreating prometaphase chromosomes with heat and then staining with Giemsa (**G-banding** technique; Figure 4-19).

About 850 G-bands can be distinguished in a human karyotype, which provides cytogeneticists with a fine degree of structural resolution. Given their intimate association with DNA, it should not be too surprising that nucleosomes can influence gene expression. Enzyme-controlled **chromatin remodeling** involves the partial or complete displacement of histones to allow access by transcription factors to promoter regions (Figure 4-20). Medical examples of chromatin remodeling and other conditions associated with the various categories of sequence complexity are discussed in Part 2.

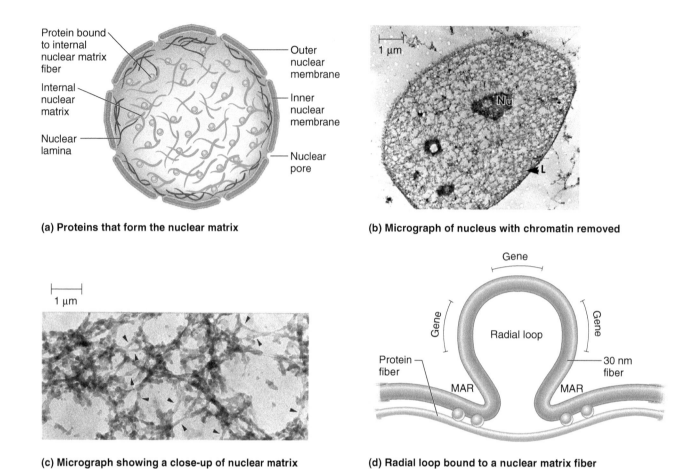

(a) **Proteins that form the nuclear matrix**

(b) **Micrograph of nucleus with chromatin removed**

(c) **Micrograph showing a close-up of nuclear matrix**

(d) **Radial loop bound to a nuclear matrix fiber**

Figure 4-17. (a-d): The nuclear matrix. (a, d: Reprinted with permission from Brooker RJ: *Genetics: Analysis & Principles*, 3rd ed. New York: McGraw-Hill, 2008. (b, c): Nickerson et al: "The nuclear matrix revealed by eluting chromatin from a cross-linked nucleus." PNAS 94: 446-4450. Figure 2ab. © 1997 National Academy of Sciences, USA.)

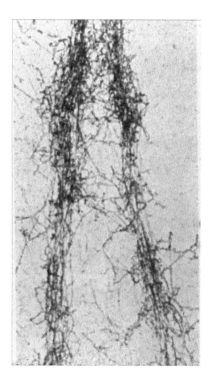

Figure 4-18. The protein scaffold of a metaphase chromosome. Banding at the level of the electron micrograph is shown.

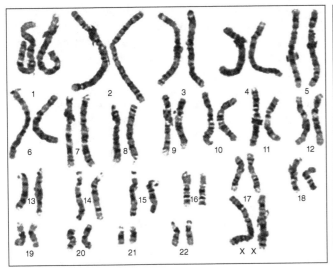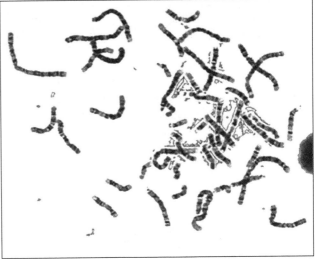

Figure 4-19. Individual patterns of density following G-banding allow cytogeneticists to identify individual chromosomes and large-scale changes in structure. The image on the left shows chromosomes arranged in homologous pairs; the right image is the way they appear in the original spread. (Reproduced with permission of Warren G. Sanger, PhD, University of Nebraska Medical Center, Omaha, Nebraska.)

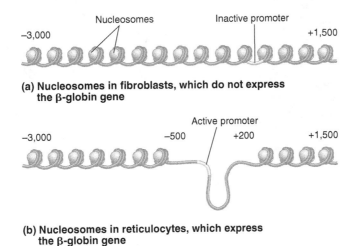

(a) Nucleosomes in fibroblasts, which do not express the β-globin gene

(b) Nucleosomes in reticulocytes, which express the β-globin gene

Figure 4-20. Partial or complete histone protein removal during chromatin remodeling. (Reprinted with permission from Brooker RJ: *Genetics: Analysis & Principles*, 3rd ed. New York: McGraw-Hill, 2008.)

Part 2: Medical Genetics

The concept that a gene exerts its effects by coding for a protein that has a specific function was first formally proposed by Archibald Garrod in 1909 in his study of the inborn error of metabolism alkaptonuria. George Beadle and Edward Tatum were awarded the Nobel Prize in Physiology or Medicine in 1958 for their experimental work in 1941 documenting the relationship between the gene and the protein (enzyme). This relationship has been described as the "one gene, one enzyme" hypothesis. This was the first identified mechanism of how a change in DNA could result in a heritable trait. For a brief time it seemed that genetics made sense.

Of course, the natural world is not that simple. Discoveries over the past several decades, as will be discussed in

detail throughout this book, have expanded the understanding of how changes in nucleic acids lead to observable differences in the physiology of the individual. Mechanisms such as epigenetic influences, posttranslational protein modifications, differential DNA processing, gene-gene interactions, gene environment interactions, gene regulation (promoters/enhancers), and so forth, all have a role in the normal workings of the organism. A common theme throughout this book is that of genotype: phenotype correlation. Specifically, by what mechanisms do changes in the genome produce human diseases?

In the first section of this chapter we discussed the many different ways that nucleic acids in the form of DNA and RNA are organized and function in the genome. The relationship is much more complicated than a straight sequence of a coding DNA that translates into a single exact protein sequence. The primary point here is that *genetics is not just about protein coding*.

A better understanding of DNA, how it is organized and arranged, what it does, what influences it, and what interacts with it leads to an enhanced understanding of disease. Many medical conditions simply cannot be understood without this knowledge base. For many conditions, the DNA relationship would never have been elucidated by an observation of the phenotype with a predictive deduction of the genotype. Powerful molecular tools have identified the genetic basis of many conditions where no physiologic clues lead to answers. For example, cystic fibrosis (CF) is a complex medical condition characterized by chronic progressive pulmonary disease and pancreatic insufficiency (Figure 4-21). The condition is still considered a lethal disorder although the life expectancy has improved dramatically from 5 years old in the 1960s to almost

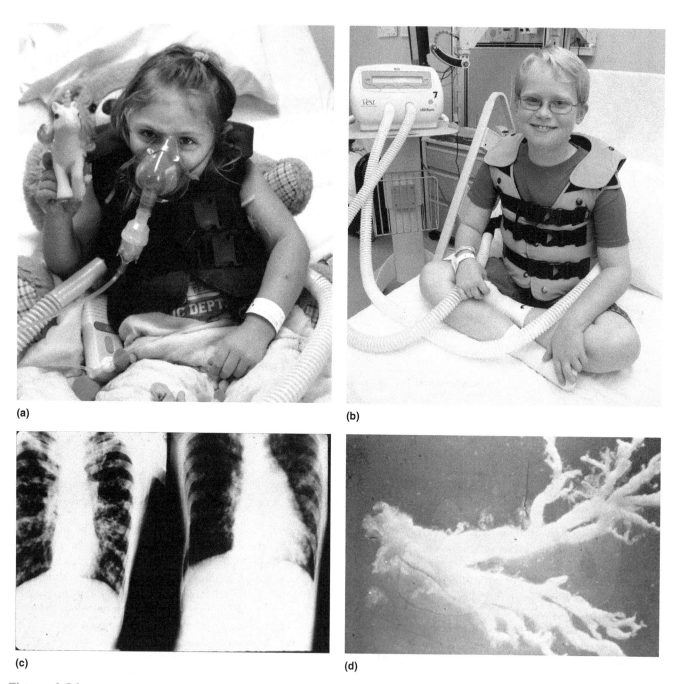

(a)

(b)

(c)

(d)

Figure 4-21. (a) Young girl with cystic fibrosis requiring oxygen therapy for chronic pulmonary disease. (b) Adolescent male with cystic fibrosis receiving aggressive pulmonary therapy. (c) Chest X-rays showing chronic obstructive pulmonary disease in patients with cystic fibrosis. (d) Mucous cast of a bronchus removed at autopsy on a patient with cystic fibrosis.

40 years old now. Cystic fibrosis is inherited as an autosomal recessive condition. It is one of the more common single gene disorders in humans with an estimated frequency of 1 per 1600 persons of Northern European descent. Early on, people had appreciated a salty taste when kissing the foreheads of babies with this condition. To this day the "sweat test," which measures sodium and chloride levels in sweat, is the gold standard diagnostic test for this condition. Many of the features of CF were suggestive of some type of problem with exocrine glands.

The pathophysiology of the condition seemed to indicate problems with inspissated mucous in these glands. Hundreds if not thousands of studies were performed to try and identify the cause of CF using these bits of information. Ultimately, the CF gene was discovered by the chance identification of genetic linkage of the condition to an unrelated enzyme, paroxynase. Sequencing of the gene and sequence homology predictions identified the gene as coding for a membrane chloride transport function. With these insights, the physiological cascade of:

1. abnormal chloride transport

2. leading to increased chloride content in the excocrine glands

3. which resulted in thickened mucous in the glands

4. leading to obstruction of the glands and impaired functions was revealed as the "cause" of CF.

It is highly unlikely that this mechanism would have been discovered in anywhere close to this time frame by nonmolecular genetic approaches.

Another critical part of the understanding of these variations on the "one gene one polypeptide" hypothesis is that many of these alternative mechanisms have a greater potential for genetic therapies than do simple changes in the code. In the example of cystic fibrosis, for example, therapy can now be targeted to the primary source of the disorder–impaired chloride transport across membranes—rather than the secondary clinical expressions. Each variation is unique and has its own implications for human health.

Table 4-3 lists some examples of human medical conditions associated with mutations in different "types" of DNA. In the text that follows we discuss a few of these in more detail. This discussion is not meant to be a comprehensive list of all such conditions, nor does it provide a detailed description of each condition. Rather we are reviewing the breadth of the medical implications in the broader context.

Changes in the DNA-Coding Sequence

It is intuitive that changes (mutations) in the DNA-coding sequence can result in disease. One way in which this may occur is if the mutation results in a missing protein product. The classic example of this would be the enzymatic defects seen in the inborn errors of metabolism (Chapter 8). Mutations that lead to poorly functioning enzymes will cause problems from the lack of normal enzymatic activity. Alternatively, changes in the coding sequence may produce a structurally abnormal product that is not deficient but that interferes with other proteins, such as in sickle cell anemia and many of the connective tissue disorders.

It is important to note that not all DNA changes—even in the coding sequence—necessarily lead to problems. Due to the "degenerative" nature of the DNA code, there is some "wobble" in protein translation in which the third position of a codon is less important than the first two in determining

Table 4-3.	Human Medical Conditions Associated With Mutations in Different Types of DNA	
Category	**Types of Disorder**	**Example(s)**
Known function		
Single-copy sequences		
Protein coding	enzyme deficiencies	phenylketonuria
	structural protein abnormality	sickle cell anemia
	changes in promoter region/ splice sites	β-thalassemia
Not protein coding	changes in miRNA	cardiomyopathy, leukemia
Multiple-copy sequences		
Protein coding	actin family	myopathy, deafness, dystonia
RNA coding	tRNA	Charcot-Marie Tooth
	rRNA	Blackfan - Diamond anemia
Noncoding	telomeres	Dyskeratosis congenita
No known function		
Single-copy sequences	pseudogenes	disease causing gene conversion
Multiple-copy sequences	repeated centromeric DNA sequences	rheumatoid arthritis, systemic lupus
	transposable elements	hemophilia
Tandem Repeats	minisatellites	myoclonic epilepsy
	microsatellites	neuromuscular disorders, hereditary non-polypotic colorectal cancer

the tRNA binding to the ribosome. Thus certain nucleotide changes will not produce changes in the expected amino acids at that position. In addition, even if an amino acid change occurs due to a mutation, there still may not be a phenotypic problem. Depending upon where in the protein the amino acid change occurs and what that amino acid is doing at that position, an amino acid substitution may not cause any appreciable alteration in the protein function. These types of silent changes are referred to as **benign polymorphisms**. Clinically benign polymorphisms present a challenge in DNA testing. The identification of a specific nucleotide change that has not been seen before (a polymorphism of "unknown significance") has to be interpreted cautiously. The identification of mutation in a gene that is associated with a specific condition is not always the cause of that condition in a particular patient. These concepts will be discussed more in Chapter 7 on Mutations and discussions on pathogenesis in Chapter 16.

Changes in the Gene Outside of the Coding Sequence

As has already been described, the components of a particular gene extend well beyond the actual coding sequence. Thus just looking at the coding sequences may not identify the cause of a genetic disorder. Sometimes the mutations may be in the promoter or enhancer regions. Recently, insights have also led to the understanding that mutations in the noncoding regions (introns) are not always benign. Changes in the intronic sequence may change such things as splice sites or other recognition points. Beta-thalassemia (Figure 4-22) is a disorder of the hemoglobin molecule. Hemoglobin is a multimeric protein composed of equal amounts of two proteins, the alpha and beta chains. The human genome has six genes (four alpha chain and two beta chain) coding for these proteins. The thalassemias represent a group of related conditions seen with a decrease in the production of one of the hemoglobin chains. The clinical presentation of thalassemias can vary from a stillborn infant to a person with mild asymptomatic anemia. Beta-thalassemia occurs with mutations that result in a decreased production of structurally normal beta-globin. Many of the mutations that lead to beta-thalassemia have been shown to be in the promoter region or at splice sites; hence a structurally normal protein is produced in decreased quantities.

Disbursed Gene Family

The actin proteins are highly conserved cytoskeletal proteins. They play a role in many cell functions such as migration, division, endocytosis, contraction, and structural integrity. Across species almost 30 different actin genes have been noted. In humans there are three major isoforms: the alpha form, which is found in muscle with different subtypes in striated and in smooth muscle, the beta form found in all cells, and the gamma form also seen in all cells. These isoforms represent a "family" of structurally and functionally related proteins.

Clinical results of various α-thalassemia genotypes

Clinical condition	Genotype	Number of functional α genes	α-chain production
Normal	HBAHBA/ HBAHBA	4	100%
Silent carrier	HBAHBA/ HBA—	3	75%
Heterozygous α-thalassemia— mild anemia	HBA—/HBA— or HBAHBA/— —	2	50%
HbH (β₄) disease— moderately severe anemia	HBA—/— —	1	25%
Homozygous α-thalassemia— lethal	— —/— —	0	0%

A β-thalassemia patient makes only α globin, not β globin.

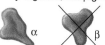

Four α subunits combine to make abnormal hemoglobin.

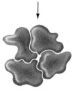

Abnormal hemoglobin molecules clump together, altering shape of red blood cells. Abnormal cells carry reduced amounts of oxygen.

Figure 4-22. Beta-thalassemia is a disorder of the hemoglobin molecule. (Reprinted with permission from Hartwell LH, et al. *Genetics: From genes to genomes.* 3rd ed. New York: McGraw-Hill, 2008.)

The genes for the different isoforms are located at different, dispersed loci.

The best explanation for the existence of these related forms is that a protein can take on slightly different functions due to mutations in duplicated copies of the gene. As each protein in a family has a different function, mutations in each specific gene will produce different clinical entities. For example, the nomenclature for actin genes is the designation of ACT. Mutations in different members of the actin family produce different phenotypes depending upon the specific gene that has been changed. Mutations in ACT A1, for example, result in various muscle diseases (myopathies). Alternatively, changes in ACT G1 produces non-syndromic deafness, changes in ACT C1 produce cardiomyopathies, and in ACT B juvenile dystonia. It is, therefore, important in genetic diagnostics that isoforms are recognized when testing is performed.

Pseudo Genes

Scattered throughout the genome are DNA sequences that are very similar to those of known functioning genes, but are nonfunctioning themselves. These sequences are referred to as "**pseudogenes.**" Pseudogenes are felt to be the historic relatives of functioning genes that have lost their coding ability or no longer express RNA. They are felt to be either duplicated or disabled copies of an original coding gene. They are thus characterized by:

1. sequence homology to a "parent gene" and

2. nonfunctionality.

The current count for human pseudogenes is around 24,000 to 25,000. The most important role of pseudogenes in medicine is that these very similar sequences can create confusion during genetic testing.

Early descriptions of pseudogenes often referred to them as part of the "junk DNA." Pseudogenes can almost be perceived as the "appendix" of the genome. As with most vestigial structures their importance may be falsely discounted. Pseudogenes may actually have a role in gene regulation and gene expression. They may in fact play a part in the regulation of protein-coding transcripts. It is also felt that some silencing RNAs (sRNA) may be derived from pseudogenes.

Tandem Repeats

As first introduced in Part 1, the term **tandem repeats** means clustered repeated nucleotides (next to each other and oriented in the same direction). They may be subcategorized as: satellites, minisatellites, or microsatellites based upon their overall size and the length of the repeated unit. The name "satellites" comes from a pattern of optical density seen on spectral analysis where DNA with tandem repeats appear as bands off of the main band (consisting of the majority of the "regular" DNA; Figure 4-23).

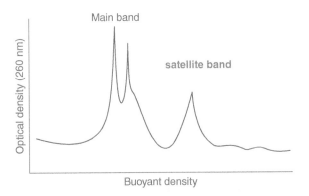

Figure 4-23. Optical density banding of nuclear DNA showing satellite bands corresponding to repetitive sequences.

Satellites

Satellite DNA ranges in size from 100 kb to over 1 Mb. Most satellites in humans are located at the centromere. The **centromere** of human chromosomes has no precisely-defined DNA sequence but in fact is largely made up of large arrays of satellite DNA. The primary centromeric repeated unit is referred to as the **alpha satellite**. The repeat unit of the alpha satellite is 171 bp and the repetitive region accounts for 3% to 5% of the overall DNA content. Centromeric DNA usually occurs in a **heterochromatic** state and is associated with a unique histone protein, CENP-A.

Deletion of the centromeric portion of a chromosome will lead to loss of further replication and migration of that particular chromosome. Some cancers have been associated with problems of centromeric function. In addition, several autoimmune diseases have been associated with anti-centromeric antibodies such as systemic sclerosis, systemic lupus erythematosis, rheumatoid arthritis, and Sjögren syndrome.

Minisatellites

Minisatellites typically are variant regions of the genome consisting of repeats rich in guanine and cytosine (GC) that range from 10 to 100 bp. The overall size of a minisatellite ranges from 1 to 20 kb. The vast majority (over 90%) of minisatellites are found in the **subtelomeric** regions of the chromosomes. Some minisatellites have an exceptionally high mutation rate approaching 20%. These hypervariable minisatellites then represent the most unstable loci of the genome.

One type of minisatellite is called **variable number of tandem repeats (VNTRs).** Individual repeats can be duplicated in or deleted from the VNTR via recombination or replication errors. This leads to variants that act as heritable alleles characterized by the different numbers of repeated DNA sequences. VNTRs are extremely useful in many settings of DNA diagnostics as a natural source of readily identifiable genomic variation between individuals. VNTRs can be used to generate an individual "**DNA fingerprint.**" Common applications using such VNTRs in molecular diagnostics include forensic investigations, paternity testing, personal identification, and population migration tracking.

Alterations in minisatellites have been associated with several human medical conditions. Minisatellites have been associated with chromosome fragile sites and are proximal to a number of recurrent translocation breakpoints. Polymorphisms in the VNTR region of certain genes have been associated with neurobehavioral disorders. VNTRs of the 5-hydroxytryptamine/serotonin transporter (5-HTT) gene have been associated with anxiety disorders and changes in the dopamine transporter 1 (DAT1) gene with attention deficit hyperactivity disorder. Unstable 15-18 minisatellite expansion in the promoter region of the glycosyltransferase 6 (GT6) gene has been shown to cause autosomal recessive myoclonic epilepsy.

Another type of minisatellite is the **telomere** of the human chromosome. All eukaryotic chromosomes are capped at the end with repeat telomere sequences that protect the ends from damage and rearrangement. The size of a telomere is about 15 kb in the germ cells. It is somewhat smaller in somatic cells. The human telomere contains the tandemly repeated sequence GGGTTA. The handling of telomeres has a specific role in the aging process with removal of telomere sequences functioning as the biologic "timekeeper" of cell cycles.

Dyskeratosis congenita (DC) is a multisystem disorder characterized by a classic triad of features that include nail dystrophy, skin hyperpigmentation, and mucosal leukoplakia (Figure 4-24). Patients also typically have bone marrow failure, premature aging, ataxia, hypoplasia of the cerebellum, and learning disabilities. Cytogenetic studies in patients with dyskeratosis congenita show shortening of the teleomeres. One form of DC is X-linked and is associated with a gene, dyskeratosis congenita 1 (DKC1). The protein associated with this protein product is dyskerin. This is a component of the small nucleolar ribonucleoprotein (snoRNA) particles. Dyskerin plays an important role in the processing of telomere complexes. The autosomal dominant form of DC is associated with mutations in the gene telomerase RNA component (TERC). The product of TERC is an RNA that is a component of the telomere that actually functions as a template. Thus the principal pathology of DC appears to be related to abnormalities of the processing of telomeres.

Microsatellites

Microsatellites represent the smallest size of tandem repeats. They may also be referred to as short tandem repeats (STRs). In humans the size of the repeated unit is 2 to 6 bp, most commonly di-, tri-, or tetranucleotide repeats. They are usually clustered in groups of 10 to 100 repeats yielding an overall size of around 100 to 150 bp.

Microsatellites play an important role in human disorders. The trinucleotide repeat disorders are a group of neurogenetic disorders that share a common pathophysiology. Abnormal expansion of normally occurring microsatellites (trinucleotide repeats) results in neurologic problems such as mental retardation, ataxia, and movement disorders (Table 4-4). These conditions demonstrate a set of novel mechanisms in the basis of genetic disorders. Most show genetic **anticipation**, i.e., a worsening of the condition as it passes through the generations. (For more details on trinucleotide repeat disorders, see Chapter 12 and the clinical correlation section that follows in this chapter.)

Lynch syndrome, also known as hereditary non-polyposis colorectal cancer (HNPCC), is a hereditary cancer syndrome associated with cancer of the colon and other abdominal/pelvic organs (Figure 4-25). HNPCC is genetically heterogeneous with five genes known to cause the condition. All five of these genes are **mismatch repair genes**—genes involved in identifying and correcting errors in DNA replication. Genetic testing for mutations in these DNA mismatch repair (MMR) genes is laborious and expensive. As a prescreen, laboratories can actually quantify the degree of **microsatellite instability** (MSI) in colonic tumor specimens. If increased microsatellite instability is identified in a tumor, there is a significantly increased risk that the patient has a mismatch repair abnormality associated with his or her cancer. This group of selected patients is thus "flagged" for further studies such as sequencing of the MMR genes. A combined strategy of immunohistochemical staining and microsatellite instability (MSI) screening is the currently recommended first-step approach for the evaluation of possible Lynch syndrome in a family.

Transposable Elements

Transposable elements are mobile segments of DNA that occur in all eukaryotic cells. They are nonrandomly distributed throughout the genome. Potentially, a third to half of the entire genome is composed of repetitive sequences that are degenerative copies of transposable elements. By the very nature of being migratory, these segments of DNA may affect an "insertional mutagenesis." In other words, they may produce mutations by disruption of a gene or by exerting affects on its promoter or enhancer. In the scope of population genetics, this is likely a prime source of generating genetic variation.

Hemophilia A is a clotting disorder due to a deficiency of a protein (factor VIII) in the clotting cascade. Factor VIII deficiency results in problems with effective blood coagulation. The gene for factor VIII is on the X chromosome, and thus the condition typically affects males. Men with this condition experience problems, often severe, with excess bleeding and bruising. If one looks at the spontaneous occurrence of hemophilia A, a 3-fold higher than expected spontaneous mutation rate is found as compared to other coding sequences. This increased mutation rate resulting in hemophilia appears related to the insertion of a truncated L1 (LINE) into the gene. Other conditions associated with a higher mutation rate felt to be related to transposable elements include neurofibromatosis and breast/ovarian cancer due to mutations in the BRCA2 gene. This is discussed further in Chapter 12 (Atypical Inheritance).

Other Changes in RNA
Transfer RNA (tRNA)

The main function of tRNA is its role in the transport of amino acids to the translational complex (RNA to protein). "Mutations" in tRNA produce problems with tRNA synthesis and coupling. Clinical conditions that have been reported with abnormalities of tRNA include Charcot-Marie-Tooth disease and other peripheral neuropathies, Alzheimer disease, Parkinson disease, and atherosclerosis.

Ribosomal RNA (rRNA)

Changes in rRNA result in defects in ribosome biogenesis. Typically, clinical disorders associated with abnormal rRNA

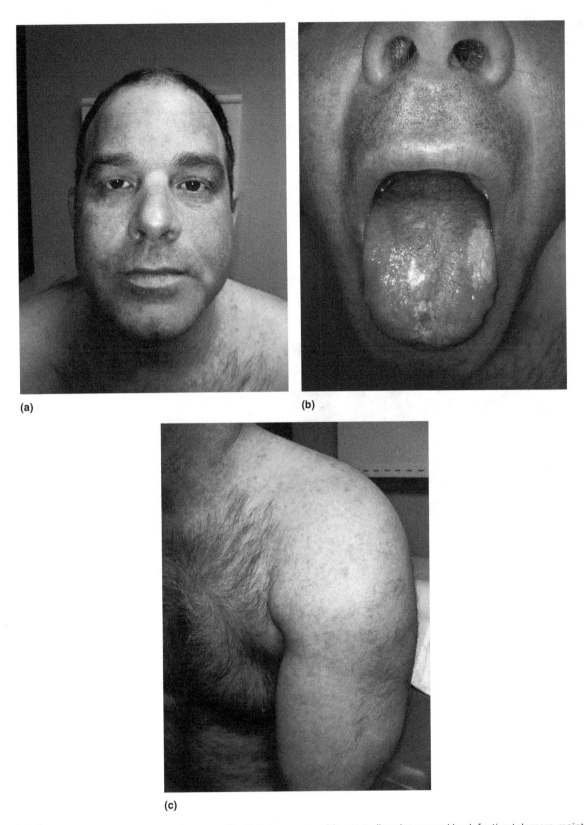

(a)

(b)

(c)

Figure 4-24. Adult male with dyskeratosis congenita. This is a rare multisystem disorder caused by defective telomere maintenance. Clinical features include abnormal 'reticular' pigmentation of the skin, ectodermal changes (brittle nails, scant hair, and poor dentition), osteoporosis, premalignant lesions of the oral mucosa, absent fingerprints, missing lacrimal ducts, hyperkeratosis of the palms, anemia, and immune deficiency. A finding of 'endoreduplication' is seen on chromosome studies.

Table 4-4.	Clinical and Molecular Characteristics of Selected of Trinucleotide Repeat Disorders				
Disorder	**Clinical Presentation**	**Trinucleotide Repeat**	**Repeat Length**		**Location of the Repeat**
			Normal	**Disease**	
Fragile X syndrome	X-linked mental retardation	CGG	29-30	>200	5' untranslated region
Myotonic dystrophy	Myotonia, cataracts	CTG	5-30	200-1000	3' untranslated region
Huntington disease	Involuntary movements Progressive neurodegeneration	CAG	11-34	39-120	open reading frame (exons)
Kennedy disease	Androgen insensitivity Spinal /bulbar muscular atrophy	CAG	11-34	40-62	open reading frame (exons)
Spinocerebellar ataxia Type 1	Progressive atrophy of cerebellum Ataxia	CAG	19-36	43-81	open reading frame (exons)
Friedreich ataxia	Ataxia, diabetes	GAA	5-33	66-1700	within

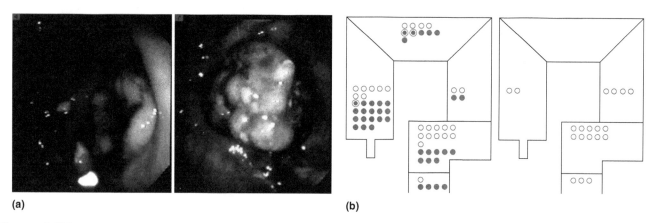

(a)   **(b)**

Figure 4-25. Lynch syndrome or hereditary non-polyposis colorectal cancer (HNPCC). (a) Endoscopic images of colorectal cancer in Lynch syndrome. (b) Diagram showing the predominance of right-sided colonic tumors in Lynch syndrome (as compared to predominantly left sided tumors in sporadic cases).

interestingly have problems with red blood cell production. Blackfan Diamond syndrome is a multiple anomaly syndrome associated with abnormal thumbs, short stature, and a congenital anemia. Over 25% of the patients with Blackfan Diamond syndrome have mutations in ribosomal protein S19. Abnormalities of rRNA have also been seen with macrocytic anemia and a predisposition to leukemia.

MicroRNAs (miRNA)

There are over 500 miRNAs described in mammals. The key feature of miRNAs are the stem loop phenomenon. They serve

as a "fine tuning" function of gene expression. Abnormalities in miRNA have been implicated in cancer, especially leukemia. Other abnormalities of miRNA include cardiac problems (cardiogenesis, hypertropic growth response, and abnormal cardiac conductance). Neurologic changes have also been seen with changes in miRNAs including a role in the pathogenesis of schizophrenia and Alzheimer disease.

Part 3: Clinical Correlation

Significant cognitive deficits (mental retardation, MR) occur in 3% to 4% of the US population. The vast majority of mental retardation can be attributed to genetic factors. In the population, MR occurs about four times as often in males as in

females. It has been known for a long time that much of this male predominance can be attributed to mutations in X-linked genes. In fact, the first report of X-linked MR in a kindred was published in 1943. Before molecular tests were readily

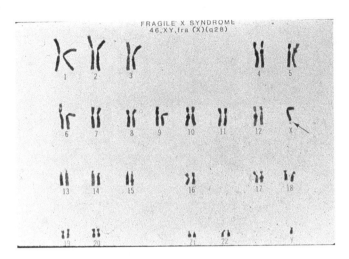

Figure 4-26. Karyotype of fragile-X syndrome. Note the "fragile" site indicated by the arrow.

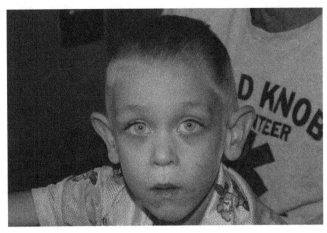

(a)

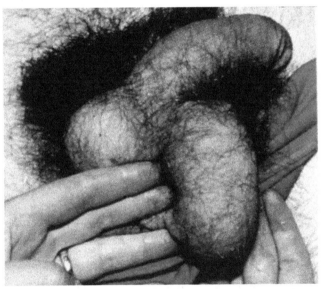

(b)

Figure 4-27. Many men with fragile-X syndrome show: (a) common characteristic facial features and (b) other traits such as macroorchidism.

available, all that the clinician could ascertain was that MR was appearing in the family in an X-linked pattern (see Chapter 6). In 1969 a laboratory directed by Dr. Herb Lubs studying X-linked mental retardation discovered a molecular marker designated as a "fragile site" on the X chromosome (Figure 4-26). This marker was only observed under specific cell culture conditions such as a folic acid deficient media. Using this marker, a subset of families with X-linked mental retardation could be identified. Thus, the clinical phenotype of fragile X syndrome was defined. Men with fragile X syndrome were noted to have cognitive deficits and mild craniofacial changes (macrocephaly in early childhood, a prominent jaw, a broad nasal bridge, large/protuberant ears, light blue irises, and epicanthal folds). Other features included large testicles (macroorchidism) after puberty, lax joints, other skeletal changes, and neurobehavioral/neuropsychiatric problems (Figure 4-27).

Further examination of kindreds with fragile X syndrome began to identify a more complex inheritance pattern. Intervening females were often found to have a partial phenotype. Many were noted to have a lesser degrees of cognitive impairment and a pattern of neurobehavioral changes as well. Some showed early ovarian failure. In addition, genetic anticipation (a worsening of the condition as it is passed through generations) was seen in a review of the pedigrees. This pattern of X-linked semi-dominant inheritance with genetic anticipation was described by Dr. Beth Sherman as what subsequently became known as the "Sherman paradox" (Figure 4-28). Ultimately, an exciting discovery was made that uncovered the mechanism of this unusual inheritance pattern. Fragile X syndrome was found to be caused by an **expanding trinucleotide repeat** (expansion of a microsatellite region) of a gene ultimately designated as FMR1 on the X chromosome at position Xq28. In the case of fragile X syndrome, the specific repeat is a CGG nucleotide triplet. The repeat region is in the 5′ untranslated region of the FMR1 gene. The typical

size of the repeat in the general population is 29 or 30 tandem copies. After an initiating event (mutation), the size of the repeat begins to expand as it progresses through the generations. In fragile X syndrome, expansion occurs only if the abnormal allele is transmitted by the mother. The expansion of the repeats can take many generations. Ultimately, when the size of the expansion exceeds 200 repeats, transcription of the FMR1 gene is turned off, the protein product of this gene is not produced, and the affected individual demonstrates clinical fragile X syndrome (Figure 4-29). But the inheritance of fragile X turns out to be even more complex. Over the past several years additional amazing insights into the pathogenesis of this condition have been reported. For more information see Chapter 12, Atypical Inheritance.

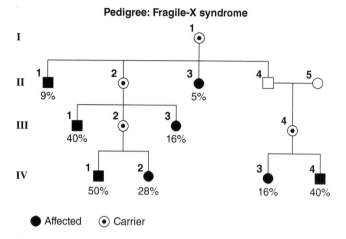

Pedigree: Fragile-X syndrome

● Affected   ◉ Carrier

Figure 4-28. A sample pedigree showing semi-dominant inheritance with genetic anticipation. This pattern illustrates the Sherman Paradox in fragile-X expression. The percentages denote the proportion of affected persons.

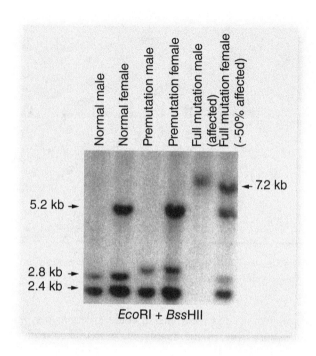

Figure 4-29. Southern blot showing differing sizes of tri-nucleotide repeats in fragile-X.

■ Board-Format Practice Questions

1. The "one-gene, one-enzyme" hypothesis as put forth by Beadle and Tatum
   A. has stood the test of time and still remains a solid working model.
   B. has been proven to be completely incorrect.
   C. has now been shown to be an overly simple representation.
   D. is true for plants, but not humans.
   E. applies to most human diseases.

2. Genes are expressed
   A. almost exclusively through protein coding.
   B. usually in isolation, not by interacting with other genes.
   C. by a variety of different mechanisms—some of which do not entail protein coding.
   D. only in the nucleus.
   E. only due to information in the coding sequence.

3. Satellite DNA
   A. is composed of tandem repeats of nucleotide sequences.
   B. excludes the centromere.
   C. are interesting genetic phenomena, but have little clinical significance.
   D. are subclassified as macro- and megasatellites.
   E. is typically very homogeneous.

4. Fragile X syndrome
   A. is caused by a change in a gene on chromosome 17.
   B. demonstrates recessive inheritance.
   C. is caused by an expanding trinucleotide repeat.
   D. is caused by folic acid deficiency.
   E. affects exclusively men.

5 Clinical Cytogenetics

C H A P T E R   S U M M A R Y

The first four chapters have taken a long-range view of the way in which genes determine a phenotype through interconnected biochemical pathways and cell interactions. In this chapter we will focus on how the genetic information packaged in chromosomes is duplicated and distributed during cell division (Figure 5-1). Then in Chapter 6, we will explore how chromosome behavior during the formation and fusion of gametes determines the predictable genetic outcomes of a mating.

The process of nuclear division is very accurate. Yet, errors do occur and can lead to changes in chromosome number and structure with often severe or even fatal consequences. It is not easy to study the genetic control of nuclear division at more than a descriptive level. This is because some of the most powerful tools available to a genetic researcher are mutations. By seeing how a mutation alters a process, one can deduce the role of the normal gene. But mutations are difficult to isolate for the molecular and biochemical events governing **mitosis**, which is the complete duplication of the genome of a cell to produce two identical cells, and **meiosis**, which is the reduction division found in egg- and sperm-forming tissue. In order to collect and analyze the roles of mutations in a given trait, one must be able to breed and manipulate them. But mutations that prevent nuclear division naturally block that approach, forcing researchers to find new ways to explore the molecular control of genetic transmission. Most medical applications, however, simply depend upon understanding the inherent logic of mitosis and meiosis and the consequences of errors or other complications that affect them. That will be our focus in this chapter.

In addition to errors in nuclear division that lead to changes in chromosome number, various agents like radiation can alter chromosome structure. Changes in structure affect a block of genes and influence many otherwise independent biochemical processes. They can also cause complicated physical interactions between chromosomes that have serious secondary consequences. In this chapter we will first discuss the normal processes of chromosomal distribution in mitosis and meiosis, and then explore the kinds of errors that affect chromosome number and structure. There are many important medical examples of each.

Part 1: Background and Systems Integration

Overview of Nuclear Division as an Information Distribution System

Some of the basic terminology used to describe the genome was introduced in the first two chapters. We know, for example, that the nucleus of a diploid (2n) cell contains two copies of each gene. The subtleties of such a statement were discussed in Chapter 4 but do not affect our understanding of nuclear division. Each gene is located somewhere on one of the numerous strands of DNA we see in the microscope as chromosomes. Each chromosome is, therefore, a separate unit of information transmission, a copy of a **linkage group**. It might contain hundreds or even several thousand genes linked in a linear array on the same strand of DNA. There are as many different linkage groups in a species as there are genetically different types of chromosome, ignoring the minor

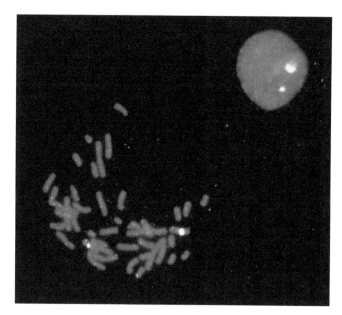

Figure 5-1. A chromosome spread (unsorted) with fluorescent probes for chromosome number 14. A nondividing cell is off to the side also showing the chromosome 14 probes. (Reprinted with permission from Brooker RJ: *Genetics: Analysis & Principles*, 3rd ed. New York: McGraw-Hill, 2008.)

differences that distinguish allelic forms of the same gene. A diploid individual carries two copies of each linkage group, i.e., a pair of **homologous chromosomes**. The goal of mitosis is to duplicate each chromosome and pass one copy of every chromosome into each of the two new nuclei of the diploid daughter cells.

The goal of meiosis, on the other hand, is more complex and in some ways more important. Meiosis is a reduction division involving two cycles. Instead of transmitting one copy of every chromosome, meiosis results in passing one copy of each *kind* of chromosome, i.e., one copy of each linkage group, to each haploid (1n) egg or sperm nucleus. The diploid (2n) nuclear composition is regenerated at fertilization, with one copy of each linkage group coming from each parent.

Although cancer, somatic mosaicism, and other outcomes involving chromosome-level changes can be significant, errors in mitosis will usually have only minor consequences, if they have any at all. The presence of one abnormal cell is hard to detect among so many normal ones in the body. Its abnormality and death go unnoticed. But an error in meiosis is far more serious, since it will affect the initial genome of the zygote produced at fertilization. Estimates range from 8% to 25% (with most authorities leaning toward the higher end of this range) of human fertilizations will result in spontaneous abortion, perinatal death, or severe developmental consequences due to changes in chromosome number from errors in meiosis or fertilization. After discussing the normal events of nuclear division, we will explore some of the consequences of errors in meiosis.

The Cell Cycle in Eukaryotes

Whether we are considering mitosis or meiosis, the phases of the cell cycle can be subdivided into two parts, **interphase** and the stages of nuclear division (Figure 5-2a, which shows the events for mitosis). Interphase is sometimes called the "resting phase," but that is a misnomer. It may be a resting stage in the sense that it occurs between rounds of active nuclear division. But functionally, it is the most active time.

During the G_1 phase of interphase, active genes are being transcribed and are controlling the biochemical life of the cell. To be accessible to the enzymes of transcription, the chromosomes are in various degrees of uncoiling. That is why a stained microscopic preparation of interphase simply looks like a dark organelle with little internal structure other than one or more **nucleoli**. At this stage, each chromosome is a single DNA double-helix molecule complexed with nucleosomal proteins. In G_1 the cell typically grows by duplicating cell contents, except for the nuclear material. Then, in response to a signal, such as cell age, reaching a critical cell size, or receiving a molecular trigger like a growth factor, a **restriction point** is reached. The cell becomes committed to make a transition into the S, or synthesis, phase. An example of activating this G_1-S checkpoint by a growth factor is shown in Figure 5-2b.

Progress through the G_1 (or G_1-S) and the later G_2 (or G_2-M) checkpoints is regulated by the formation of complexes of specific cyclins and cyclin-dependent kinases (CDKs). CDKs regulate the activity of other proteins by phosphorylating them, thereby either activating or inactivating them, depending on the function of the target protein. The specific cyclins determine which target proteins are acted on. At the G_1-S checkpoint, the cyclin-CDK complex activates proteins needed for DNA replication. At the later G_2-M checkpoint, a different cyclin-CDK complex activates proteins responsible for condensation and other chromosomal changes. If damage such as a DNA break is detected, a checkpoint protein like p53 inhibits the formation of an active cyclin/CDK complex.

In some cell lineages, a division restriction point is delayed or stops. A nucleus can be temporarily inactive (Figure 5-3) so it is not preparing for a new cell division cycle, or it might be terminally differentiated and will never divide again. Such a cell is described as being in the G_0 phase.

In the S (synthesis) phase, DNA replication occurs. To accomplish this complex task, the chromosomes must of course remain uncoiled, or uncondensed. But if we could visualize them in a microscope, we would see that the two single-stranded templates of the replicating parent DNA molecule separate and a pair of new complementary strands is constructed as described in Chapter 2. The two strands remain connected at the centromere, so when they condense during nuclear division, we are able to see the two copies for the first time (Figure 5-4) as **sister chromatids**. From here to the middle of nuclear division, each chromosome has twice the usual amount of DNA.

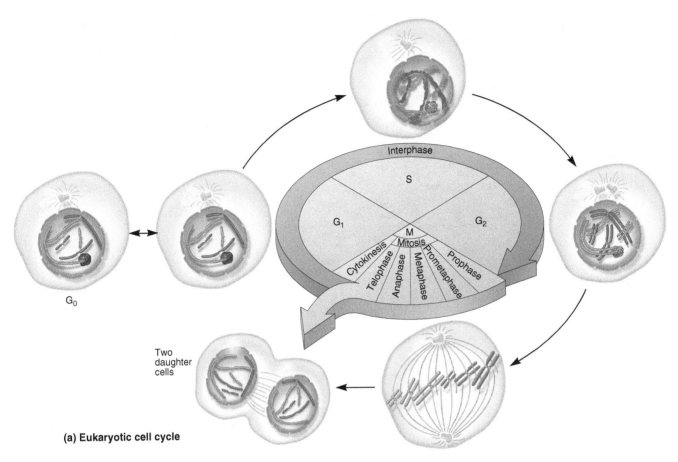

(a) Eukaryotic cell cycle

Figure 5-2a. The growth-duplication cycle of mitosis. (Reprinted with permission from Brooker RJ: *Genetics: Analysis & Principles*, 3rd ed. New York: McGraw-Hill, 2008.)

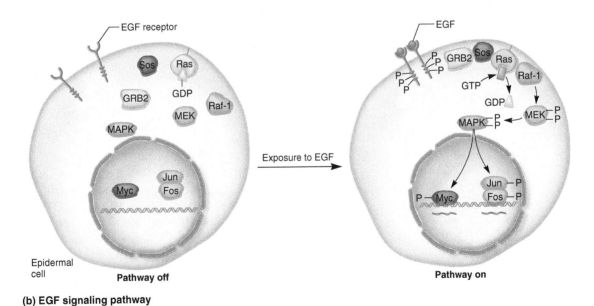

(b) EGF signaling pathway

Figure 5-2b. Activation of cell division by epidermal growth factor (EGF). EGF binds a pair of EGF receptors and causes them to form an active dimer and become phosphorylated. This attracts the GRB2 and other proteins intracellularly, ultimately activating the Ras protein by forming a Ras/GTP (i.e., guanosine triphosphate) complex. This complex activates the Raf-1 protein kinase that phosphorylates MEK, which then phosphorylates MAPK. This MAPK then activates transcription factors that initiate cell division. (Reprinted with permission from Brooker RJ: *Genetics: Analysis & Principles*, 3rd ed. New York: McGraw-Hill, 2008.)

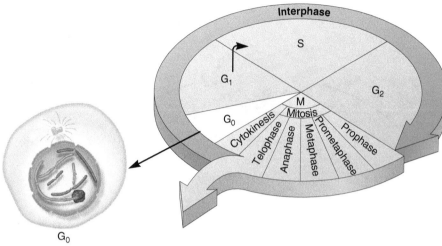

Interphase

S

G₁

G₂

M

G₀

Mitosis

Cytokinesis

Telophase

Anaphase

Metaphase

Prometaphase

Prophase

G₀

Temporarily paused or
terminally differentiated

Figure 5-3. The G₀ phase represents a cell that is no longer dividing, as in case of a terminally differentiated cell lineage. (Reprinted with permission from Brooker RJ: *Genetics: Analysis & Principles*, 3rd ed. New York: McGraw-Hill, 2008.)

The terminology concerning chromosome number and DNA content during this transition can be confusing, but it is simplified if one keeps a key definition in mind. The term "chromosome" literally means "colored body." No matter how many chromosome arms it carries, anything connected together at the same centromere is one unit and, thus, one chromosome. To count chromosomes, you must simply count the number of centromeres. Chromosome number does not change between the beginning and the end of interphase. What changes is the amount of DNA in the nucleus. The **C**

value is the amount of DNA in a haploid (1n) nucleus. The diploid cell at G₁, therefore, has a DNA content of 2C. During S, this doubles to 4C. Nuclear division reduces it back to 2C in each of the two daughter cells at the end of mitosis or to 1C in each of the four nuclei that result from the meiotic reduction division to produce haploid eggs or sperm.

During G₂, the cell makes final preparations for division of the nucleus and cytoplasm. A key event that continues from S into G₂ is the error correction in DNA repair. The checkpoint between G2 and mitosis or meiosis (M) is not passed until repair activities have been completed. Timing of the substages of interphase will differ among species and as a function of how actively the tissue is dividing, with the period of interphase before S being the most variable. One estimate for dividing mouse fibroblasts is 9.1 hours for G₁, 9.9 hours for S, 2.2 hours for G₂, and 0.7 hours for mitosis (M).

Mitosis: Somatic Cell Division

The stages of mitosis (Figure 5-5) are defined for the convenience of talking about the details of the process. Keep in mind, however, that it is actually a continuous process. At the start, the DNA and chromosomal proteins have already duplicated in interphase, and the two sister chromatids of each replicated chromosome are still attached at the centromere (Figure 5-4). An additional cell organelle also comes into play. The **centrosome** containing a pair of **centrioles** is located in the cytoplasm near the nucleus. They produce the array of microtubules that move chromosomes during nuclear division.

Prophase is a preparatory phase (*pro* = before). The chromosomes coil or condense into compact structures that can move easily within a cell and that can begin to be seen microscopically. The nuclear membrane breaks down, and the centrosomes divide and begin moving to opposite poles of the cell. As they separate, they generate an array of microtubules called the **spindle**, which is composed of tubulin.

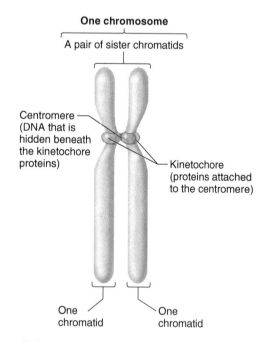

One chromosome

A pair of sister chromatids

Centromere
(DNA that is
hidden beneath
the kinetochore
proteins)

Kinetochore
(proteins attached
to the centromere)

One
chromatid

One
chromatid

Figure 5-4. Chromosomes become highly coiled, or compacted, during early nuclear division (metaphase) and clearly show the position of the centromere attachment of the copies or the separation of the sister chromatids. (Reprinted with permission from Brooker RJ: *Genetics: Analysis & Principles*, 3rd ed. New York: McGraw-Hill, 2008.)

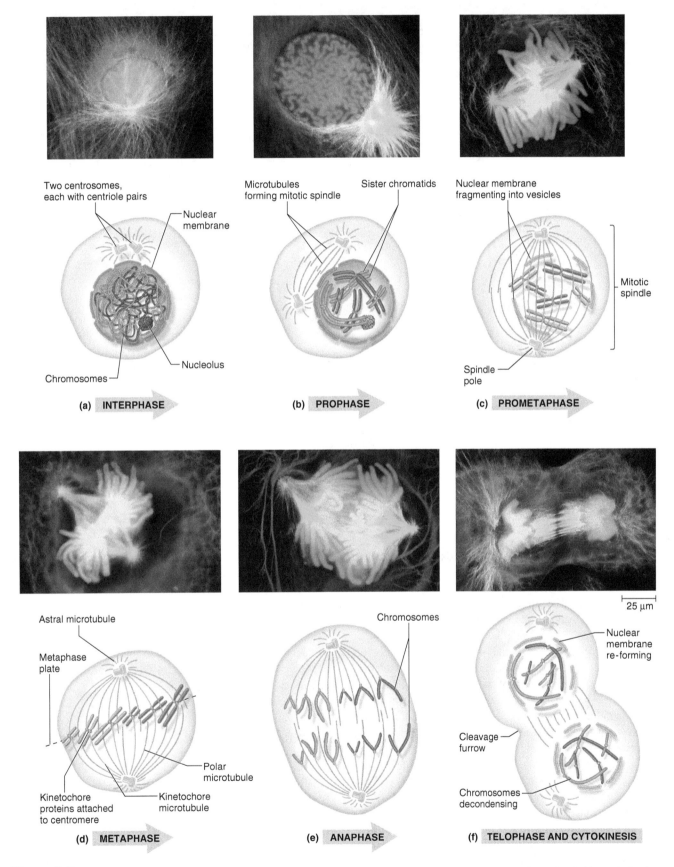

Figure 5-5. Stages of mitosis. (Photomicrographs © Dr. Conly L. Rieder, Wadsworth Center, Albany, New York 12201-0509. Reprinted with permission from Brooker RJ: *Genetics: Analysis & Principles*, 3rd ed. New York: McGraw-Hill, 2008.)

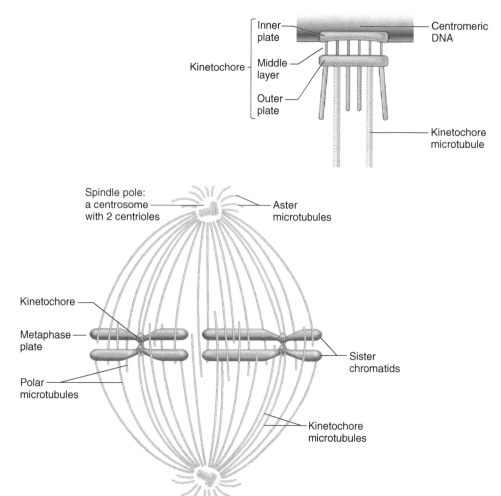

Figure 5-6. The mitotic spindle is made up of kinetochore microtubules that bind to the chromosome's kinetochore and polar microtubules that help keep the poles separate and the spindle in position. The kinetochore is made up of the centromeric DNA and two layers of kinetochore proteins that bind the kinetochore microtubules. (Reprinted with permission from Brooker RJ: *Genetics: Analysis & Principles,* 3rd ed. New York: McGraw-Hill, 2008.)

In **prometaphase**, the sister chromatids become attached to the spindle by means of the kinetochore microtubules that extend from the **kinetochore**, a group of proteins that binds the centromeric DNA region (Figure 5-6). The microtubules from the spindle, called the polar microtubules, overlap near the equator of the cell and help keep the spindle poles separate. One reason this phase is important in medical genetics is that current cytogenetic standards use prometaphase chromosomes to establish the **karyotype,** or chromosome picture (e.g., Figure 5-23), for clinical evaluation. The chromosomes are less condensed then than they will be at later stages, so more detail can be seen with certain kinds of staining treatments.

During **metaphase**, the chromosomes line up at the equator between the centrosome poles. The chromosome still has two attached sister chromatids, with each attached to the opposite pole. **Anaphase** begins when the centromere divides and each chromatid is now a separate chromosome. Chromosome number has temporarily doubled, e.g., from 46 chromosomes (each with a pair of sister chromatids) to 92 in humans. The kinetochore microtubules shorten by dissociation of their tubulin subunits, so the chromosomes move toward the poles a bit like pieces in the classic *Pac-Man* computer game.

In **telophase**, generally the briefest phase of mitosis, events opposite to those of prophase occur. The chromosomes decondense; the spindle breaks down; and two new nuclear membranes form around the chromosomes at each pole. In addition, division of the cytoplasm, called **cytokinesis**, occurs when a contractile ring that includes actin and the motor protein myosin constricts the cell membrane to distribute the cytoplasm and its organelles into the two daughter cells (Figure 5-7).

Meiosis: Producing Haploid Egg and Sperm Nuclei

In contrast to mitosis, which passes one duplicate copy of every chromosome to each of the daughter cells, meiosis reduces chromosome number by half. It does this in two cycles of division: prophase I, metaphase I, anaphase I, telophase I, followed by a second round with prophase II, and so forth (Figure 5-8). But it is not sufficient simply to cut chromosome number in half. Each haploid gamete must have one copy of each kind of chromosome, i.e., one copy of each linkage group. The process that allows this to occur centers on

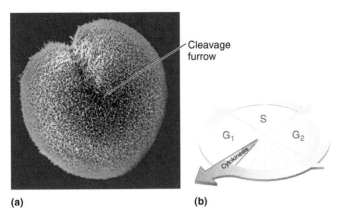

Cleavage
furrow

S

G₁   G₂

Cytokinesis

(a)   **(b)**

Figure 5-7. Division of the cytoplasm in cytokinesis is seen in the formation of a cleavage furrow produced by a ring of actin filaments and myosin motor proteins. Cytokinesis divides the cytoplasm and its internal organelles into two daughter cells.
(b: Reprinted with permission from Brooker RJ: *Genetics: Analysis & Principles*, 3rd ed. New York: McGraw-Hill, 2008.)

events in **prophase I**. In prophase I, as in the beginning of mitosis, the spindle forms, chromosomes condense, and the nuclear membrane breaks down. But instead of each chromosome attaching independently to the spindle microtubules, the homologous chromosomes pair together to form a **bivalent**. The process of pairing is called **synapsis** and involves the creation of a **synaptonemal complex** (Figure 5-9) that only forms between the chromatids of different homologous chromosomes. They do not form between sister chromatids. Consequently, there will be one bivalent for each type of chromosome, i.e., one bivalent for each linkage group. It is the bivalent that binds to the spindle so that at anaphase I, one of the chromosomes (still with the two sister chromatids attached at the centromere) moves to one pole while the other homologous chromosome moves to the opposite pole. Thus, chromosome number is reduced from the diploid set of chromosomes (2n) to two haploid (1n) nuclei by the end of the first meiotic division.

Synapsis has at least two important functions in prophase I. First, it puts all of the copies of each linkage group into a separate cluster. This enables the cell to distribute one complete set of genetic information to each cell at the end of the first division. Synapsis keeps the homologous chromosomes together in a group. Second, there is an exchange between homologous chromosomes, called **crossing over** or **recombination**, which shuffles the alleles that are carried by the two homologues. Recombination is a powerful force in generating the enormous range of genetic variation that can be found among the offspring from each pair of parents. Since so many important events occur during prophase I, it is divided into subphases described in detail in Figure 5-10.

Following prophase I, the chromosomes move to the equator of the cell in metaphase I (Figure 5-11), and the homologous chromosomes are pulled to opposite poles in anaphase I. As we will see in Chapter 6, this separation, or **segregation**, of any genetic differences in the alleles carried by homologues is the basis of one of the fundamental Mendelian rules of genetic

transmission. After a brief telophase I and cytokinesis, the second division proceeds as in mitosis, except that chromosome number is now haploid. The reduction division occurs during the first meiotic division. In humans, the result from each primary cell is four haploid sperm nuclei in **spermatogenesis** or one haploid egg nucleus plus three small haploid **polar bodies** in oogenesis (Figure 5-12).

The Karyotype

A karyotype is a picture of chromosomal makeup (Figure 5-13). Chemicals like colchicine and its synthetic equivalent colcemid will bind and unassemble the microtubules of the spindle. Without a functioning spindle, cell division is halted at prometaphase and metaphase. Their condensed shapes clearly show relative chromosome sizes and centromere placements. These characteristics can then be used to arrange pairs of homologous chromosomes into a standardized pattern called a karyotype.

Additional information can come from modifying the basic staining protocols before the chromosomes are visualized microscopically. Giemsa is a polychromatic stain that darkens chromatin material uniformly. Chromosomes in dividing cells show up clearly, but modifications of technique can enhance structural detail. One example is G-banding, mentioned in Chapter 4 (Figure 4-19), which involves pretreating the chromosomes with the proteolytic enzyme trypsin before staining with Giemsa. The resulting dark bands are areas of heterochromatin, which is highly condensed chromosomal material. The intervening light bands are euchromatin. This produces a chromosome-specific pattern of dark and light bands that allows some degree of resolution for intrachromosomal changes in structure. Although small changes cannot be detected with these techniques, information about the karyotype of an individual can identify changes in chromosome number and large changes in chromosome structure that have clinical significance.

Overview of Changes in Chromosome Number and Structure

Species differ in the way their genomes are distributed among chromosomes. There is no correlation between the number of chromosomes and the developmental complexity of an organism. Likewise, genes of similar function are scattered among the chromosomes. There is no correlation between a particular chromosome and a particular body part or metabolic process. Chromosomes are simply the structures that link together and distribute genetic information from one cell generation to the next during mitosis and meiosis. **Euploid** is the normal chromosomal makeup of an individual (*eu* = true or normal; *ploid* = multiple). Deviations involving the loss or gain of one or more chromosomes are **aneuploid**, or "not true" multiples. A **polyploid** has "many" multiples of chromosomes, e.g., 3n triploids and 4n tetraploids. When they occur, changes in

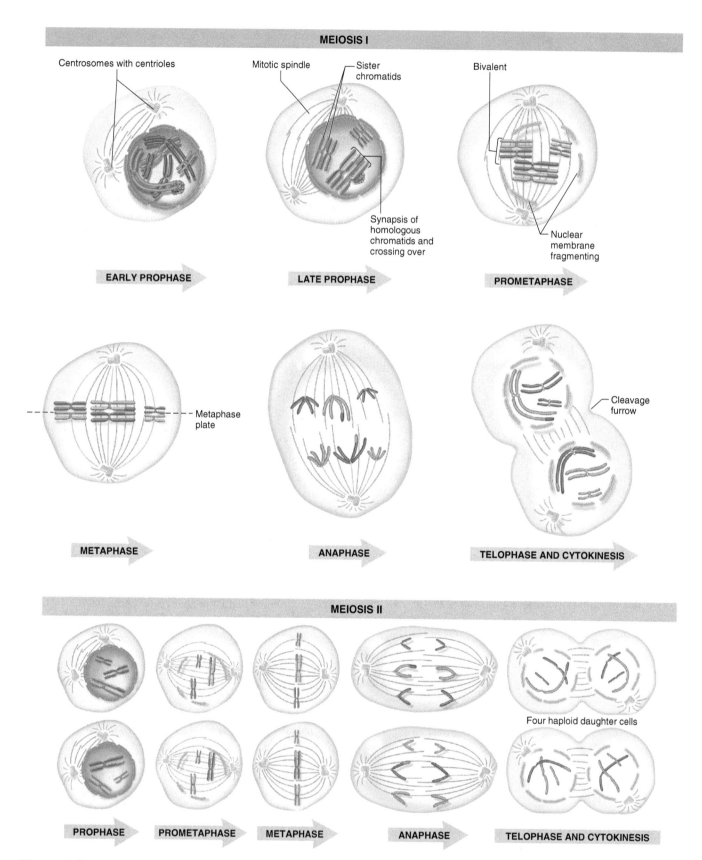

Figure 5-8. Meiosis involves two rounds of division and yields four haploid nuclei, each carrying one copy of each type of chromosome. Key events occur in prophase I of the first cycle including synapsis, or pairing, of homologous chromosome copies and recombination between them. (Reprinted with permission from Brooker RJ: *Genetics: Analysis & Principles*, 3rd ed. New York: McGraw-Hill, 2008.)

Figure 5-9. In prophase I, the synaptonemal complex forms between homologous chromosomes. (a) An electron micrograph of a synaptonemal complex. (b) Diagram of the elements that make up the synaptonemal complex between chromatids. (Reprinted with permission from Brooker RJ: *Genetics: Analysis & Principles*, 3rd ed. New York: McGraw-Hill, 2008.)

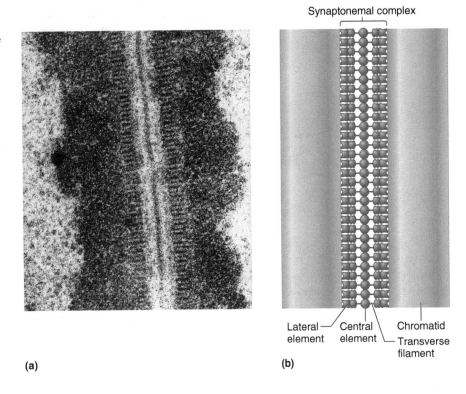

(a)

Synaptonemal complex

Lateral element   Central element   Chromatid   Transverse filament

(b)

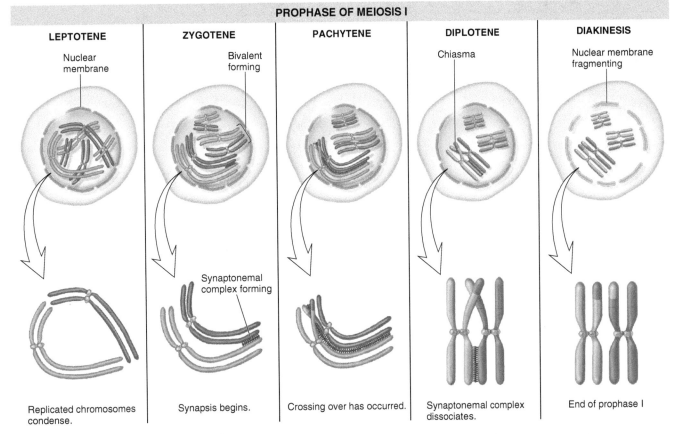

PROPHASE OF MEIOSIS I

LEPTOTENE	ZYGOTENE	PACHYTENE	DIPLOTENE	DIAKINESIS
Nuclear membrane	Bivalent forming		Chiasma	Nuclear membrane fragmenting
	Synaptonemal complex forming			
Replicated chromosomes condense.	Synapsis begins.	Crossing over has occurred.	Synaptonemal complex dissociates.	End of prophase I

Figure 5-10. Events that occur during prophase I of meiosis include synapsis and recombination. (Reprinted with permission from Brooker RJ: *Genetics: Analysis & Principles*, 3rd ed. New York: McGraw-Hill, 2008.)

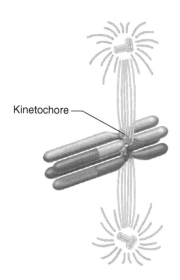

Figure 5-11. The kinetochore microtubules from one pole are attached to only one of the chromatid pairs in a bivalent Thus, the chromosomes in a homologous pair are attached to different poles. (Reprinted with permission from Brooker RJ: *Genetics: Analysis & Principles*, 3rd ed. New York: McGraw-Hill, 2008.)

chromosome number are almost always much more serious than a single gene, or point, mutation, because so many different genes, and thus many biochemical processes, are involved. Chromosome number can also be altered by fusion or fission of the centromeric regions, although this phenomenon is typically of more importance when comparing chromosome arm homologies in related species.

Chromosome aberrations, or changes in structure, occur when the linkage of genes within and between chromosomes is altered (Figure 5-14). Changes in chromosome structure are most commonly due to breaks that are incorrectly repaired during replication. Chromosome breaks are very common. One estimate is that an average of 55,000 single-strand breaks and 9 double-strand breaks occur in DNA molecules in each nucleus each day. The vast majority of these are repaired, but if several affected strands are near each other, the broken ends can be reattached incorrectly.

Three types of aberrations can affect the genetic content of an individual chromosome. If two breaks are repaired so that the intervening segment is left out, a portion of the chromosome is no longer attached to a centromere and is lost from the nucleus the next time it divides. This yields a **deletion**

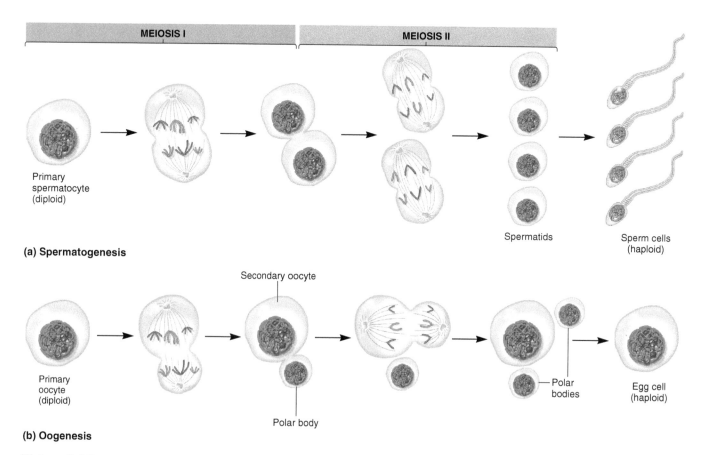

(a) Spermatogenesis

(b) Oogenesis

Figure 5-12. Comparison of: (a) spermatogenesis, which can yield four haploid sperm, and (b) oogenesis, which yields one haploid egg cell and up to three haploid polar bodies, which degenerate. (Reprinted with permission from Brooker RJ: *Genetics: Analysis & Principles*, 3rd ed. New York: McGraw-Hill, 2008.)

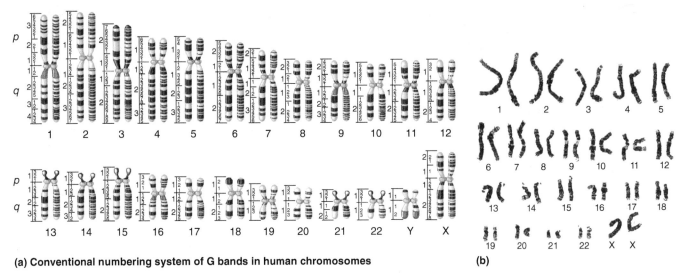

(a) Conventional numbering system of G bands in human chromosomes

(b)

Figure 5-13. Karyotypes are ways of organizing and presenting the chromosomal makeup of an individual. (a: Reprinted with permission from Brooker RJ: *Genetics: Analysis & Principles,* 4th ed. New York: McGraw-Hill, 2012. b: Reprinted with permission, Dr. Warren G. Sanger, University of Nebraska Medical Center.)

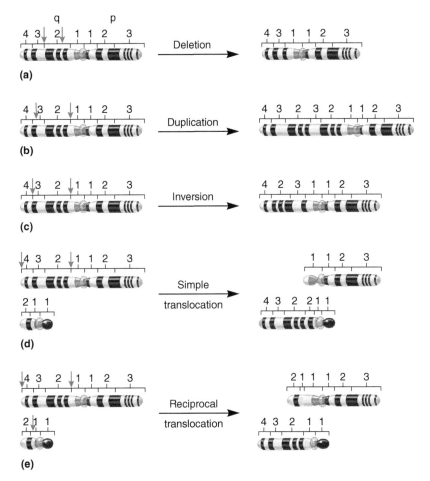

Figure 5-14. Chromosome aberrations are changes in chromosome structure. (a) Deletion is the loss of a segment of chromosome. (b) Duplication is the insertion of a section of chromosome so that two copies of each affected gene are present. (c) Inversions can occur when two breakpoints are reattached at alternate ends. (d) Simple translocation is the movement of a section of one chromosome to a different linkage group. (e) Reciprocal translocation involves the exchange of sections between nonhomologous chromosomes.
(Reprinted with permission from Brooker RJ: *Genetics: Analysis & Principles,* 3rd ed. New York: McGraw-Hill, 2008.)

or **deficiency**. Various mechanisms can cause a portion of the chromosome to be present twice, **duplication**. The order of genes along a chromosome can also change. For example, if two breaks in the chromosome are repaired so that alternate ends are attached, the intervening segment is now reversed, creating an **inversion**. In addition to the obvious changes in genetic content caused by these aberrations, especially in duplications and deficiencies, point mutations occur if the DNA breakpoints happen to be within the coding region of a gene. Furthermore, topological relationships among synapsed chromosomes in prophase I of meiosis can cause secondary consequences for the genetic composition of a fertilized egg. These are described in more detail later.

Finally, aberrations can affect more than one chromosome at a time. When a portion of one chromosome is reattached to a chromosome from a different linkage group, the result is called a **translocation**. Simple translocations involve the movement of a piece of one chromosome to another. When this translocated chromosome is passed to an offspring, there are extra copies of the genes carried in the translocated region. **Reciprocal translocations** involve the complementary exchange of segments between two nonhomologous chromosomes. If both translocated chromosomes are passed to the offspring, there is no overall change in genome content. But if only one of them is passed on, the offspring will carry an unbalanced genome content. Thus, translocations change how genes are arranged in linkage groups and can have secondary

consequences due to the way the altered chromosomes segregate in meiosis. We will look at the consequences of these abnormalities in more detail next.

Aneuploidy: Errors in Segregation

Aneuploidy is a deviation from the normal chromosome complement involving less than a full haploid set of chromosomes. The breakdown of a spindle microtubule, delayed division of the centromere connecting two sister chromatids, and other events can lead to the failure of chromosomes to segregate properly to opposite poles during division. Although this can occur in both mitosis and meiosis, our focus here will be on meiotic errors.

Failure to separate, or "segregate," normally can occur at either the first or the second meiotic division (Figure 5-15). The term used to describe this kind of error, **nondisjunction**, is actually a double negative. "Junction" (to join) means to go together, so *dis*junction is *not* to go together, i.e., to separate. *Non*disjunction is, therefore, *not* to separate, thus go together. The result is a gamete with either two copies or no copy of one or more chromosomes. When such a gamete combines with a normal gamete at fertilization, the resulting genome will be unbalanced by having abnormal numbers of active genes coding for their protein products. This will affect a large number of independent developmental and physiological processes. Most such affected embryos will die early.

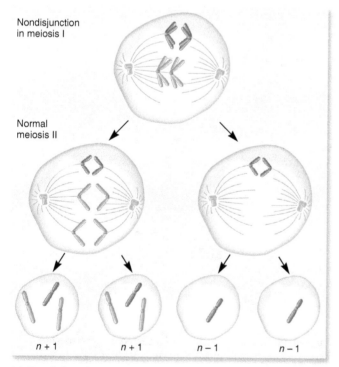

(a) Nondisjunction in meiosis I

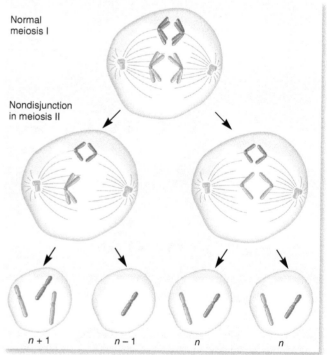

(b) Nondisjunction in meiosis II

Figure 5-15. Nondisjunction is a failure of the separation of homologues at the first or second meiotic division to yield cells that are missing or have extra copies of a chromosome. (Reprinted with permission from Brooker RJ: *Genetics: Analysis & Principles*, 3rd ed. New York: McGraw-Hill, 2008.)

If an extra copy of a chromosome is present, there will then be three copies of that linkage group, a **trisomic** ("tri" is three, "som" is body). Alternatively, if the abnormal gamete has lost its copy of that chromosome, fertilization will result in only one copy of the linkage group, a **monosomic** ("mono" is one), coming from the normal gamete fertilizing the gamete that is deficient. In humans, most trisomics and all but one type of monosomic typically die early in development. Most special cases involve aneuploidy of the X or Y chromosomes. Since females carry two X chromosomes but males have only one, it is normal to have a difference in the copy number, or dosage, of all X-linked genes when comparing the two genders. One mechanism that compensates for this difference in copy number, X-chromosome inactivation, will be discussed next. Here we will simply point out that the mechanism that allows males and females to develop normally with different numbers of X chromosomes can also allow development to proceed fairly normally if aneuploidy of a sex chromosome occurs.

X-chromosome Inactivation in Mammals

In mammals, the number of copies of X-linked genes will differ between males (with one X chromosome) and females (with two). To balance this difference, i.e., to accomplish "dosage compensation," almost all genes on one X chromosome in a cell are inactivated (Xi) by a process called **Lyonization** after its discoverer, Mary Lyon. Important exceptions will be discussed later. Lyonization involves the tight coiling of all X chromosomes except for one that is left genetically active (Xa). X inactivation is permanent in the somatic cells but has to be reversible in the development of the germ cells. In summary, X inactivation occurs early in embryogenesis, it is random, and it is clonal in that, once inactivated, that same X chromosome remains inactive in somatic daughter cells.

In interphase nuclei, the inactivated X can be seen as a dark spot or Barr body, named for Murray Barr, who first described them in cells from female cats. If additional X chromosomes are present due to errors in segregation, they are also Lyonized to produce additional Barr bodies. The nucleus shown in Figure 5-16, for example, has three Barr bodies in an abnormal cell containing a total of four X chromosomes in addition to the normal 22 pairs of autosomes ($2n = 48$).

X-chromosome inactivation is an example of **epigenetic modification**. In this phenomenon, a gene or in this case a chromosome becomes inactivated during an individual's lifetime. X inactivation is passed on to daughter cells during cell division, yielding patterns like the black and orange patch pattern seen in calico cats (Figure 5-17). Inactivation occurs randomly, so a female is really a patchwork of genetic expressions, a "functional mosaic," for any genes that differ between her two X chromosome copies. But in a broader context, one should be careful when using the term "mosaic," because in medical genetics it is usually reserved to describe differences in genetic makeup, not simply expression.

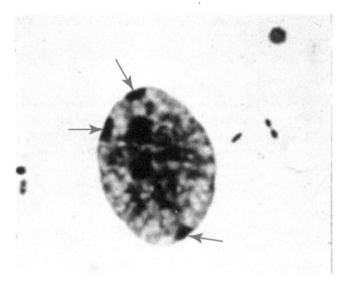

Figure 5-16. Three Barr bodies in an abnormal cell containing a total of four X chromosomes. Barr bodies are formed by the tight coiling, or Lyonization, of all except one X chromosome, so normal female nuclei have one Barr body.

The mechanism of X inactivation involves a limited amount of blocking factor protein that binds to an X chromosome and blocks its inactivation. All other X chromosomes are left unprotected and are inactivated. The **X inactivation center** (XIC) is thought to control this chromosomal silencing process by binding the blocking factor protein. Indeed, if

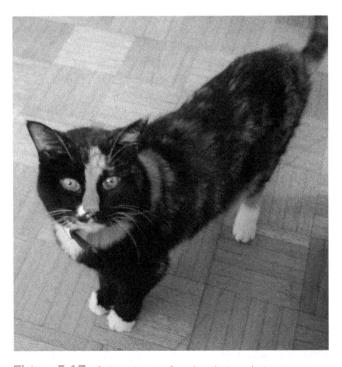

Figure 5-17. Calico cats are females that are heterozygous for black and orange alleles carried on randomly inactivated X chromosomes to yield patches of orange and black fur, respectively. (Courtesy of Sarah M. Granlund.)

the XIC is translocated to an autosome, that autosome will become inactivated.

Polyploidy

Polyploidy is a change in chromosome number that involves multiples of a full haploid set. It is commonly found in plants, where it is an important mechanism for speciation. Many crop plants are polyploids derived from wild ancestors. Examples include coffee (4×, 6×, 8×), bananas (3×), bread wheat (6×), and common tobacco (4×). Agricultural geneticists can artificially induce polyploidy to combine genomes from different plant species. For some reason, polyploidy is tolerated much less well in animal development. In humans polyploidy is usually fatal at an early stage of development. Among the possible causes, polyploidy will result if more than one sperm enters the egg simultaneously or if there is a failure of separation of haploid nuclei during meiosis in the developing egg cell.

Changes in Chromosome Content: Deletions and Duplications

The terms "deletion" and "deficiency" are interchangeable and refer to the loss of a section of DNA that can range in size from simply affecting a region of one gene to encompassing tens or even hundreds of linked genes. If it is limited to a single gene, it may be difficult to tell a deletion from a nucleotide substitution or other point mutation. One way to identify them is by DNA sequencing or measuring the size of fragments amplified by the **polymerase chain reaction**, PCR (see Chapter 2). A small deletion will yield an amplified DNA fragment that is smaller than one from a simple base substitution mutation in which all nucleotides are present.

Figures 5-18 and 5-19 show some of the ways a change can be made in chromosome content. Typically, homozygosity

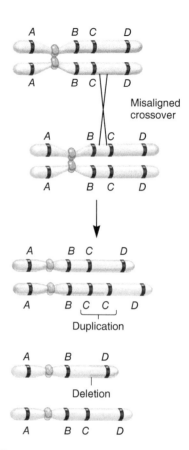

Figure 5-19. Crossing over between two improperly aligned homologues can generate deletions and duplications by recombination. (Reprinted with permission from Brooker RJ: *Genetics: Analysis & Principles*, 3rd ed. New York: McGraw-Hill, 2008.)

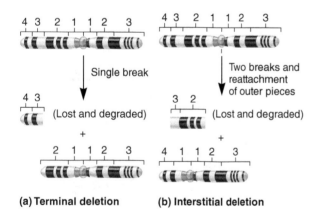

(a) Terminal deletion   **(b) Interstitial deletion**

Figure 5-18. Loss of genetic material can occur from (a) terminal deletions in which the broken end of a chromosome is lost, or (b) interstitial deletions involving two breaks and the loss of the intervening section of the chromosome. (Reprinted with permission from Brooker RJ: *Genetics: Analysis & Principles*, 3rd ed. New York: McGraw-Hill, 2008.)

for a deletion is lethal (it is equivalent to being homozygous for a large number of damaging point mutations), and heterozygosity can have severe effects on development. A deletion can also affect the phenotype if it happens to be heterozygous with a recessive mutant allele on the "normal" homologue. Since the dominant is missing in the deleted chromosome, the sole recessive allele is expressed phenotypically. This phenomenon is sometimes called **pseudodominance**. In experimental organisms like *Drosophila*, deletion mapping is a powerful tool for analyzing linkage relationships and for manipulating developmental processes.

Duplications are regions of a chromosome that occur twice, so that the diploid has a total of three copies of each gene in the duplication. The duplicated copies can be directly adjacent, called **tandem duplications**, or can be located at a distance from each other as **dispersed duplications**. On balance, a duplication generally has a smaller effect on development than does a deletion of the same size. But in both cases, deletions and duplications essentially alter the **gene dosage**, which changes the amount of protein produced when the genes are active. This can cause an imbalance in biochemical processes throughout the body.

Changes in Chromosome Organization: Inversions

As is true for all aberrations, there are several mechanisms that will cause a change in the order of genes on a chromosome. One way is for two simultaneous breaks to occur on portions of a chromosome that happen to be coiled next to each other in the interphase nucleus. A change in order will occur if the broken ends are misattached (Figure 5-20). If the two breaks are in different arms so that the centromere is included within the inverted region, it is called a **pericentric inversion** (*peri* = around, as in *perimeter*). If both endpoints of the inversion are in the same arm, it is a **paracentric inversion** (*para* = beside, as in *paramedic*). A pericentric inversion will change chromosome appearance if the breaks are not symmetrical around the centromere. Other than possible point mutations at the breakpoints, the genetic content of the chromosome is not altered in either type. But that does not mean that inversions are without consequences for the carrier. The consequences are expressed in a different way, specifically as a reduction in genetically normal gametes. This is due to the physical looping of one chromosome to allow its genes to pair with their homologous copies on the other chromosome in an inversion heterozygote during synapsis. This will result in chromosome anomalies if crossing over occurs within the synapsed inverted region in prophase I of meiosis (Figure 5-21).

As we saw earlier, at synapsis in prophase I, the synaptonemal complex forms between the identical regions of the non-sister chromatids all along the length of the paired chromosomes. The only way for that to happen in an inversion heterozygote is for one of the strands to form a loop as shown in Figure 5-21. Recombination occurs during synapsis. So, if a recombination event occurs within the inversion loop, the strands become attached so that deleted and duplicated chromosomes are produced. You can demonstrate this yourself by tracing one of the chromosome strands beginning at the top arrow of Figure 5-21a; at the recombination point, the path

crosses to the other chromosome and ends at the second arrow. The result is a chromosome that is duplicated for the normal sequence to the left of the first breakpoint and deleted for the region to the right of the second breakpoint. If the inversion is paracentric (Figure 5-21b), the centromere will be duplicated in one of the crossover products yielding a **dicentric chromosome** that forms a bridge between the separating nuclei when the centromeres move to opposite poles in anaphase I. The other crossover product has no centromere and is considered an **acentric fragment**, which is left behind when the nucleus divides. Neither type of gamete will yield a viable zygote, so fertility is reduced in inversion heterozygotes.

Translocations

Translocations are the main type of chromosome aberration affecting two different chromosomes at the same time. If the exchange is reciprocal, so that a fragment from the first chromosome becomes attached to the centromere-bearing second chromosome, and vice versa, the genetic content of the cell is not affected except for possible point mutations at the breakpoints as in an inversion. But, as in inversion heterozygotes, reciprocal translocation heterozygotes can suffer severe reductions in fertility due to segregation in meiosis. The mechanism behind this is illustrated in Figure 5-22 and is not as complicated as it may initially appear. It essentially comes down to how the centromeres happen to attach to the meiotic spindle.

In our earlier discussion of meiosis, we pointed out that independent assortment is the result of the randomness with which different pairs of synapsed chromosomes attach to the spindle. If one bivalent is heterozygous *Aa* and a second bivalent is heterozygous *Bb*, the two sets of centromeres could attach so that the two dominant alleles are toward the same pole. In that case one gamete gets both dominant alleles, *AB*, and the other gets both recessive alleles. Or they could attach with the dominant-carrying strands facing opposite poles, so each gamete gets one dominant allele and one recessive, that is, they will be either *Ab* or *aB*. Think of segregation of centromeres in a reciprocal translocation heterozygote the same way.

To interpret Figure 5.22, you must imagine that the centromeres are attached to the spindle and that the poles are at the top and bottom of the figure. The left-hand portion of the figure is equivalent to one bivalent, and the right-hand side is a second bivalent. They interact because parts of their structures are synapsed to different homologues, but the key is how the centromeres attach to the spindle and segregate. Let us consider the case of **adjacent segregation** first (central panel of Figure 5-22). That is what will result if the centromeres are laid out as in the top part of the figure. The upper centromere of each bivalent will move to the top pole and the lower centromere of each bivalent will move the opposite direction. At the end of that first meiosis, each haploid nucleus has one normal and one translocated chromosome, thus being duplicated for some regions and deficient for others. These will not

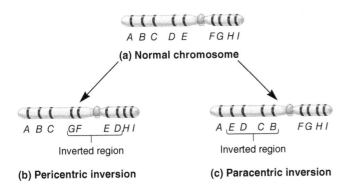

(a) Normal chromosome

A B C D E   F G H I

(b) Pericentric inversion

A B C   G F   E D H I

Inverted region

(c) Paracentric inversion

A   E D C B   F G H I

Inverted region

Figure 5-20. Inversions occur when the ends of chromosome segments are reattached incorrectly. The products can be classified as (a) pericentric or (b) paracentric, depending on whether the centromere is included or not included in the inversion. (Reprinted with permission from Brooker RJ: *Genetics: Analysis & Principles*, 3rd ed. New York: McGraw-Hill, 2008.)

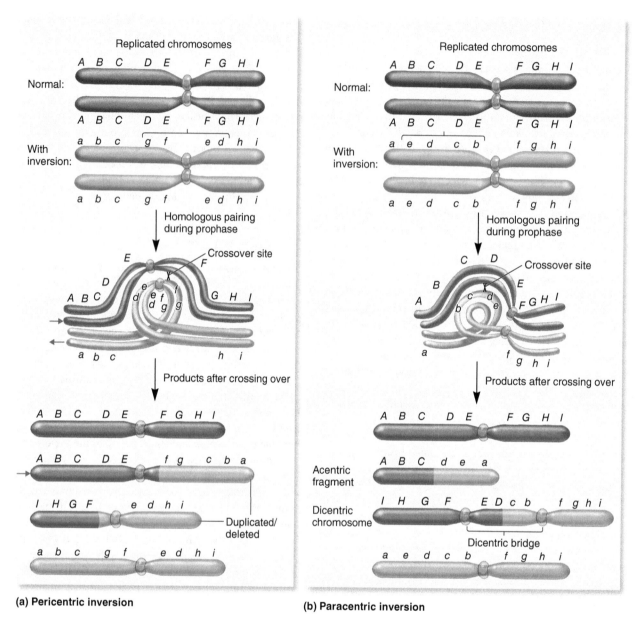

Figure 5-21. Crossing over in an inversion heterozygote yields deletions and duplications in half the haploid products of meiosis. In a paracentric inversion heterozygote, the centromere will be included in the segment that is either duplicated or deleted. This will result in dicentric bridges or acentric fragments, respectively. (Reprinted with permission from Brooker RJ: *Genetics: Analysis & Principles*, 3rd ed. New York: McGraw-Hill, 2008.)

yield viable zygotes. But now imagine that the centromeres of one of the bivalents are flipped, so that the upper left centromere segregates along with the lower right centromere, and the lower left goes with the upper right. This is **alternate segregation** and results in one haploid having the two normal chromosomes and the other haploid getting both of the translocated chromosomes. The genetic content is balanced and the zygotes they create will each have a complete diploid genome.

An important example of this type of aberration is the **Robertsonian translocation,** in which two nonhomologous **acrocentric** or **telocentric** chromosomes become fused at their centromeres to produce one linkage group. This results

in a reduced chromosome number that may or may not have a phenotypic effect, depending on whether any coding DNA is lost in the fusion.

Somatic Mosaics

The changes in chromosome makeup described so far in meiosis affect every cell in the offspring's body. But changes in chromosome number and structure can also occur during mitosis. The effect of such somatic changes will be limited to the lineage of cells that derive from the original error. They lead to an individual that is a cellular mosaic of different genotypes.

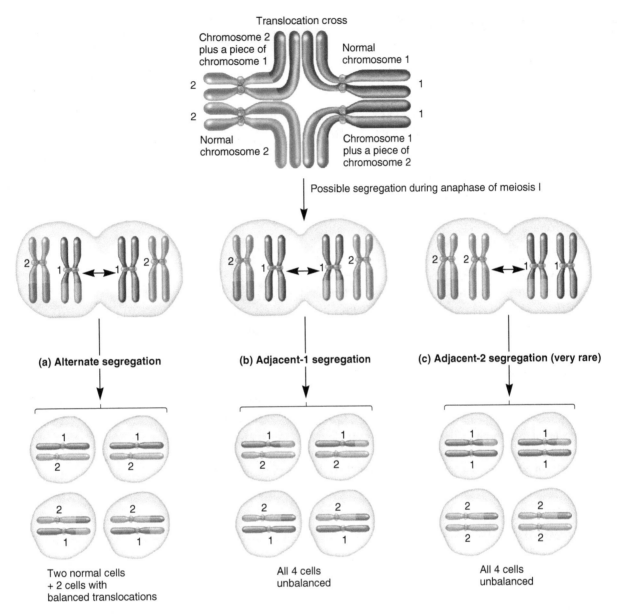

Figure 5-22. Translocation products depend on how the homologous centromeres attach to the spindle during meiosis. (Reprinted with permission from Brooker RJ: *Genetics: Analysis & Principles*, 3rd ed. New York: McGraw-Hill, 2008.)

Indeed, at some level, we are all probably mosaics of slight genetic differences that have occurred during our development. Most will involve point mutations of genes that may not even be transcribed in the specialized cell type in which they are found. A few will involve changes in chromosome number or structure that can cause serious medical conditions like certain cancers.

Another related phenomenon should be mentioned here. It is autonomous gene expression.

"Autonomous" means self-contained. In the context of gene expression it refers to a gene that affects only the biochemical activities of the cell in which it acts. Its gene product is not diffusible, so mutant cells in such a mosaic patch cannot be helped by normal tissue surrounding them. The phenotype for a visible trait would, therefore, be a mosaic spot or patch.

The Unique Nature of the Y Chromosome

Comparatively few genes are located on the human Y chromosome. Those that are unique to the Y, so-called **holandric** genes, include the *Sry* (sex-determining region Y) gene that is necessary for normal male-specific development. It specifies testis determination and promotes the synthesis of testosterone. In addition, a few genes are found in small areas of homology between the X and Y chromosomes called **pseudoautosomal regions**. These promote pairing of the X and Y to assist in proper segregation during meiosis. Like genes on the human X chromosome, those in the pseudoautosomal region of the Y can show recombination. But they do not undergo Lyonization, or X chromosome inactivation, so this small region of X and Y homology behaves like an autosomal region.

Introduction

Mitosis and meiosis are intricate and coordinated. Like most biological systems, however, things may not happen perfectly. The discipline of cytogenetics is the study of what happens when the processes of mitosis or meiosis do not go according to design or plan.

Cytogenetic abnormalities are important conditions to know about, because of their historic standing as well as the relative frequency of these conditions in general. The determination of the human chromosome count at a modal number of 46 was only correctly assigned in 1956. Shortly thereafter in 1959, trisomy 21 (an extra, i.e., third, copy of chromosome 21) was associated with Down syndrome as the first identified genetic marker of a medical condition. Thus, cytogenetic anomalies became the first genetic abnormalities that were understood at an etiologic level. Advances in cytogenetic technology have occurred at a rapid pace (Refer to Tables 1-3 and 1-4 for an overview). For the medical student, cytogenetic abnormalities are also important as frequently asked questions on board examinations. A student should be aware of the (historically) major chromosomal syndromes. This chapter will provide brief descriptions and highlights of these conditions; however, these descriptions are not meant to be comprehensive. Specifically, this is not a dysmorphology textbook. For more details on any given condition, you are referred to the most recent edition of any of several good references at the end of this chapter.

Chromosome Abnormalities

Chromosomal abnormalities are relatively common (Table 5-1). Prior to conception 5% of sperm and 50% of oocytes have abnormal chromosome complements. Not surprisingly, then, 50% of conceptions are expected to have an abnormal chromosome makeup. At the time of live term births, however, only 0.8% of infants will have a chromosome abnormality. As these numbers clearly suggest, chromosome abnormalities have a strong association with early pregnancy loss (Tables 5-1 and 5-2). In fact, 95% of all chromosomal abnormalities present at conception are not live-born.

By way of definition, pregnancy loss at less than 6 weeks post conception would be classified as an "early loss." Losses between 6 and 22 weeks are termed "miscarriage" or "spontaneous abortion." Losses later than or equal to 23 weeks are best classified as "stillborn" infants. Other terms would include intrauterine fetal death and/or products of conception in reference to the tissue that is lost with a spontaneous miscarriage.

Cytogenetic analysis of first trimester products of conception show 65% will have an abnormal chromosome count. In contrast, only 1.5% are abnormal by mid gestation (approximately 20 weeks), and, as mentioned above, only 0.8% of live-born children will have a chromosome imbalance.

Recurrent pregnancy losses may sometimes be perceived as infertility, because the conceptions are actually not recognized and the pregnancy is lost early. A chromosome analysis of the couple is part of the workup for infertility. Likewise, in the case of recognized miscarriages, any couple who has experienced three or more spontaneous miscarriages should be offered chromosomal analysis. In this setting, 10% of the time, one of the partners carries a balanced chromosome rearrangement.

The occurrence of chromosome imbalances has a strong association with advanced maternal age (Table 5-3). As mothers

Table 5-1.	Estimated Frequencies of Chromosome Abnormalities (Perinatal)
Preconception Spermatozoa Oocyte	4%-7% 50%
Couples with ≥ 3 miscarriages	10%-15%
At conception	50%
At first trimester miscarriage	65%
At mid-gestation	1-3%
Stillborn infants/perinatal death	5%-6%
At birth	0.8%

Table 5-2.	Estimated Frequencies of Chromosomal Anomalies	
Condition	First Trimester Miscarriage	Live Births
45, X	10%	1/5000 (0.02%)
Other sex chromosome XXX Klinefelter XYY	1%	1% 1/700 females (0.14%) 1/500 (0.2%) 1/800 males (0.14%)
Trisomy 16	15%	0
Other trisomies Down syndrome Trisomy 13 Trisomy 18	32%	(0.5%) 1/600 (0.17%) 1/5000 (0.02%) 1/3500 (0.03%)
Triploidy/tetraploid	11%	1/10,000 (0.01%)
Structural rearrangements	12%	Unknown (maybe 0.5%)

Table 5-3.	Frequency of Down Syndrome in Association With Maternal Age	
Maternal Age	Frequency of Down Syndrome (live births)
<25	1/1600
25-29	1/1100
30-34	1/700
35-39	1/250
40-42	1/80
>42	1/40

the longer period of time that these cells stay in this suspended state predisposes to a greater chance of nondisjunction when the process is finally allowed to proceed. The rise in nondisjunction is first noticed with maternal ages in the mid thirties, and rises asymptotically after 40.

Although the association of an advanced maternal age with the occurrence of Down syndrome is well known, it should be pointed out that this association holds true for all types of nondisjunction. It is also important to point out that this increase occurs on a *per pregnancy* basis. Thus, nondisjunction occurs more often in older mothers per pregnancy. As there are many more pregnancies in younger mothers, there are actually more children born with Down syndrome and other chromosome abnormalities to younger mothers.

age, there is an increase in abnormalities due to chromosomal nondisjunction. These meiotic errors are presumably related to the normal status of human oocytes. Human female fetuses typically have several million oocytes around mid-gestation. By term birth, this number has been culled down to a few hundred thousand functional cells, although only about 400 will actually be released at ovulations through the reproductive life of the female. These oocytes have started meiosis, but are arrested mid-process at the specialized stage called dictyotene in prophase I. Meiosis I is not completed until ovulation, and meiosis II is not accomplished until fertilization. Presumably,

Laboratory Diagnosis of Chromosome Abnormalities

As described earlier, a **karyotype** is a conventional representation of chromosome structure and number (Figure 5-23). The method used in most clinical diagnostic settings is G banded chromosomes. The current standard is what is referred to as high resolution or prometaphase chromosomes. This typically would represent 700 to 800 recognizable bands on the karyotype.

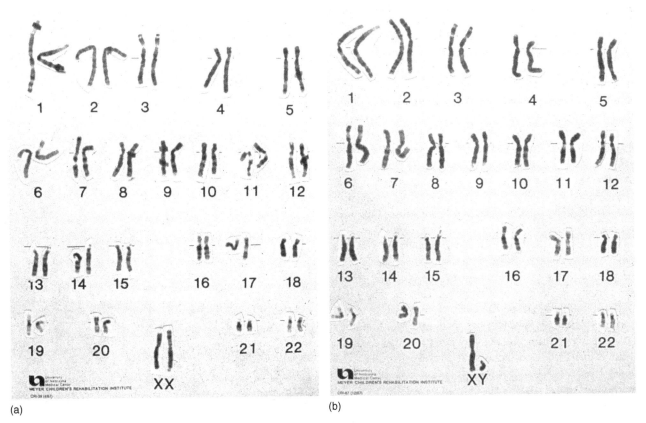

(a) (b)

Figure 5-23. Normal karyotypes. G banded. High resolution (prometaphase). (a) Female (b) Male. (Courtesy of Dr. Warren G. Sanger, University of Nebraska Medical Center.)

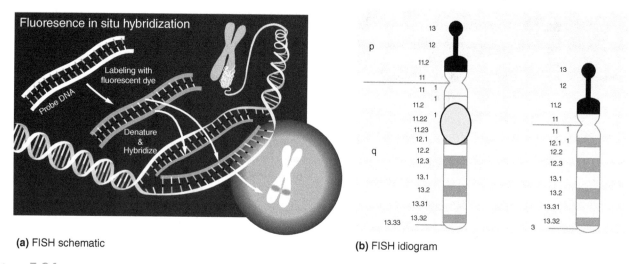

(a) FISH schematic

(b) FISH idiogram

Figure 5-24. Flourescent *in situ* hybridization (FISH). (a) Schematic of process. (b) Idiogram showing a deletion on chromosome 22.

Recent advances in cytogenetics have sprung from the advancement of a technology known as **fluorescent** *in situ* **hybridization** (FISH). Basically FISH utilizes a synthesized probe that is composed of the complementary sequence to a known segment of DNA. The probe is attached to a fluorescent marker. The probe strand is then applied to the patient's DNA. If the complementary strand is present, the two will hybridize. The presence of the hybridization can then be detected by the presence of fluorescence as seen under the microscope (Figure 5-24).

Fluorescent *in situ* hybridization technology has truly revolutionized the practice of clinical genetics. The first readily available clinical uses of this technique were single locus FISH. These studies led to the description and definition of the etiology of specific recognizable conditions due to duplications or deletions too small to be detected by even high resolution chromosome studies (Figure 5-25). Collectively, these disorders may be called **contiguous gene syndromes**. These conditions are characterized by recognizable patterns of multiple malformations and anomalies due to the duplication or deletion of several genes that are situated together at a particular chromosomal locus. These are discussed in more detail later.

Fluorescent *in situ* hybridization technology has a myriad of other applications in the clinical setting. An assembly of FISH probes that provide coverage of entire chromosomes may be used for chromosome painting. This may be quite helpful in sorting out complex rearrangements, identifying the origin of marker chromosomes, and so forth. A significant advantage of FISH technology over standard karyotype analysis is that FISH does not require actively dividing cells. In order to create a traditional karyotype, living cells must be allowed to divide. Then cell division must be stopped by biochemical methods to halt further progression. In order to visualize a "chromosome," the cell cycle must be stopped somewhere between metaphase and prophase. But FISH studies can be performed on any target nucleic acid segment regardless of what point of the cell cycle it is in. It can be used for any segment of nucleic acid, even for those outside a cell. This offers a great advantage in the clinical realm allowing for its application in many different settings and providing more rapid diagnostics (Figure 5-26).

The areas underneath the telomeres of the chromosomes are regions prone to rearrangements and mismatches. Further expansion of the applications of FISH studies led to the expansion from single locus FISH to what was known as **sub-telomeric FISH** panels (Figure 5-27). This panel, developed around 1998 to 1999, included approximately 40 probes that corresponded to the sub-telomeric regions of the chromosomes (note, there are not 46 probes since the acrocentric chromosomes do not have telomeres for a short arm).

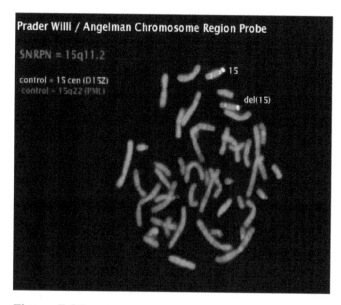

Figure 5-25. FISH study demonstrating a 15q deletion in the Prader-Willi/Angelman syndrome region. (Courtesy of Dr. Warren G. Sanger, University of Nebraska Medical Center.)

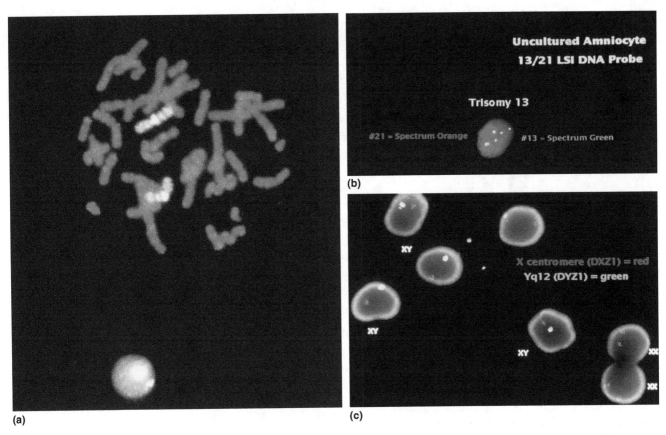

Figure 5-26. Different applications of FISH technology. (a) Whole chromosome painting. (b) Interphase (amniocentesis) FISH showing Trisomy 13. (c) Interphase (amniocentesis) FISH showing XX/XY mosaicism. (Courtesy of Dr. Warren G. Sanger, University of Nebraska Medical Center.)

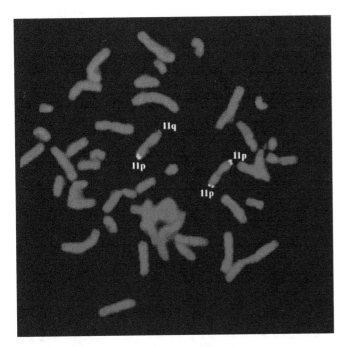

Figure 5-27. Sub-telomeric FISH study with chromosome 3 example. (Reprinted with permission from Clarkson B, Pavenski K, Dupuis L, et al. Detecting Rearrangements in Children Using Subtelomeric FISH and SKY. *American Journal of Medical Genetics* 107:267-274, 2002.)

The advent of a sub-telomeric FISH is now only of historic interest as it has already been supplanted by further refined techniques. But at the time it was introduced, it represented an important advancement in cytogenetic diagnostics. Published studies around 1999 to 2000 or so, showed the diagnostic yield of sub-telomeric FISH (chances of finding a positive result) in mental retardation was 7.4% for moderate levels of mental retardation and 0.5% for mild mental retardation, with an average around 3%. This made sub-telomeric rearrangements the most common identifiable cause of moderate mental retardation in humans (i.e., a calculated incidence in the general population of 0.22% as compared to the incidence of Trisomy 21 at 1 in 800 [0.13%]).

Further expansion of FISH technology beyond the sub-telomeric FISH panel included the development of a technology called **array comparative genomic hybridization (aCGH)**. Array comparative genomic hybridization refers to the process of comparing sample DNA to known reference DNA and looking for changes in copy numbers (either duplications or deletions). Application of aCGH technology on small microscopic slides with multiple imbedded wells is referred to as a microarray (Figure 5-28). Hence array comparative genomic hybridization (aCGH) refers to the use of aCGH on a microarray platform. This technology is an ever-evolving one. The original aCGH platforms had approximately 400 probes

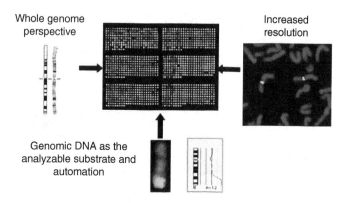

Figure 5-28. Microarray-based comparative genomic hybridization. (Reproduced with permission of Warren G. Sanger, PhD, University of Nebraska Medical Center, Omaha, Nebraska.)

Table 5-4.	Conventional Chromosomal Syndromes		
Condition	Eponym		Description of Chromosomal Change
Polyploidy			
	Triploid		69, XXX or XXY or XYY
Trisomy			
	Trisomy 13	Patau syndrome	47, +13
	Trisomy 18	Edwards syndrome	47, +18
	Trisomy 21	Down syndrome	47, +21
Sex Chromosome			
	Monosomy X	Turner syndrome	45, X
	XXY	Klinefelter syndrome	47, XXY
	XXX		47, XXX
	XYY		47, XYY
Deletion			
	4p deletion	Wolf-Hirschhorn syndrome	4p-
	5p deletion	Cri-du-chat syndrome	5p-

but were rapidly replaced by platforms that included 2000, then 40,000, then 105,000. Now a few laboratories offer aCGH panels of 180,000 probes. These platforms offer coverage of less than 1 megabase (Mb) intervals across the entire genome, although the intervals are not actually distributed evenly. To put this in perspective, the size of the single *dystrophin* gene is approximately 1.8 Mb. Still, it would not surprise anyone if, as you read this, these numbers are already outdated. In fact on the horizon aCGH technology may even be replaced by emerging technology such as whole exonic sequencing.

With these advances in technology, the boundaries between molecular genetics and cytogenetics have blurred. Currently this hybrid discipline is referred to by many as **molecular cytogenetics.** Array CGH and related modern whole genome screening techniques are discussed in additional detail in Chapter 11.

Chromosome Aneuploidy

Aneuploid literally means "not the correct multiple or number." **Aneuploidy** then is the state of being aneuploid. Thus, chromosomal aneuploidy refers to the situation in which an individual possesses an abnormal chromosome number. Table 5-4 lists some of the more important or common human chromosomal aneuploidy syndromes. These conditions are important to recognize for several reasons. As mentioned earlier, historically these were the first described conditions with an identifiable genetic etiology. The general public is well aware of some of these conditions—and often has significant misconceptions. And, not least important, they appear frequently in questions on standardized examinations.

One variant of chromosome number is referred to as **polyploidy. Triploidy** means 69 chromosomes with a full three copies of every chromosome (Figure 5-29). It is a very common occurrence in conceptions. But, as with most chromosome imbalances, the vast majority of such conceptions result in a spontaneous miscarriage (Table 5-2). In fact, it is estimated that approximately 11% of all spontaneous miscarriages have a

triploid karyotype. Occasionally there is a live birth of an individual with a triploid chromosome count. This is much more likely if the individual is mosaic for this change (Figure 5-30). Overall it is estimated that approximately 1 in 10,000 live births may have this abnormality. The karyotype in triploid individuals can be 69, XXX, 69, XXY or 69, XYY. Triploidy most often results from a single egg being fertilized by two sperm (**dispermy**), resulting in an extra set of chromosomes

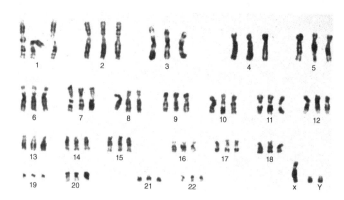

Figure 5-29. Karyotype with Triploid count (69 XYY). Likely due to dispermy. (Reproduced with permission of Warren G. Sanger, PhD, University of Nebraska Medical Center, Omaha, Nebraska.)

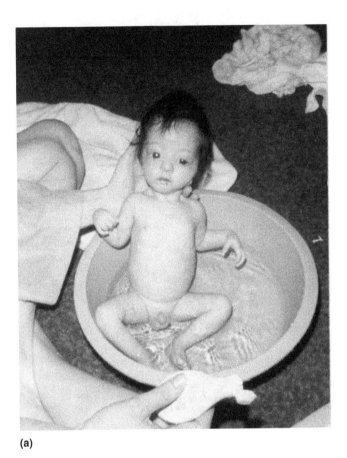 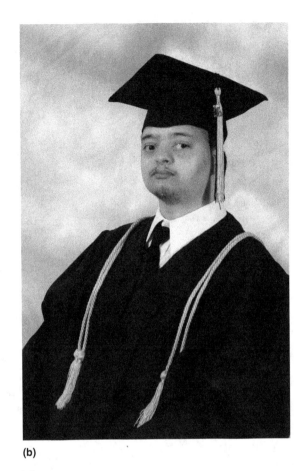

(a)   (b)

Figure 5-30. Patient with diploid/triploid mosaicism. (a) Infant. (b) Young adult.

from the father (**diandry**). It can also occur from **digyny**, in which the full extra set is from the mother.

Fetuses with dygyny tend to have a relatively small placenta with a better developed fetus. Conversely, fetuses with dyandry are less well developed, and there is a large abnormal placenta. These variations in clinical expression can be explained by differences in what is known as imprinting. For further information on imprinting, please refer to Chapter 12, which addresses Atypical Inheritance.

Tetraploidy (92 chromosomes) is common in spontaneous miscarriages but is typically not found in live born infants.

Sex chromosome aneuploidy

Because of the unique nature of the sex chromosomes, aneuploid situations are better tolerated. Specifically, sex chromosome aneuploidy is seen more commonly in live born infants than is autosome aneuploidy. At conception, the occurrence is likely similar, but autosome aneuploidy is more likely to be lost as a spontaneous miscarriage.

1. *Turner syndrome.* A missing X chromosome (45, X) is the only whole chromosome **monosomy** that is compatible with postnatal life in humans. The phenotype was described by Henry Turner in 1938 with the condition

now having the eponym of Turner syndrome. The initial description was that of girls with short stature, pubertal failure, cubitus valgus and webbed neck (Figure 5-31). Other features may include a broad chest with wide spaced nipples and angulated nails. A variety of structural anomalies may occur. The two most important ones to note are coarctation of the aorta and a "horseshoe" kidney. Many of the clinical features in Turner syndrome can be assigned as being secondary to congenital lymphedema (Figure 5-32). The discovery of a missing X chromosome as the cause of Turner syndrome was made by Charles Ford in 1959.

Depending on the presentation of a particular girl, the diagnosis of Turner syndrome may be made at various points in her life. On occasion, infants with Turner syndrome can be recognized due to the presence of suspicious somatic features. The congenital lymphedema may persist after birth and show up as edema of the dorsum of the hands and feet (Figure 5-33). Differential pulses may indicate a coarctation of the aorta, which, if present in a newborn female, may warrant further investigation into possible Turner syndrome. But many girls with Turner syndrome will not have any identifiable features at birth. The most consistent clinical features seen in individuals

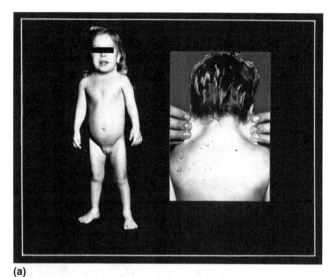

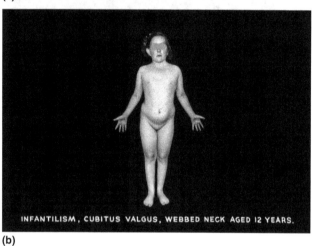

Figure 5-31. Turner syndrome. These photographs were taken from the original pictures used by Dr. Henry Turner in his 1938 publication. Black and white photographs were cut and pasted on black cardboard. Hand lettering was with a white ink pen. (Courtesy G.B. Schaefer; originals donated to the archives of the Endocrine Society of America.)

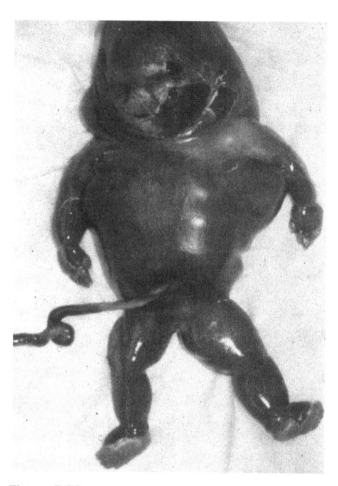

Figure 5-32. Spontaneous miscarriage of fetus with Turner syndrome. Note striking lymphedema, which can explain most of the somatic features associated with Turner syndrome.

with a 45, X karyotype are short stature and primary ovarian failure. Both of these would obviously present later in life.

This offers a situation in which early proactive awareness by a physician can have significant benefits for the patient. It is important to recognize Turner syndrome early, because of the advantages of using growth hormone to increase final adult height. Therefore, even in the absence of any physical features, girls with an otherwise unexplained short stature should have a karyotype performed (Figure 5-34).

In general, and contrary to what is reported in the older literature, Turner syndrome is associated with normal intelligence. These women have distinct neuropsychological changes, including consistent problems

with visual–spatial integration and often difficulties in mathematics.

The Turner syndrome phenotype may be associated with several chromosomal imbalances. Approximately half of the girls with Turner syndrome have a straight 45, X karyotype (Figure 5-35). Another 25% have some form of sex chromosome mosaicism, with the remainder having a variety of other chromosomal rearrangements including isochromosome Xq, deletion Xq, or deletion Xp. Turner syndrome is estimated to occur in 1 in 2500 live births.

2. *Klinefelter syndrome.* Klinefelter syndrome (Figure 5-36) is a disorder found in males associated with a 47, XXY karyotype (Figure 5-37a). The major clinical features of Klinefelter syndrome are attributable to hypogonadism (primary testicular failure). Because of the primary testicular failure, these individuals often present with gynecomastia, infertility, and a "eunichoid habitus." Hypo-mentation (decreased IQ) is relatively common in this condition; however, many individuals

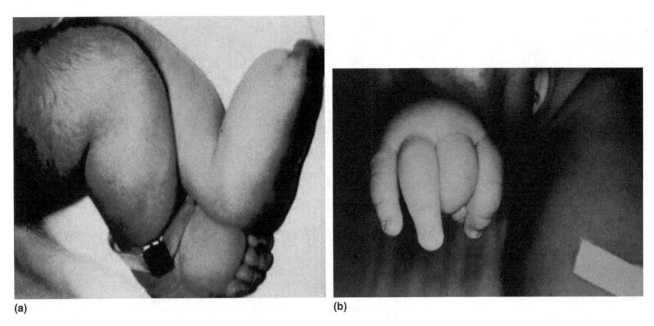

(a)   (b)

Figure 5-33. Dorsal edema of the (a) feet and (b) hands in two infants with Turner syndrome.

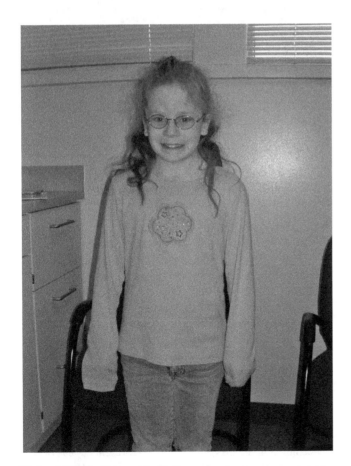

Figure 5-34. Young girl with Turner syndrome; no appreciable dysmorphic features of Turner syndrome.

with this condition have normal intellect. The overall mean IQ with Klinefelter syndrome is around 90. This condition occurs in approximately 1 in 600 newborn males.

It is important to note that 40%-50% of males with Klinefelter syndrome have no discernable physical features. They only present as male infertility due to azoospermia (no production of sperm). For that reason, a semen analysis with a follow up karyotype is indicated as part of the infertility workup.

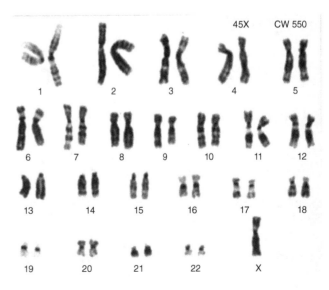

Figure 5-35. Karyotype 45, X. (Reproduced with permission of Warren G. Sanger, PhD, University of Nebraska Medical Center, Omaha, Nebraska.)

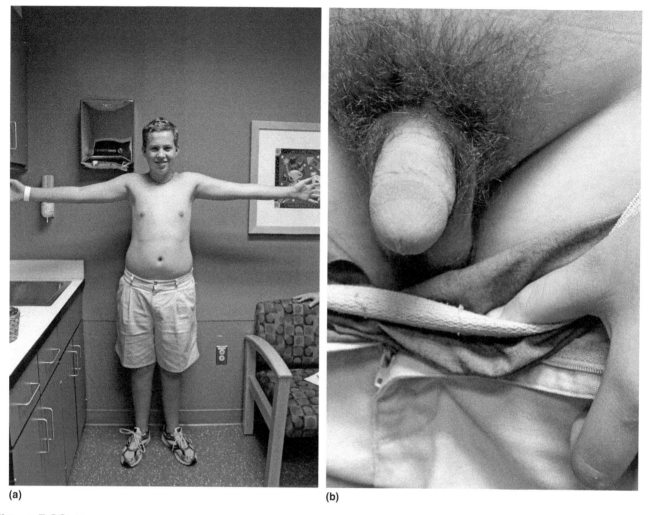

(a)   (b)

Figure 5-36. Young man with Klinefelter syndrome. (a) Tall stature with "eunichoid habitus"; (b) Small testes.

Variants of Klinefelter syndrome include 48, XXXY (Figure 5-37b) and 49, XXXXY. In general, these individuals have a Klinefelter-like phenotype. The primary differences are that with an increasing number of X's, there is an increase in growth restriction and decrease in IQ. Many individuals with these variants may have some mild craniofacial and skeletal changes not otherwise seen in 47, XXY Klinefelter syndrome.

3. *XXX Syndrome.* Women with a 47, XXX karyotype (Figure 5-38) are typically reported as having "no pattern of malformations." Pubarche and fertility are felt to be typically normal. As compared to the general population, females with 47, XXX tend to be a little taller and have a slightly decreased average head circumference. As a group they tend to have a slightly higher incidence of learning disabilities, developmental disabilities, discoordination, and an increase in behavioral problems (Figure 5-39).

Variants of the 47, XXX syndrome include 48, XXXX and 49, XXXXX. Again, as the number X's increases, the overall IQ decreases. Some individuals who have

XXXX and XXXXX have been reported to have facies not unlike that seen in Down syndrome.

4. *XYY.* Individuals with a 47, XYY karyotype (Figure 5-39) have been reported to have subtle features of slightly taller than expected stature, discoordination, speech delays, behavior differences, and learning disabilities. These men have normal fertility. Occasionally reported features include large teeth, prominent glabella, long arms and legs, and difficult to control acne. The overall incidence is felt to be 1 in 700 to 1 in 1000 males. Early reports in the 1970s showed an increased incidence of XYY karyotype in men that were incarcerated. Socio-biological interpretation raised the question of an XYY karyotype being associated with a "criminal phenotype." It has been shown that this condition is not associated with a criminal phenotype, but in fact the increased incidence noted in the prison population represents a bias of ascertainment—presumably not due to increased chances of committing crime, but, of being caught. They are tall, clumsy, and mentally slow.

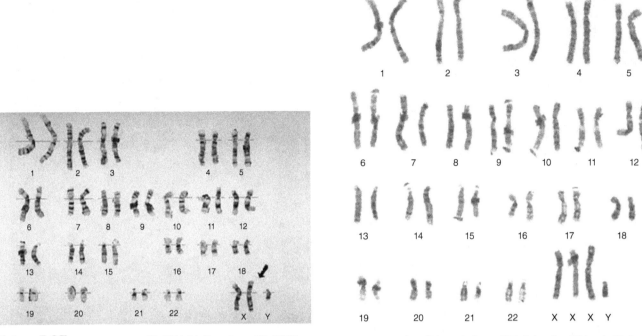

Figure 5-37. (a) Karyotype 47, XXY. (b) Karyotype 48, XXXY. (Reproduced with permission of Warren G. Sanger, PhD, University of Nebraska Medical Center, Omaha, Nebraska.)

Trisomies

Trisomy refers to the presence of a single extra full chromosome. Trisomies of all autosomes occur with a relatively high frequency in conceptions, but most are lost as miscarriages. Only three whole chromosome (non-mosaic) aneuploidies are compatible with postnatal life in humans. These are Trisomy 13, 18, and 21.

1. *Trisomy 21 (Down syndrome).* Down syndrome was described by Langdon Down in 1866. Individuals with Down syndrome have a readily recognizable facial appearance described as flattening of the facial profile,

small nose, epicanthal folds, and Brushfield spots (focal areas of dysplasia on the iris). They may have notably short fifth fingers, a wide gap between the first and second toes, and single transverse palmar creases (Figure 5-40). In 1959, the karyotypic association of Trisomy 21 in association with the phenotype of Down syndrome was described (Figure 5-41). Down syndrome is estimated to occur at 1 in 800 live births.

The vast majority (95%) of individuals with Down syndrome have whole chromosome aneuploidy (trisomy 21) as the etiology. Another 4% have a variety of translocations, most importantly a 14:21 Robertsonian

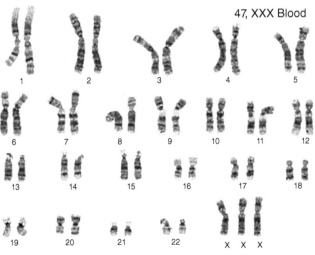

Figure 5-38. Karyotype 47, XXX. (Reproduced with permission of Warren G. Sanger, PhD, University of Nebraska Medical Center, Omaha, Nebraska.)

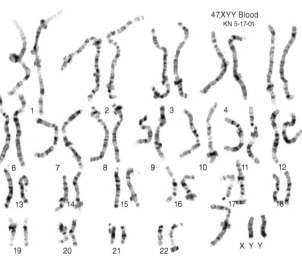

Figure 5-39. Karyotype 47, XYY. (Reproduced with permission of Warren G. Sanger, PhD, University of Nebraska Medical Center, Omaha, Nebraska.)

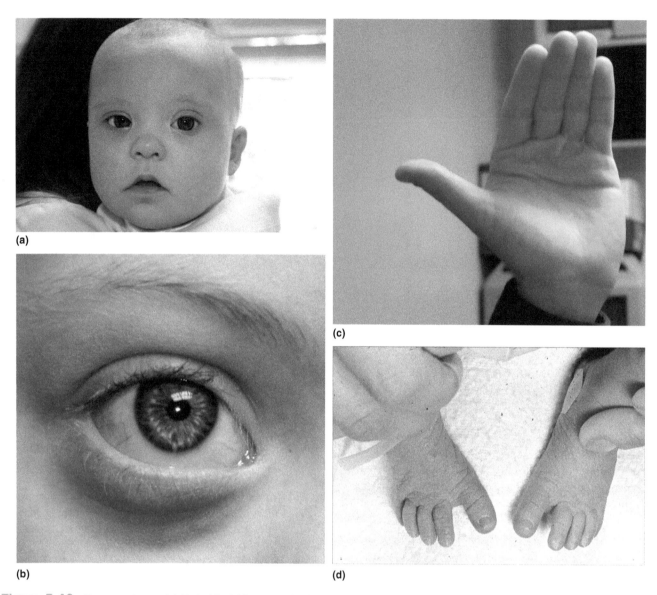

Figure 5-40. Down syndrome. (a) Typical facial features. (b) Eye showing Brushfield spots (small light colored spots within the iris due to focal dysplasia of the connective tissue). (c) Single transverse palmar (simian) crease. (d) Wide gap between first and second toes.

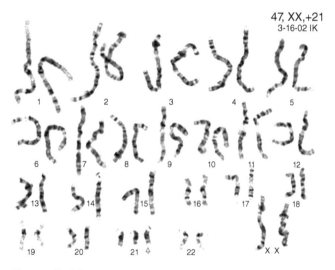

47, XX,+21
3-16-02 IK

Figure 5-41. Karyotype 47, XX, +21. (Reproduced with permission of Warren G. Sanger, PhD, University of Nebraska Medical Center, Omaha, Nebraska.)

translocation. Approximately 1% of individuals with Down syndrome have mosaicism.

Individuals with Down syndrome have a variety of health issues that are important to be aware of. These issues need to be addressed as a condition-specific series of recommended additions to the "typical" health care maintenance regimen as these patients are followed in their medical home.

- Individuals with Down syndrome have a variety of neurologic problems. These can include lower than average IQ, Alzheimer disease, low muscle tone (hypotonia), and vision and hearing problems.
- Congenital heart malformations occur in about 50% of the cases. The most common heart anomaly is an atrial-ventricular canal which, if large enough, may have no associated cardiac murmur. Thus, an echocardiogram is recommended for all people with

Down syndrome at the time of diagnosis, regardless of the presence or absence of a murmur.

- Other structural changes in Down syndrome include atlanto-occipital instability of the spine and a variety of different GI obstructions. Acquired hypothyroidism occurs much more often in these individuals.

- The overall incidence of leukemia is approximately 11-fold greater than in the general population.

2. *Trisomy 13 (Patau syndrome).* Trisomy 13 is associated with multiple congenital abnormalities and severe cognitive impairments. Structural changes include cleft lip and cleft palate, microphthalmia, polydactyly, microcephaly, and congenital heart disease (Figure 5-42). The etiology is either nondisjunction or an inherited translocation of chromosome 13 (Figure 5-43). The incidence is estimated at 1 in 5000 births.

3. *Trisomy 18 Edwards syndrome.* A similar phenotype is seen in Trisomy 18 (Edwards syndrome). Clinical features include severe growth deficiency, mental retardation, clinched fist with overlapping fingers, "rocker bottom" feet, and congenital heart disease (Figure 5-44). The etiology is also nondisjunction or inherited translocation, but of the 18th chromosome (Figure 5-45). The estimated incidence is 1 in 3000.

From a management standpoint, the most critical issue for Trisomy 13 and 18 is a decrease in the overall life expectancy. Table 5-5 summarizes the reported data on the longevity expectations of these two conditions. It is important to highlight that the last column shows that death by year one is estimated to be about 90% for both conditions. It is critical that the clinicians working with families who have newborns with these severe conditions be aware of the fact that 90% is not 100%. Long-term survival with Trisomy 13 and 18 have been reported on occasion in almost every genetic practice. It is, therefore, important to give the family the most accurate information. One should not downplay the ominous statistics, but yet be aware of the correct statistics.

Chromosome Mosaicism

Chromosomal changes due to mitotic errors that occur after conception can result in chromosomal mosaicism i.e., not every cell has the same chromosome makeup. (The concept of mosaicism is discussed in additional detail in Chapter 12 Atypical Inheritance). The number and distribution of the chromosomally abnormal cells in an individual will vary depending upon the timing and on which progenitor cells the abnormality begins with. It follows that the phenotype can be strikingly variable from being almost the same as "the full blown" condition to a non-expressed one. Figure 5-46 shows a young girl who was evaluated for mild developmental delays. Her cytogenetic testing revealed mosaicism for Down syndrome (7 out of 30 cells tested). As can be seen from the picture, her craniofacial features truly do not bear a resemblance to the phenotype

of Down syndrome. In fact, the only appreciably abnormal physical feature seen was a wide gap between her first and second toes. Undoubtedly, however, this mild mosaicism is the cause of her developmental delays.

Another important feature to highlight is the association between chromosomal mosaicism and skin pigmentary changes. This arises from the embryology of the neural crest cells. After separating from the neural tube, some of the neural crest cells migrate extensively and give rise to many different types of differentiated cells. These cell types include neurons and glial cells of the nervous systems, medulla cells of the adrenal gland, the melatonin producing cells of the epidermis, and skeletal and connective tissue components of the craniofacial complex. This known association may provide the critical clue in defining an etiology of a particular problem. Specifically, skin pigmentary changes that follow a pattern known as **Blaschko lines** may indicate an underlying chromosomal mosaicism. Hence, part of the diagnostic work-up of individuals with neurologic problems (seizures, mental retardation, and so forth) and skin pigmentary changes includes a skin biopsy to obtain cultured fibroblasts for karyotypic analyses on another tissue (Figure 5-47).

Changes in Chromosome Structure

Not all chromosome imbalances are changes in the number of entire chromosomes. Partial changes in chromosome structure include duplications, deletions, and translocations. The phenotype associated with partial structural chromosomal changes (duplications/deletions) depends on many factors, including the size of the change, which region of which chromosome is involved, and the particular genes present in the affected region. In general, duplications may not be as problematic as deletions. While these factors intuitively make sense, there is much variation that cannot be explained by these factors alone. Many other modifiers are also likely at work.

Translocations may be either balanced or unbalanced. Balanced translocations are defined as those rearrangements in which there is a change in the *position* but not the actual *amount* of genetic material. Conversely, unbalanced translocations occur when there are changes in both the amount and location. In theory, persons carrying balanced translocations should have no clinical effects from the rearrangement. The major implication of carrying a balanced translocation is the possibility of passing on an unbalanced rearrangement to the next generation. As explained in the first section, the possible outcomes in the offspring of a carrier of a balanced translocation would be:

1. normal chromosomes

2. unbalanced rearrangement, or

3. a balanced rearrangement like the parent.

The clinical sequelae of an unbalanced translocation are that of producing a deletion or duplication—with the same implications for these imbalances as noted earlier.

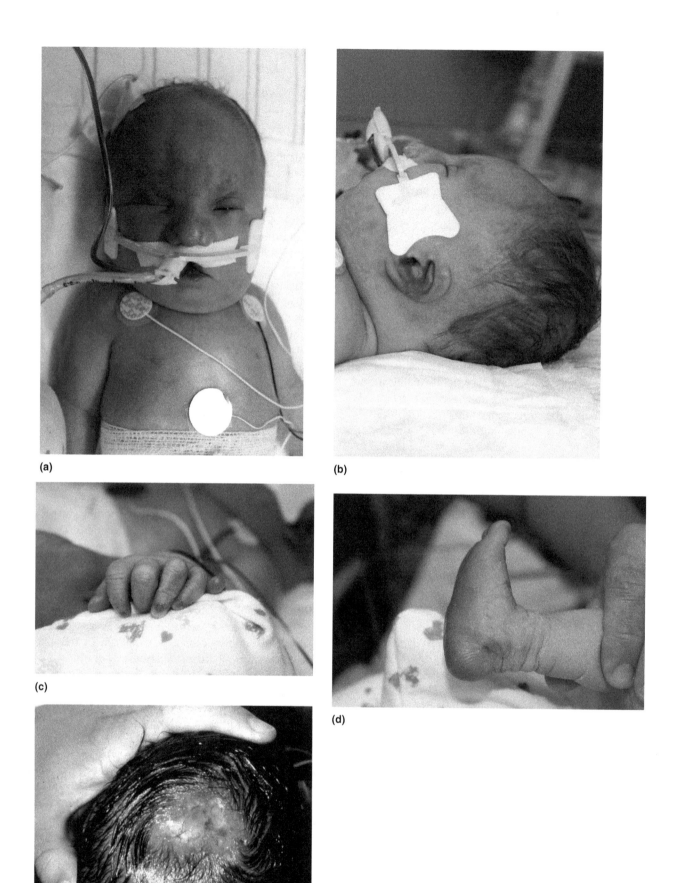

(a)

(b)

(c)

(d)

(e)

Figure 5-42. Two day old girl with Trisomy 13 (Patau syndrome). (a) Craniofacial features include microcephaly with sloping forehead, supraorbital creases, and broad triangular nose. (b) Low set pinnae with abnormal helices. (c) Postaxial polydactyly. (d) "Rocker bottom feet" (prominent calcanei). (e) Another child Trisomy 13 with cutis aplasia of the scalp.

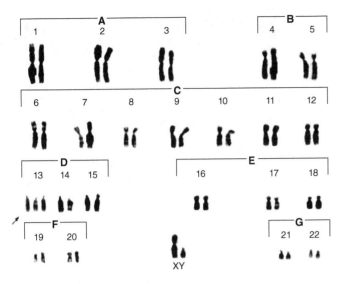

Figure 5-43. Karyotype 47, XY, +13. (Reproduced with permission of Warren G. Sanger, PhD, University of Nebraska Medical Center, Omaha, Nebraska.)

Figure 5-45. Karyotype 47, XY, +18. (Reproduced with permission of Warren G. Sanger, PhD, University of Nebraska Medical Center, Omaha, Nebraska.)

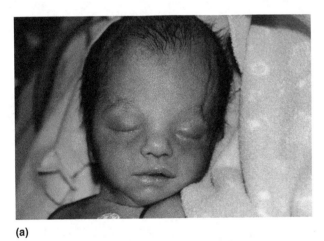

(a)

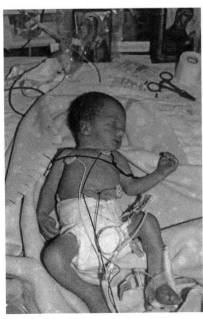

(b)

Figure 5-44. Patient with Trisomy 18 (Edward syndrome).

Table 5-5.	Published Longevity Statistics for Trisomy 13 and Trisomy 18	
	Trisomy 13	Trisomy 18
Mean life expectancy	130-180 days	60 days
Median life expectancy (40-48 days if no major cardiac/GI malformations)	7-10 days	4 days
Death by 1 month	45%	
Death by 6 months	70%	
Death by 1 year	82%-90%	90%

When individuals are identified with chromosome rearrangements (either balanced or unbalanced) as part of a diagnostic evaluation, it is absolutely indicated to do a karyotype on the parents. In the situations of chromosome structural changes, there is a possibility that one of the parents is a carrier of a balanced translocation. Up to 10% of the time, one of the parents of a child with an unbalanced translocation may themselves have a balanced translocation. Particularly important are certain rare abnormalities such as tandem duplication of chromosomes. Figure 5-48a shows a 13:13 translocation present in a newborn male with features of Trisomy 13. Even though this individual has 46 chromosomes, he is functionally trisomic for 13 and had the full array of clinical features. Karyotypic analysis of this individual's parents showed that the mother had 45 chromosomes with one of the chromosomes being the 13:13 hybrid chromosome. Thus, the only possible reproductive outcomes for this individual were either to have a child that was monosomic for 13 (and invariably would miscarry) or have a child with Trisomy 13 (Figure 5-48b).

An important observation has been noted by clinicians in this regards for decades. A child might have been seen for an evaluation because of multiple congenital anomalies,

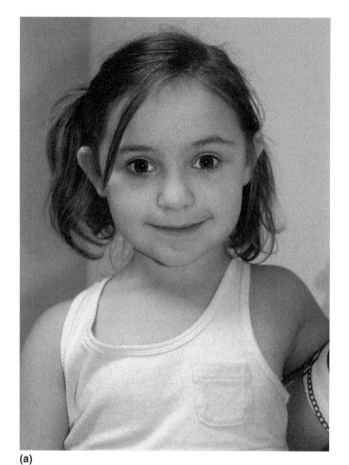

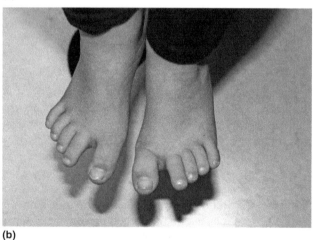

Figure 5-46. (a) Young girl with mosaicism for Trisomy 21 (7 of 30 cells in peripheral blood with trisomy). She presented with mild developmental delays. (b) The only physical feature of Down syndrome was a wide gap between the first and second toes.

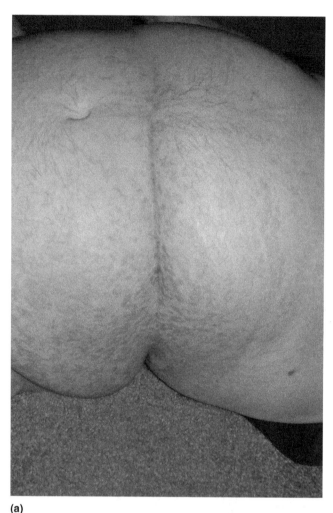

(a)

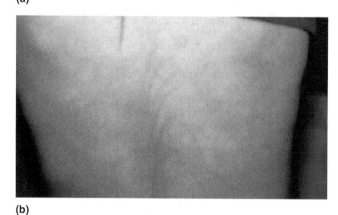

(b)

Figure 5-47. Hyperpigmented skin patches associated with chromosomal mosaicism. (a) large clonal patches of pigment. This patient has diploid/triploid mosaicism. (b) Hyperpigmented swirls on back. This patient has mosaicism for tetrasomy 12p. Both patients had normal blood chromosome studies.

dysmorphic features, and/or cognitive deficits. As part of that evaluation, cytogenetic studies were performed, and the child was noted to have a balanced translocation. In order to clarify this abnormality, the next step was to perform parental studies. Not infrequently, one of the parents (with no clinical

abnormalities) would be found to have the same balanced rearrangement. The logical interpretation would be that this was a coincidental finding unrelated to the child's problems, since an unaffected parent had the same chromosome change. However, this situation was seen all too commonly

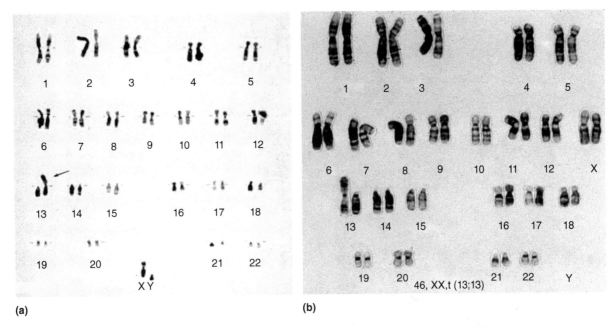

(a)   **(b)**

Figure 5-48. Two karyotypes with Trisomy 13 due to a 13:13 translocation (both from amniocentesis). (Courtesy Dr. Warren G. Sanger, University of Nebraska Medical Center.)

in these types of evaluations, leading many clinicians to suspect that the situation was not as straightforward as it seemed. With advances in molecular techniques, it has now become apparent the transmission of an apparently balanced rearrangement from a parent to the child may involve further changes, such as small duplications or deletions around the breakpoints (or elsewhere), that were too small to detect at the resolution of a karyotype.

Structural rearrangements involving the X chromosome can influence the process of Lyonization. As such, different patterns of expression may be seen. In the event of a structurally abnormal X chromosome (i.e., one with a deletion), the abnormal X is preferentially inactivated, leaving the normal X active. But with balanced X-autosome translocations, the *normal* X chromosome is the one that is usually inactivated. It has been hypothesized that this is because inactivation of the X-autosome translocated chromosome is probably lethal. These differing patterns are observed phenomena, not events that could be predicted.

Chromosome Structural Changes Associated with Well-Described Syndromes

Prior to FISH, a handful of conditions were identified with specific structural chromosomal imbalances big enough to see in karyotypes. These conditions had a recognizable phenotype that allowed the identification of a described syndrome in association with the specific chromosome imbalance. Historically, two are worth mentioning.

1. *Wolf-Hirschhorn syndrome (4p-).* Deletion of the terminal end of the short arm of chromosome 4 has been associated with a condition known as Wolf-Hirschhorn syndrome (Figures 5-49 and 5-50). Patients with

Wolf-Hirschhorn syndrome have microcephaly, a "characteristic" facial appearance due to a very prominent nasal bridge, mental deficiency, and cleft lip with or without cleft palate. This can either be *de novo* or inherited.

2. *Cri-du-chat (5p-) syndrome.* Figure 5-51 shows an individual with a deletion of the terminal portion of the short arm of chromosome 5 (Figure 5-52). This particular deletion has been associated with a unique phenotype (syndrome) known as Cri-du-chat, which is the French term for "cry of the cat." This cry is distinctive and truly reflective of its name. This condition can sometimes be suspected upon hearing the characteristic cry. Other physical features include low-birth weight, microcephaly, hypertelorism, rounded facies, micrognathia, and severe cognitive deficits. This may be a *de novo* or inherited abnormality.

Contiguous Gene Syndromes

Wolf Hirschhorn syndrome and Cri-du-chat syndrome represent well-described "contiguous gene syndromes" (Table 5-6). Such disorders are conditions that have a recognizable phenotype with an associated structural chromosome change. The changes may be large enough to be seen on a karyotype or small enough that a molecular cytogenetic testing modality (such as FISH) is needed to identify it. The multiple genes involved sometimes can actually predict phenotypes. The clinical manifestations can be attributed to multiple genes that are located in tandem on the chromosomes which are either deleted or duplicated. Sometimes knowledge of the genes involved may provide direct insight into the

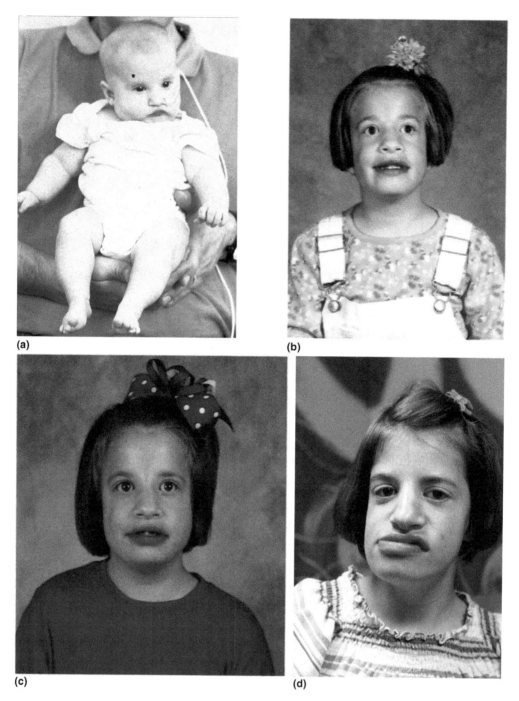

Figure 5-49. Young girl with Wolf-Hirschhorn syndrome (4p-). (a) 9-months old. (b) 6-years old. (c) 9-years old. (d) 18-years old.

phenotype. More often, however, it is not possible to predict the phenotype based upon the genes involved.

The characteristics of contiguous gene syndromes are:

1. They have a recognizable phenotype.

2. Typically the individual is heterozygous for the genetic change.

3. The condition shows familial transmission that looks Mendelian in nature (dominant transmission).

4. They typically show markedly variable expression.

A classic example of a contiguous gene syndrome is Williams syndrome. Williams syndrome has a recognizable phenotype associated with short stature, pixie or "elfin like" facial features, a stellate pattern to the iris, hypercalcemia, and a variety of vascular changes (Figure 5-53). The facial features are somewhat subtle. In the pre-FISH era, the clinical diagnosis could often be difficult. Ultimately, Williams syndrome has been shown to be associated with a deletion at 7q11.23 (Figure 5-54). One gene in this region is the elastin gene which codes for a protein that, as the name would imply, gives elasticity to connective tissues. Many of the somatic

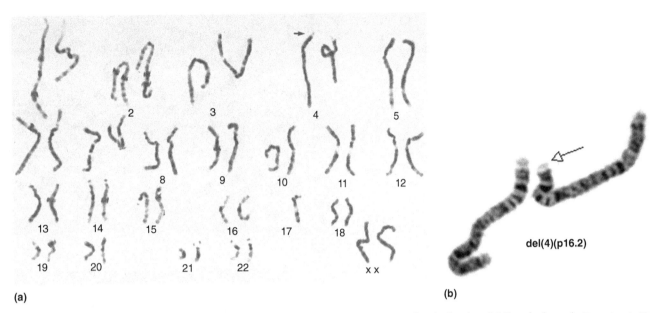

(a)

(b)

Figure 5-50. (a) Karyotype 46, XX, deletion 4p. (b) High resolution chromosome 4 pair showing deletion 4p (arrow). (Reproduced with permission of Warren G. Sanger, PhD, University of Nebraska Medical Center, Omaha, Nebraska.)

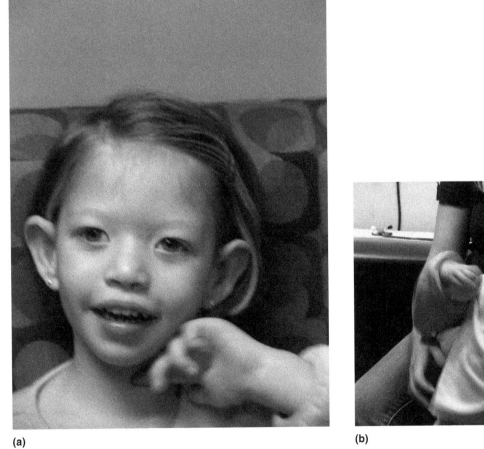

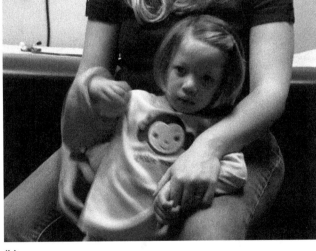

(a)

(b)

Figure 5-51. Young girl with Cri-du-chat syndrome (5p-). (Reprinted with permission from Brooker RJ: *Genetics: Analysis & Principles*, 3rd ed. New York: McGraw-Hill, 2008.)

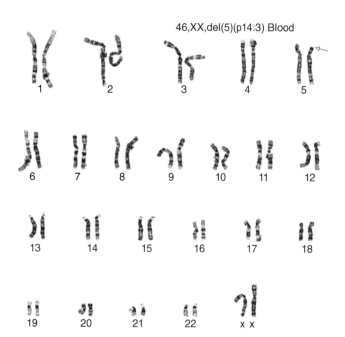

46,XX,del(5)(p14.3) Blood

Figure 5-52. Karyotype 46, XX, del 5p. (Reproduced with permission of Warren G. Sanger, PhD, University of Nebraska Medical Center, Omaha, Nebraska)

Table 5-6.	Important Contiguous Gene Syndromes	
Eponym	**Chromosomal Change**	**Major Clinical Features (not including developmental delays)**
Prader-Willi	del 15q12	Obesity, hypotonia, mental retardation, small hands/feet
Angelman	del 15q12	Ataxia, hypertonia, inappropriate laughter
Williams	del 7q11.23	Hypercalemia, "elfin like" facies, supravalvular aortic stenosis
DiGeorge	del 22q11	Conotruncal heart defects, hypoparathyroidism (hypocalcemia), aplasia/hypoplasia of thymus
Shprintzen	del 22q11	Palatal abnormalities, conotruncal heart defects, characteristic facies
Miller-Dieker	del 17p13.3	Type 1 lissencephaly, characteristic facies
Smith Magenis	del 17p11.2	Brachycephaly, short hands/feet, self injurious behavior
Langer-Giedeon	del 8q23.3	Multiple bony exostoses, large nose, sparse hair
none	del 1q21	Cardiac defects, limb anomalies
none	del or dup 16p11	Autism

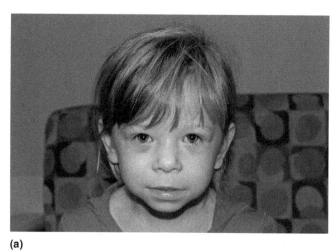

(a)

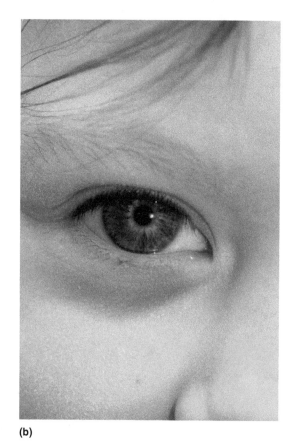

(b)

Figure 5-53. A young girl with Williams syndrome. (a) Note classic facial changes. (b) "Stellate" pattern of the irises.

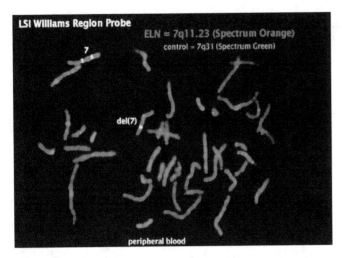

Figure 5-54. FISH study showing 7q deletion seen with Williams syndrome. (Reproduced with permission of Warren G. Sanger, PhD, University of Nebraska Medical Center, Omaha, Nebraska.)

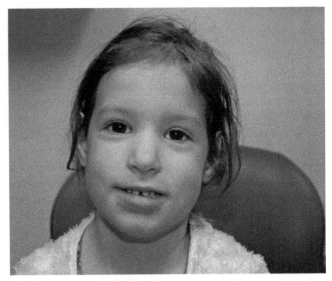

(a)

changes seen in Williams syndrome can be attributed to the deletion of the elastin gene. Other deleted genes in this region are related to the other changes, such as cognitive and behavioral abnormalities, seen in these patients.

The advent of microarray comparative genomic hybridization has greatly expanded the list of identifiable contiguous gene disorders. An interesting phenomenon is now frequently encountered that is an important issue for families. Microarray studies are now identifying conditions that bear no eponymic designation, i.e., there is no name to the syndrome. For these conditions, the actual "name" is the cytogenetic description. Surprisingly, this has turned out to be concerning to some families. One such example is the 1q21.1 deletion. This particular micro-deletion was first described in 2008. With microarray technology, it has been found to be a relatively common deletion in patients with mild neurodevelopmental disorders or congenital heart malformations. The phenotypic range is broad and includes speech and language delays, behavioral changes, mild dysmorphic facies, and congenital heart malformations in some (Figure 5-55a). The gene for thrombocytopenia-aplasia of the radius (TAR) is in this region. Depending on the size of the abnormality, it may be deleted as part of this change. If the TAR gene is deleted, patients have been noted to have variable expression of radial anomalies and/or thrombocytopenia (Figure 5-55b). There is no eponym associated with this condition. The actual designation is "1q21.1 deletion."

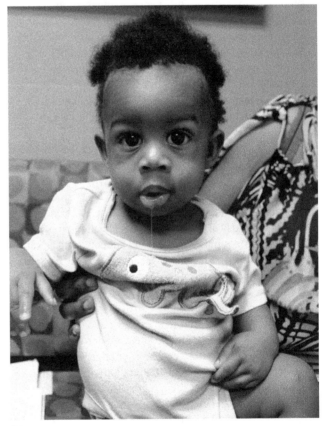

(b)

Figure 5-55. Two patients with a 1q21.1 deletion discovered on microarray studies. (a) Middle-aged girl who presented with mild developmental delays and behavioral problems. (b) Young boy with 1q21.1 deletion with developmental delays, hypotonia, and radial hypoplasia.

Part 3: Clinical Correlation

DiGeorge syndrome (DGS) was described by the pediatric endocrinologist Angelo DiGeorge in 1968. The condition represents a **field defect** of the developing third and fourth branchial arches of the human embryo. The pattern of anomalies seen in DiGeorge syndrome reflects the embryological derivatives of this region. Patients with DGS have hypoplasia or aplasia of the parathyroid glands with subsequent hypocalcemia. Absence of the thymus produces a T-cell deficiency with immune dysfunction. The third and fourth branchial arches contribute to the "upper heart", with disruption of this part of development leading to congenital heart malformations classified as conotruncal heart anomalies. Minor changes of the lower face and ears may also occur (Figure 5-56a).

Robert Shprintzen, a speech-language pathologist, and colleagues described the syndrome that bears his name in 1978. Shprintzen syndrome is also called velo-cardio-facial syndrome, describing the major features of the condition. Changes in the development of the palate are common. This includes structural malformations such as cleft palate and functional defects such as velo-palatal insufficiency. Other features include conotruncal heart malformations and characteristic facial features including a distinctive nasal appearance. Patients with Shprintzen syndrome (Figure 5-56b) have a high incidence of learning disabilities and neuropsychiatric problems as well.

With advances in cytogenetic techniques in the early 1980s, several reports began to appear of patients with either DiGeorge or Shprintzen syndrome with deletions in the 22q1 region. With the introduction of FISH studies, 90% of patients with either condition were found to have deletions in the region 22q11.2. Subsequent investigations found 22q11.2 deletions in a smaller number of patients with a variety of other described syndromes such as Opitz BBB syndrome, CHARGE syndrome, and Cayler cardiofacial syndrome (also known as asymmetric crying facies). Even more fascinating, it was discovered that almost 30% of patients with isolated (non-syndromic) conotruncal malformations have a 22q11.2 deletion. To date over 180 different malformations have been reported in association with this contiguous gene disorder. Given the association with so many different syndromes and anomalies, it is best at this point in time to refer to the spectrum of 22q11.2 deletions as the overriding designation. It is estimated that 1 in 4000 individuals may have a 22q11.2 deletion.

As this deletion is transmitted through the generations, there is marked inter-familial and intra-familial variability. The inheritance pattern is best described as looking like autosomal dominant inheritance with variable expression and incomplete penetrance. A discussion of these terms in the next chapter, Chapter 6 on Mendelian Inheritance, will clarify this relationship and build on this introduction.

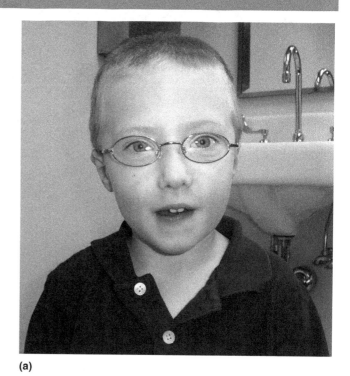

(a)

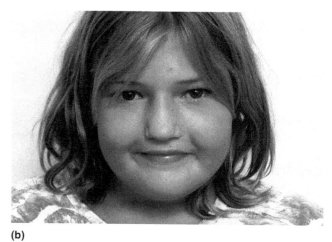

(b)

Figure 5-56. Two patients with 22q11.2 deletions. (a) Phenotype = partial DiGeorge syndrome. (b) Phenotype is that of velo-cardio-facial (Shprintzen) syndrome. She has typical facial changes, palatal cleft and conotruncal heart defect. (a: Courtesy of Dr. Nancy Mendelsohn, Children's Hospitals and Clinics of Minnesota)

■ Board-Format Practice Questions

1. In regards to chromosome aneuploidies in humans:
   A. They are rare at the time of conception.
   B. They are seen more often as pregnancy progresses.
   C. If present at conception, they most often end in a miscarriage.
   D. All whole chromosome trisomies are incompatible with postnatal life.
   E. All whole chromosome monosomies are incompatible with postnatal life.

2. The incidence of chromosome abnormalities at the time of conception is:
   A. 1/120
   B. 1/75
   C. 1/65
   D. 1/10
   E. 1/2

3. Turner Syndrome:
   A. is the only whole chromosome monosomy seen in live births in humans.
   B. the most common congenital heart disease is a ventricular septal defect.
   C. is milder in boys.
   D. girls with this condition are usually tall for age.
   E. is more accurately described as Turner's syndrome.

4. In regards to chromosome disorders in humans:
   A. they occur rarely and are not of major clinical importance.
   B. they may show a paternal age effect.
   C. aneuploidies for the sex chromosomes occur more commonly than for the autosomes in live births.
   D. whole chromosome aneuploidies can be seen in patients for any of the 23 pairs.
   E. the most common clinical outcome in a chromosome abnormality is a newborn with a birth defect.

5. In regards to contiguous gene syndromes:
   A. Clinical syndromes are usually associated with homozygosity of the deletion.
   B. They usually track through a family like an autosomal recessive trait.
   C. They usually occur sporadically, but may be familial.
   D. Because they occur on the same part of the chromosome, there is very little variability in the phenotype.
   E. Diagnosis by chromosome analysis is more sensitive and practical than FISH testing.

Supplementary Readings

Cassidy, S., and J. Allanson. *Management of Genetic Syndromes*, 2nd ed. Hoboken, NJ: Wiley-Liss Publishing; 2004.

Gardener, R. and G. Sullivan. *Chromosome Abnormalities and Genetic Counseling*, 3rd ed. Oxford: Oxford University Press; 2004.

Hennekam, R., J. Allanson, and I. Krantz. *Gorlin's Syndromes of the Head and Neck*. Oxford: Oxford University Press, 2010.

Jones, K. *Smith's Recognizable Patterns of Human Malformations*, 6th ed. Philadelphia: Elsevier, Saunders Publishing, 2005.

Shprintzen, R. *Genetics, Syndromes and Communication Disorders*. San Diego: Singular Publishing Group, 1997.

chapter

6 Mendelian Genetics: Patterns of Gene Transmission

CHAPTER SUMMARY

Gregor Mendel (1822-1884) is heralded as the Father of Genetics, although he would not recognize that title, since the term "gene" was not coined until 1909. At the time of Mendel's experiments on plant hybrids (Figure 6-1), a prevailing theory of trait transmission was blending inheritance, in which traits are mixed and altered in the offspring. His training in physics and mathematics was unusual for a biologist of his time. It gave him a quantitative outlook on natural laws that enabled him to detect relationships in his results that other biologists had overlooked.

Mendel carried out carefully controlled experiments in which he cross-pollinated true-breeding strains (we would now call them "homozygous") and protected the experimental plants from accidental pollination by insects or the wind. Strains of the garden pea, *Pisum sativum*, were available with distinctly differing traits like yellow *versus* green seeds and white *versus* purple flowers. He kept careful records of results, from which he was able to identify predictable patterns in the frequency of traits among large numbers of offspring. The proportions he found required an assumption that challenged the contemporary idea of blending inheritance. Mendel's assumption of "unit factor inheritance" was that the determinants of traits (today's "genes") were distinct factors that occur in pairs in each individual (today's "diploid"). Furthermore, only one of the two copies was passed by each parent to an offspring. Building on this theoretical foundation, he was able to deduce from his data the three rules of transmission that are often called the Mendelian Laws. The mathematical logic behind his assumption of unit factor inheritance and the significance of the regular patterns of factor transmission were not fully understood by his colleagues, and his work went unnoticed until his publications were independently rediscovered in 1900 by Carl Correns, Hugo de Vries, and Erich von Tschermak. Experimental exploration into the rules of hereditary transmission dates from that rediscovery. Now extensive datasets can be created, even from purely historical data, to show the hereditary relationships among related individuals.

The Mendelian Laws of genetic transmission are, however, not laws in the scientific sense of that word. A natural law is a tested theory that has been shown to be universally true. But, in contrast to this highest level of authority, each of the Mendelian "Laws" has important exceptions that affect the way patterns of inheritance are expressed. In this chapter we will discuss the mechanisms behind the three classical Mendelian Rules of transmission and some of the important ways in which a gene's contributions to a phenotype can alter the appearance of the underlying patterns of inheritance.

Part 1: Background and Systems Integration

Mendelian Rules of Transmission

Mendel's key experiments on plant hybridization were published in 1866. The quality of biological microscopy and nuclear staining techniques did not improve to the point where chromosomes could be seen and studied until the 1880s. Thus, the relationships that Mendel described were deduced from patterns he saw in his data. But at least in the case of two of his principal rules, **segregation** and **independent**

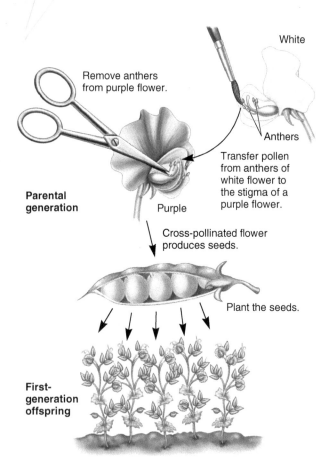

Remove anthers from purple flower.

White

Anthers

Transfer pollen from anthers of white flower to the stigma of a purple flower.

Parental generation

Purple

Cross-pollinated flower produces seeds.

Plant the seeds.

First-generation offspring

Figure 6-1. Gregor Mendel established a controlled breeding plan to trace the transmission of simple traits using plants like the garden pea. (Reprinted with permission from Brooker RJ: *Genetics: Analysis & Principles*, 3rd ed. New York: McGraw-Hill, 2008.)

Heterozygous (Yy) cell from a plant with yellow seeds

Meiosis I
Prophase

Metaphase

Anaphase
Telophase

Meiosis II

Haploid cells

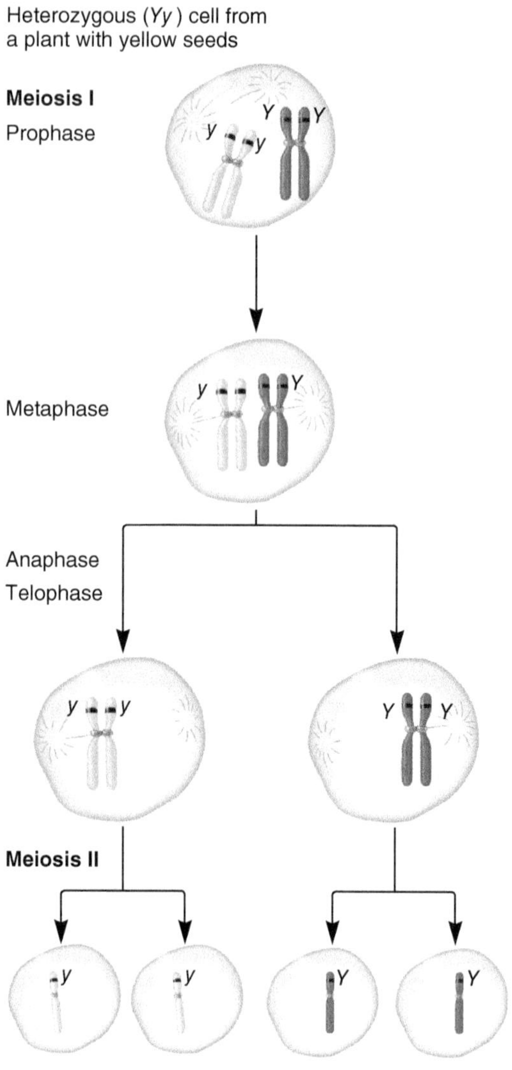

Figure 6-2. An abbreviated summary of key events in meiosis. In this example, the homologous chromosomes carry different alleles for the Y gene. At metaphase I, they line up in the center of the spindle, and at anaphase I one homologue and its allele (y) moves to the left and the other homologue and its allele (Y) separates from the first and moves to the right. This separation is the basis of the Mendelian Rule of segregation. (Reprinted with permission from Brooker RJ: *Genetics: Analysis & Principles*, 3rd ed. New York: McGraw-Hill, 2008.)

assortment, he was actually describing the behavior of chromosomes during meiosis.

From our earlier discussion of meiosis, you will remember that each chromosome replicates during the S phase of interphase. Chromosomes then coil, and homologous pairs synapse during prophase I of meiosis (Figure 6-2). Each synapsed pair, or bivalent, becomes attached to kinetochore microtubules of the spindle. At anaphase I the homologous chromosomes separate, reducing chromosome number from the diploid to the haploid in each of the two resulting cells. This separation of homologous chromosomes in the first meiotic division is the mechanism behind Mendel's rule of segregation.

If we follow two pairs of homologous chromosomes that are heterozygous for genes Y and R (Figure 6-3), we can see that the way in which one pair lines up at metaphase I is independent of the way the other lines up. Half the time we expect the two dominant alleles to line up on opposite sides of the metaphase plate, and half the time they will be on the same side. When the homologous chromosomes separate from each other, the segregation of Y and y is at random with respect to the segregation of R and r. For that reason, gametes carrying the four possible allele combinations, YR, Yr, yR, and yr, are

in equal frequency. This is the mechanism that explains Mendel's rule of random, or independent, assortment.

The third Mendelian rule, **dominance** and **recessiveness**, is unrelated to chromosome behavior. As mentioned earlier, dominance is simply a function of the way in which biochemical regulation of phenotypes can buffer against the deleterious influence of a recessive mutation. If one normal copy of a gene makes enough products that the phenotype is expressed normally, the mutant allele will be masked, i.e., it will be recessive to the dominant allele. Although it is true that most new mutations are recessive, there are many exceptions. Indeed, it is the exceptions to all three Mendelian rules

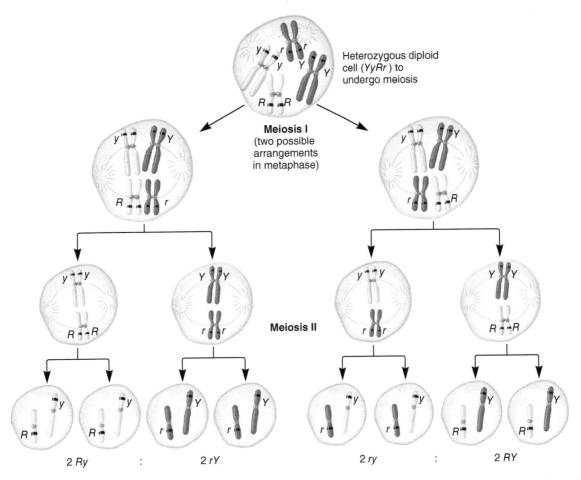

Figure 6-3. Events of meiosis in which we follow the behavior of two different pairs of chromosomes. (Reprinted with permission from Brooker RJ: *Genetics: Analysis & Principles*, 3rd ed. New York: McGraw-Hill, 2008.)

that make the interpretation of genetic transmission such an interesting array of puzzles.

Transmission Probabilities and Recurrence Rates

When the genotypes of the parents and the nature of a gene's expression are known, one can easily predict the probabilities of each genotypic and phenotypic outcome. The segregations of alleles from each parent are independent events. So, according to the product rule of probability, you simply multiply the independent probabilities to determine the overall likelihood of a given outcome. The likelihood of a particular allele being inherited from the father is multiplied by the likelihood of a particular allele from the mother. For example, since half of the alleles from a heterozygous *Rr* father or mother will be *R*, the overall probability of the first child being homozygous *RR* is ½ × ½ = ¼ (Figure 6-4). Such outcomes are often summarized in a table called a Punnett square after the pioneer geneticist, R.C. Punnett, who first used it.

Being able to predict the probability of a typical genetic outcome is one of the most powerful foundations of genetics. If you are focusing on only one gene and both parents

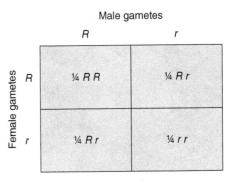

Figure 6-4. Punnett square for a simple monohybrid cross, showing the basis of a 1:2:1 genotypic segregation pattern (¼ *RR*, ½ *Rr*, ¼ *rr*). If the *R* allele is fully dominant, the phenotypic ratio in this monohybrid cross is 3:1, i.e., ¾ *R* – and ¼ *rr*.

are heterozygous, as in Figure 6-4, then the genotypic ratio in the next generation is ¼:½:¼, or 1:2:1. With complete dominance, the phenotypic ratio is ¾:¼ = 3:1. Adding a second segregating gene simply expands the probability calculation. For example, consider offspring from a dihybrid cross of *Aa Bb* × *Aa Bb*, where the dash indicates that the second allele in a genotype with one dominant could be either a dominant or recessive without changing the phenotype. According to product rule, we simply multiply the probabilities of each gene combination:

$$\begin{array}{ccc} & \tfrac{3}{4}\,A- & \tfrac{1}{4}\,aa \\ \times & \tfrac{3}{4}\,B- & \tfrac{1}{4}\,bb \\ \hline \end{array}$$

9/16 A– B–   3/16 aa B–   3/16 A– bb   1/16 aa bb, or in short form, 9:3:3:1.

For three independently-segregating genes, you simply add another cycle of multiplication by 3:1, giving eight different types in a ratio of 27:9:9:9:3:3:3:1. But the examples of most interest are those in which some other factor is influencing the expression of these genes. If one allele is not completely dominant over the other, for example, the phenotypic ratio will be the same as the genotypic ratio.

$$\begin{array}{ccc} & \tfrac{1}{4}\,AA & 2/4\,Aa & \tfrac{1}{4}\,aa \\ \times & \tfrac{1}{4}\,BB & 2/4\,Bb & \tfrac{1}{4}\,bb \end{array}$$

yields a 1:2:1:2:4:2:1:2:1 ratio, with the most common (at 4/16) being the dihybrid (2/4 Aa × 2/4 Bb = 4/16 Aa Bb). Of course, if the genes are located near each other on the same chromosome, they will tend to be inherited together and the patterns of transmission prediction must be modified.

On the surface, then, the rules governing gene transmission are fairly straightforward. It is one reason that genetics has such useful predictive power. But as we have already seen, genes code for products that can interact in complex ways with each other and with environmental conditions. A simple example is **incomplete dominance** seen, for example, in the pigmentation of some flowers (Figure 6-5). One allele does not produce enough active enzyme to catalyze as much red pigment in the heterozygote as two alleles do in the homozygote. Such incomplete dominance affects the ways in which genotypes are expressed phenotypically. It is a common exception to the classical Mendelian Rule of dominance.

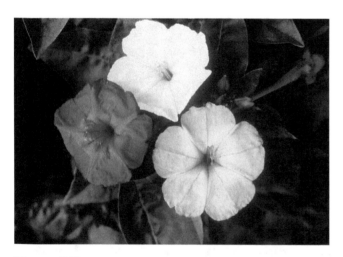

Figure 6-5. Flower color provides a classical example of incomplete dominance. In this case, let us call the genotype that produces red flowers *RR* and the genotype for white flowers *rr*. The heterozygote, *Rr*, produces less red pigment, so flower color is an intermediate, pink. The intensity of flower pigmentation and copies of the functional (*R*) allele show a dosage effect. (© Robert Calentine/Visuals Unlimited.)

Thus, while inheritance patterns form the working foundation, each trait's phenotypic assessment is often the primary focus in day-to-day applications of medical genetics.

Special Cases: An Overview

For traits with medical implications, recurrence rates are an important consideration. These are based on both the pattern of Mendelian inheritance and on the way the alleles are expressed during development of the phenotype. But even if the genes are not contributing to development with equal weight, gene interactions can influence the phenotypic outcome in complex ways. In the following sections, we will introduce the genetic and biochemical basis underlying some common ways in which genetic outcomes can be expressed. Specific medical examples will be the focus of Parts 2 and 3.

Exceptions to the Rule of Dominance and Recessiveness

The concept of dominance was conceived before it was possible to measure the biochemical events underlying the development of a trait. As we saw with the example of flower color in Petunias, some alleles contribute to the phenotype with a dosage effect. This yields incomplete dominance of one allele over another. Each allele adds a certain amount to the trait's intensity, and the heterozygote can, therefore, be distinguished from either homozygote. Indeed, many genes have a small, cumulative phenotypic effect like this. Furthermore, dominance is sometimes influenced by the techniques we apply to measure phenotypes. An example of this idea is seen in starch production in peas (Figure 6-6). On a

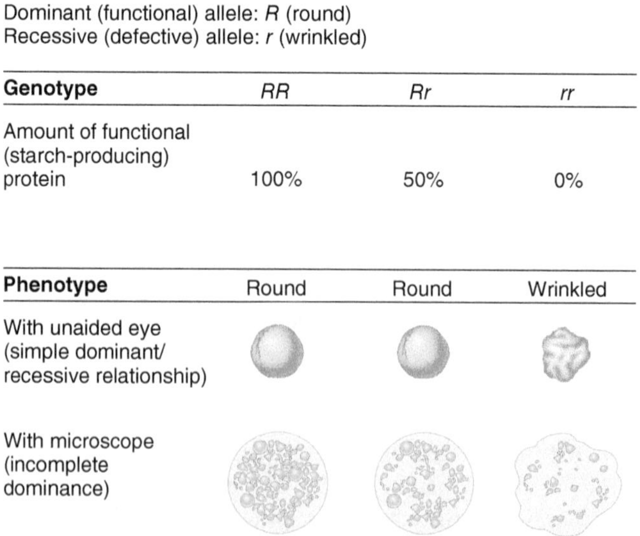

Dominant (functional) allele: *R* (round)
Recessive (defective) allele: *r* (wrinkled)

Genotype	*RR*	*Rr*	*rr*
Amount of functional (starch-producing) protein	100%	50%	0%

Phenotype	Round	Round	Wrinkled
With unaided eye (simple dominant/recessive relationship)			
With microscope (incomplete dominance)			

Figure 6-6. The distinction between complete and incomplete dominance is often a function of the level of magnification or the precision of information we have about a phenotype. In this example, microscopic examination of pea seeds that are heterozygous for the *r* allele have markedly fewer starch grains than those that are homozygous *RR*. (Reprinted with permission from Brooker RJ: *Genetics: Analysis & Principles*, 3rd ed. New York: McGraw-Hill, 2008.)

	A B	A b	a B	a b
A B	A A B B	A A B b	A a B B	A a B b
A b	A A B b	A A b b	A a B b	A a b b
a B	A a B B	A a B b	a a B B	a a B b
a b	A a B b	A a b b	a a B b	a a b b

(a)

	A B	A b	a B	a b
A B	A A B B	A A B b	A a B B	A a B b
A b	A A B b	A A b b	A a B b	A a b b
a B	A a B B	A a B b	a a B B	a a B b
a b	A a B b	A a b b	a a B b	a a b b

(b)

Figure 6-7. Dihybrid Punnett square showing: (a) 9:3:3:1 dihybrid ratio for coat color and spot number. (b) 12:3:1 modified dihybrid ratio due to dominant epistasis, when the dominant *A* allele masks segregation at the *B* locus. Consider, for example, an animal that is normally light brown with yellow spots. A 12:3:1 phenotypic ratio is produced if the *A* mutant produces complete melanism, so no yellow spots can be seen. Melanism masks the expression of any segregating gene that would otherwise influence yellow appearance.

superficial phenotypic level, both the dominant homozygous and the heterozygous seeds have the same round appearance. But biochemically, the heterozygous seeds have significantly less starch. At the visual level, round is dominant to wrinkle. But at the biochemical or histological level, it is easy to distinguish the heterozygotes from either of the homozygous genotypes, and the trait is incompletely dominant. Indeed, at the biochemical level, almost all traits are probably incompletely dominant to some extent.

Gene Interactions

Although individual genes can have a large phenotypic effect, they seldom if ever act in complete developmental isolation. Gene interactions are more the rule than the exception. But the outcomes are no less predictable. This can be illustrated by a few simple examples based on dihybrid phenotypic patterns. When two genes affect the same or a closely-related trait, the 9:3:3:1 dihybrid segregation pattern is modified in predictable ways. As shown by the example in Figure 6-7, interactions merge segregating categories, depending on how the genes work together on the same trait. Some common examples are summarized in Figure 6-8.

The typical dihybrid ratio will be modified as a function of how the genes interact in forming the phenotype. For example, **epistasis** (literally, to "stand above") is a situation in which one gene masks the expression of a second gene. By analogy, having a completely shaven head masks the expression of genes that determine hair color, so complete baldness is epistatic to, it "stands above," hair color (Figure 6-9). Similarly, Mexican hairless dogs do not express the genes that

	A-B-	A-bb	aaB-	aabb
Typical dihybrid	9/16	3/16	3/16	1/16
Dominant epistasis	12/16		3/16	1/16
Recessive epistasis	9/16	3/16	4/16	
Either dominant is sufficient for the trait	15/16			1/16
Both dominants are required for the trait	9/16		7/16	

Figure 6-8. Modified dihybrid ratios due to some common kinds of gene interaction.

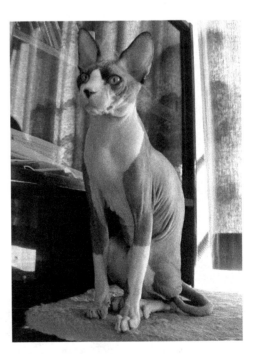

Figure 6-9. The absence of hair, whether due to a hair stylist or a mutation, is epistatic to (it masks) the genes coding for hair color and curliness. The Sphynx is a hairless breed of cat. (Photograph by M. Minderhoud. Licensed under GFDL, http://www.gnu.org/copyleft/fdl.html or CC-BY-SA-3.0, http://creativecommons.org/licenses/by-sa/3.0/, via Wikimedia Commons).

would otherwise define hair texture or curliness. By masking the segregation of other genes affecting the same trait, the overall phenotypic ratios will be altered. The expected phenotypic ratios will depend on whether the epistatic gene acts through a dominant or a recessive phenotype.

Genes in the same, or a closely related, pathway also interact in ways that can modify the predicted phenotypic ratios. Consider the situation in which a trait is affected by a dominant mutation of either the *A* or the *B* gene. Only in the 1/16th of the offspring that are homozygous recessive *aabb* will the alternative trait appear. The modified ratio is, therefore, 15:1. On the other hand, if the trait can be blocked by homozygous recessive genotypes at either locus, the resulting phenotypic ratio will be 9:7. Other combinations of interaction are also possible. The key idea, therefore, is to think about genetic applications on two levels: the underlying genetic segregations and the ways the resulting allele combinations influence development.

Genotype × Environment Interactions

Just as some genes will affect the phenotypic expression of other genes, environmental influences also play a key role in developmental expression. Indeed, **genotype × environmental interactions** are probably more often the rule than the exception, especially for environmental variables like temperature that can affect molecular stability or the rate of a biochemical reaction. A classic example is the pigmentation pattern seen in Himalayan rabbits and cats (Figure 6-10). In this case, the enzyme for synthesizing melanin is inactivated in the warmer parts of the body so they are lightly pigmented. Only in the cooler areas like the ears, tip of the nose, and feet does the enzyme work normally. Not surprisingly, genotype × environment interactions can be limited to a specific time period or developmental stage if they are associated with genes that are only transcribed for a defined period.

In an earlier chapter, we briefly discussed sickle cell anemia as an example of a simple Mendelian trait. It is also the basis of a phenotype that is affected by environmental conditions. Sickling of the red blood cells (RBCs) takes place when oxygen (O_2) concentrations in the blood are low, and hemoglobin

begins to crystallize in the cells. This can happen during high physical activity in which O_2 levels in the muscles decline or during travel by air or to high elevations when atmospheric pressure is lower. But by carefully monitoring conditions like these, individuals with sickle cell anemia can live normally. Similarly, phenylketonuria (PKU), one of the first human traits shown to follow Mendelian transmission, has a severity that is affected by environmental factors. Individuals with PKU lack functional phenylalanine hydroxylase. If their dietary phenylalanine levels are not restricted, its buildup can cause a variety of serious phenotypic effects including mental retardation. But by following a diet restricted in phenylalanine, their development can be normal. Understanding how an individual's genotype interacts with their environment is critical to many treatment protocols.

Penetrance and Expressivity

We saw earlier that most, if not all, traits actually show incomplete dominance if one measures the level of biochemical activity in each genotype. There is an underlying, sometimes hidden, stepwise gradation of cellular and biochemical genetic effects. Dominance is essentially a phenomenon caused by the architecture of biochemical pathways that allows variation among common genotypes so that the heterozygote is still effective enough to produce a normal outcome. That same gradation in gene action underlies a separate, but related, pair of phenomena: **incomplete penetrance** and variable **expressivity** (Figure 6-11).

A trait is completely penetrant if each individual expresses his or her own individual genotype. But sometimes a particular genotype is inherited, but the trait it determines is not expressed. In those instances, the genotype is partly masked, or incompletely penetrant into the phenotype. To quantify the degree of penetrance, it is necessary to evaluate a large number of individuals who are known to have the appropriate genotype. Given such population data, the percent penetrance can become a tool, i.e., an independent probability of expression,

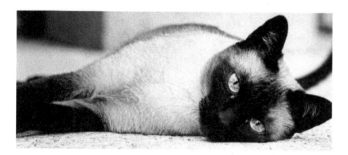

Figure 6-10. The pigment pattern in Siamese cats is caused by a gene that codes an enzyme which is most active at cooler temperatures. (Photograph by Telekokopelli. Licensed under CC-BY-SA-3.0 (http://creativecommons.org/licenses/by-sa/3.0), via Wikimedia Commons.).

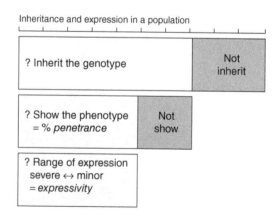

Figure 6-11. This graphical representation shows the relationships between inheriting the genotype for a trait (top), exhibiting that trait if it is incompletely penetrant (middle), and the severity when it is expressed (bottom).

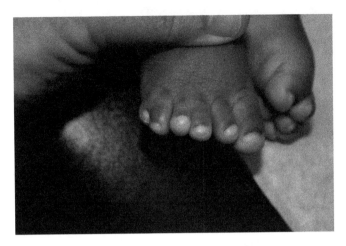

Figure 6-12. Polydactyly is a dominant trait with variable expression. This foot shows postaxial polydactyly with duplication of the 5th toe.

in predicting the expected outcome in a birth or a pedigree. For example, assume that two parents are heterozygous for a recessive condition that has 70% penetrance. What is the probability that their first child will show the trait? From two heterozygous parents, there is a ¼ chance that the child will be homozygous. But among such homozygotes only 0.7 will actually express the trait. The overall probability of a *phenotypically* affected child in this case is, therefore, ¼ (0.7) = 17.5%.

Phenotypic variability goes even further. Not all individuals will express a trait with equal severity. In some cases a trait will be strongly expressed and in other cases it can be mild. Thus, among those showing a trait, variation is seen in the range of **expressivity**. Indeed, penetrance and expressivity may only be different faces of the same phenomenon—variable outcomes in the development of a sensitive characteristic. Polydactyly (Figure 6-12), for example, is an incompletely penetrant trait that is also variable in its expressivity. An individual inheriting this dominant mutation may have five normal fingers and toes

(incomplete penetrance). But if the mutation is shown phenotypically, the degree of expression can range from a small additional digit on only one hand or foot to well-formed extra digits on all of them (variable expressivity).

Lethal Alleles

When it can be traced to a genetic cause, "death" is a phenotype. In fact, gene mutations that cause death in homozygotes are the most common type of genetic change. At first this may seem hard to believe. But if we take a moment to think about all of the biological processes of cells and our general physiology that are indispensable to us, it begins to become less surprising. Although dominant lethal mutations might occur, they immediately kill the carrier, so they are not inherited. Thus, only recessive lethal mutations play a role in genetic assessment. The most relevant are probably those with both homozygous lethality and some separate physical or developmental phenotype in the heterozygote. In these instances, the physical or developmental phenotype will be dominant since it will be expressed in the heterozygous carriers, and lethality will be recessive because it is expressed in the homozygote.

For a recessive lethal mutation that has a phenotypic effect in heterozygotes, the expected Mendelian ratios among offspring will be modified. Consider the shortened tail in Manx cats (Figure 6-13). The tail is short in heterozygotes, and homozygotes for the tail mutation die early in development. If two Manx cats produce offspring, the resulting phenotypic ratio will be 2:1, i.e., 2/3 will have short tails and 1/3 will be normal. Thus, while the underlying Mendelian segregation ratio is unchanged, the data are changed by the elimination of one of the genotypic classes.

Multiple Alleles

In the examples discussed so far, we have focused on fairly direct connections between a genotype and a phenotype. Often, there are two fairly distinct phenotypes associated with

Figure 6-13. A tail-less Manx, named Silverwing, photographed in 1902. The shortened tail of a Manx cat is caused by a mutation that is homozygous lethal. The dihybrid 1:2:1 Mendelian ratio is, therefore, modified to a 2:1 ratio of shortened tail to normal tail. (A: Originally appeared in *Cats and All About Them* by Frances Simpson, published by Frederick A. Stokes Company Publishers, September 1902. B: Reprinted with permission from Brooker RJ: *Genetics: Analysis & Principles*, 3rd ed. New York: McGraw-Hill, 2008.)

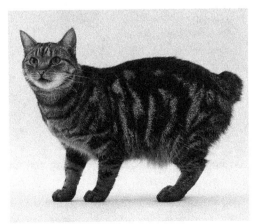

(a) A Manx cat

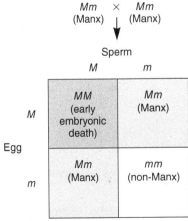

(b) Example of a Manx inheritance pattern

normal *versus* abnormal development, even when a variety of alleles are present in a population. For that reason, it is common to simplify genotypic models to two alleles. But the increasingly available data about proteins and DNA sequences must often be interpreted with multiple allele models. Familiar examples of multiple allelism include the vast genetic diversity seen at the histocompatibility loci determining tissue types and the common polymorphism for cell surface antigens that is known as the ABO blood type (Figure 6-14). A key thing to keep in mind when analyzing traits like this is that a gene pool can carry several different alleles at some moderate frequency, but each individual in that population carries at most two of them.

Consider, for example, the paternity suit of a woman with blood type A against a man with blood type B. The child has blood type O. Can the man be excluded as being the child's father? A and B blood types are detected with specific antibodies, and the inability to detect either of these yields a third alternative, the recessive O blood type. The A blood type is due to the I^A allele, and the B blood type to the I^B allele. The O blood type has neither and is represented as a recessive homozygote, $i\,i$. We can evaluate this problem using a Punnett square organized like the one in Figure 6-14. First, we realize that the blood types of the adults are only phenotypes and, thus, give us only partial information about their genotypes. For example, the man with blood type B could have either of two genotypes: $I^B I^B$ or $I^B i$. The mother must have at least one I^A allele and the male must carry I^B. But for the child to have the O blood type ($i\,i$), both parents must be heterozygous for the i allele. On the basis of the available information, the male cannot be excluded in this case. His genotype could possibly be $I^B i$. But if additional evidence showed that his parents were both $I^A I^B$, for example, then he can be excluded, because he must be homozygous $I^B I^B$ and could not have passed an i allele to the child.

Legal cases now frequently use multiple-allelic DNA markers. But until the advent of DNA markers as forensic evidence, blood type was often employed. One famous case

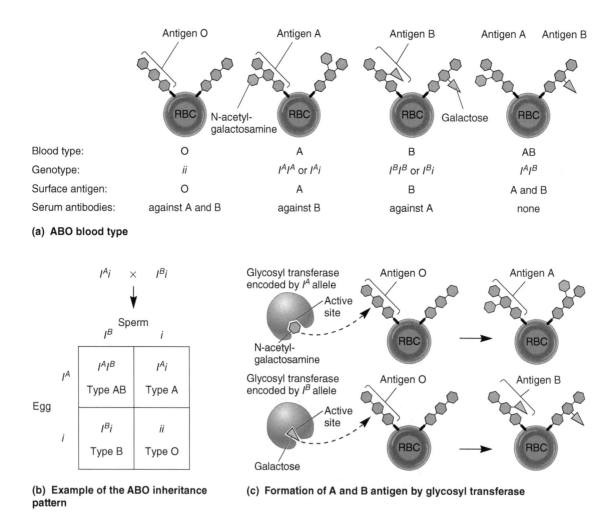

Figure 6-14. ABO blood type is due to a surface antigen and the complementary serum antibodies. (a) Antigens on the RBC surfaces and the associated antibodies in the blood serum. (b) To predict offspring genotypes and phenotypes, one must relax the assumption that only two alleles are segregating in a mating. (c) Glycosyl transferase alleles encoded by the I gene recognize and bind different sugars to the carbohydrate tree. (Reprinted with permission from Brooker RJ: *Genetics: Analysis & Principles*, 3rd ed. New York: McGraw-Hill, 2008.)

in 1943 involved the actor Charlie Chaplin who was accused of fathering a child with the actress Joan Barry. She sued for child support, but blood tests definitively excluded him. When the court did not admit this evidence, he was forced to pay child support anyway. This eventually led to new laws, and the legal system continues to advance slowly as it recognizes the uses and limitations of new technologies to improve the value of evidence.

Contrasting Sex-linked, Sex-limited, and Sex-influenced Expression

Sex-linkage and the mechanisms we call **sex-limited** and **sex-influenced** expression are three quite different phenomena. The main thing they have in common is some kind of relationship with the distribution of genes on the sex-determining chromosomes or developmental effects that differ between females and males. Thus, a careful fitting of information about inheritance and mechanism of gene function is needed to interpret these superficially-related phenomena properly.

Authorities actually differ in the way they use the term "sex-linkage." For some, it is synonymous to X-linkage, with the content of the Y chromosome providing a special case of its own. For others, "sex-linkage" applies to any gene on either sex chromosome and is then subdivided into the X-linked and the Y-linked categories. Since most genes are located on the X, this difference in terminology is almost never a source of confusion. For this discussion, however, the key point is that the X chromosome (and the Y chromosome for that matter) carries many genes that have nothing to do with gender differences *per se*.

In contrast, sex-limited and sex-influenced characters are clearly gender related. A sex-limited character is one that determines a phenotype that is found in only one of the two sexes. Genes responsible for sperm formation in males or a prolapsed uterus in females are examples. Sexually dimorphic animals like chickens show gender differences in traits like body proportions and feathering. The genes for such traits can be found on any chromosome. As expected, most are autosomal. Sex-influenced characters, on the other hand, are those that have a statistically higher frequency of being expressed in one sex than in the other. Examples include a higher frequency of cleft lip and gout in males and a higher frequency of cleft palate, spina bifida, and breast cancer in females. Pyloric stenosis is more common in males, especially firstborn males, than in females. Although the reason for these differences in frequency is often not known, the traits are not gender-specific.

When analyzing traits like these, and indeed anytime one is exploring the genetic mechanisms behind an observation, always remember the rules of probability. Simply having several males with a certain trait appearing in a family pedigree does not necessarily tell us anything concrete about the mode of inheritance or its expression. But patterns of expression in the pedigree can offer the key. Still, rare occurrences cannot be ignored. As is true for many aspects of medicine, the process of diagnosis combines information about both probability and people.

Part 2: Medical Genetics

Introduction

The work of Gregor Mendel in the late 1800s ushered in the modern era of the science of genetics. His work on segregation identified the basic principles of uni-factorial inheritance. His description of the patterns of inheritance provided the basis for what we now understand to be single gene transmission of traits. In fact, conditions exhibiting single gene inheritance patterns are often referred to as **Mendelian traits**. In this era of medical practice, every practicing health care provider should have a solid working knowledge of basic inheritance patterns. The standard of care is that a 3-generational pedigree is part of the medical records of each and every patient (see Chapter 9, Family History). Every practitioner should readily be able to look at a patient's pedigree and identify familial conditions and determine the most likely mode of inheritance of that condition. In the section above, the basic principles of single gene inheritance have been reviewed. Now we will discuss the clinical characteristics, special considerations, and exceptions to the rules associated with each inheritance pattern.

Before we move into a discussion of specific inheritance patterns, a few definitions and concepts should be discussed. A genetic **locus** (plural **loci**) refers to the specific location of a particular segment of DNA, i.e., on which chromosome and where on that chromosome does a segment reside. When tracking traits through a family, the most common application of the term locus refers to the location of a particular **gene**. For example, the CFTR gene which is associated with the condition cystic fibrosis is found on the long arm of chromosome 7. Thus, the locus for the cystic fibrosis gene is designated 7q31.2 (Figure 6-15). Still, it should be emphasized that, although the typical use of the term locus in medical practice is for the location of a functioning gene, all other segments of DNA still have a physical position which is the locus for that designated segment.

Each gene has an expected (normal or **wild type**) sequence. Although humans demonstrate tremendous variability in their phenotypes, it is important to note that over 99.9% of genetic code among people is exactly the same. For most genes, an alternative form is simply not compatible with viability. If a **polymorphism** (literally "multiple forms") does exist for a given gene, the different sequence is termed an **allele.** It is estimated that there is 1 **single nucleotide polymorphism (SNP)** per 1000 base pairs in the human genome. This translates into approximately 3 million SNP's per individual person. Most SNP's are inconsequential as far as clinical expression.

Chromosomal location of a gene

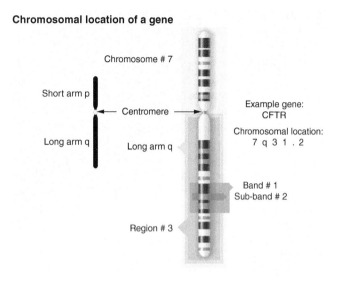

Figure 6-15. The chromosomal location (locus) for the CFTR gene on chromosome 7q31.2. Mutations in this gene cause the genetic condition cystic fibrosis. (From Genetics Home Reference. US National Library of Medicine. *Handbook: Help Me Understand Genetics.* Available at: http://ghr.nlm.nih.gov/handbook. Accessed August 21, 2012.)

But these "benign" SNP's are very important as markers of variation in people and can be used for linkage assessment. The small subgroup of SNP's that do have clinical implications account for much of the observed human diversity.

A person is said to be **homozygous** for a specific gene if both copies of that gene have the same sequence; i.e., the two copies are of the same allele. Likewise, if the two copies of a gene have different sequences, the person is **heterozygous** for that gene; i.e., there are two different alleles. In describing the association of the genotype to the person, a reference could be made to the person being a **homozygote** or a **heterozygote** for that condition. Genetic **homogeneity** for a particular disorder means that a single polymorphism (mutation) only causes that condition. In actuality, genetic homogeneity is rare. In fact, we can only think of one example of a human disorder that exhibits genetic homogeneity. A single nucleotide polymorphism

(SNP) in the beta hemoglobin gene on chromosome 11 causes sickle cell anemia (SSA). The SNP that causes SSA is a change from an adenosine (A) to a thymidine (T) at nucleotide position 334 (this SNP has been designated rs334). This nucleotide change results in an amino acid switch in the hemoglobin molecule where a valine amino acid is substituted for a glutamate at the sixth position in the protein chain. Only this change in the hemoglobin molecule results in sickle cell. This makes sickle cell anemia one of the very few conditions in humans that exhibit genetic homogeneity (Figure 6-16).

When discussing disease-causing mutations, almost all other human conditions exhibit **genetic heterogeneity**. Genetic heterogeneity means that different mutations cause an identical, or very similar, phenotype. Two different types of genetic heterogeneity can occur. **Allelic heterogeneity** refers to different mutations within the same locus producing the same condition. While the CFTR gene is the only gene known to be associated with cystic fibrosis (CF), several different mutations of this one gene can all produce the condition. About 75% of all CF mutations are a specific change designated deltaF508 (a deletion of a phenylalanine at amino acid position 508). Analysis of the different mutations seen in persons with CF has led to the development of CF gene "panels." These panels test for mutations selected for their relative frequency in a given population. For example, a panel of the 12 most common mutations will identify 85% of alleles. A panel of 34 common mutations will detect 90% of alleles. These panels offer an alternative to the more expensive and cumbersome process of sequencing the entire gene. For now this is a desirable first approach given that it is quicker and significantly less expensive. But advances in sequencing techniques are likely to change this situation in the very near future.

Alternatively, some conditions exhibit **locus heterogeneity**. Locus heterogeneity refers to mutations at completely different loci producing the same phenotype. Spinocerebellar atrophy (SCA) is an inherited disorder characterized by a progressive degeneration of the brainstem and cerebellum (Figure 6-17). Most of the families reported with SCAs demonstrate autosomal dominant inheritance. In the mid-1980s,

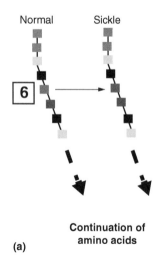

(a)

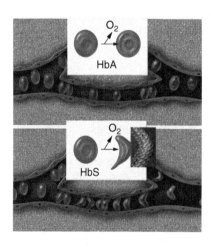

(b)

Figure 6-16. (A, B) A single unique nucleotide polymorphism (SNP) in the beta hemoglobin gene on chromosome 11 causes sickle cell anemia (SSA).

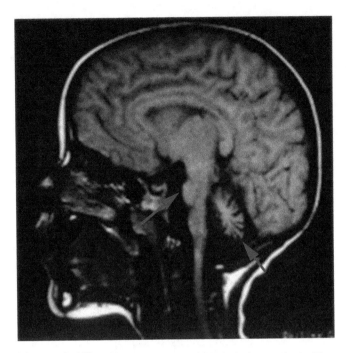

Figure 6-17. Sagittal MRI scan of the brain in a patient with spinocerebellar atrophy. The arrows point out the small size of the brainstem and cerebellum associated with atrophy of these structures.

Table 6-1.	Locus Heterogeneity in Spinocerebellar Atrophy (SCA)
Spino-cerebellar atrophy Type	Locus
1	6p23
2	12q23
3	14q24.3
4	16q22.1
5	11p11
6	19p13
7	3p21.1
8	13q21
9	Not Known
10	22q13
11	15q14
12	5q31
13	19q13.3
14	19q13.4
15	3p26.1–25.3
16	8q22.1
17	6q27
18	7q22-32
19	1p21–q21
20	11p13–q11
21	7p21.3–p15.1
22	Same as type 19
23	20p13–p12.3
24	Now SCAR4
25	2p21–p13
26	19p13.3
27	13q34
28	18p11
29	3p26
30	4q34.3–q35.1
31	16q21

linkage studies suggested that dominant SCA was linked to the major histocompatibility (HLA) locus on chromosome 6p. Further investigation revealed that this was true for only some families. Subsequently, other loci were discovered that also caused SCA. At the present time, over 30 different loci have been identified as being linked to dominant SCA (Table 6-1). Thus, dominant SCA demonstrates striking locus heterogeneity.

Clinical Aspects of Mendelian Inheritance

In these times, most students have had significant exposure to the concepts of single gene inheritance. Often biology classes in junior high school (or even earlier) have discussed the basic concepts of Mendelian transmission of traits. The introductory part of this chapter provides a targeted overview of the basics of Mendelian principles. As with most things, further understanding of the basic principles usually leads to "exceptions to the rules." Such is the case with single gene inheritance. All health care providers should first have a solid understanding of Mendelian principles. Yet equally important, they will need to appreciate all of the potential nuances that can be introduced in the clinical realm. In the sections below we take each major single gene inheritance pattern and provide information about it in three categories:

1. Classic characteristics.

2. Recurrence risks.

3. Special inheritance considerations.

Autosomal Inheritance

Mendelian traits that are transmitted by genes that lie on the autosomes (the numbered 22 pairs of non-sex chromosomes) demonstrate autosomal inheritance. Autosomal inheritance is characterized by the transmission of the two alleles segregating independently in the same manner by both males in females. It is important to note that transmission is not the same as expression. Thus, while autosomal conditions are transmitted in the same manner in males and females, expression may be different between the two sexes (see more detailed discussion in Part 1).

Depending on the pathogenesis of the genetic change (see Chapter 16), a condition may demonstrate **autosomal dominant** or **autosomal recessive** inheritance.

Autosomal Dominant (AD) Inheritance

1. *Classic characteristics.* For an allele to be characterized as dominant, only one copy of the abnormal gene is required for the individual to be affected. Both males and females are affected and may transmit the gene to offspring of either sex. Dominant conditions demonstrate "vertical transmission." A review of the pedigree shows the trait of interest passing from one generation to the next; or in the vernacular, "down the line."

Most people understand the concept of a trait being genetic if it "runs in the family." If a trait is found in a parent and is subsequently seen in their child, it tends to make sense. What is often very confusing to families is the concept of a condition being genetic when there is no other affected person in the family. This is particularly true for dominant conditions. For dominant conditions, affected offspring typically have affected parents. There are several clinical scenarios, however, in which a person is seen with a known autosomal dominant condition without an affected parent. In these settings, careful review of the family history and examination of key persons in the family may be necessary to sort things out.

In some cases, there is no affected parent, because there is a new mutation in the child (truly the first occurrence in the family). The occurrence of new (sporadic) dominant mutations has been reported in association with an advanced paternal age in many human genetic conditions. For example, achondroplasia is a rare skeletal dysplasia (Figure 6-18). The condition is associated with a disproportionately short stature described as rhizomelic shortening (the upper segments are more shortened) of the limbs. Persons with achondroplasia also have a relative macrocephaly. Achondroplasia is known to be an autosomal dominant condition. It is caused by mutations in a gene called fibroblast growth factor receptor 3 (FGFR3). When it is familial, typical vertical transmission in keeping with autosomal dominant inheritance is observed. But, 80% of children born with achondroplasia do not have an affected parent. In this setting it has been shown that this is due to the occurrence of new, sporadic mutations of the FGFR3 gene in the offspring. The occurrence of new mutations in achondroplasia is now known to be correlated with an advanced paternal age. Achondroplasia is not the only autosomal dominant (AD) condition shown to have a paternal age affect (Table 6-2). In fact, it is likely that sporadic mutations at all loci are increased with aging fathers. It is just that the AD conditions are more readily observed events.

The increased occurrence of new mutations with an advanced paternal age bears additional discussion. First, it is important to note that the new occurrence of abnormal genetic events increases with an advanced *parental* (both sexes) age. The association of an increased chance of *chromosomal non-disjunction* seen with an *advanced maternal age* was discussed in Chapter 5, Cytogenetics (Figure 6-19). Here we have discussed the increased chance of *single gene mutations* in association with an

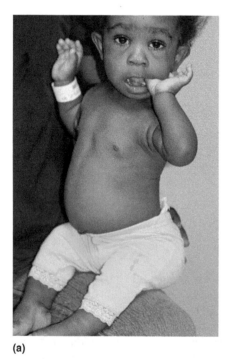

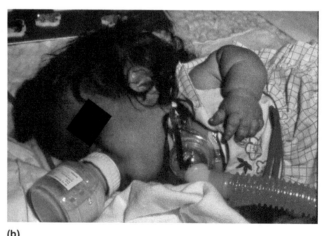

Figure 6-18. (a) Young girl with achondroplasia; (b) Female infant with homozygous achondroplasia.

Table 6-2.	Examples of Dominant Conditions With Documented Paternal Age Effect*

Achondroplasia

Apert syndrome

Marfan syndrome

Neurofibromatosis

Treacher–Collins syndrome

Crouzon syndrome

Progeria

*This phenomenon is probably true for all loci, but is most easily observed in dominant syndromes; Thompson, J.N., G.B. Schaefer, M.C. Conley, and C.G.N. Mascie-Taylor: Parental Age Can Affect the Severity of an Inherited Human Trait. (Letter) New Engl. J. Med., 314(8):521, 1986.

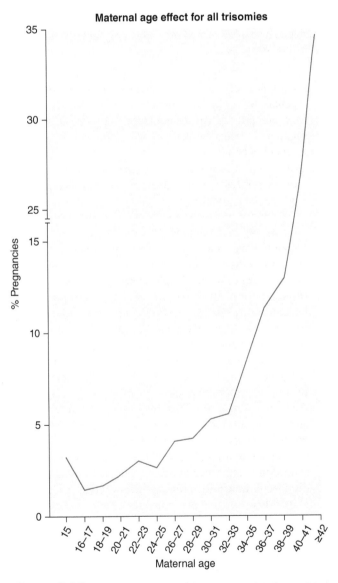

Figure 6-19. Increasing incidence of births with infants with all trisomies correlated with mother's age at the time of delivery. (Reprinted with permission from Crow JF, *Nat Rev Genet* 2000;1:40.)

advanced paternal age (Figure 6-20). Simply put, as the parent get older, the chances of genetic abnormalities in the offspring increases. In reality, the occurrence of birth defects as it relates to parental ages is a somewhat "J" shaped curve (Figure 6-21). There is an increased incidence of birth defects in particularly young parents—presumably due to different mechanisms. The lowest incidence of congenital anomalies is seen with parents who are between 18 to 30 years old. As the ages of the parents go beyond 30, the chances of birth defects starts to increase. Beyond 40 years old, the incidence rises asymptotically.

As we discussed earlier, the nature of the difference in genetic changes seen in men *versus* women lies in the physiology of gamete formation (Figures 6-22 and 6-23). A newborn female infant has only a few hundred thousand in her ovaries. These oocytes have started into meiosis, but have stopped the process in meiosis I. Meiosis I is not completed until ovulation, and meiosis II is not accomplished until fertilization. Thus, as mothers age their oocytes have remained in this state of suspended chromosome division for long periods of time. This presumably leads to a greater chance of meiotic error. Alternatively, men do not make mature sperm until puberty. Spermatozoa are made in the millions with a turnover rate around 60 days. Thus, the more sperms that are made, the greater the chance of a copy (transcription) error.

Besides the occurrence of spontaneous mutations, there are other reasons that a child affected with an AD condition may not have an affected parent. Possibilities include the parent carrying the gene but not expressing it (see incomplete penetrance below), or a parent having gonadal (germ line) mosaicism for a dominant mutation (discussed further in Chapter 12, Atypical Inheritance).

2. *Recurrence risks.* Consider the matings of an affected heterozygote for an autosomal dominant condition and a normal homozygote. There is a 50% chance that any given offspring will be affected and a 50% chance that it will be unaffected. Since the trait is autosomal, both sexes have the same probabilities.

For the rare matings of two affected heterozygotes, the recurrence risks for each offspring are as follows:

- 25% chance affected homozygote
- 50% chance affected heterozygote
- 25% chance normal homozygote
- Total recurrence risk for an affected child: 75%

3. *Special inheritance considerations.* In general, affected individuals of autosomal dominant conditions are heterozygotes. Since homozygous affected individuals are typically quite rare, the usual mating in dominantly inherited diseases is between a homozygous normal and a heterozygous affected individual. But, if the allele is sufficiently common in the population, matings between two heterozygous affected parents resulting in homozygous affected offspring are seen. **True (complete) dominance** implies that an identical phenotype is seen

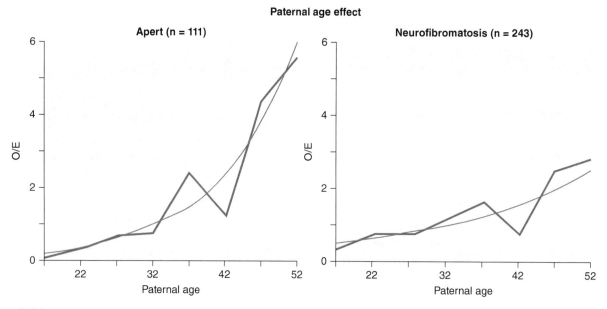

Figure 6-20. Graphs of increasing incidence of Apert syndrome and neurofibromatosis correlated with father's age at the time of delivery. O/E = observed / expected. (Reprinted with permission from Crow JF, *Nat Rev Genet* 2000;1:40.)

in those who are heterozygous or homozygous for the mutation. In other words, having only one copy of the abnormal allele produces the "full" phenotype. In the realm of human genetic conditions, few actually demonstrate complete dominance. Huntington disease (HD) is an autosomal dominant neurodegenerative condition. It is characterized by adult onset degeneration of the basal ganglia (Figure 6-24a). Correlated with these brain changes, patients with Huntington disease exhibit progressive neurologic symptoms that include involuntary and abnormal (choreiform) movements. Over time the progressive neurologic problems result in an early death. Studies in unique populations in which HD occurs in a high frequency have shown that HD demonstrates a true dominance pattern of inheritance. Another condition that has been shown to exhibit true dominance in its

inheritance is Best disease—also known as vitelliform macular dystrophy. Best disease (Figure 6-24b) is associated with progressive accumulation of lipofucsin in the pigmentary retinal epithelium with resultant vision loss. Evaluation of a large Swedish kindred dating back to the 17th century has also confirmed true dominance–with no identified differences in expression seen between heterozygotes and homozygotes.

The above examples, however, are the exceptions. In humans, affected homozygotes for dominant conditions typically have a more severe phenotype than do the heterozygotes. Achondroplasia, for example, is an autosomal dominant skeletal dysplasia briefly described earlier (Figure 6-18a). Heterozygotes with achondroplasia have the bony changes described for the condition, but have normal intelligence and a normal life expectancy. In the rare event that two individuals with achondroplasia mate, there is a 1 in 4 chance that the conception will result in homozygosity for the FGFR3 mutation for this condition. In homozygosity for achondroplasia, the bony changes are much more severe (Figure 6-18b) and are most often associated with death in infancy. In the strictest sense, then, achondroplasia is not a true dominant condition, but would be better described as semi-dominant. Since almost all human dominant conditions are transmitted this way, convention is simply to call them autosomal dominant.

Another variation on the theme of dominant inheritance is that of **co-dominance**. Co-dominance refers to the simultaneous expression of both alleles in a **compound heterozygote**. In this setting it is again important to remember the distinction between genotype and phenotype and to be aware of the level at which the phenotype is defined. Some of the better examples of co-dominance

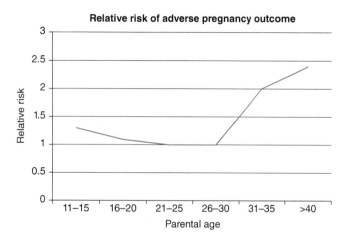

Figure 6-21. Overall incidence of birth defects with advancing parental age.

Figure 6-22. Diagram of ontogeny of male and female germ lines.

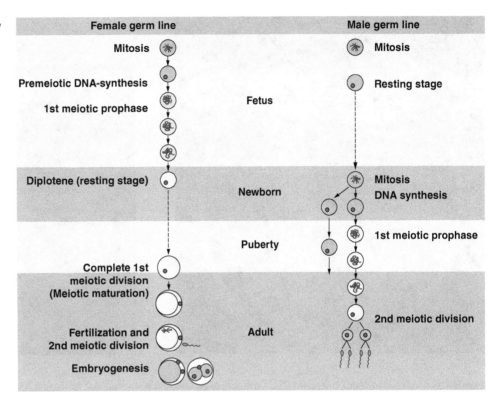

in plants and animals involve different genes that control coloration. In humans, examples of co-dominance are rare. In fact, the ABO and MN blood types as phenotypes are among the few conditions that have been shown to be co-dominant phenotypes in people.

Dominant conditions typically show some degree of **variable expression**. There are many possible causes

of variable expression including environmental factors, modifier genes, varying genetic backgrounds, and so forth. Variable expression (or **variability**) simply refers to the severity of the condition, i.e., to what degree is the person affected with the condition or "how much" the condition is manifest. The degree of variability differs from condition to condition. Some show a wide range

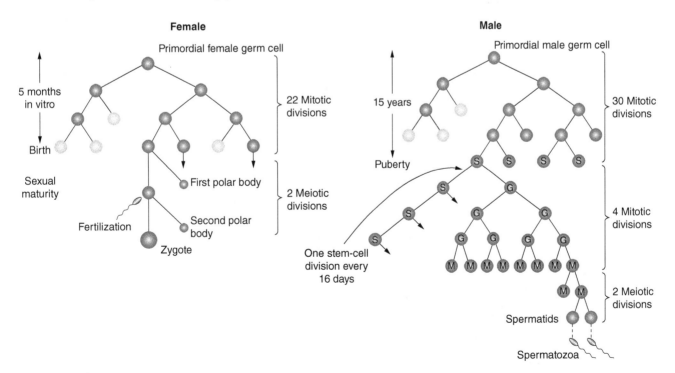

Figure 6-23. Cell divisions and gametogenesis. (Reprinted with permission from Crow JF, *Nat Rev Genet* 2000;1:40.)

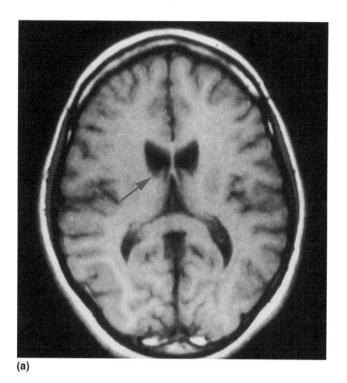

(a)

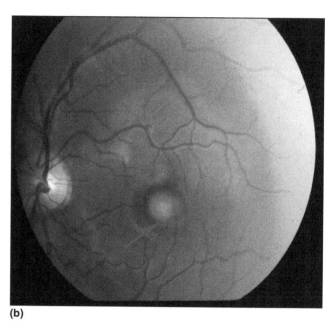

(b)

Figure 6-24. Two examples of conditions exhibiting 'true' dominant inheritance. (a) Brain MRI of a patient with Huntington disease. Arrow is pointing to area of marked degeneration of the basla ganglia. (b) Retinal photograph of a patient with Best disease (vitelliform macular degeneration). Arrow points to characteristic retinal abnormality—deposits of fatty material in the sub-retinal space, which creates a characteristic lesion resembling an egg yolk.

of variability, others much less. A given condition may also differ in the variability seen within a family (**intra-familial variability**) as compared to between different families (**inter-familial variability**).

As a side note, it is important to distinguish variable expression from **pleiotropism**. Although the terms refer to two distinctly different concepts, they are often confused. Pleiotropism (or pleiotropic effects) refers to having several different clinical manifestations of a single genetic change. For instance, Marfan syndrome is a heritable disorder of connective tissue (Figure 6-25). Marfan syndrome is caused by mutations in the gene that

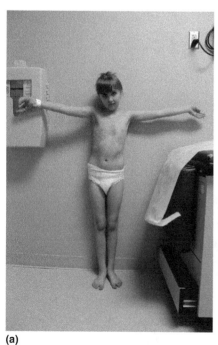

(a)

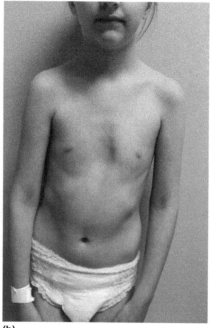

(b)

Figure 6-25. Young girl with Marfan syndrome.

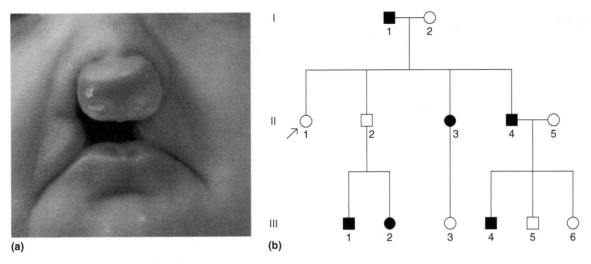

Figure 6-26. (a) Young child with van der Woude syndrome. Note the bilateral cleft lip and the lower lip pits. (b) Pedigree of a family with van der Woude syndrome. See text for details about incomplete penetrance.

codes for the protein fibrillin. Fibrillin is a microfibrillar protein that is a major component of the connective tissue of structures such as bones, eyes, skin, and larger blood vessels. As such, persons with Marfan syndrome can have problems with all of these tissues. They have a disproportionately tall stature, with the excessive length being in the limbs as compared to the trunk. They can have ocular changes, such as severe myopia, retinal detachments, and dislocations of the lenses. Their skin is hyperextensible, bruises easily, and exhibits poor wound healing. The most serious complication of the condition is progressive dilation of the root of the aorta, which if severe enough can lead to rupture and sudden death. In fact, in patients with untreated Marfan syndrome, the average life expectancy is under 30 years. All of the different problems listed above are due to the one genetic change (fibrillin mutation) and represent the pleiotropic effects seen from this mutation.

An individual who has the genotype for a disease may not exhibit the disease phenotype at all, even though he or she can transmit the disease gene to the next generation. As discussed in an earlier section, this is referred to as **incomplete penetrance**. Thus, incomplete penetrance represents the far extreme of variable expression, i.e., it is so mildly expressed that it is not even detectable. Some conditions are completely penetrant meaning that if you have the genotype you will definitely express the condition. But if a trait is incompletely penetrant, the degree of penetrance cannot be reasoned out or inferred. It must be determined by examining a large number of families to calculate what proportion of known heterozygotes (autosomal dominant, AD) or homozygotes (autosomal recessive, AR) develop the disease phenotype. With enough family data, a penetrance rate can be determined for a particular condition. A condition that is found to be 60%

penetrant, for example, means that 60% of persons with the mutant genotype will actually show clinical expression. The remaining 40% will have the same genotype without any clinical signs or symptoms of the condition.

Van der Woude syndrome (Figure 6-26a) is an autosomal dominant condition that has lower lip pits and clefting as major features. Both features are variably expressed. From extensive family data, the condition is also reported to be 80% penetrant. Figure 6.26b shows a pedigree of a family with van der Woude syndrome. First inspection of the pedigree suggests autosomal dominant transmission, which is in fact correct. But closer inspection of the pedigree shows an interesting phenomenon. Individual II.2 is an unaffected person but has two affected children. This person must then carry the van der Woude mutation but not be expressing it, i.e., showing incomplete penetrance.

In this particular family, an interesting question then came from individual II.1 (noted by the arrow on the pedigree). This lady wanted to know what her chances were of having a child affected with van der Woude syndrome. It would have been tempting to give her a recurrence risk of zero since she was unaffected. However, what she observed in her brother and his children made her realize that this is, in fact, was not the correct answer. So what is correct? To get to the correct answer, you need to apply logic, knowledge of inheritance patterns, and all available information about the condition. Since her father (I.1) is affected, she has a 50% chance of inheriting the gene. Since she is unaffected, she could only have an affected child if she has the mutation *and* is non-penetrant. Diagram out the possibilities if you need to. The chance that she inherited the mutation and does not show it is 1/6 (0.167). If she carries the gene, then there is a 50% chance that any of her children would inherit

Table 6-3.	Genetic Profiles (Descriptions) of Inheritance Characteristics of a Few Select Conditions		
Condition	Penetrance	Inter-Familial Variability	Intra-Familial Variability
Neurofibromatosis	Complete	High	High
Marfan syndrome	Complete	High	Limited
Split-hand/foot	Incomplete	High	High

the mutant gene, giving an overall probability of $0.167 \times 0.5 = 0.0835$. Finally, even if the child inherits the gene, the condition is only 80% penetrant. The actual risk of her having an affected child is $0.0835 \times 0.8 = 0.067$. So her risk for an affected child is 6.7%, not zero!

In order to provide families with the best available information, counseling must be based on the knowledge of all of the above parameters for the condition, although we grant that, for rare conditions, this information may be incomplete. Still, when counseling with families, information about expression and penetrance needs to be included. Each condition has its own specific "profile" of how it is typically transmitted. Table 6-3 gives just a few examples.

Autosomal Recessive (AR) Inheritance

1. *Classic characteristics.* As a group, recessive conditions are less common and show less variability in their expression than do dominant conditions. In contrast to dominant conditions, recessive conditions typically show "horizontal transmission." This means that the condition may be found in multiple individuals in the same generation, but are noted to be passed down the generations. Because the risk is only 1 in 4 that a child will be born to two carrier parents, and because most American families are small (2-3 children), most affected individuals with AR disorders will appear to be sporadic cases (only 1 case in a kindred). The most common presentation is one where the parents of an affected individual are both unaffected. Assessment of the genotypes would show that both parents are heterozygotes, or carriers of the condition. The family history would be negative except for the possibility of affected siblings, or the possibility of affected relatives due to consanguinity in the family.

2. *Recurrence risks.* For two heterozygotes, the recurrence risk to have an affected child is 25% per conception. The phenotypically normal siblings of an affected child have a 2/3 chance of carrying the recessive allele. This probability may not be immediately evident, but you need to understand the answer completely. It is an important clinical concept, and it appears frequently on standardized tests. It may be helpful to visualize a Punnett square. The reason that the answer is 2/3, instead of 2/4, is that one of

the possibilities (i.e., being affected and thus homozygous recessive) has already been eliminated, because of the information that the sib is phenotypically unaffected. Thus, of the three possible outcomes for each unaffected child, there is 1 out of 3 chance that the child will inherit neither abnormal allele and a 2 out of 3 chance of inheriting one copy, i.e., of being a carrier.

Occasionally a heterozygote (carrier) may mate with an affected homozygote. In this case each offspring has a 50% risk to be affected and a 50% risk to be a carrier. The pedigree in this situation would actually resemble autosomal dominant inheritance. This has been termed **quasi-dominance**. Quasi-dominant inheritance is more likely to occur with common autosomal recessive genes or in the case of parental consanguinity.

The mating of two affected homozygotes results in 100% of the offspring being homozygous affected. This situation is more likely to occur in situations of assortative mating, i.e., mating of phenotypically similar individuals. For example, the most common genetic cause of non-syndromic neurosensory hearing loss is an autosomal recessive mutation in any one of several genes. Persons that are deaf or hard of hearing often tend to find each other because of targeted social networking. As such, it is not at all uncommon for two deaf/hard of hearing persons to have children together. If the etiology of the hearing loss in both parents is caused by the same recessive gene, all of their children will have hearing loss as do their parents.

3. *Special inheritance considerations.* It is estimated that humans have approximately 22,000 functioning genes. It is also predicted that on average every person carries recessive mutations in 5 to 8 of these genes. In the case of random matings, then, the chance that both members of a couple happen to carry a recessive mutation of the same gene is relatively small. This then is the reason that recessive conditions tend to be seen less commonly than dominant conditions (Table 6-4). Still, there are a

Table 6-4.	Frequencies of a Few Selected Genetic Conditions
Dominant Condition	Prevalence
Neurofibromatosis	1:4500
Familial hypercholesterolemia	1:500
AD Polycystic kidney disease	1:200 to 1:1000
Marfan syndrome	1:5000
Recessive Condition	Prevalence
Phenylketonuria	1:17,000
Smith-Lemli-Opitz syndrome	1:30,000
AR Polycystic kidney disease	1:10,000 to 1:40,000
Cystic fibrosis	1:16,000

few situations in which recessive conditions occur more frequently than would be expected.

Consanguinity is defined as the mating of individuals with a close relationship by descent from a common ancestor. In simpler terms, it refers to the mating of closely related individuals. There are many important issues to consider in regards to consanguineous matings. There is, and always has been, a strong social stigma against consanguineous matings. Although there is probably no such thing as a universally accepted moral or ethical principle, consanguinity comes close. It is probably the nearest thing to a universal taboo that exists. Given the sensitive nature of the situation, the clinician must remain non-condemning if such information is revealed. Consanguinity as an event does not occur in an evenly-distributed manner. "Pockets" exist across the United States and the world in which consanguinity occurs at a significantly increased rate. Often geographic, cultural, or religious factors limit the pool of possible mates, making a consanguineous union much more likely.

Intuitively, it can be reasoned that the closer the degree of relationship exists for a couple, the more likely that a recessive condition might occur in their offspring. In defining the relative risk of consanguinity, one must first determine how close the relationship is. How closely persons are related can essentially be described by the number of intervening meioses between them (degrees). Thus, first degree relatives have only one meiosis between them. Figure 6-27 provides a graphic representation of degrees of relationship. This will be discussed in more detail in Chapter 9 on Family History and Pedigree Analysis. Mathematically, the degree of relationship can be expressed in several different ways. The **coefficient of inbreeding** (F) is the probability that an individual is homozygous at a given locus that is inherited from a common ancestor. For a pair of individuals, the **kinship coefficient** (φ) is equal to the

F of their offspring. The **coefficient of relationship** (R) estimates the proportion of genes shared by individuals with at least one common ancestor. Figure 6-28 demonstrates these concepts. While it is unlikely that the non-geneticist will spend time calculating these coefficients, it is helpful for any practitioner to understand the basic concepts of relatedness.

The major biological impact of consanguinity is to increase the risk of genetic abnormalities in the offspring. When defining relative risk, one must of course start at the baseline. For most purposes, a baseline risk of 4% can be used for the occurrence of congenital anomalies and 3% for mental retardation. In the event of a consanguineous union, published risks over these baselines are:

1. Third degree relative (e.g., first cousins): There is a 2% to 3% risk of mental retardation or a serious genetic condition in the offspring. These numbers come from recent data. This risk is significantly lower than the 10% estimates that were previously reported.

2. Second degree relative (e.g., half-siblings, uncle-niece): There is a 5% to 15% chance of "genetic abnormalities."

3. First degree relative (e.g., father-daughter, brother-sister): There is a:

   - 40% chance of an offspring with any "significant abnormality"
   - 12% chance of an autosomal recessive disorder
   - 16% chance of a congenital anomaly
   - 10% to 15% chance of significant cognitive impairments

Some recessive conditions occur at a higher frequency than would be predicted, because of a **heterozygote advantage.** A heterozygote advantage is seen when the carriers of a recessive disorder have a selective reproductive advantage, i.e., they are more likely to reproduce. Thus, even though the recessive disorder seen in the homozygotes may be serious or even fatal, the condition is perpetuated at a relatively high frequency in the population. The most commonly purported heterozygote advantage is that of sickle cell anemia (SSA). Patients who are affected with sickle cell (homozygote recessive) have a serious medical condition associated with abnormal hemoglobin molecules that result in an altered shape of the RBCs from the normal "donut" shape to a curvilinear or sickle-shaped cell (hence the name). The abnormally shaped RBCs do not flow smoothly through the small capillaries and produce multiple micro-infarcts in the tissues. Clinical symptoms due to these vascular occlusions include severe, incapacitating pain, congestion and destruction of the spleen, multiple somatic symptoms and poor growth. Sickle cell anemia occurs at a high frequency in people of African and Mediterranean descent. There is good evidence to suggest that the higher incidence of SSA in these groups is due to a heterozygote advantage. Although SSA is a serious condition, the heterozygous carriers (who typically

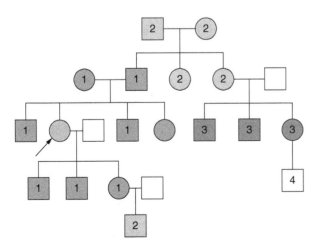

Figure 6-27. Sample pedigree demonstrating degrees of relationship to the proband (arrow).

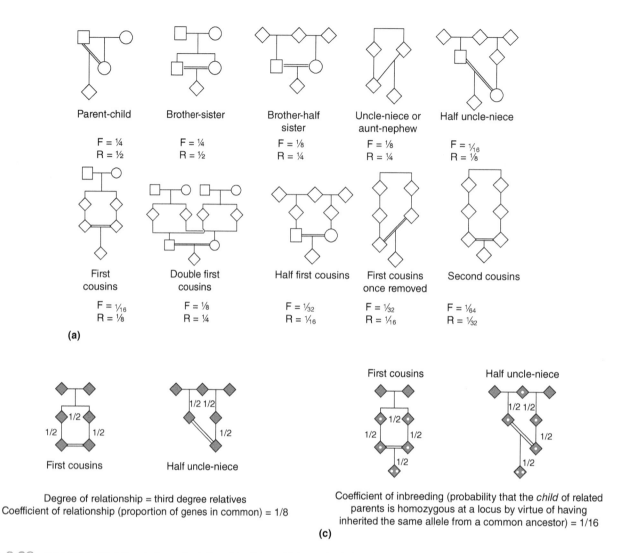

Figure 6-28. Examples of (a) the degree of relationship, (b) coefficient of relationship (R), and (c) coefficient of inbreeding (F) for selected consanguineous matings.

have no symptoms) appear to have an increased resistance to malaria and, thus, are more likely to reproduce in locations where malaria is endemic. Some other examples of heterozygote advantage that have been suggested are listed in Table 6-5. Recessive disorders may also occur at a frequency higher than would be predicted because of a **founder effect.** The founder effect refers to the over-representation of a particular allele seen in a population that originates from a relatively small group in which the allele frequency is not representative of the overall population.

Table 6-5.	Proposed Examples of Heterozygote Advantage (see text for explanation)			
Recessive Condition	**Gene**	**Gene Function**	**Heterozygote Advantage**	**Affected Populations**
Sickle cell anemia	β-Hemoglobin	Oxygen transport	Resistance to malarial infections	African, Mediterranean
Cystic fibrosis	CFTR	Chloride transporter	Resistance to secretory diarrhea Resistance to tuberculosis	Northern European
Smith-Lemli-Opitz syndrome	Dehydrocholesterol reductase	Cholesterol metabolism	Better vitamin D metabolism	Northern European
Homozygous lethal	Triosephosphate	Glycolysis isomerase	Resistance against oxidative stress	Eastern European
Carnitine-palmtyl	CPT1A	Transport of fatty acids (speculated)	Resistance to high fat diet	Potentially all Native Alaskans

The founder effect may also apply to dominant conditions. All of these concepts will be discussed in more detail in Chapter 15 in the discussions on population genetics.

Sex-Linked Inheritance

Sex-linked inheritance refers to the inheritance patterns that are different than those described earlier for autosomal inheritance, due to the fact that the locus in question resides on either the X or the Y chromosome. These differences are due to variant structure and functions of these two chromosomes as compared to the 22 autosomes (see Chapter 5). **Y-linked inheritance,** also referred to as **holandric inheritance**, is of limited clinical significance. The Y chromosome contains few functioning genes. Most of these are genes that have something to do with sex determination. That is, they are genes which, if present, will shift gonadal differentiation from the default ovarian development to testicular development. The nature of this is, therefore, that a transmittable trait typically does not occur. To date there has not been a true Y-linked phenotypic feature seen in humans. The often purported example of "hairy ears" is more likely an autosomal trait with sex-limited expression. If a Y-linked condition were identified, the hallmark inheritance pattern would be that of exclusive male-to-male transmission.

X-linked inheritance is seen when the locus in question resides on the X chromosome. The X chromosome is one of the larger chromosomes and contains hundreds of functioning genes (estimated at 900–1400). In humans, the fact that females have two X chromosomes and males only one leads to a difference in expression of X-linked conditions between the sexes. Mutant alleles on the X chromosome are fully expressed in males, who have only a single X chromosome, i.e., are **hemizygous** for X-linked genes. Thus, for almost all X-linked conditions, males exhibit a more severe phenotype than females carrying the same mutation. This phenomenon is also part of the reason that certain conditions, such as mental retardation, occur much more often in males than in females (males have four times the incidence of mental retardation than females).

Lyonization (X-chromosome inactivation, see Chapter 5) is an important determinant of the degree of phenotypic expression of X-linked mutations in females. Functionally, women are mosaic for the expression of X-linked genes. For each cell the expression is dependent on which X chromosome is active and which is not. In general, the process of X-inactivation occurs early enough in embryogenesis that pattern of expression is actually clonal (in patches). Depending on the genetic change in question, the pattern of X-chromosome inactivation can sometimes actually be mapped (Figure 6-29). An example of this is hypohydrotic ectodermal dysplasia, a disorder caused by mutations of an X-linked gene EDA1 (Xq12-13). In this condition, changes in the ectodermal derivates cause problems with the skin, hair, teeth, and nails. The most serious medical consequence of this condition is that affected males will have a paucity of sweat glands. Inadequate sweating can lead to dramatic overheating of the core body temperature resulting in brain

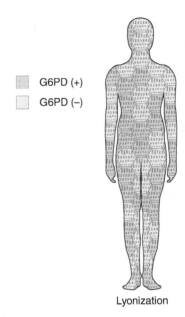

☐ G6PD (+)
☐ G6PD (–)

Lyonization

Figure 6-29. Schematic showing an expression map of glucose-6-dehydrogenase deficiency in female carriers of this X-linked disorder.

injury or death. Using a simple staining technique, sweat glands can be visualized (Figure 6-30). Female heterozygotes of this condition can be shown to have clonal patches of normal and abnormal density of sweat glands (the normal being around 250 pores per square centimeter).

In theory, Lyonization should be random. If so, the ratio of expression of the two X chromosomes should be on average 1:1. As discussed in Chapter 5, certain situations can produce a **skewed X-chromosome inactivation** ratio (i.e., significantly deviating from the expected 1:1 ratio). If a female heterozygote happens to have a significantly skewed inactivation ratio such that a larger proportion of the X chromosome containing the *normal* allele is inactivated, she will tend to exhibit clinical findings beyond what is usually seen. The higher the degree of skewing that occurs, the closer the phenotype approaches that of an affected male. Duchenne muscular dystrophy (DMD) is an X-linked muscle disease. Boys with this condition show a progressive degeneration of muscle that leads to weakness (Figure 6-31). Worsening weakness leads to problems with ambulation, then respiration, and ultimately an early death with an average life expectancy that is currently around 20 years old. One of the hallmark clues to the diagnosis is a marked elevation in a serum enzyme known as creatine phosphokinase (CPK or CK). Elevations of this enzyme correlate with the degree of muscle deterioration. Many men with DMD will also have a dilated cardiomyopathy; the heart being an additional muscle involved. Duchenne dystrophy has been known for decades as exhibiting X-linked recessive inheritance. Traditionally it has been characterized as being asymptomatic or non-expressing in carrier females. Clinical experience in following these families over time has, however, shown that partial expression can occur in carrier

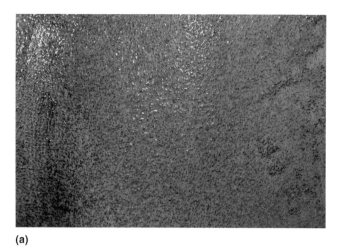

(a)

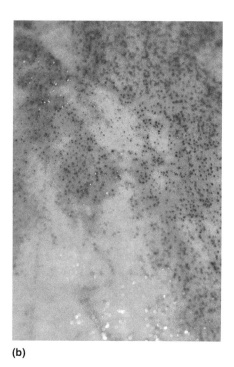

(b)

Figure 6-30. (a) Iodine-starch painting of the skin in a normal female. The black "dots" represent individual sweat glands. Note the well developed and evenly distributed placement of the sweat glands. (b) Iodine-starch painting of the skin in a female heterozygous for a mutation in the gene EDA1. Note the clonal patches of skin showing decreased numbers of sweat glands.

females. Some may exhibit a cardiomyopathy with middle age onset. Others may have milder elevations in their CK levels with a few even demonstrating muscle weakness or wasting. The partial expression of signs and symptoms in female carriers of DMD is explained, at least in part, by skewed X-inactivation.

A few other important principles of sex-linked inheritance are worth mentioning here. When reviewing a pedigree in attempting to define the likely mode of inheritance, one of the first things to note is the pattern of transmission related to the sexes of the parents and offspring. Fathers must transmit their Y chromosome to their sons; thus, there is no male-to-male transmission of X-linked genes. Again, Y-linked inheritance is highly unlikely to present as a clinically significant issue. As with autosomal traits, X-linked conditions may be recessive or dominant depending on the phenotypic threshold

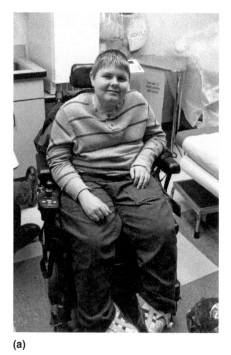

(a)

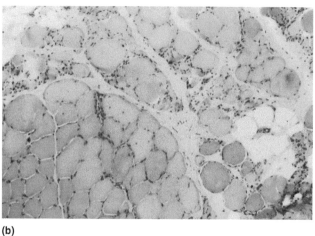

(b)

Figure 6-31. (a) Young boy with Duchenne muscular dystrophy. (b) Muscle biopsy of Duchenne muscular dystrophy. Muscle shows "dystrophic" changes with variable fiber size and staining. Centrally located nuclei are also seen.

that is defined. One important clinical question that arises has to do with the new occurrence of a condition that is known to be X-linked. In other words, what about the situation of a male in the family affected with an X-linked condition in which there are no other affected individuals? Where did the mutation originate? One obvious possibility is that the mutation is a new event in the egg responsible for his conception.

Alternatively, the mutation could be present in the mother and she is asymptomatic. In this case the mutation could have started with her, or even in the generation(s) before her. Empiric data have shown that in the event of a new X-linked mutation in an affected male in the family, there is a 2/3 chance that the mother is a carrier, and, of course, a 1/3 chance that the affected male represents a new (sporadic) mutation.

X-linked Recessive (XLR) Inheritance

1. *Classic characteristics.* As noted above, the nature of X-linked conditions is such that expression in females typically is less severe than for males. There are, however, a few notable exceptions as will be discussed in the Clinical Correlation section. X-linked recessive conditions, then, are those in which the threshold for expression is such that the condition is rarely expressed clinically in heterozygous females, but full expression is seen in males; i.e., only males are affected.

2. *Recurrence risks.* In the usual mating between a heterozygous carrier female and a normal male, the risks for offspring are as follows:

   - 25% chance affected male
   - 25% chance unaffected male
   - 25% chance carrier female (unaffected)
   - 25% chance noncarrier female (unaffected)
   - Total risk for an affected child: 25%

   Another type of mating that might occur is between an affected male and a homozygous normal female. The risks for offspring of this mating are as follows:

   - All males unaffected
   - All females obligate carriers
   - Total: 50% chance normal male, 50% chance carrier female

3. *Special inheritance considerations.* A classic characteristic of X-linked recessive disorders is that females are unaffected. There are, however, special circumstances under which a female may actually express such a condition. There are several known reasons for the observation of the rare expression of X-linked recessive traits in females.

   - If the abnormal allele is common enough in the population, female homozygosity for an X-linked mutation may occur.
   - Female hemizygosity of an X-linked mutation can occur in women with Turner syndrome.

   - In the event of an X-chromosome/autosome translocation with resulting deleted X-chromosome material, there is preferential inactivation of the normal X. This results in the woman being hemizygous for the deleted region.
   - If there is random significant skewed Lyonization of the X bearing a normal allele, a female heterozygote may show variable degrees of expression that correlates with the relative proportion of normal X's expressed.
   - A female may appear to be affected due to an autosomal **phenocopy** of the X-linked disorder (locus heterogeneity).

X-linked Dominant (XLD) Inheritance

1. *Classic characteristics.* In X-linked dominant conditions, males and females can both be affected. Within kindreds, the number of affected individuals should be equal between the two sexes. Typically the clinical expression is more consistent and severe in hemizygous males than in heterozygous females. In heterozygous females, the variability of expression is often quite broad. Depending on the condition, the severity of expression in males can be that of lethality (incompatible with postnatal life). In these kindreds no affected males are seen, but a disproportionate number of live-born females are seen. For example, Aicardi syndrome (Figure 6-32) is an X-linked dominant condition. The condition demonstrates male lethality. Affected females present with no dysmorphic features, marked neurodevelopmental delays, and difficult to control seizures. Evaluation of these girls shows agenesis of the corpus callosum and markedly abnormal ocular findings. Reported ocular findings include optic atrophy, optic nerve coloboma, chorioretinopathy, chorioretinal lacunae, retinal detachment, cataract, and nystagmus.

2. *Recurrence risks.* X-linked dominant inheritance segregates according to the X chromosome with dominant (single abnormal allele) inheritance.

   In the mating of an affected male with a normal female, assuming no male lethality:

   - All daughters will be affected.
   - All sons will be normal.

   In the mating of an affected female with a normal male:

   - Each daughter and each son has a 50% chance of being affected.

3. *Special inheritance considerations.* The distinction between dominant and recessive inheritance patterns may not always be clear. This is particularly true for X-linked conditions. In some X-linked conditions, mild expression in carrier females is common, and is sometimes referred to as "semi-dominance." Hypohydrotic ectodermal dysplasia is a disorder of the derivatives of

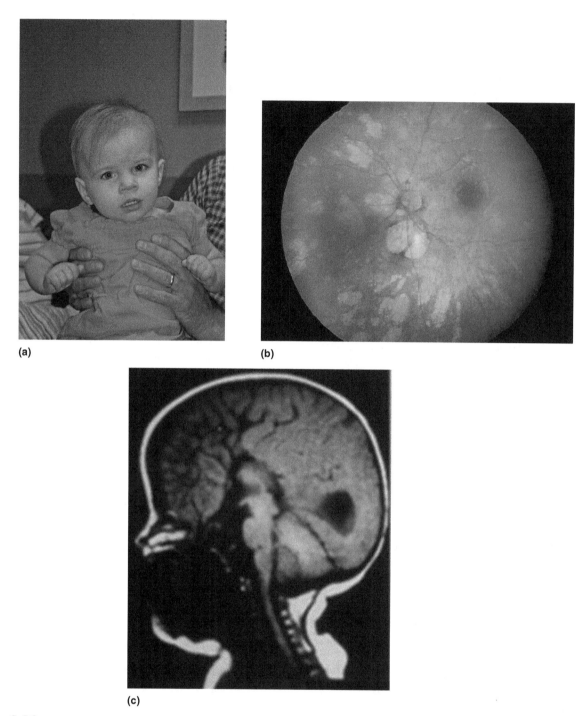

Figure 6-32. Young girl with Aicardi syndrome. She has severe developmental delays and difficult to control seizures. (a) Normal facies (i.e., not dysmorphic). (b) Retinal photograph showing multiple retinal abnormalities. (c) Sagittal MRI of brain showing agenesis of the corpus callosum.

the embryonic ectoderm (skin, hair, nails and teeth). The condition is genetically heterogeneous, the most common form being due to mutations in an X-linked gene, EDA1. The condition is typically classified as an X-linked recessive disorder. Males with this condition exhibit full expression with poor growth and function of the affected tissues. If female carriers of this condition are carefully evaluated, subtle findings of this condition are often detected. They may be noted to sweat less than expected (somewhat subjective) and often have dental abnormalities. This makes the classification of the condition as XLR debatable. It might better be described as XLD (X-linked dominant), but it is not at all clear where to "draw the line"!

Craniofrontonasal dysplasia (CFND) is a disorder primarily seen in females. The phenotype is quite dramatic (Figure 6-33). The fully expressed phenotype is pleiotropic with multiple somatic manifestations. As the name of the condition implies, the craniofacial features are a key set of findings. Affected females have a short skull base (brachycephaly), premature fusion (synostosis) of the coronal cranial sutures, extremely wide-spaced eyes (hypertelorism), a protruberant forehead (frontal bossing), a "widow's peak" configuration to the frontal hairline, down-slanting angle to the eyes, and a wide or bifid nasal tip. Other reported anomalies include oro-facial clefting and peripheral skeletal changes (short neck, sloping shoulders, Sprengel anomaly, brachydactyly and/or syndactyly [short and/ or fused digits]). Patients with CFND have normal intelligence.

Although there may be genetic heterogeneity for this condition, most of the cases can be shown to be due to mutations in

a gene designated as Ephrin-B (EPHB1). This gene is a member of the Eph family of receptor protein-tyrosine kinases. The gene is on the X chromosome at location Xq21.

A fascinating aspect of this condition is that even though this is due to an X-linked gene, males who have a (hemizygous) mutation of the Ephrin-B gene have a phenotype that is actually milder than that seen in females. Indeed, males with EPHB1 mutations may have no somatic features whatsoever. Some may have subtle facial features similar to, but milder than, females. Interestingly, there are a few features seen in males that do not occur in the females, such as short stature, pectus excavatum, anomalies of the clavicles, minor genital anomalies, and diaphragmatic hernias.

The nature of the X-linked basis of this is often evident on review of the pedigrees of some larger families (Figure 6-34).

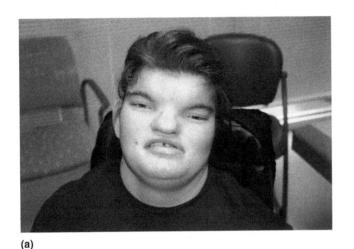
(a)

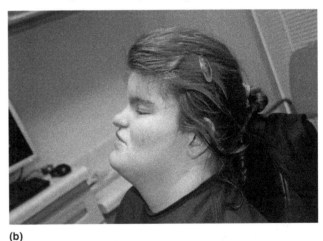
(b)

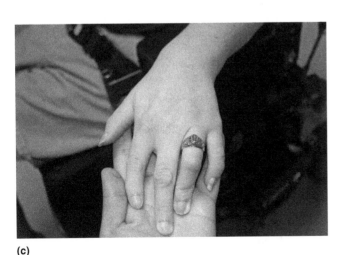
(c)

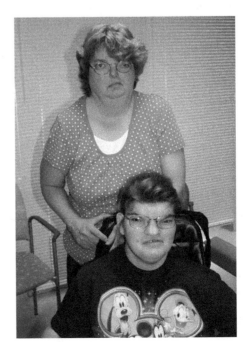
(d)

Figure 6-33. (a – c) Adolescent female with craniofrontonasal dysplasia demonstrating classic facial and digital changes. This young lady has a documented EPHB1 mutation. (d) Patient and her affected mother.

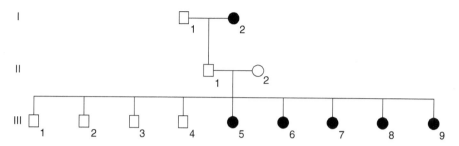

Figure 6-34. Pedigree of a kindred with craniofrontonasal dysplasia. Note that individual II.1 is an obligate hemizygous carrier. He has no discernable phenotypic features. The outcomes in his children are completely reflective of the gene being X-linked. All of his daughters and none of his sons were affected.

Apparently unaffected males who do have an EPHB1 mutation will show the expected outcome of having all of their daughters affected and none of their sons affected.

To date, no known explanation has been put forth to explain this unique pattern of inheritance of X-linked dominant inheritance with female predominant expression.

■ Chapter 6 Board-Format Practice Questions

1. In chickens there is a known gene that determines the type of tail and neck plumage. *Cock-feathering* is more long and curved, while *hen-feathering* is more short and rounded. This gene is not on a sex chromosome. The genotype–phenotype relationship is described below:

Genotype	Phenotype in females	Phenotype in males
HH	Hen-feathered	Hen-feathered
Hh	Hen-feathered	Hen-feathered
hh	Hen-feathered	Cock-feathered

In this example, the inheritance that most likely exhibits cock feathering is
A. recessive with sex-limited phenotype.
B. dominant with sex-limited phenotype.
C. semi-dominance.
D. co-dominance.
E. mitochondrial.

2. Parental age effects on the incidence of genetic disorders include
A. lower incidence of genetic disorders in the offspring of older parents.
B. increased incidence of chromosome aneuploidy with advanced paternal age.
C. increased incidence of single gene mutations with advanced maternal age.
D. increased incidence of non-disjunction with advanced maternal age.
E. decreased incidence of transcription errors with advanced paternal age.

3. Patients with Smith-Lemli-Opitz (SLO) syndrome exhibit many clinical features including mental retardation, an unusual facial appearance, genital abnormalities, and syndactyly (fusion of the digits). Patients with SLO tend to be similar in their features. SLO is an autosomal recessive condition. All heterozygotes will have expression. There is only one gene known to be responsible for this condition. This condition shows
A. highly variable phenotype.
B. locus heterogeneity.
C. pleiotropism.
D. thresholding.
E. Lyonization.

4. The one feature that is most helpful in determining in a pedigree if a particular condition, which was occurring in multiple generations of a family is likely to be X-linked dominant rather than autosomal dominant is
A. females affected more severely than males.
B. lack of female-to-female transmission.
C. more males affected than females.
D. all daughters of affected males are affected.
E. condition not appearing in any descendants of affected males.

5. Although there are exceptions to every rule, certain generalizations do apply to inheritance patterns. When comparing disorders that have dominant inheritance compared to those that have recessive inheritance, it is generally true that
A. dominant conditions occur less frequently.
B. dominant conditions show more variability of expression.
C. incomplete penetrance is a characteristic of recessive disorders.
D. pleiotropism only occurs in dominant conditions.
E. dominant conditions are often holandric in nature.

Mutation

CHAPTER SUMMARY

In earlier chapters, we saw how genes produce the enzymes that control specific biochemical reactions. Normal development depends on these information coding and regulatory systems working properly. But DNA replication is not perfect. Biochemical mistakes happen. Most replication errors are corrected by repair enzymes, but those that are missed become new mutations. In the broadest sense, then, a mutation is a heritable genetic change passed from one cell to another. For that reason, the biochemical correction mechanisms that work in parallel with replication are important for biological continuity.

Unfortunately, repair systems themselves can mutate, as in a patient with xeroderma pigmentosum (Figure 7-1). These patients have an increased mutation rate, as seen for example in higher rates of skin cancer, because of an inability to repair genetic damage caused by ultraviolet radiation. Other kinds of mutation repair deficiency are also known. Clearly, mutation rate is not a mathematical constant. Mutation rates can change.

Consider the following question. Would it be good if the process of mutation could be reduced? Would it be better if no new genetic changes ever occurred again? At first thought, the logical answer would probably be "yes." Eliminating mutation would be good. When you consider the many who must deal with developmental or physiological disabilities due to harmful mutations, it is easy to see the negative side of the process. But the environment in which we live is not constant. We continue to face new biologic challenges. Exposure to novel disease pathogens is only one obvious example. Physiological processes allow us to respond to changes in the environment. But genetic diversity adds another mechanism of response. In theory, therefore, the genetic diversity created by mutation may be fundamentally good—at least for the long-term survival of the species.

One way to think about this question is to consider biochemical pathways controlled by proteins under **allosteric** regulation. Binding with cofactors can change protein conformation within limits affected by environmental variables like temperature. A heterozygote for a key regulatory step can produce alternate protein forms with slightly different temperature optima. For that reason, a heterozygote is better able to handle the range of environmental conditions it naturally encounters. This can lead to the establishment of a **polymorphism** (literally "poly," many or multiple; "morph," forms). In such situations, there is not just one single form that is truly the "normal" or "wild type," since different forms may be best for different geographical conditions or seasons. Without mutation to generate new variation, the diversity of a gene pool will deteriorate. In fact, many species are on the verge of extinction, because their population size is so small that rare mutation can no longer replace the genetic diversity eroded by random processes.

Mutation is fundamentally intrinsic to the imperfect mechanism of DNA replication. But can the spontaneous **mutation rate** change? It might surprise you to learn that the answer is "yes," an answer that would have surprised most geneticists even a short time ago. The biochemistry of DNA replication is complex. Errors occur. We have already mentioned the important role that genetic repair enzymes play in correcting some of these errors. But in addition to loss of function by mutation, as in xeroderma pigmentosum, our repair mechanisms themselves can vary in efficiency so mutation rates change. Experimental evidence comes from many sources, including the improved efficiency in DNA repair found in organisms that live in highly mutagenic environments like the radioactive waste near uranium mines. Thus, mutation rate can be modified to some degree by influencing repair efficiency.

Clearly, there is a long-term benefit to the population from producing a low background level of genetic variation by mutation. But typically our medical focus is on the harmful consequence of mutations for a patient. In this chapter we will explore some of the common molecular mechanisms that lead to heritable genetic change.

Part 1: Background and Systems Integration

Types of Mutation

Mutations are heritable genetic changes. They occur both in the nuclear genome and in the DNA of organelles like mitochondria. Mutations of chromosome structure have already been discussed in Chapter 5, so our focus here will be on **point mutations**, that is changes at the base pair level within a gene or its control regions (Table 7-1). Such mutations can be viewed from different perspectives, like the type of nucleotide change or the effect of that change on coding outcomes.

There are several ways to change a nucleotide pair (Figure 7-2), so that one base is substituted for another.

A **transition** mutation occurs when one purine is replaced by the other purine (A ↔ G), or one pyrimidine is replaced by the other pyrimidine (T ↔ C). In a **transversion** mutation, on the other hand, a purine is replaced with a pyrimidine, or vice versa. Because of the degeneracy of the genetic code we discussed earlier, a transition mutation at the third position may often have no effect on the amino acid that is incorporated into the final protein. Such a mutation can be called a **silent mutation**. In contrast, transversion mutations usually cause a change in the amino acid. Since any change is more likely to be bad than it is to be good, transversion mutations are less

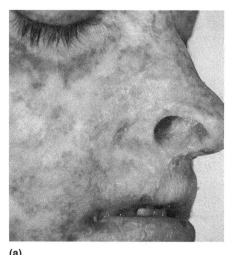

(a)

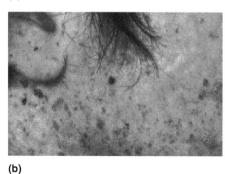

(b)

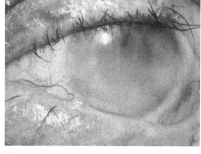

(c)

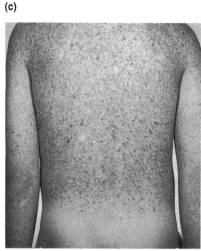

(d)

Figure 7-1. An individual showing the effects of xeroderma pigmentosum, a defect in one of the genes involved in the process of nucleotide excision repair. Individuals with this condition are unable to repair UV-induced mutations, which gives them a predisposition to skin cancer and related problems. (Reprinted with permission from Rünger TM, DiGiovanna JJ, Kraemer KH: Chapter 139. Hereditary Disorders of Genome Instability and DNA Repair. In: Goldsmith LA, Katz SI, Gilchrest BA, Paller AS, Leffell DJ, Dallas NA, eds. *Fitzpatrick's Dermatology in General Medicine*. 8th ed. New York: McGraw-Hill; 2012.)

Table 7-1.	Types of Point Mutations
Type	**Example**
Base substitution	5′ – C T T A **G** C T A G – 3′ → 5′ – C T T A **A** C T A G – 3′ 3′ – G A A T **C** G A T C – 5′ 3′ – G A A T **T** G A T C – 5′
Transition	one purine is changed to the other purine, or one pyrimidine is changed to the other pyrimidine; the example above is a transition mutation (G to A)
Transversion	a purine is changed to a pyrimidine, or vice versa
Base addition	5′ – C T T A G C T A G – 3′ → 5′ – C T T A G **A** C T A G – 3′ 3′ – G A A T C G A T C – 5′ 3′ – G A A T C **T** G A T C – 5′
Base deletion	5′ – C T T **A** G C T A G – 3′ → 5′ – C T T G C T A G – 3′ 3′ – G A A T C G A T C – 5′ 3′ – G A A C G A T C – 5′

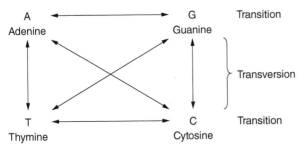

Figure 7-2. Transition mutations involve substituting one purine for the other, or one pyrimide for the other. Transversion mutations occur when a purine is substituted for a pyrimidine or vice versa.

likely to remain long in the population. A base change that translates as a change in an amino acid is called a **missense mutation**. They change the encoded information. A base change that results in a stop codon (UAA, UAG, or UGA) is called a **nonsense mutation**.

A base deletion or base addition involves the loss or gain, respectively, of one or more nucleotides. If the affected number of nucleotides is not divisible by three (in other words, if it does not involve one or more complete codons), the triplet reading frame is shifted for the remainder of gene translation. Such a **frameshift mutation** can dramatically alter the amino acid makeup of the protein. It also often results in a stop triplet (a nonsense mutation) soon after the point of the frameshift and leads to early termination of translation.

Mutations that change an amino acid in a protein can differ in the impact they have on development. At the least severe end of the spectrum, the amino acid change does not alter the protein's function in any important way. A change from one small hydrophilic amino acid to another in a non-active part of the protein is a real change, but it is unlikely to have much impact. That can be described as a **neutral mutation**. Sometimes the change is expressed under some conditions, but not others; its expression is **conditional**. The altered protein might change in the way it works in different temperatures or different chemical environments. The mutations that have medical significance, however, generally alter biological function in

critical ways. They are classed as **deleterious mutations**. At the most extreme are those that affect such a critical aspect of biological function that life cannot continue. **Lethal mutations** cause death at a point in development where their function becomes crucial. Many act very early in development, but some act fairly late or even into adulthood.

As we saw in our earlier discussions of gene expression, a developmental step often involves the interaction of more than one protein. Occasionally a second mutation can balance, and thus essentially "repair," the effect of the first. Compensating, or **suppressor**, mutations can even occur within the same gene. The combination of potential changes is almost endless. For that reason, one must keep an open mind to the events that might explain a particular case. The relationship between genes and phenotypes is complex.

Frequency versus Rate

The terms "mutation frequency" and "mutation rate" are often used interchangeably. That is a mistake. They refer to two distinctly different things. **Mutation frequency** refers to the proportion of alleles of a given type in the gene pool. One might say, for example, that the frequency of melanism (black color) in Malasian leopards is almost 50%. Depending on the context, a statement like this could refer either to the proportion of alleles of that type in the gene pool or how often the trait is seen in members of the population. Typically, the reference will be clear from the context. **Mutation rate**, on the other hand, refers to the rate at which new mutant alleles are formed, and it is reported at different scales. One can talk about the mutation rate per nucleotide, per gene, per gamete, per generation, or some other molecular level or developmental scale. Thus, mutation frequency is a measure of existing genetic diversity and is generally easier to measure than mutation rate. The effects of selection pressure, population size, magnitude of developmental effect, and other factors mean that mutation frequency and mutation rate are not necessarily even correlated.

The first direct measure of a human mutation rate was based on DNA sequence comparisons from the human Y chromosome: one mutation per 30 million base pairs (3.3×10^{-8} mutations/bp). This is in the same range as estimates from more traditional surveys of mutant phenotypes. Although different genes have slightly different mutation rates that can range in magnitude because of factors like gene size (number of base pairs that can change), a typical average rate is about 1×10^{-5} to 1×10^{-6} mutations per gene per generation. In addition to gene size, the measurement of mutation rate can be affected by factors like mutational hotspots, which are areas of increased mutational activity. But even these cases do not paint a complete picture of the difficulties encountered in mutation detection. Silent, neutral, and conditional mutations, by definition, are not clinically obvious. Mutation tests are not done on people who meet the definition of being normal or healthy. Thus, the detection of mutant phenotypes generally uncovers only a portion of the real underlying genetic diversity of the gene pool.

Sample estimates of mutation rate in humans include achondroplasia, 4.2 to 14.3×10^{-5}; aniridia, 0.5×10^{-5}; and retinoblastoma, 1.2 to 2.3×10^{-5}. In contrast, the rate for the dystrophin gene, which is mutated in Duchenne and Becker muscular dystrophies, is as high as about 1×10^{-4}. This high rate is not surprising when one realizes this is one of the largest genes known.

Several factors complicate the estimation of mutation rates. For example, retinoblastoma has a penetrance of 80% or less, so there is a problem of ascertainment involved in its detection. When a mutation is not expressed in some individuals, it may only be identified in pedigrees. Other altered phenotypes, indeed perhaps most of them, are due to several different loci with similar phenotypic expressions. For that reason, data about which specific gene has mutated may be unreliable without molecular support. But the range of rates cited here will at least give us a working basis on which to discuss predictive models.

There is another interesting factor that can affect mutation. Its rate may not be the same in both sexes. Indeed, this is known to be true in experimental organisms like *Drosophila*. But in humans, it is difficult to measure mutation rate accurately in most parts of the genome. Mutations are rare and, especially if they are recessive, they may be hard to detect. Yet, careful studies of the pseudoautosomal region shared by the human X and Y chromosomes show that mutation rate may be higher in males than in females.

Before passing from this general discussion of mutation rate and frequency into more specific aspects of genetic instability, we should take another look at the concept of mutation rate. Superficially, this is a straightforward measurement of the occurrence of a new mutation. But this seemingly simple concept is actually much more complex. One can begin to appreciate this by considering the genetic events that can occur between the establishment of the germ-line cells in embryonic testes and ovaries and the eventual gametes produced in the sexually mature adult (Figure 7-3). If we think for a moment about mutation as a genetic error, there are actually three different phases to consider. The literature sometimes confuses things by equating them. But they are definitely not the same.

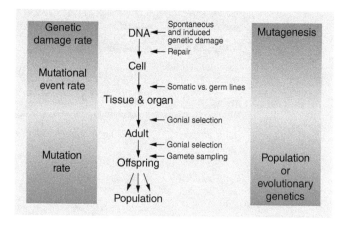

Figure 7-3. Three different levels at which one can assess mutation: the "genetic damage rate" during DNA replication has many errors, but most are repaired; the unrepaired changes are the measured as the "mutational event rate"; and the changes that actually enter the gene pool are represented in the classical "mutation rate," which can include multiple identical copies of an earlier genetic change, a cluster, due to mitotic replication in the germ cell line. (Reprinted from Thompson et al: *Environ. Molec. Mutagenesis* 1998;32:292-300).

First, the **genetic damage rate** is the rate at which errors occur during the process of DNA replication. Mispairing of nucleotides and single- and double-strand DNA breaks are very common. But efficient repair mechanisms identify and correct most of the errors. The **mutational event rate** measures what is left after repair has taken place. Many people incorrectly assume that this is the rate of new mutation that is estimated experimentally from population data and pedigrees. But in fact, a new mutation occurring early in the growth of testis and ovary tissue (i.e., long before meiosis begins) can be replicated during cell division so that many cells in the growing gonad carry the same new mutation. Then, when meiosis finally begins, many eggs or sperm may carry a copy of the same original new mutation (gonadal mosaicism). **Mutation rate** is typically measured by counting the number of new members of a population that carry a particular genetic change. The measured mutation rate will, therefore, be higher if a single early premeiotic mutation event has been duplicated into a number of gametes yielding a cluster of related individuals carrying the same new mutation. Clusters of mutation have now been documented in humans and in many other organisms. Thus, the genetic damage rate, the mutational event rate, and the traditional mutation rate can be very different. They vary independently as a function of mutation-generating factors and repair efficiency.

What Is a Polymorphism?

We highlight this question, because there is an important difference in the way the concept of **polymorphism** is interpreted in specialty areas of genetics. Being aware of this can help avoid serious confusion. The term "polymorphism" was first used to describe genetic diversity studied by population geneticists. In that field, by definition, a polymorphism occurs when the most common allele is at a frequency of less than 99%. That cut-off value is important. Mathematically, it is unlikely for a mutant allele to have a frequency of 1% or more unless it has some advantage under some environmental conditions. When a population geneticist finds a polymorphism, the next question is "What advantage keeps the rare form so common?"

On the other hand, in a clinical setting, the term is used in a more general way. There, "polymorphism" can refer to any gene or nucleotide in which more than one form is found in the population. Frequency is not important. In a clinical laboratory report, an identifiable genetic change from the accepted standard sequence will be defined as a "benign polymorphism" having no clinical relevance, a "mutation," or a "change of unknown clinical significance." The focus is on individual patients, rather than on the population or gene pool. The takeaway lesson is, therefore, to be aware of the context of usage and not be confused if different sources use the term in ways that appear inconsistent.

Measurement of Mutation Rate in Model Organisms

It is difficult to measure mutation rate directly in humans. Pre-existing genetic diversity in our gene pool and the inability to carry out definitive experimental matings are limiting factors, as is the length of our life cycle. Obviously, one cannot argue such an experimental approach seriously. It is not surprisingly, therefore, that most of our understanding of the mutation process comes from studies in model organisms. To illustrate the approaches that are possible in the large field of mutagenesis, we will explore the logic behind three classical methods: the Ames test with bacteria, the X-linked lethal assay in *Drosophila* that led to a Nobel Prize for H.J. Muller, and the seven-locus test in mice. The key to an effective assay system is, of course, that a lot of data can be collected efficiently and inexpensively. Even enhanced mutation rates are rare phenomena.

The Ames test (Figure 7-4) uses back-mutation in bacteria to assess the mutagenic effect of a chemical treatment. A test chemical is added to a culture of bacteria that have a nutritional deficiency, such as the inability to synthesize histidine. The purpose of the screen is to measure back-mutation from the abnormal to a normal gene function. How well can treated mutant bacterial cells grow on medium that lacks their nutritional requirement? Given the large number of bacterial cells that can be tested for reversion, this is a very effective assay for potential mutagenic agents.

Muller was awarded the Nobel Prize in 1946 for demonstrating with *Drosophila* that X-rays are mutagenic. *Drosophila* males with their one X chromosome are mated to genetically marked females, such as *Basc*, with X chromosomes carrying a dominant eye shape mutation and inversions that reduce crossing over. Each first-generation female is then mated to genetically marked males, and their offspring are screened for survival. If a new lethal mutation occurs on the parental male's X chromosome during gamete formation, it will be passed to his non-*Basc* second generation male off-

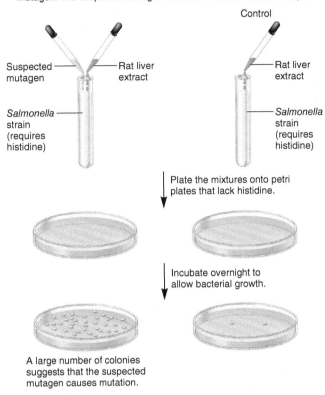

Mix together the *Salmonella* strain, rat liver extract, and suspected mutagen. The suspected mutagen is omitted from the control sample.

Control

Suspected mutagen — — Rat liver extract

Rat liver extract

Salmonella strain (requires histidine)

Salmonella strain (requires histidine)

Plate the mixtures onto petri plates that lack histidine.

Incubate overnight to allow bacterial growth.

A large number of colonies suggests that the suspected mutagen causes mutation.

Figure 7-4. The Ames test uses a strain of the bacterium *Salmonella typhimurium* to test chemicals for their mutagenicity. (Reprinted with permission from Brooker RJ: *Genetics: Analysis & Principles*, 3rd ed. New York: McGraw-Hill, 2008.)

spring. A significant increase in the absence of this genetic class is confirmation that a new lethal mutation was produced by the treatment. This assay continues to be used to screen for hazardous mutagenic chemicals from industrial by-products and for other experimental questions.

The mouse seven-locus test begins with an inbred strain that carries seven easily identifiable recessive mutations. These are mated with mice treated with a potential mutagen or control condition. If a new mutation occurs at one of these seven representative genes, the offspring will be homozygous for the recessive and show the mutant trait. Although the conclusions from this mammalian assay may be most closely associated with human biology, the cost for experiments is much higher than for work with bacteria or *Drosophila*. Insights into the mutagenic effect of suspected chemicals are, therefore, aided by conclusions drawn from all experimental systems.

Mechanisms for Spontaneous Mutation

Several different types of chemical change can occur in DNA spontaneously. The most common is a **depurination** (Figure 7-5), in which either an adenine or a guanine base is removed from a nucleotide, leaving the sugar-phosphate backbone intact, and the partner nucleotide temporarily unpaired. When the DNA then replicates after such a change,

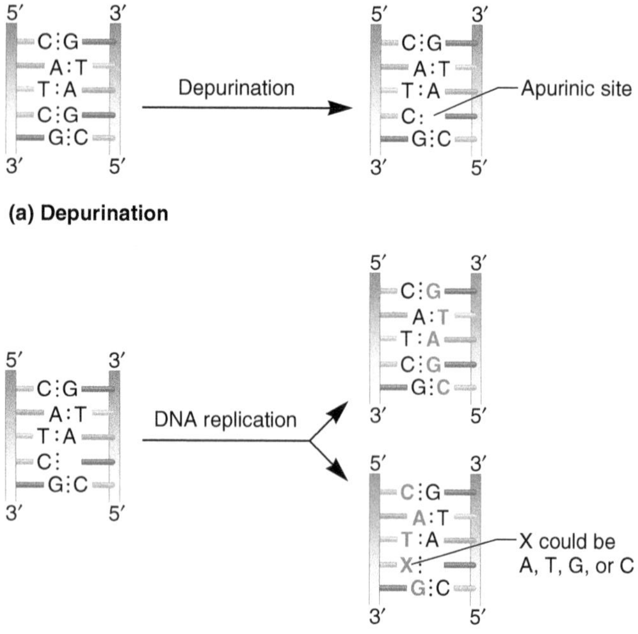

(a) Depurination

(b) Replication over an apurinic site

Figure 7-5. Depurination. (a) The guanine base is released from the deoxyribose backbone leaving a site with no purine, i.e., an apurinic site. (b) In the absence of a pairing partner during DNA replication, any of the four possible nucleotides can become incorporated into the new chain. (Reprinted with permission from Brooker RJ: *Genetics: Analysis & Principles*, 3rd ed. New York: McGraw-Hill, 2008.)

any nucleotide can be inserted opposite this vacated position. Only a quarter of the times, therefore, will the originally correct nucleotide be incorporated, so depurination can lead to a mutational substitution 75% of the time.

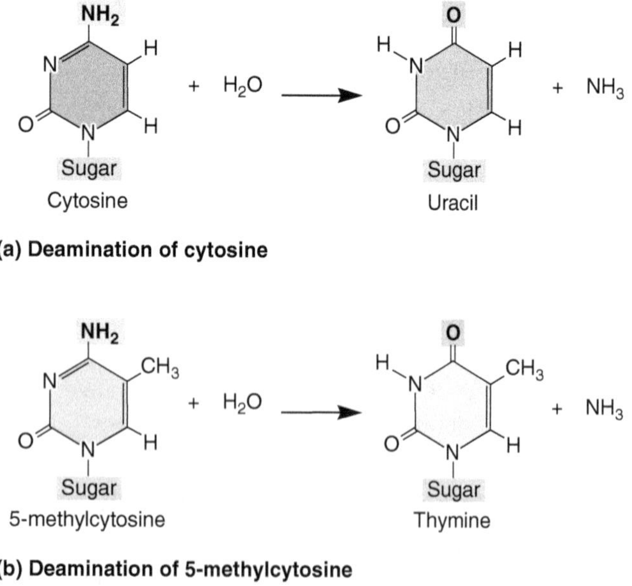

(a) Deamination of cytosine

(b) Deamination of 5-methylcytosine

Figure 7-6. Spontaneous deamination. (a) Removal of the NH_2–amino group yields uracil. (b) Removal of the amino group from 5-methylcytosine yields thymine. (Reprinted with permission from Brooker RJ: *Genetics: Analysis & Principles*, 3rd ed. New York: McGraw-Hill, 2008.)

Another common chemical change occurs when an amino group is removed from cytosine. This **deamination** (Figure 7-6) produces uracil, which will then pair with adenine during DNA replication and lead to a replacement of a C-G pair with a T-A pair after a complete cycle. Often the presence of uracil in DNA will be recognized as an error and be corrected by repair enzymes. If not repaired, however, a base pair substitution mutation results. In a similar process, methylation of cytosine occurs commonly. If 5-methylcytosine is deaminated, a thymine nucleotide will result. This may be corrected less efficiently, since it is a normal base in DNA.

Tautomeric shifts are also common sources of spontaneous mutation. A tautomeric shift (Figure 7-7) involves a reversible change in hydrogen that alters the nucleotide base to a different isomer. The base pairing we assume when predicting DNA structure is altered if a base is in its rare tautomeric form. Tautomeric shifts can, therefore, cause atypical pairing of nucleotides (such as T with G, or C with A) that lead to base pair substitution mutations after one further cycle of replication.

Damage by Mutagens

Many chemicals can cause mutations by altering the structure or base pairing of DNA. The Environmental Protection Agency (EPA) screens chemical by-products of industry and other sources of potentially harmful chemicals to reduce their passage into our environment. To illustrate this large and important area of environmental health, we will look at some examples of common mutagenic agents.

Both chemical and physical agents can cause mutations. They elevate the rate of mutation above the baseline that results from normal chemical events like those described in the previous section. Furthermore, many chemicals that cause mutation are also potent carcinogens. A couple of examples will illustrate the ways these agents can work.

One way that mutagens work is by modifying the nucleotide base so it mispairs, similar to the natural mispairings that we saw can occur because of tautomeric shifts. For example, nitrous acid removes the amino group from adenine or cytosine (Figure 7-8), causing them to pair incorrectly at replication. Base analogues like 5-bromouracil (5BU) are chemicals that can become incorporated in the new DNA strand, but then undergo tautomeric shifts and mispair. 5BU, for example, undergoes a tautomeric shift at a fairly high rate so it mispairs with guanine instead of adenine (Figure 7-9). After a second round of replication, the original A-T base pair has been replaced by a G-C base pair.

Additions or deletions can be caused by chemicals that insert (i.e., intercalate) into a strand and distort the normal pairing between bases. This leads to a frameshift mutation that affects the product of translation. Acridine dyes cause mutations this way.

Thymine dimers were discussed earlier. They form when two adjacent thymine bases absorb increased energy from ultraviolet light and bond each other, rather than binding the matching adenines on the complementary strand (Figure 7-10). At replication these do not pair with new

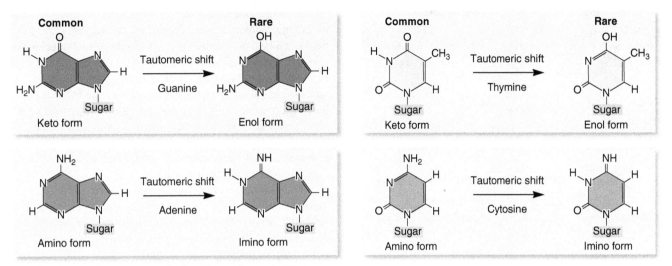

(a) Tautomeric shifts that occur in the 4 bases found in DNA

(b) Mis–base pairing due to tautomeric shifts

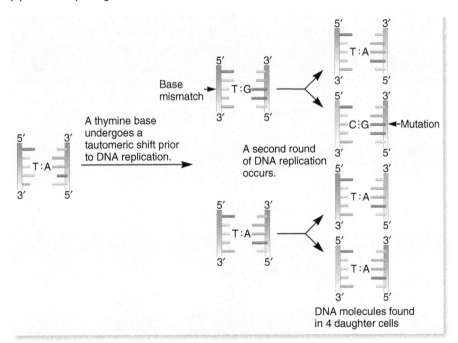

(c) Tautomeric shifts and DNA replication can cause mutation

Figure 7-7. Tautomeric shifts change common forms of a nucleotide base into a rare form. (a) Tautomeric shifts are shown for each of the nucleotide bases. (b) Tautomeric shifts lead to mispairing of the nucleotides. (c) If not repaired, a tautomeric shift like this one causing the base pairing of thymine to guanine will result in a new mutation in which C-G replaces the original T-A. (Reprinted with permission from Brooker RJ: *Genetics: Analysis & Principles*, 3rd ed. New York: McGraw-Hill, 2008.)

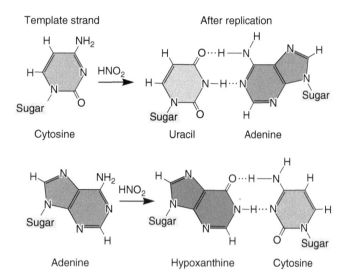

Figure 7-8. The mutagen nitrous acid replaces amino groups with keto groups, thus converting cytosine into uracil or adenine into hypoxanthine. The pairing of these modified bases leads to a mutation when the strand replicates. (Reprinted with permission from Brooker RJ: *Genetics: Analysis & Principles*, 3rd ed. New York: McGraw-Hill, 2008.)

nucleotides and the new strand is shortened by two bases, thus shifting the reading frame.

DNA Repair

More than 100 genes are involved in DNA repair, one of the only biological molecules that routinely undergoes such a process instead of simply being replaced. Without highly efficient repair, the information content of DNA would be so degraded that the existence of complex biological systems is probably not possible. DNA repair mechanisms will be illustrated by several examples.

In some cases, an error can be repaired directly, such as having a thymine dimer repaired by breaking the bond between adjacent thymine bases. A more common mechanism is base excision repair, in which the incorrect base is removed and then replaced (Figure 7-11). For example, in many species an enzyme called N-glycosylase removes the incorrect base leaving an apurinic or apyrimidinic site. In a process called nick translation, a second enzyme, AP endonuclease, recognizes the abnormal site and makes a nick on the 5′ side. DNA polymerase then removes it and replaces it with a new nucleotide. Ligase completes the bond.

Nucleotide excision repair can correct many different kinds of genetic damage by removing and replacing a short segment of the DNA molecule. Enzymes recognize and remove a series of nucleotides on the mismatched strand, and correct nucleotides are then inserted using the complementary sequence. These and other ways of identifying and correcting errors in the DNA molecular help minimize the number of inherited changes transmitted to the next generation. Clearly, they do not correct all errors, but their efficiency is a critical element of the stability of the DNA molecule from one generation to the next.

Transposable Elements and Trinucleotide Repeats

When recognized as a common element of the genome, transposable elements were nicknamed "jumping genes." But mobile genetic elements were an unsettling addition to the events that influence genome organization. One of the earliest to identify this unusual genetic activity was Barbara McClintock, who received the Nobel Prize for her work on transposable elements in maize in 1983. The significance of her work went unrecognized for many years. Her story

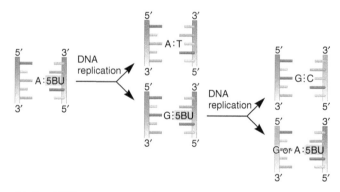

(a) Base pairing of 5BU with adenine or guanine

(b) How 5BU causes a mutation in a base pair during DNA replication

Figure 7-9. The action of 5-bromouracil (5BU), an analog of thymine, as a mutagen. (a) In its keto form, 5BU pairs with adenine and no change occurs. But in its enol form, 5BU pairs with guanine. (b) When it pairs with guanine, a mutation can result after the next round of replication. (Reprinted with permission from Brooker RJ: *Genetics: Analysis & Principles*, 3rd ed. New York: McGraw-Hill, 2008.)

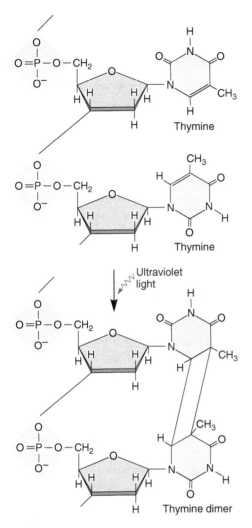

Figure 7-10. In a thymine dimer, the energy absorbed by adjacent thymine nucleotides causes them to bind to each other, rather than to the adenine nucleotides of the complementary strand. (Reprinted with permission from Brooker RJ: *Genetics: Analysis & Principles*, 3rd ed. New York: McGraw-Hill, 2008.)

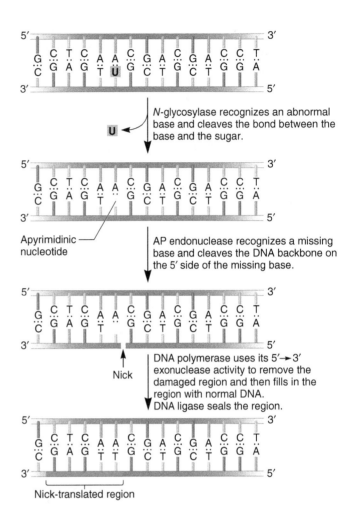

Figure 7-11. Excision repair occurs when the enzyme N-glycosylase recognizes an incorrect base and removes it from its sugar. In this example, the uracil is removed leaving an apurinic site. AP endonuclease acts on this site by breaking the 5′ connection of the sugar-phosphate DNA backbone. DNA polymerase removes nucleotides in the region and replaces them, followed by the formation of the final bond by DNA ligase. (Reprinted with permission from Brooker RJ: *Genetics: Analysis & Principles*, 3rd ed. New York: McGraw-Hill, 2008.)

should resonate with all who pursue new knowledge. Do not be intimidated into silence by the current authorities in your field. Be open to new ideas. Be rigorous in employing good scientific standards. Transposable elements changed our understanding about genome stability. Human elements like the *Alu* sequence were discussed in Chapter 4. Active transposable elements are important mutation-generating factors in many species. We bring them back into our discussion here to emphasize the role that mobile genetic elements can play in generating new mutations.

Although unrelated to transposable elements, trinucleotide repeats offer another example of how elements of genome structure can affect genetic stability. Several human diseases, such as Huntington disease (CAG repeat, more than about 27 times), fragile X syndrome (CGG or GCC repeats, more than about 200 times), and myotonic muscular dystrophy (CTG repeat, more than about 200 times), have been traced to variations in repeat number. In many cases, the repeated

sequence increases the number of glutamine amino acids in the translated protein, which causes the proteins to accumulate. In other cases, like the **CpG islands** generated in fragile X syndrome, methylation of the islands can lead to reductions in transcription.

Germinal versus Somatic Mutation

The focus of this chapter has been on heritable changes, **germinal** (or germ-line) **mutations**, passed in eggs or sperm to affect development of an offspring. But the mutational mechanisms we have discussed can also cause mutations in cells within the body well after birth. **Somatic mutations** may be limited to a small cell population, but they can have a life-changing effect on the carrier. Many cancer tumors, for example, show genetic differences from other cells of the body.

Other examples include patches of tissue, like a spot of white hair or of differently pigmented skin, with a phenotype distinct from the rest of the body.

If the somatic mutation occurs early enough in embryonic development, the cells it produces can include germ-line tissue. In that case, a mutation that originated in early somatic cell lineages can be passed to offspring and may be indistinguishable from a normally inherited germ-line mutation. This will be discussed further in Chapter 12, Atypical Inheritance.

Paternal Age Effect

Since mutations accumulate in somatic cells, it is clear that the nuclear genetic content can gradually change as an individual ages. One special example is the accumulation of mutations in the premeiotic cell lineage of germ tissue, like the testes of human males. As mentioned in the discussion of parental age effects in a previous chapter, premeiotic mutations do not accumulate in the human female germ line, because the cells are arrested in prophase I during fetal development. But in males there are many cycles of mitotic division during which new mutations can occur before the final meiosis.

Another interesting possibility is that the phenotypic similarity between fathers and offspring may actually increase as a function of the father's age. This may be indirectly due to reduced developmental homeostasis. The logic is a bit involved, but essentially it is proposed that, as compensating mechanisms of homeostasis are degraded by these new mutations, an extreme genotype can be expressed more accurately. They are less effectively buffered toward normal. Thus, more extreme phenotypes may appear in the offspring of older male parents. Without effective phenotypic compensation from homeostasis, these later offspring may express extreme phenotypes shared with their father that would otherwise have been at least partly masked. Thus, heritability as measured by the similarity of father and offspring increases. Heritability will be discussed in more detail in Chapter 10 on gene × environment interactions.

Genetic Variability: The Role of Mutation in Replenishing Genetic Resources

DNA biochemistry is a complex topic. Spontaneous errors in DNA replication will occur because of normal changes in the structure or bonding of nucleotide bases. Most such errors are corrected by repair enzymes that work during the G_2 phase prior to nuclear division. But the efficiency of repair enzymes can vary, and some environmental conditions might activate even more accurate or sensitive repair enzyme alternatives. Whatever the mechanisms at work in a given situation, it is clear that mutation is a normal background event in all living systems, and mutation rates vary among genes and from one biological system to another.

On top of that, of course, is the increased mutation that occurs from the action of mutation-creating agents in our environment. Environmental mutagens are a potent source of health problems like cancer. Actions that we take as a society to recognize and reduce exposure to mutagens are repaid by safer, longer, healthier lives. Still, it is an awareness we can never take for granted. Chemicals in our environment are changing constantly. Furthermore, we are living longer than we did 100 years ago, so the risk of mutation in a lifetime is higher.

On the other hand, mutation, at least in producing minor allelic or quantitative variation, is also a prime contributor to developmental mechanisms like **allosteric** flexibility at rate-controlling biochemical steps. An ability to survive successfully in a cycling, changing environment depends in part on well-understood mechanisms like this. The success of life in a changing environment stands on a balance between the good and the bad, between the subtle and the severe. Mutation has consequences that are both harmful and beneficial. Its effects are often sad for individuals, but we cannot live without it as a species. This multifaceted view of such a central process of all biology should not surprise anyone who recognizes the dynamic nature of life.

Part 2: Medical Genetics

By far, the most common application of genetics in the practice of medicine is in the realm of diagnostics. Patients will have specific medical signs and symptoms or a significant family history. The question posed is "Why?" "What is the cause?" "What are the implications for the family?" The diagnostic approach in genetics may involve a special type of physical examination, the **dysmorphologic** exam, to make a specific diagnosis based on physical characteristics. Therein can be found the root of clinical genetics. But with the frequent advances now seen in readily available molecular techniques, genetic testing is increasingly becoming a mainstay of genetic diagnostics. The crux of clinical genetic testing is the identification of specific mutations that can be linked to medical problems, confirming or making the diagnosis. It is thus crucial that all physicians

have a solid understanding of mutations—what they are, what they do, how they occur. This is particularly important in accurately interpreting the results of clinical genetic testing. The practitioner must understand the results and interpretations of the tests and be able to decipher the nomenclature in which they are provided.

What Is a mutation?—The Medical Perspective

As we saw in the first section of this chapter, a **mutation** in the purest sense is simply a heritable change (somatic or germ-line) in the genomic sequence that causes it to vary from the "normal" or "wild type" sequence. **Polymorphism** refers to having multiple forms of a gene. In population genetics, this term is reserved for those mutations that occur with a high enough frequency (in at least 1% of the general population).

For medicine, the central question regarding mutations is "what are the clinical consequences?" Just because a genetic change occurs, it is not necessarily true that an abnormality will result. Once again, the concepts of genotype and phenotype must be emphasized. The genotype refers to the genetic code. A mutation as noted earlier is simply a genotypic change—as compared to the reference (normal) sequence. The phenotype is an observable feature in the individual. The phenotype may be defined at any of many different levels. A phenotype can be a biochemical measurement, a physiologic state, an antigenic presence, or a physical feature. An abnormal phenotype, then, is any deviation from that typically seen in the general population. It is also important to note that caution must be used in designating a phenotypic change as abnormal; consideration has to be given to normal population variation.

So to return to our earlier discussion, all changes in the DNA code that differ from the wild type (normal) sequence are abnormal and would be termed mutations. The most important subsequent question is "what effect does the mutation have on the individual?" Many changes in gene sequences produce phenotypic changes by changing the function of the gene. These are simply **pathogenic mutations**.

However, some genetic changes produce no discernible clinical effects. So how does this happen? Why don't all mutations produce clinical problems? There are several possible explanations for this:

1. Certain nucleotide changes will not alter the amino acid sequence in the translated protein because of the degenerate nature of the genetic code. The presumption is that this would not have any effect on the structure or function of that protein.

2. Changes in the DNA sequence may occur in a non-coding region of the gene, i.e., within an intronic section of the gene. In theory such changes would not be predicted to cause problems. (Recent studies, however, have clearly shown that this is not always the case. Certain intronic changes, while not altering the coding sequence, may have other secondary consequences, such as altering splice sites, and thus still have adverse phenotypic effects.)

3. A specific mutation may change the gene function somewhat, but not enough to exceed the biologic threshold needed to tip the balance toward clinically apparent problems.

4. Along these same lines, a problem may not be readily apparent at one point in time. There may still be an effect that is yet to come and be identified as a "late-onset" disorder.

Regardless of the mechanism, the common outcome is a mutation that does not produce a phenotypic change. These are collectively referred to as **benign variants**.

It is important that these concepts are understood when reviewing reports from genetic tests. As certain genes are repeatedly sequenced, labs will develop a library or inventory of identified changes. If a variant is identified on a clinical test, the laboratory will report the specific change and provide an interpretation based on experience and the existing medical literature. An identified variant will typically be reported as:

1. Normal sequence

2. Variant present. If present, it will be classified as:
   • Known pathogenic (disease causing) mutation
   • Known benign variant
   • Variant of unknown/uncertain significance

In the vernacular, the term "mutation" carries a negative connotation. But in reality, a mutation is just an observable change in the genomic sequence. Some changes may actually be beneficial. In fact, in evolutionary theory these must occur. In the brief history of medical practice, however, relatively few beneficial mutations have been reported. Clinically, most polymorphisms identified in a person have no effect or are deleterious. Still, there are notable exceptions. A 32-base pair deletion in the chemokine receptor type 5 (CCR5) confers resistance to HIV infections in homozygotes and delays progression of an HIV infection to clinical AIDS in heterozygotes. Likewise, some mutations may be deleterious in homozygotes affected with a recessive disorder but actually be advantageous in heterozygotes (see Chapter 6 on Mendelian inheritance).

To prevent confusion some have advocated not even using the terms mutation and polymorphism, but instead neutral terms like "sequence variant," "alteration," and "allelic variant". For us, "mutation" is a valid term with strong historical and practical use. For the purposes of this book, we will typically limit the term "mutation" to disease-causing variants.

Frequency of Mutations

Most people intuitively think of mutations as being rare events. This is largely due to the historical observations of dramatic, easily observable consequences of mutations. The genetic bases of conditions like congenital anomalies, genetic syndromes, and neuro-developmental disorders were among the first to be defined. Thus, the association of rare observable conditions with an identifiable correlating mutation led to the assumption that mutations were rare events. In reality, nothing could be further from the truth. It is true that a specific mutation event will be rare. But cumulative evidence over the past four decades has led to the clear conclusion that mutations as a group occur with an amazingly high frequency—if one simply knows where to look.

Mutation rates vary greatly across species. The measured rates of spontaneous mutation per genome under research settings are remarkably similar within broad groups of organisms, but they differ strikingly among the groups. Since unprotected DNA has a higher mutation rate, the more complex organisms have structural modifications of their DNA, such as bundling into chromosomes with further protection by

Table 7-2.	Mutation Rates for Selected 'Hotspots' in the Human Genome*		
Gene Symbol	**Gene Product**	**Associated Disorder**	**Mutation Rate**
NF1	Neurofibromin	Neurofibromatosis	5×10^{-3}
PKD1	Polycystin1	Polycystic kidney disease	6×10^{-3}
DMD	Dystrophin	Duchenne muscular dystrophy	1×10^{-4}
FGFR3	Fibroblast growth factor 3	Achondroplasia	1.8×10^{-4}
PAX6	Paired box 6	Aniridia	0.5×10^{-5}
RB1	p105-Rb	Retinoblastoma	1.5×10^{-5}
HemA	Factor VIII	Hemophilia A†	2.5×10^{-5}

*Note the average mutation rate of 1×10^{-6} mutations per locus.

†Hemophilia A demonstrates a sex difference in mutation rates with the rate being 5 times higher in males

chromatin, histone proteins, and other factors, which buffer against mutations. In humans, mitochondrial DNA is not protected like chromosomal DNA and, thus, has a much higher mutation rate. This is discussed further in Chapter 13, Disorders of Organelles.

A large body of literature exists on the frequency of mutations in humans. In order to get a better grasp on the genetic diversity among people, one must look at these other lines of documented evidence. We will summarize these to put the answer to the question about human mutation load into a clinically relevant context.

1. *Changes in DNA transmitted to the next generation.* Current estimates for a human genome is that there are 2.5×10^{-8} mutations per base per generation and 1×10^{-6} per gene per generation. Every time human DNA is passed from one generation to the next, it accumulates 100 to 200 new mutations, according to a DNA-sequencing analysis of the Y chromosome. Given a current estimate of 22,000 genes in the human genome, this suggests at least 1 in 20 persons is expected to inherit a clinically significant gene change (germinal mutation) from one or the other parent.

2. *Prevalence of identifiable polymorphisms in an individual.* For 20 million coding base pairs, there are an estimated 60,000 single nucleotide polymorphisms (SNPs) in humans. It is estimated that everyone has 5 to 15 genes in our approximately 22,000 gene makeup that are functionally "abnormal," i.e., possess recessive mutations. James Watson, of Watson and Crick DNA structure fame, allowed his genome to be sequenced. He had 12 identified recessive mutations, which is consistent with estimates of the mutation load of a typical individual. As the genetic basis of common disorders is worked out, none of us may be "free" from genetic disease.

3. *Somatic mutations.* As an individual lives out his/her life, the natural history of an individual includes the accumulation of mutations. Somatic mutations occur

with a frequency of "certainty" in every individual. They will occur. The accumulations of these mutations are then responsible for much of the commonality of the human experience including aging, adult onset disorders, and effects on longevity.

Simply put, mutations are common events. A closer look at mutations and at how and when they occur reveals several important observations about the nature of mutations in general. New mutations are not evenly distributed across the genome. Distinct **mutation "hot spots"** exist. Certain areas of the genome clearly have a higher mutation rate than the observed baseline. Examples of these are provided in Table 7-2. There are several possible reasons why one particular gene (locus) may show a higher mutation rate. In general, it is not surprising that larger genes have a higher mutation than smaller ones. The presumption is that if there are more nucleotides, there is a greater chance of a change occurring in one of them. Research observation confirms this assumption.

Many of the other known explanations for the occurrence of mutation hot spots are sequence specific. For example, a particular sequence may be close to a transposable element, be a site recognized for viral incorporation, or be prone to recombinant loops. In the realm of immunogenetics, a unique mutational phenomenon is observed. In the genes that code for immunoglobins and their associated proteins, somatic hyper-mutation is noted in the immune response. In order to generate as much diversity in antibody production as possible, the immune-responsive genes have an inherent mechanism for generating genetic changes.

A few loci are even known to have a lower than average mutation rate. For instance, von Hippel-Lindau (vHL) syndrome is a familial cancer syndrome characterized by predisposition to several malignant and benign tumors, most frequently in the eyes, CNS, and abdomen. The estimated mutation rate for vHL is about 1×10^{-7}. Finally, some loci may show sex differences in mutation rates. Hemophilia A is an X-linked disorder of factor VIII of the clotting cascade. For this locus, the mutation rate in males is significantly higher than in females, estimated at a ratio of 9:1.

Types of Mutations

There are several ways to alter genetic material. Small-scale changes can be classified by various schemes. One method is to classify them by the effect of the change on gene structure. This is reviewed in the first section of this chapter and summarized in Table 7-1. Alternative schemes include grouping by the effect on function, i.e., on pathogenesis (further discussed in Chapter 16), or in populations by the effect on fitness.

Genetic changes can be complex and can occur in a variety of ways. For that reason there is a clear need for convention in describing the changes. As such, standard nomenclature has been developed to denote specific changes uniformly. It is important to note that the description can be at multiple levels. The first parameter is to define what biochemical is being described. A single letter is used to designate which compound is being referenced:

- "c." for a coding DNA sequence (cDNA, complementary to a mature mRNA molecule)
- "g." for a genomic sequence
- "m." or "mt." for a mitochondrial sequence
- "r." for an RNA sequence
- "p." for a protein sequence

For DNA changes, further descriptors include:

1. Which of the nucleotides is changed [adenine (A), guanine (G), thymine (T), and cytosine (C)]. The first letter represents the wild-type nucleotide, and the second letter represents altered nucleotide (for example, A > G).

2. The position or location within the gene is numbered, starting with the first nucleotide at the 5′ end of the sequence as number 1.

3. Specific symbols to designate the type of change [for example '>' for a nucleotide substitution or 'Δ' (delta) for a deletion].

So, for example, c.76A > T would describe a nucleotide substitution in which the adenine at the 76th position is replaced by a thymine in the cDNA. This is read as "seventy-six A to T." Sometimes there may be confusion over the different nomenclatures. For instance, there are times when description of the change in the *protein sequence* is preferable to describing that of the *nucleotide* change. In those situations, a similar but different convention is used.

1. The 20 amino acids are designated by an alphabetical letter. Table 7-3 lists the assigned letters for each amino acid.

2. The position number begins with methionine (the translation initiator) numbered as + 1.

3. Symbols are used to describe the different type of changes:
   - > for substitution
   - Del or Δ for deletion

- Dup for duplication
- Ins for insertion

The most common mutation seen in cystic fibrosis is a 3-nucleotide deletion that results in a missing phenylalanine at amino acid position 508. This would be designated p.ΔF508.

Details of the rules for generally accepted sequence variant nomenclature may be found on the Human Genome Variant Society website (http://www.hgvs.org/mutnomen/).

The clinically focused physician might ask why so much attention is paid to the type of mutation. Isn't it enough simply to know that there is a mutation in the gene of interest? As will be detailed in the Clinical Correlation section of this chapter, knowing the type of mutation and the mechanism by which it exerts its effect is critical for developing potential therapies and interventions.

Causes of Mutations

Traditionally, the causes of mutations are felt to be either spontaneous or induced. A spontaneous mutation is one that arises "naturally," rather than being the result of exposure to mutagens. These are hypothesized to be random mistakes usually due to errors in the normal functioning of cellular mechanisms like DNA replication, i.e., the system malfunctions without external influence. These could be errors anywhere along the normal course of mitosis, meiosis, or DNA replication and repair. The assumption is that over time, with enough replications, a mistake will eventually occur for no apparent reason. This phenomenon can be referred to as **molecular decay**. An intriguing question remains. Is there really such a thing as a spontaneous mutation *or* are these simply occurrences in which the causative agent or event has not been discovered?

Induced mutations occur when an eliciting agent is directly responsible for observed DNA changes. These agents are referred to as **mutagens**. As the name would imply, mutagens are any agent that can induce or increase the overall rate of new mutations. Here, it is worth making a couple of definition distinctions. A **carcinogen** is an agent that can induce or increase the risk of cancer. While many mutagens also act as carcinogens, the two lists are not identical. Some mutagens do not lead to cancer and some carcinogens are not mutagens. Likewise, **teratogens** are external agents that can result in congenital anomalies if a developing fetus receives a significant exposure. While exposures to mutagens during pregnancy can readily cause birth defects, many of the clinically important teratogenic agents produce effects by mechanisms other than the generation of mutations.

The best understood mutagens are:

1. Electromagnetic radiation
   - Increased mutation rates are associated with shorter wave lengths. Longer waves (light, radio, microwave) are less mutagenic. But, the association of the ultraviolet waves from sunlight exposure and skin cancer is strong.
   - X-rays and gamma rays are highly mutagenic.

Table 7-3.	Listing of Codes Used in Description of Protein Sequence Variants		
One Letter Code	**Three Letter Code**	**Amino Acid**	**Associated Codons**
A	Ala	Alanine	GCA, GCC, GCG, GCT
B	Asx	Asparagine or Aspartic acid	AAC, AAT, GAC, GAT
C	Cys	Cysteine	TGC, TGT
D	Asp	Aspartic acid	GAC, GAT
E	Glu	Glutamic acid	GAA, GAG
F	Phe	Phenylalanine	TTC, TTT
G	Gly	Glycine	GGA, GGC, GGG, GGT
H	His	Histidine	CAC, CAT
I	Ile	Isoleucine	ATA, ATC, ATT
K	Lys	Lysine	AAA, AAG
L	Leu	Leucine	CTA, CTC, CTG, CTT, TTA, TTG
M	Met	Methionine	ATG
N	Asn	Asparagine	AAC, AAT
P	Pro	Proline	CCA, CCC, CCG, CCT
Q	Gln	Glutamine	CAA, CAG
R	Arg	Arginine	AGA, AGG, CGA, CGC, CGG, CGT
S	Ser	Serine	AGC, AGT, TCA, TCC, TCG, TCT
T	Thr	Threonine	ACA, ACC, ACG, ACT
V	Val	Valine	GTA, GTC, GTG, GTT
W	Trp	Tryptophan	TGG
X	X	stop codon	TAA, TAG, TGA
Y	Tyr	Tyrosine	TAC, TAT
Z	Glx	Glutamine or Glutamic acid	CAA, CAG, GAA, GAG

Reprinted with permission from the Human Genome Variation Society.

- In clinical medicine, it is extremely important to protect patients from as much radiation as possible.

2. Chemicals
   - The first identified chemical mutagen was nitrogen mustard, which was used as a toxic weapon in World War II.
   - Chemicals may be mutagenic by affecting DNA reassembling, altering DNA replication at various stages, or by altering DNA structure by causing breaks or abnormal cross links.
   - Oxidative stress

3. Viral agents
   - Not surprisingly, double-stranded DNA viruses that insert their own genome into the human host DNA are the most mutagenic.

4. Transposable elements

DNA Repair

The human genome possesses multiple complex mechanisms for DNA repair. The fact that mutations are such common events essentially makes these mechanisms necessary for the survival of complex organisms. Early clues to the existence of these mechanisms were found in a group of rare genetic syndromes. A list of some of these syndromes is provided in Table 7-4. These conditions are linked by common clinical features that include predisposition to cancer, skin rashes or sensitivity to sunlight, immune deficiencies, premature aging, brittle hair, dysmorphic facies, structural congenital anomalies, bone marrow depression, short stature, cognitive dysfunction, and neurosensory abnormalities. The individual conditions exhibit their own specific combination of a subset of these features as well as other unique features that help define them as separate entities (Figures 7-12 and 7-13). The common feature of these conditions is genomic instability. The association of clinical findings such as genomic instability in the context of elevated cancer risks, premature aging, bone marrow suppression, and immune deficiencies are highly suggestive of abnormalities in DNA repair. Ultimately, the discovery of the gene(s) associated with these conditions has provided great insight into the mechanisms of normal DNA repair.

Gene(s)	DNA Repair Mechanism Affected	Syndrome	Major Clinical Features
Table 7-4.	**Rare Genetic Syndromes Caused by Mutations in Genes Involved in DNA Repair**		
ERCC6 ERCC8	Excision repair	Cockayne syndrome	Dwarfism, premature aging, pigmentary retinal degeneration, optic atrophy, deafness, marbled epiphyses, sensitivity to sunlight, mental retardation, joint contractures
MLH1 MSH2 MSH6 PMS1 PMS2 TGFB3 MLH3	Mismatch repair	Hereditary non-polyposis colorectal cancer (HNPCC) also known as Lynch syndrome	Early onset of colorectal tumors; predominantly right-sided (proximal) tumors
RecQ3	Unwinding DNA to allow repair to occur DNA ligase activity impaired (2^0)	Bloom syndrome	Short stature, narrow face with prominent nose, high-pitched voice, 'butterfly'-shaped facial rash, increased susceptibility to infections
ATM	Phosphorylation of key substrates involved in DNA repair	Ataxia-telangiectasia also known as Louis-Bar syndrome	Chromosome breakage, ataxia, telangiectasias, immune dysfunction
XPA-XPG ERCC 2,3,4,5	Excision repair	Xeroderma pigmentosa	Abnormal response to UV damage; includes hair and skin abnormalities
FAA - FAM	Replication fork	Fanconi anemia	Pancytopenia, cardiac, renal, limb malformations, pigmentary change

Current understanding of DNA repair mechanisms shows that different types of repair exist to fix different types of damage. The most common forms of damage actually have devoted repair enzymes, i.e., there can be direct repair of a specific change. O^6-methylguanine is the major mutagenic lesion in DNA induced by alkylating agents. The methylguanine-DNA methyltransferase (MGMT) enzyme can remove the methyl group from O^6-methylguanine, directly reversing the abnormal modification. More complex repair mechanisms exist for more complex abnormalities. Excision repair mechanisms will correct missing or altered bases with changes on only one strand. Mismatch repair systems correct the situation where both bases are "normal" but the combination of the two is not. Finally, interstrand cross-link or double-stranded break repair

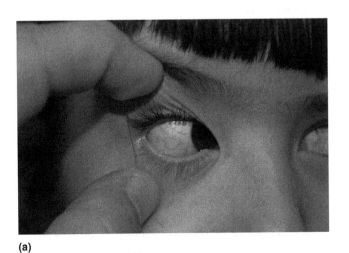

(a)

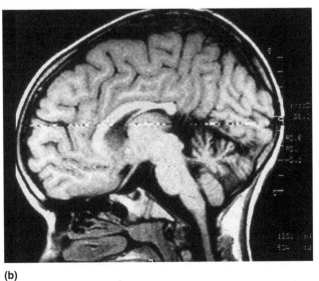

(b)

Figure 7-12. Young girl with ataxia-telangiectasia. (a) Note the telangiectasias (small, dilated blood vessels) on the sclera. (b) Note cerebellar atrophy on the MRI. This is the source of the ataxia. This condition is caused by a mutation in the ATM gene, a major component of the mechanism for double-stranded DNA repair.

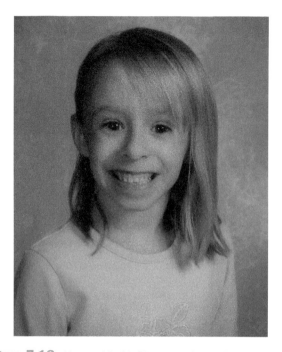

Figure 7-13. Young girl with Bloom syndrome. This condition is characterized by short stature, sun-sensitivity, pigmentary skin changes, chromosome instability, and an increased propensity to malignancies. This child had spontaneous chromosome break-age noted on a karyotype. Subsequent testing showed compound heterozygosity for mutations in the DNA helicase RecQ protein-like 3 gene.

mechanisms are needed when both strands are damaged. This is a particularly tricky "fix," because if both strands are damaged, there is no template for repair. Specific disorders have now been associated with malfunction of these different systems. This information is also included in Table 7-4.

Impact of Mutations

Political and public health analyses of health care often talk about cost estimates of a specific condition. It is helpful to know the magnitude of the impact of a problem on the overall health system. In actuality, however, it is practically impossible to make an accurate estimate of the scope of the impact of mutations on human health. Given the way in which they might be classified, mutations potentially have a role in all human medical conditions. Their impact goes well beyond the standard parameters of illness, lost productivity, and quality of life. On the other hand, as we discussed earlier, the complete absence of mutation is likely to be a detriment to the long-term health and well-being of a population. The ratio of benefits to harm of genetic change in populations *versus* individuals is not the same. For now, however, the study of medical genetics continues to focus on the occurrence of harmful mutations and their role in human disease—as best it can be grasped.

Part 3: Clinical Correlation

As mentioned earlier, knowledge about the underlying nature of a mutation responsible for a specific disorder is likely to have direct implications for therapy. Different types of mutations affect their changes in different ways. This, then, may lead to differential responses to therapy.

For most common disorders, the gene(s) responsible for the disorder have been identified. Study of the mutations found in these conditions usually identifies significant genetic heterogeneity. For a given condition, patients may be seen who have mutations of any conceivable type. Two common conditions [cystic fibrosis (CF) and Duchenne muscular dystrophy (DMD)] exhibit these characteristics. Cystic fibrosis (Figure 4-21) is an autosomal recessive disorder characterized by clinical symptoms secondary to the obstruction of exocrine glands by inspissated (i.e., having a thickened or dried consistency) mucous excretion. It has been shown that the primary defect is in a chloride transport gene called the cystic fibrosis transmembrane receptor (CFTR) that causes increased chloride concentrations in the exocrine secretions. A hyperviscous mucous results from high chloride concentrations. Obstruction of the exocrine glands results in pancreatic insufficiency and chronic progressive obstructive lung disease as the primary symptoms. Currently, patients with CF have an average life expectancy in the 30s and continuing to increase. Duchenne muscular dystrophy (Figure 6-31) is an X-linked

muscle disorder caused by mutations in a gene called *dystrophin*. Dystrophin functions as a biologic "shock absorber" for muscle contractions by anchoring to the sarcolemmal membranes. Missing or poorly functioning *dystrophin* leads to a progressive muscle disease due to an underlying mechanical destruction of the muscle fibers. Clinically, patients with DMD exhibit progressive weakness, cardiomyopthy, and ultimately death by the late teens or early 20s.

Nonsense mutations change the genetic code by producing a premature stop codon. This results in a shortened (truncated) protein. This shortened protein typically is partly or completely dysfunctional. Genetic testing for both CF and DMD has indeed shown marked genetic heterogeneity. Salient to this discussion, 10% to 15% of patients with DMD and 10% of patients with CF are found to have disease caused by nonsense mutations. Sequence analysis (not just deletion/duplication analysis alone) is needed to identify mutations that lead to premature stop signals in these patients.

In the study of antibiotics and their effects on microbes, it was discovered that the antibiotic gentamycin could induce "read-throughs" of nonsense mutations. In other words, it would allow the transcription mechanism to skip over the ectopically placed stop codon. The use of gentamycin as a drug to treat genetic mutations is not feasible, since the concentrations required to have a reasonable effect proved to be too toxic. Using this information, a drug was subsequently developed that had the same effects on nonsense mutations as gentamycin, but without the toxicity. This drug was originally called PTC124 during its time as an early investigational drug (Post-Transcriptional Control = PTC of the regulatory processes that occur after mRNA molecule has been made). Later the trade name Atrulen was given to this drug. This medication is odorless and tasteless. It is taken orally as a powder that can be dissolved in water or milk. The mechanism of action is to allow ribosomes to read through premature stop codons. In doing so, the stop codon is replaced with a random amino acid, not necessarily the correct one. A point of caution is that a drug will not generally be gene-specific. It also has the potential to turn on something it should not.

This drug is well advanced into clinical trials. It is being studied as a potential therapy for nonsense mutation mediated genetic disease, with the first clinical trials being conducted with patients with DMD and CF. It is not yet known how effective these trials may be. Still, this type of approach is clearly marking the current era as being on the threshold of true genetic therapies—actually correcting genetic mistakes. In addition, this example highlights the importance of knowing *which type* of mutation is present. In the case of Atrulen, it specifically identifies which subgroup of patients would benefit from this type of therapy. If this fails to excite you, maybe you are not ready for 21st-century medicine!

■ Board-Format Practice Questions

1. A common clinical feature seen in persons affected with a disorder of DNA repair is
   A. albinism.
   B. predisposition to cancer.
   C. excess stability of the genome.
   D. hyperproduction of immune globulins.
   E. delayed aging.
2. A patient is suspected of having a specific medical condition. A DNA sequencing test is performed to confirm the clinical diagnosis. In the report, the laboratory says that a change in the DNA sequence was found. The report also states that this particular change has been seen in several other individuals, none of whom have had the suspected condition. The best interpretation of this is that the genetic change is a
   A. normal sequence.
   B. known pathogenic mutation.
   C. known benign polymorphism.
   D. polymorphism of unknown significance.
   E. codon malalignment.
3. Which is the correct statement regarding mutations?
   A. Mutations are rare events.
   B. Mutations occur at a rate evenly distributed across the genome.
   C. Spontaneous mutations are typically more severe than induced mutations.
   D. Because mutations are set in the DNA, therapy is not possible.
   E. Mutations may occur in either germ-line or somatic cells.
4. Agents that are known to induce mutations (mutagens):
   A. often are also carcinogenic (i.e., induce cancer).
   B. cannot be teratogenic (i.e., induce birth defects).
   C. are mostly man-made (i.e., are not naturally occurring).
   D. are typically unavoidable.
   E. typically produce a mut^0 phenotype.
5. Mutations
   A. occur less often in unprotected DNA.
   B. may be induced by bacterial infections.
   C. may occur in the movement of transposable elements.
   D. designated by the Δ sign are more likely to occur around rivers.
   E. have a large impact on the health of the population that is quantified by the National Cost Estimates survey.

chapter 8

Metabolism

CHAPTER SUMMARY

Even the simplest cell may house thousands of individual chemical reactions. But the number of different kinds of chemical reaction is surprisingly small. In fact, we saw the same underlying pattern in our discussion of genetic regulation. While the specific details of the vast array of regulatory events may be complicated, only a fairly small number of different principles are needed to explain the essential mechanisms at work in an organism. There is often a surprising degree of simplicity underlying the seemingly complex events of life. As we will see in this chapter, the genetic control of metabolism is no different. But we can never lose sight of the fact that it is the understanding of the specific processes, in all their complexity, that actually makes the difference for an individual patient.

The study of metabolism focuses on function. Metabolism is made up of the biochemical reactions with which a living system obtains energy from the environment and stores it or uses it for growth and other biological activity. As we saw in Chapter 2, the study of so-called "inborn errors of metabolism" gave Garrod and other early researchers their first insight into how our genetic makeup controls life processes. One of the earliest recognized human metabolic diseases, phenylketonuria (PKU; Figure 8-1), provides a good prototype of the way our current understanding of the genetic control of metabolism is applied in practice.

The recessive condition PKU was first described in 1934 by A. Fölling, based on his study of two siblings. This brother and sister showed mental retardation. They also had a characteristic musty odor to their urine, where Fölling discovered phenylpyruvic acid. A special diet low in phenylalanine, adopted in 1955, was the first effective therapy for this condition. Soon after that, a blood screening test was developed, and states began to adopt laws requiring newborn children to be tested before they were discharged from hospitals. Today, about 300 newborn children are diagnosed with PKU each year, and mental retardation is prevented by early implementation of a low-phenylalanine diet. As microarrays and other biochemical assays enter the field, designing better-tailored treatment regimens can benefit future patients. But few will probably be as directly treatable as this dietary approach to a comparatively simple metabolic disorder.

As we learn more about individual metabolic disorders, the conditions that were once grouped together as examples of the same defect are often found to be functionally related but biochemically separable. After all, metabolism is a sequential process of reaction steps toward a shared outcome. But even when the underlying biochemistry is well-understood, the treatment regimen may not be easy to implement. Even in the relatively straightforward example of PKU, a low phenylalanine diet is not one that affected individuals willingly follow for the rest of their lives. In this chapter we will focus on examples of metabolic disorders and on how to think about the processes at work. But understanding the impact of these conditions and their treatment options on the lifestyles of affected individuals is also important.

The Basic Chemistry of Metabolism

Enzymes are protein-based catalysts that accelerate chemical reactions. These reactions define the changing structure and biochemistry of events that occur at all levels of biological activity. Enzymes work by lowering the activation energy needed for a targeted chemical reaction to occur. By definition, an enzyme speeds up a chemical reaction without being permanently changed by the reaction. In other words, enzymes are not chemical reactants. That means that a small amount of a given enzyme can have a potentially large effect on the biochemical reaction it catalyzes. For most biological reactions, the amount of enzyme is produced in excess. This serves to buffer critical developmental steps against the effects of environmental changes and other potential sources of functional variation. For that reason, a clinically diagnosable disease is often not apparent until the level of the key enzyme is at 5% or less of its normal concentration.

Often a cofactor will help an enzyme work more efficiently. A **coenzyme** is an organic molecule that acts as a donor or acceptor of molecular groups added to or taken from a substrate molecule. For example, water-soluble vitamins like members of the vitamin B complex and vitamin C act in this way.

Metabolism is a network of chemical reactions. When viewed from the perspective of genetics, our focus may be upon one specific mutation. But we should never forget the overall context of its function. With that in mind, there are

several recurring patterns that can help create the landscape of metabolic interactions. First, the activity of a relevant enzyme is generally more important than the level of its substrate. Certain steps in a biochemical pathway, especially steps that are not reversible, can serve as regulatory control sites. **Allosteric control** at these steps is the key to their regulation. Allosteric control refers to the reversible changes in protein shape, and thus functions, of active sites that can be produced when the enzyme binds to a small molecule. The small molecule thus acts as an allosteric effector. Allosteric interactions can either enhance or inhibit the enzyme's catalytic ability and thus induce or repress its activity temporarily.

In addition to allosteric interactions, some proteins are also affected by **covalent modification**. Examples include phosphorylation and adenylation at key steps in a metabolic pathway. The pathways can, therefore, be rapidly activated or inhibited by small changes. Changes in enzyme amounts and levels of activity can also affect metabolism, as can the partitioning of key metabolic processes in different cellular compartments, like the cytosol or the mitochondrial matrix.

The Logic of Mapping Biochemical Pathways

A mutation can cause a problem in a metabolic pathway in at least two ways. The mutation can cause a missing or deficient product, or it can cause the buildup of an earlier precursor. Both mechanisms may have serious phenotypic consequences. Knowledge of the effect of each mutation will ultimately allow researchers to map the relationship between steps in a biochemical or developmental pathway and the gene, and thus the active enzyme, responsible for each catalytic reaction. George Beadle and Edward Tatum shared a Nobel Prize for their work with the simple bread mold, *Neurospora crassa*. In their studies, mutations became powerful tools with which to dissect a biochemical pathway. A short description of their approach will illustrate the logic that is applied today in a wide array of organisms. Even though the specific techniques now employed can be quite diverse, the underlying logic has the same roots.

As we have seen, an enzyme catalyzes the conversion of one molecule into another, with a series of enzymes carrying out the sequential steps to form an ultimate product. Using *Neurospora*, for example, colonies can be grown by replicate plating of cells onto a series of petri dishes (Figure 8-2a). If the petri dish medium is "complete," it contains all of the basic nutrients needed for both normal and defective cells to survive. Minimal medium, however, has only those basic precursor nutrients from which all other nutritional requirements can be produced by a normal cell. Thus, if a cell can survive on complete medium but not on minimal medium, it must have a mutation in some critical biochemical pathway.

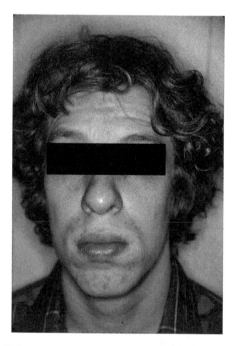

Figure 8-1. Adult male with PKU. This patient was born before the advent of newborn screening. His diagnosis was not made until he was 23 years old. He has severe cognitive impairments.

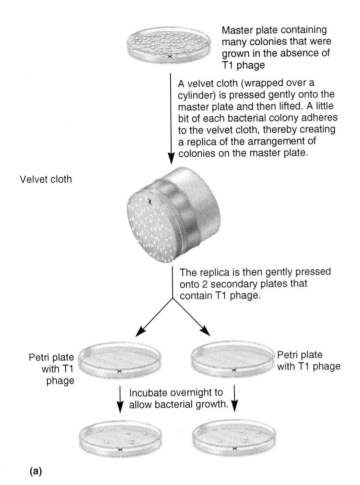

Master plate containing many colonies that were grown in the absence of T1 phage

A velvet cloth (wrapped over a cylinder) is pressed gently onto the master plate and then lifted. A little bit of each bacterial colony adheres to the velvet cloth, thereby creating a replica of the arrangement of colonies on the master plate.

Velvet cloth

The replica is then gently pressed onto 2 secondary plates that contain T1 phage.

Petri plate with T1 phage

Petri plate with T1 phage

Incubate overnight to allow bacterial growth.

(a)

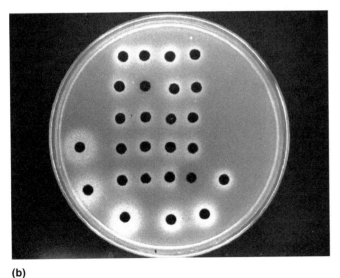

(b)

Figure 8-2. Microbial inhibition assay for metabolic disorders. (a) Schematic of process using the fungus *Neurospora*. (b) Photo of a plate used for the "Guthrie test." This was a bacterial inhibition assay for phenylketonuria. This methodology allowed for the mass screening of newborns for PKU. (Reprinted with permission from Brooker RJ: *Genetics: Analysis & Principles*, 3rd ed. New York: McGraw-Hill, 2008.)

In 1963, Robert Guthrie's Bacterial Inhibition Assay for Phenylketonuria (PKU) was the first application of this screening technique for disorders in human newborns (Figure 8-2b). Within a decade it was adopted as the first newborn screen in large populations.

To dissect the biochemistry of a specific pathway, the first step is to collect a series of mutations with a shared nutritional deficiency. These cells can grow on complete medium and on medium supplemented with a specific end product, such as the amino acid phenylalanine. But they cannot grow on minimal medium. Such nutritional mutants are called **auxotrophs**; genetically normal cells are called **prototrophs**. The next step is to replica plate auxotrophs onto a series of petri dishes containing minimal medium that has been supplemented with specific chemicals in the biosynthetic pathway. In the sample of growth results shown in Table 8-1, a plus sign indicates that the plated cells are able to grow and form a colony, while a minus sign indicates lack of growth. Strains and intermediates are presented at random in this first table, as would be the case for a collection of initial laboratory data.

The logic for interpreting these data is straightforward. Consider one sample step. If a specific mutation produces a defective enzyme incapable of converting intermediate molecule B into C (shown by the broken arrowhead in the following sequence), then it cannot grow if given supplements of B or any other molecules that occur earlier in the pathway. But it can grow if given supplements of C or of molecular intermediates that occur later in the sequence of biochemical steps.

Earlier Precursor → → → B ⏌ C → → → End Product

These results are reflected in the first row of Table 8-1. Cells plated onto petri dishes supplemented with chemicals A or B cannot convert those into the next molecule in the sequence. But supplementation with any later molecule can allow the sequence of reactions to continue normally. By arranging the sequence of precursor molecules and mutant growth characteristics so that the plusses are grouped at the right end of each line and the mutant strains are ranged from most to least successful in supplementation, the pathway can be read directly from the table. The example of randomly-collected data in Table 8-1 is followed by an organized sequence of mutation steps and intermediate molecules in Table 8-2. In this hypothetical case the sequence of intermediate molecular steps is:

Earlier Precursor → A → B → C → D → E → End Product

In the case of the conversion of molecule C into D, either there are two separate molecular steps controlled by enzymes #3 and #4 with an unknown intermediate, or these two mutants affect the same gene and are allelic.

Although this classical example using *Neurospora* focuses on a specific experimental design, the logic can be applied broadly. In the next section we will take an overview of the evaluation of inborn errors of metabolism in humans, and **Part 2: Medical Genetics** will discuss important clinical examples.

| Table 8-1. | Growth (+) or Absence of Growth (−) of Six Different Auxotroph Mutations for a Hypothetical "End Product" in a Biochemical Pathway. By Evaluating the Ability of Each Mutant Strain to Grow on Minimal Medium (Min), or Minimal Medium Supplemented With an Intermediate Molecule in the Pathway, the Mutants Can Be Mapped in Terms of Their Role in the Pathway |

Mutant Strain	Min	Min + C	Min + E	Min + A	Min + D	Min + B	+ End Product
1	−	+	+	−	+	−	+
2	−	−	+	−	−	−	+
3	−	−	+	−	+	−	+
4	−	−	+	−	+	−	+
5	−	+	+	−	+	+	+
6	−	+	+	+	+	+	+

| Table 8-2. | Data From Table 8.1 Reordered in Terms of the Sequence of Functional Intermediates and the Mutant Blocks in This Biochemical Pathway. (Min = Minimal Medium) |

Mutant Strain	Min	Min + A	Min + B	Min + C	Min + D	Min + E	+ End Product
6	−	+	+	+	+	+	+
5	−	−	+	+	+	+	+
1	−	−	−	+	+	+	+
3	−	−	−	−	+	+	+
4	−	−	−	−	+	+	+
2	−	−	−	−	−	+	+

Mutations and the Level of Phenotypic Discernment

In classical studies of metabolic defects, the enzymatic activity was completely absent. A **null allele** is one in which the enzyme is nonfunctional. But we now know many examples in which the enzyme is functional, but kinetically weakened. Such so-called "leaky" mutations yield a protein with lowered enzyme activity or which has an activity that is conditionally affected by changes in some environmental variable.

Differences in the level of enzyme activity can, but will not always, cause a phenotypic change. Such variation is expressed in terms of phenotypic discernment (Table 8-3), that is, the "ability to detect." If the mutation has no activity in homozygotes, the phenotype of the individual is expected to show the consequences of that absence. But as noted earlier, there is a large excess production of many enzymes, and a leaky mutant with only 5% of the normal enzyme activity may be phenotypically normal or have a mild to severe phenotypic expression.

Table 8-3.	Sample Levels of Phenotypic Discernment		
Genotype	aa	Aa	AA
1. Null mutation (no "a" allele activity)			
Enzyme activity	0%	50%	100%
Phenotype	affected	unaffected	unaffected
2. Leaky mutation ("a" allele has half normal activity)			
Enzyme activity	50%	75%	100%
Phenotype	normal	normal	normal
3. Leaky mutation ("a" allele has 1/20th normal activity)			
Enzyme activity	5%	52.5%	100%
Phenotype	mild or normal	normal	normal

An increasing number of metabolic diseases can be diagnosed by screening newborns. Gas chromatography or mass spectrometry assays, DNA microarrays, and other techniques can be used for screening. But screening tests that have been in common use for decades often draw attention to cases where these more precise techniques can be employed efficiently. This is clearly an area in which pediatric genetics will change rapidly as new techniques become increasingly available.

Part 2: Medical Genetics

Introduction

In 1902 Archibald Garrod defined a category of genetic disorders that he referred to as "inborn errors of metabolism." These conditions have their origin in human biochemistry. Inborn errors of metabolism (IBEMs) occur when there is a block in a metabolic pathway due to an inherited defect in an enzymatic protein. They thus represent the clinical sequelae of abnormalities of normal metabolic pathways. They are of great clinical importance for several reasons:

1. They were the first conditions in which a specific genetic change could be linked to an altered protein (i.e., to an enzyme) and the change in the protein could be linked to associated pathophysiological abnormalities.

2. The first large scale population screening efforts for genetic conditions were screening newborns for IBEMs. Screening newborns for selected genetic disorders remains one of the great success stories in public health. This will be discussed in detail in Chapter 11 on Genetic Testing and Screening.

3. Effective therapies exist for many IBEMs. The success of therapy is highly dependent on the early recognition and intervention of the disorder.

4. Although these conditions are individually somewhat rare, collectively they are encountered regularly in the general practice of medicine.

5. The range of clinical signs and symptoms seen in IBEMs is extremely broad—so much so that they should be considered in the differential diagnosis of almost any clinical feature. The presentations can range from prenatal (hiccups) to adult psychiatric problems.

The topic of inborn errors of metabolism is extremely broad. Various large multivolume texts provide comprehensive lists of conditions with detailed discussion of the biochemistry, pathophysiology, molecular genetics, and clinical aspects of these disorders. For this chapter, we have selected the salient features of the more common conditions. We provide general information about the disorders and outline clinically important features. For more detailed discussions, the reader is referred to any one of several excellent books listed at the end of this chapter in the Resources section.

Phenylketonuria (PKU) is an inborn error of metabolism that results from a problem with converting the amino acid phenylalanine to tyrosine. More is known about this condition than any other IBEM. As such we will use PKU as our example frequently throughout the rest of this chapter to highlight the unifying principles. In addition, the Clinical Correlation section of this chapter focuses on the medical problems and treatment issues in PKU.

Basic Principles of Inborn Errors of Metabolism

The primary understanding of IBEMs requires a review of human biochemistry. Chemical reactions in living organisms are typically facilitated by enzymes. Enzymes are simply biochemical catalysts. These chemical reactions are such that kinetically they would occur spontaneously, albeit slower (Figure 8-3a). Enzymes (catalysts) "push" natural reactions along at an accelerated rate (Figure 8-3b). Some enzymes may also have their activity enhanced by the presence of **cofactors** (Figure 8-3c). Cofactors (sometimes called **coenzymes**) act in concert with an enzyme. Cofactors are typically nonprotein compounds that bind to the enzymatic protein. They may be organic or inorganic compounds. Vitamins are typically organic cofactors. The enzyme by itself is referred to as an **apoenzyme**. The enzyme coupled with the cofactor is the **holoenzyme**. For some enzymes, a deficiency of cofactor will reduce its activity, for others, the enzyme may not function at all without it. Some enzymes will require multiple cofactors for effective functioning.

An interesting biological phenomenon was mentioned earlier but is important to emphasize. For most human enzyme systems there is apparently a tremendous excess of enzyme above what is needed for normal functioning. In fact, the excess is so significant, that for many conditions, an abnormality or disease may not occur until the enzyme activity falls below 5% of "normal." Thus, most IBEMs are inherited in a recessive manner with close to null allele function for both copies. The majority of IBEMs are autosomal recessive with a few being X-linked recessive.

Pathophysiology of Inborn Errors of Metabolism: How Do Enzymatic Blocks Cause Disease?

An understanding of the pathophysiology of a disorder is central to developing appropriate therapies and interventions. It is not enough simply to say that a mutation changes an enzyme and causes the enzyme not to work. More importantly, the question is what happens when the enzyme does not work?

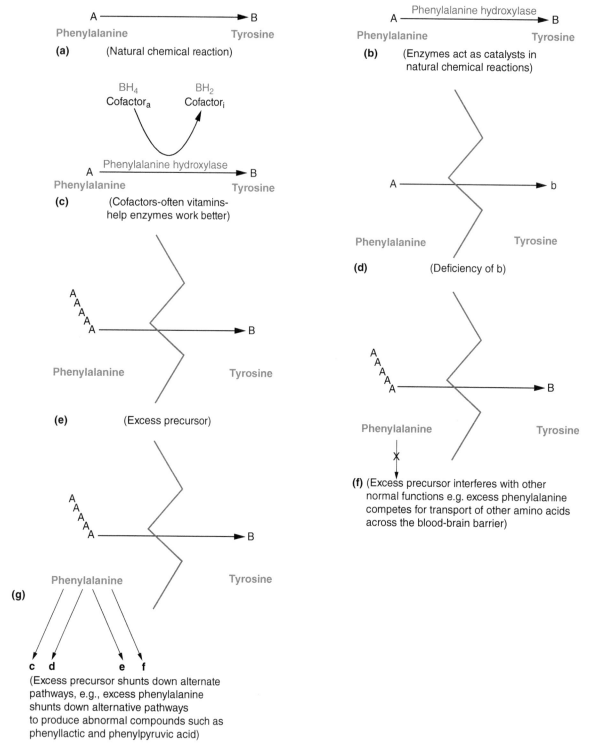

Figure 8-3. (a) Naturally occurring chemical reaction. Enzyme kinetics favor the spontaneous conversion given the right substrates. The example here is the conversion of phenylalanine (phe) to tyrosine (tyr). (b) The enzyme phenylalanine hydroxylase acts as a catalyst in the conversion of phe to tyr. (c) Biopterin (BH4) acts as a cofactor that enhances phenylalanine hydroxylase activity. (d) Deficiency in an enzyme slows down the enzymatic process. This results in the decreased production of the product (tyr) of the reaction. (e) Deficiency in an enzyme slows down the enzymatic process. Another result is the buildup of the precursor (phe) in the reaction. (f) One result of an excess of precursor can be the interference with other normal processes. Excess phenylalanine will interfere with the transport of other large neutral amino acids across the blood-brain-barrier. (g) Another result of an excess of precursor is shutting down alternative (not typical) pathways. The end result is the generation of compounds not usually present in significant quantities. These compounds can themselves produce physiological problems.

What are the metabolic consequences of this abnormality? How does this translate into actual symptoms for the patient?

The intuitive answer to these questions is that an enzymatic block will result in a *deficiency of the product* of the enzymatic reaction. This is an important consideration. In our example of PKU, genetic changes that disable the enzyme phenylalanine hydroxylase disrupt the conversion of phenylalanine to its related amino acid tyrosine. This leads to decreased amounts of tyrosine, which in turn produces several problems (Figure 8-3d). In PKU, deficiency of tyrosine can lead to impaired protein production in general, due to the fact that there is not enough tyrosine for the synthesis of any protein. In addition, tyrosine is a precursor in the synthesis of the neurotransmitters L-dopa, dopamine, norepinephrine, and epinephrine. Low tyrosine levels will thus result in decreased production of these important chemicals with subsequent neurological problems. Also, tyrosine is in the metabolic pathway of melanin synthesis. This correlates with a long-standing observation that people with PKU tend to be lightly pigmented (Figure 8-4).

Equally important, there are other pathophysiological consequences of an enzymatic block. Besides a deficiency of the product of the reaction, a block will also lead to an *accumulation of excess precursor* (Figure 8-3e). Intuitively, one might wonder what possible problems might result from having "extra" phenylalanine in the system. The answer is actually "quite a bit." The large neutral amino acid transporter (LAT1) is a membrane transport protein that preferentially transports neutral branched amino acids (valine, leucine, isoleucine) and aromatic amino acids (tryptophan, tyrosine) across the blood-brain barrier. In PKU, excess amounts of phenylalanine compete with these other amino acids for transport across

the blood-brain barrier resulting in deficiency of these other amino acids in the brain (Figure 8-3f). It is this deficiency that is thought to be one of the primary sources of problems in untreated PKU in older individuals. Another problem with having an excess of a precursor is that the something has to be done with the extra. Often, excess precursor shunts down alternate biochemical pathways in ways that would not naturally occur (Figure 8-3g). In PKU, excess phenylalanine is shunted into other pathways with resultant excess of phenyllactic acid, phenylpyruvic acid, and phosphoethanolamine. The excess secretion of these compounds and their metabolites in the urine is responsible for the "phenylketones" in the urine from which the condition gets its name. The increased amount of phenylpyruvic acid is the source of musky smell associated with untreated patients. Finally, excess phosphoethanolamine has a variety of effects, one of which may be CNS excitation, which has been postulated to be associated with the hyperactivity seen in persons with poor control.

Presenting Features of IBEMs

As mentioned earlier, IBEMs may show a plethora of presenting symptoms—so much so that they can appropriately be placed in the differential diagnosis of almost any human malady. For instance, there are solid data that suggest that upward of 25% of neonatal deaths attributed to overwhelming infection (septicemia) in which an infectious agent cannot be identified are actually due to undiagnosed IBEMs. With advances in newborn screening (see Chapter 11), it is hoped that this number will decrease. At the other end of the spectrum, there are many adults with primary psychiatric diagnoses who in reality have

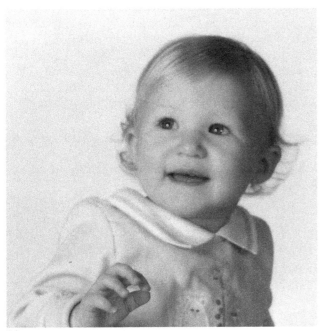 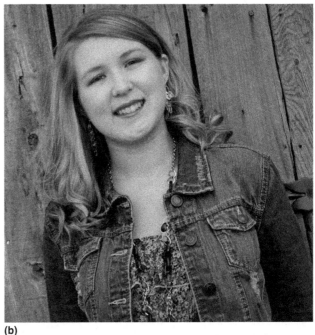

(a) (b)

Figure 8-4. Young lady with phenylketonuria. (a) Infancy (b) Early adolescence. Note lighter pigmentation.

Table 8-4.	Presenting Clinical Symptoms of Metabolic Disorders: Prenatal

Fetal hiccups

Fetal seizures (may be perceived by mother as "hard kicking" or "dancing" in the womb

Abnormal fetal growth

Abnormal ultrasound (*e.g.*, structural anomalies, cardiomyopathy)

Maternal HELLP syndrome (H – hemolysis; EL – elevated liver enzymes; LP – low platelet count)

a metabolic disorder as the cause of their mental illness. The mantra is "if you don't think about it, you will miss it."

It is helpful to think about the presenting features of metabolic disorders in terms of where in the life cycle they may present. But it is also important to remember that these groupings are not absolute. Most metabolic disorders have a spectrum of presentations depending upon the severity of the metabolic defect. As such, many IBEMs have clinically defined subtypes (i.e., infantile, juvenile, adult). These designations are helpful in the clinical realm in that they provide the family with some general prognostic information. Tables 8-4 to 8-7 provide lists of common symptoms that could suggest an IBEM listed by periods of the life cycle when they would likely occur. Still, it is important to remember that these are actually artificial designations of what is in fact a continuum of clinical outcomes.

One special category of presentation of IBEMs worth mentioning is structural congenital anomalies. There are several described multiple anomaly syndromes that ultimately have been shown to have an IBEM as the basic etiology.

Table 8-5.	Presenting Clinical Symptoms of Metabolic Disorders: Neonate

Newborn screening (may sometimes identify maternal IBEM)
  "Sterile sepsis"
  Hypoglycemia/hyperglycemia
  High anion gap acidosis
  Recurrent vomiting
  Poor feeding/FTT
  Abnormal smell
    Sweet smelling urine (organic acidemias)
    Maple syrup urine (branched chain disorder, MSUD)
    Sweaty socks (isovaleric acidemia)

Liver dysfunction

Conjugated or unconjugated hyperbilirubinemia

Hepatosplenomegaly

Neurologic symptoms
  Developmental delay
  Regression
  Seizures
  Nystagmus
  Dystonia
  Abnormal movements
  Lethargy/coma
  Strokes

Table 8-6.	Presenting Clinical Symptoms of Metabolic Disorders: Older Infant/Child

Cardiomyopathy/myopathy
  Exercise intolerance
  Rhabdomyolysis
  Muscle pain/spasms

Metabolic Reye syndrome with hypoketotic hypoglycemia and/or hyperammonemia

Food aversion/failure to thrive/episodic acute illnesses

Impairment of senses
  Vision (cataracts, RP)
  Hearing impairment

Mental retardation

Autism

Cerebral palsy

Skeletal dysplasia

Electrolyte abnormalities

Renal symptoms

RTA/Fanconi syndrome

Dysmorphic features

Table 8-8 lists many of these. One example is Smith-Lemli-Opitz syndrome. Smith-Lemli-Opitz syndrome (SLO) is a well-described multiple anomaly syndrome characterized by facial, digital, and genital abnormalities (Figure 8-5).

These individuals also have marked neurodevelopmental disabilities and autistic behaviors (over half will meet standardized diagnostic criteria for autism). Years after the description of this syndrome, several clinicians noticed an unexpected finding on general laboratory testing. They noted that many of the patients with SLO had significantly lower serum cholesterol levels. Prompted by this finding, subsequent investigations demonstrated that the cause of SLO was an enzymatic defect of an enzyme called 7-dehydrocholesterol reductase (Figure 8-6). It is now known that deficiency of this enzyme results in a deficit of cholesterol production and an increase

Table 8-7.	Presenting Clinical Symptoms of Metabolic Disorders: Adult

Weakness (often progressive)

Neurological changes/deterioration

Dementia

Psychiatric symptoms

Psychosis, depression

Paroxysmal disorders

Seizures

Movement disorders

Birth defects (in offspring)

Table 8-8.	Examples of Metabolic Disorders Associated With Structural Congenital Anomalies

Lysosomal storage disorders
    Dysostosis multiplex
    Hepatosplenomegaly

Connective tissue disorders
    Joint laxity
    Fragile skin with poor recoil
    Aneurysms
    Heart valve problems
    Scoliosis
    Disproportionately long limbs

Peroxisomal disorders
    Cerebral dysgenesis
    Congenital heart malformations
    Bone dysplasias
    Hypospadius
    Pyloric stenosis
    Renal cysts

Congenital disorders of glycosylation
    Nonimmune hydrops
    Inverted nipples
    Cerebral dysgenesis
    Congenital heart malformations
    Joint contractures
    Hepatosplenomegaly
    Coloboma
    Palatal defects

Sterol metabolic disorder
    Orofacial clefts
    Congenital heart malformations
    Polydactyly/syndactyly
    Genital anomalies
    Renal malformations
    Pyloric stenosis/gut malrotation
    Skeletal dysplasias

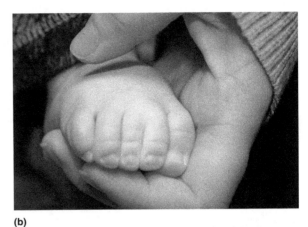
(b)

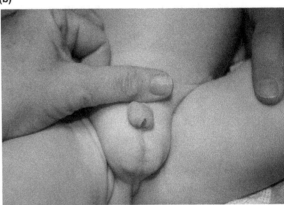
(c)

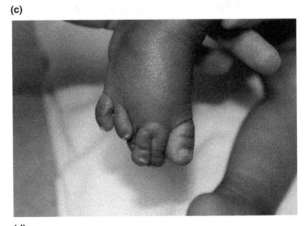
(d)

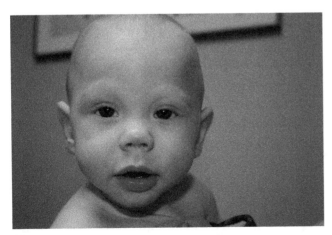
(a)

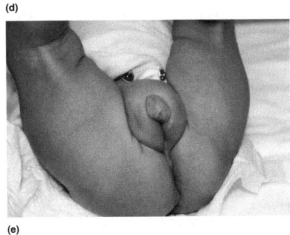
(e)

Figure 8-5. Two children with Smith-Lemli-Opitz syndrome demonstrating the key facial, digital, and genital findings of this condition.

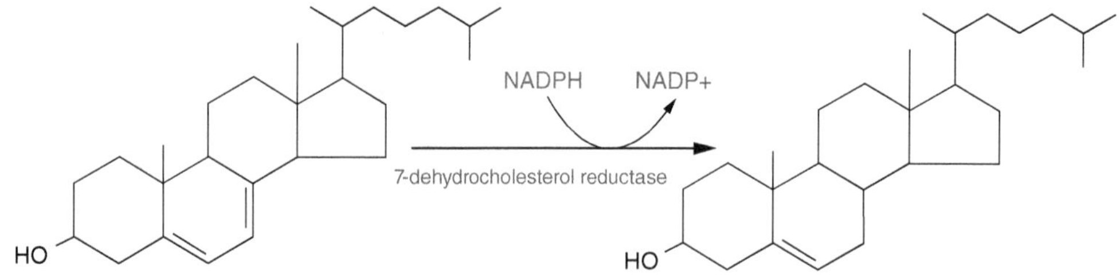

Figure 8-6. The terminal step in cholesterol synthesis is the conversion of 7-dehydrocholesterol to cholesterol. The block of this step due to reduction of the activity of the 7-dehydrocholesterol reductase enzyme results in Smith-Lemli-Opitz syndrome.

in the precursor 7-dehydrocholesterol. The pathophysiology of SLO is in part due to an overall deficiency in cholesterol and all of the many metabolic derivatives of it.

Diagnosis of IBEMs

Within the realm of clinical medicine, metabolic disorders will often have a mystical folklore about them. Nongenetic physicians typically do not go back and review their notes from biochemistry class. Referrals are often made with the request "Something is not right, could it be one of those metabolic things." Although the vast majority of readers of this text will not go on to careers in metabolic genetics, it is still important that you be aware of such conditions. Recognition and intervention—at least at the general level—of a metabolic condition can be crucial to a better outcome in the time before a metabolic consultant arrives. The astute clinician should always be alert to the possibility of an IBEM particularly since there are effective treatments available for many of them. They should also be very familiar with the symptom and associations listed in Tables 8-4 to 8-7. If a metabolic disorder is suspected, appropriate laboratory tests can be obtained immediately. Table 8-9 lists important selected routine laboratories and specific metabolic laboratories that will be helpful in a diagnostic evaluation.

Key Metabolic Disorders

As noted earlier, detailed discussions of all known metabolic disorders require several volumes of quite large books (see Supplementary Readings list at the end of this chapter). And information is growing. Still, there are certain clinical "pearls" that are important for all physicians to be aware of. As such we have selected several conditions for brief discussions. Those selected below were chosen for any of several reasons: conditions that are relatively common, conditions that require quick recognition and intervention to prevent morbidity and mortality, and a few that simply show up frequently on the board examinations. Hopefully, much of this has been covered in a prior medical biochemistry course. Table 8-10 provides a frame work for thinking about IBEMs by category.

While there are many different ways to subgroup these conditions, we prefer to think along the lines of chemical "families." We have organized the conditions to be discussed

later according to these categories. While these discussions may seem cursory, they at least provide a frame of reference for critically important issues related to the IBEMs. For detailed discussions, the reader is referred to the Reference section of this chapter for a listing of key metabolic texts.

1. *Disorders of amino acid metabolism*. Historically, the disorders of amino acid metabolism have received more attention than probably any other category of IBEMs.

   Alkaptonuria was one of the first metabolic conditions described—being one of Garrod's original four conditions described in his Croonian Lectures of 1902. It is caused by a defect in phenylalanine and tyrosine catabolism. It results in the accumulation of homogentisic acid, an intermediary metabolite in the degradation of tyrosine. The hallmark diagnostic feature of this disorder is that homogentistic acid in the urine darkens upon standing exposed to air. The black appearing urine is striking and

Table 8-9.	Testing for Metabolic Disorders

Selected Routine Labs

Liver function studies

CBC

UA (look at and smell the urine yourself)

CPK

Audiogram

Ophthalmologic exam

Selected imaging: CXR, brain MRI

Metabolic Labs	Disorders
Urine reducing substances	Galactosemia, fructosemia
Plasma amino acids	Aminoacidopathies
Urine amino acids	RTA, Lowe syndrome
Urine organic acids	Organic acidemias
Serum lactate/pyruvate ratio	PDH, PC, mitochondrial
Serum ammonia	Urea cycle defects
Serum acyl-carnitine profile	Fatty acid oxidation
Serum very-long chain fatty acids/phytanic acid	Peroxisomal disorders

Table 8-10. Major Inborn Errors of Metabolism—Organized by Category

Disorders of Amino Acid Metabolism
- Hyperphenylalanemias (includes phenylketonuria)
- Alkaptonuria
- Branched chain amnioacidopathy (maple syrup urine disease)
- Transsulfuration defects (homocystinuria)
- Non-ketotic hyperglycinemia
- Albinism

Disorders of Carbohydrates
- Galactosemia
- Fructosemia

Urea Cycle Defects
- Ornithine transcarbamylase (OTC)
- Carbamyl palmotyl synthetase (CPS)
- Arginase
- Arginosuccinate acid synthetase
- Arginosuccinase

Organic Acidemias
- Proprionic acidemia
- Methylmalonic acidemia
- Isovaleric acidemia
- Glutaric acidemia
- Glycerol kinase deficiency

Disorders of Terminal Energy Metabolism
- Lactic acidemias
- Mitochondrial disorders
- Fatty acid oxidation defects
- Disorders of oxidative phosphorylation or respiratory chain

Lysosomal Storage Disorders
- Glycogen storage diseases
- Mucopolysaccharides (storage of glycosaminoglycans)
- Mucolipidoses
- Glycoprotein disorders (Mannosidosis, Fucosidosis, Sialidosis)
- Acid Lipase deficiency (Wolman)
- Ceramidase deficiency (Farber)
- Sphingomyelinase deficiency (Niemann-Pick)
- Glucocerebrosidase deficiency (Gaucher)
- Galactosylceramide deficiency (Krabbe)
- Metachromatic leukodystrophy/multiple sulfatase deficiency
- α-Galactosidase (Fabry)
- GM1 and GM2 Gangliosidosis

Lipoprotein Disorders
- Hyperlipidemias
- Bile acid biosynthesis disorders

Disorders of Heme Metabolism
- Porphyrias
- Hereditary hyperbilirubinemias

Disorders of Trace Metals
- Menkes
- Wilson
- Hemachromatosis

Peroxisomal Disorders
- Zellweger
- Adrenoleukodystrophy/adrenomyeloneuropathy
- Refsum disease

Disorders of Nucleic Acids
- Lesch-Nyhan syndrome
- Adenosine deaminase (ADA) deficiency
- Gout
- Adenylosuccinate lyase (ADSL) deficiency
- Phosphoribosylpyrophosphate (PRibPP) synthetase superactivity

Disorders of Vitamins/Cofactors
- Folate
- Cobalamin
- Biotin
- Vitamin D

Coagulation Cascade
- von Willebrand
- Hemophilias

Membrane Transport Systems
- Cystinuria
- Renal tubular acidosis
- Fanconi
- Lowe
- Hypophosphatemic rickets
- Cystic fibrosis

Disorders of Sterol Metabolism
- Smith-Lemli-Opitz syndrome
- Conradi Hunermann
- CHILD (Congenital hemidysplasia with ichthyosiform erythroderma and limb defects)
- Desmosterolosis

often heralds the diagnosis prior to the appearance of symptoms (i.e., pigment staining of connective tissue causing a disorder known as **onchronosis**, coronary artery disease, and kidney stones).

Homocystinuria is a disorder of sulfated amino acids (methionine) due to cystathionine beta synthase (CBS) deficiency. Affected individuals have physical features suggestive of a connective tissue disorder. One such feature is spontaneous dislocation of the lenses of the eyes. It is fascinating to note that when this happens, the dislocation is always in the inferior and medial directions, in contrast to Marfan syndrome where the dislocation is superior and laterally (Figure 8-7). This metabolic block produces an increased homocystine level, which has the effect of increasing the cohesiveness of platelets. The

tendency for "sticky platelets" leads to an increased risk for pathologic thrombotic events. This can contribute to cognitive changes and can cause significant medical problems and reduced longevity. While homocystinuria is an autosomal recessive disorder, carriers (heterozygotes) for the condition also appear to have an increased risk of pathologic vascular occlusion.

A deficiency of an enzyme complex known as branched-chain ketoacid dehydrogenase causes a buildup of the branched-chain amino acids (leucine, isoleucine, and valine) and their metabolites. The excess metabolites of this disorder are organic acids, which have a distinctive odor that can be identified in an affected infant's urine. This odor truly smells like maple syrup, with the condition thus being called maple syrup

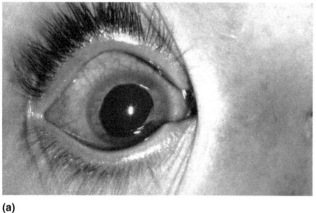
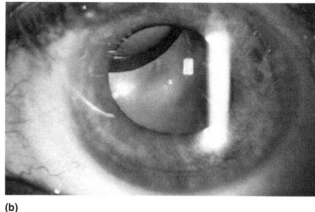

(a) **(b)**

Figure 8.7. (a) Lens dislocation (medial and inferior) in the eye of a patient with homocystinuria. (b) For comparison note the superior and lateral lens dislocation in a patient with Marfan syndrome.

urine disease (MSUD). Patients with MSUD typically present as seriously ill infants with vomiting, lethargy, metabolic acidosis, and neurological compromise.

Disruption of the catabolism of other amino acids results the accumulation of other organic acids. Isovaleric academia is due to abnormal leucine metabolism. Affected infants have presenting symptoms similar to other organic acidemias such as vomiting, metabolic acidosis, and neurological compromise (seizures, stupor, and coma). Infants with isovaleric academia are reported to have an odor reminiscent of "sweaty socks."

2. *Disorders of carbohydrate metabolism.* Galactosemia and fructosemia are disorders of the metabolism of the sugars galactose and fructose, respectively. Infants with these conditions have similar symptoms that include vomiting, liver dysfunction, renal failure, and overall systemic collapse if not treated. Infants with galactosemia are at high risk for *Escherichia coli* sepsis. Both conditions are caused by enzymatic defects that render the person incapable of adequately metabolizing the respective sugar. The onset of the conditions differs with the introduction of the sugar in the diet. Galactose, which is derived from lactose, is often present in the infant diet in the first few days of life. Fructose is usually introduced later (4-6 months) with the introduction of fruits into the diet or with the first dose of a sucrose containing medication. Careful attention to the diet history and notice of the timing of dietary changes can be invaluable in arriving at a rapid diagnosis. The mainstay of treatment for both conditions is the elimination of the offending sugar from the diet.

The glycogen storage disorders (GSDs) are a group of conditions that share in common some disturbance of glycogen metabolism—either synthesis or degradation. GSDs are mostly characterized by a fasting hypoglycemia. Thus, infants typically do not present until their diet is modified toward times of more extended fasting. Some may have impressive hepatomegaly (Figure 8-8). Pompe

disease is somewhat unique in this group as it presents with early severe infantile hypotonia and cardiomyopathy (Figure 8-9). The defective enzyme, acid maltase (acid alpha-glucosidase), is a scavenger enzyme in the lysozymes that rapidly degrade glycogen in a non-directed fashion. Physiologically it is much more like other lysosomal storage disorders (see below).

3. *Urea cycle disorders.* The catabolism of protein ultimately results in the generation of ammonia, an extremely toxic compound. Excess levels of ammonia will result in severe and irreversible neurological damage. Patients may present with seizures, stupor, or coma. In less severe cases, symptoms may include fluctuating sensorium and/or psychiatric disturbances. The urea cycle exists to eliminate ammonia quickly from the body. Inborn errors of any of the five reactions of the cycle will lead to varying degrees of hyperammonemia and the resultant symptoms. Because ammonia is so toxic and the damage is irreversible, it is crucial that

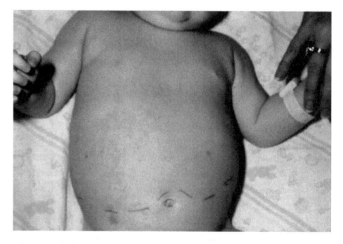

Figure 8-8. One-year-old child with glycogen storage disease type III. The line drawn on the abdomen delineates the lower margin of the liver.

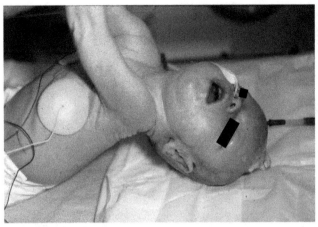

(a)

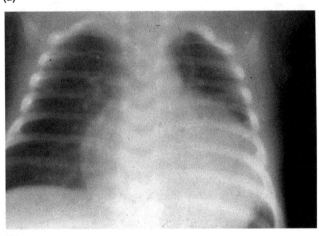

(b)

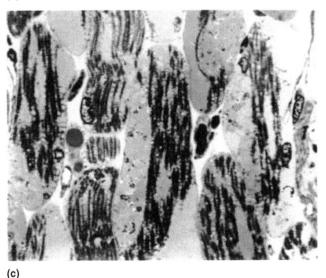

(c)

Figure 8-9. Newborn with Pompe disease. (a) Note severe hypotonia. (b) Striking cardiomegaly. (c) Muscle biopsy at 2 months old. Note tremendous glycogen stores disrupting muscle fibers. (c: Reproduced, with permission, from Amalfitano A, Bengur AR, Morse RP, Majure JM, Case LE, Veerling DL, Mackey J, Kishnani P, Smith W, McVie-Wylie A, Sullivan JA, Hoganson GE, Phillips JA 3rd, Schaefer GB, Charrow J, Ware RE, Bossen EH, Chen YT. Recombinant human acid alpha-glucosidase enzyme therapy for infantile glycogen storage disease type II: results of a phase I/II clinical trial. Genet Med. 2001 Mar-Apr;3(2):132-138.)

clinicians consider a hyper-ammonemic disorder in any patient with unexplained neurological changes.

Ornithine transcarbamylase (OTC) deficiency is an X-linked disorder. It is due to an error in the second reaction of ammonia detoxification. Affected males usually present with an early severe neonatal encephalopathy. Rapid intervention is critical in preventing morbidity and mortality. Female heterozygotes of OTC deficiency will present with a wide range of symptoms depending upon the degree of inactivation (Lyonization) of the X chromosome carrying the mutation. Symptoms in carrier females can range from completely unaffected to self-assigned protein restriction to fluctuating sensorium and/or psychiatric symptoms.

4. *Disorders of fatty acid oxidation.* Fatty acid oxidation is a complex process of mobilizing stored fat to meet increased energy demands. The major components of this process are the mobilization of free fatty acids via the lipolysis of diacylglycerols in the adipocytes mediated by lipases, uptake of the free fatty acids by the cells, activation of the fatty acids into acyl-CoA derivatives by fatty acyl-CoA ligase, transport of the fatty acyl-CoA complex into the mitochondria facilitated by carnitine palmitoyltransferases, and beta-oxidation of the fatty acids within the mitochondria. Different types of fatty acid molecules are processed by different enzymes specific to the type and size of the particles. Interruption of any portion of this process will result in significant reductions in energy production.

   Medium chain acyl-CoA dehydrogenase *(MCAD)* deficiency is an autosomal recessive disorder that results in abnormalities of the beta-oxidation of medium-sized fatty acids. MCAD is one of the most common IBEMs. In fact it is the most common metabolic condition on the typical newborn screening panel. The major clinical symptom is hypoglycemia. It is important to note that it is one of the specific causes of hypoketotic hypoglycemia. Other symptoms include lethargy and seizures. The presentation of MCAD varies greatly from a sudden infant death (SIDs) picture in infants, to a metabolic Reye syndrome in children, to episodic unexplained weakness in adults.

5. *Lysosomal storage disorders (LSDs).* The lysosomes are subcellular organelles that carry on a variety of catabolic processes via acid hydrolases. Various acid hydrolases are specific to their own category of biochemicals. The typical presentation of LSD is a person who is normal as an infant, but at some later point in life begins to experience progressive problems related to the accumulation of uncleared biochemicals. The LSDs comprise about 40 different disorders categorized by the type of biochemical that accumulates (e.g., mucopolysaccharides, complex proteo-lipids, mucolipids, and glycoproteins). As noted earlier, GSD type II (Pompe disease) is also LSD (Figure 8-9).

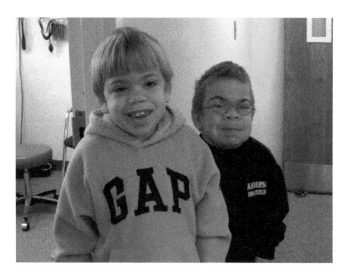

Figure 8-10. Brothers with Hunter syndrome (mucopolysaccharidosis type II).

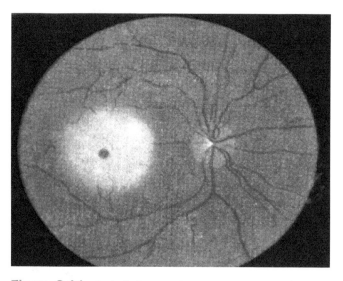

Figure 8-11. Retinal photograph in a patient with Tay-Sachs disease demonstrating the finding described as a "cherry red macule."(de Aragão REM, Ramos RMG, Pereira FBA, et al: "Cherry red spot" in a patient with Tay-Sachs disease: case report. *Arquivos Brasileiros de Oftalmologia.* 2009;72(4):537-539.)

An increased awareness of the LSDs and their early recognition has occurred over the past several years. This has been prompted by the advent of targeted therapies. Enzyme replacement either by direct infusion or transplanted cells has recently been developed for several LSDs. Clinically available therapies for Pompe disease, Hurler syndrome, Hunter syndrome (Figure 8-10), Fabry disease, Maroteaux-Lamy disease, and Gaucher disease exist. Therapies are involved and quite expensive, but they still represent the first wave of hope for patients with these devastating progressive conditions. Given the possibility of treatment, there is a heightened emphasis on early detection.

Tay-Sachs disease is a lysosomal storage disorder characterized by the buildup of GM2 ganglioside. It is an autosomal recessive disorder. Clinically, infants with Tay-Sachs are normal as infants. At around 4 to 5 months of age, they begin to have neurological regression due to neuronal loss from the accumulation of the gangliosides. Infants will begin to lose skills and their hearing, begin to have seizures, and many develop a characteristic exaggerated "startle response." Fundoscopic examination often reveals a "cherry red macule" (Figure 8-11), which is typical of this condition but not unique—being seen also in a handful of other storage disorders. Tay-Sachs is also notable for being one of several conditions that occur much more frequently in persons of Eastern European (Ashkenazi) Jewish descent (this will be discussed more in Chapter 15 on Population Genetics).

6. **Disorders of trace metals.** Trace metals (iron, copper, zinc, manganese, cadmium, and so forth), as the name implies, occur in minute quantities (parts per million) in the body, and yet they play significant roles in the overall health of the individual. Trace metals typically function as cofactors for enzymes. Nutritional deficits of these metals produce well-recognized symptom complexes (e.g., acrodermatitis enteropathica with zinc deficiency). In addition there are known IBEMs of trace metal metabolism that are expressed as their own clinical entity.

Menkes disease is a disorder of copper transport. The primary pathological consequence is poor delivery of copper to the subcellular compartments where it is needed (deficiency). It is an X-linked disorder. The condition is characterized by neurological dysfunction/degeneration. Because of the copper deficiency, connective tissue processing is impaired. Thus, patients with Menkes disease will have connective tissue disorder-like findings, such as tortuous blood vessels, bony abnormalities, and "sagging facies" (Figure 8-12a). Earlier descriptions called the condition "Menkes kinky hair disease" describing the abnormal hair of these patients. Because of the copper deficiency, the hair is hypopigmented, brittle, and quite curly. Under the microscope the hairs shafts have distinct angulations called "pili torti" (Figure 8-12b).

Wilson disease (also known as hepatolenticular degeneration) is another disorder of copper metabolism. It is an autosomal recessive condition. The responsible gene has been identified, but the exact pathophysiological mechanism has yet to be completely worked out. The observable end result, however, is copper overload, which seems responsible for the symptoms. One observable feature of this is brown circumferential rings on the periphery of the iris called Kayser–Fleisher ring (Figure 8-13).

Hemochromatosis is a disorder of iron metabolism. It is one of the most common known human genetic disorders. It is estimated that about 1 in 250 people in the United States have this condition. It is an autosomal recessive that has genetic heterogeneity. The "classic" form of hemochromatosis is caused by changes in a gene called HFE at chromosome locus 6p21.3. Although the

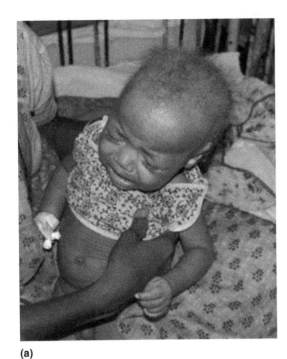

(a)

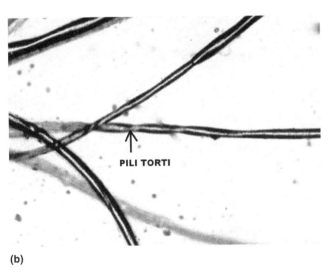

PILI TORTI

(b)

Figure 8-12. (a) Infant with Menkes syndrome—a disorder of copper metabolism. (b) Hair shaft from a patient with Menkes disease showing the "kinked" lesion in the shaft (pili torti). (Reprinted with permission from Datta AK, Ghosh T, Nayak K, et al: Menkes kinky hair disease: A case report. *Cases J.* 2008;1:158.)

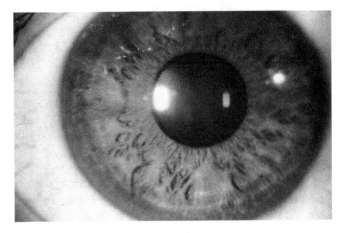

Figure 8-13. Kayser-Fleischer ring in a patient with Wilson disease.

exact pathogenetic mechanism is not known, it is clear that the responsible genes play critical roles in iron transport. The end results are a variety of symptoms due to iron overload. This includes liver problems (cirrhosis and tumors), diabetes, gonadal dysfunction, joint pains, and cardiomyopathy. Treatment is designed to decrease iron intake and to chelate excess iron from the body. Hemochromatosis is a condition that demonstrates a sex-influenced phenotype. As an autosomal recessive disorder, it occurs at an equal frequency in males in females. Males, however, are more severely affected. It is presumed that this is in part due to the female menstrual cycle, which naturally provides a mechanism for eliminating iron from the system.

7. *Disorders of nucleic acids.* There are several reported disorders of nucleic acid metabolism. The most well-known condition is Lesch-Nyhan syndrome. Lesch-Nyhan syndrome is characterized by a phenotype of severe neurobehavioral symptoms. The most striking features are cognitive deficits, movement disorders, and dramatic self-injurious behaviors (severe biting with mutilation of the lips and fingers). It is an X-linked recessive disorder. It is caused by changes in the hypoxanthine-guanine phosphoribosyl transferase enzyme (HgPRT), which plays a central role in purine metabolism. Another metabolic defect of nucleotide metabolism is adenosine deaminase (ADA) deficiency, which produces severe combined immune deficiency (SCID). Adenylosuccinate lyase (ADSL) deficiency and phosphoribosylpyrophosphate synthetase (PRibPP) superactivity are defects of nucleotide metabolism that have been seen in patients with non-syndromic mental retardation and/or autism.

8. *Vitamins and cofactors.* Many metabolic disorders have been reported due to abnormalities of the vitamins or cofactors associated with specific enzymatic reactions. Biotinidase deficiency is a disorder of the recycling of the cofactor biotin. This results in biotin deficiency. Patients with this disorder will have progressive symptoms of dystonia, eczema-like rash, cognitive deficits, and seizures. The treatment is easy and effective–simply supplement biotin.

Clinically, the cofactor abnormality often mimics the actual enzyme deficiency. Still, there are typically significant differences in the implications for therapy. Such is the case for the disorders of biopterin metabolism, which clinically resembles phenylketonuria (with BH_4 being the cofactor for PKU) but has significant differences in outcome and therapy.

It is also important to note that some cofactors operate with multiple enzyme systems. Thus, a defect in cobalamin metabolism produces characteristic abnormalities of two different enzymatic defects: methylmalonic acidemia and homocystinuria.

9. *Disorders of sterol metabolism.* Despite all of the bad press that cholesterol receives, it is a critical compound. It is a major component of cell membranes and a key precursor in the synthesis of biochemicals such as steroids, vitamin D, bile acids, and so forth. The synthesis of cholesterol starts with acetyl-CoA, which then proceeds through more than 15 enzymatic steps until the end product of cholesterol is achieved. Blocks in many of these steps have been described in association with recognizable clinical syndromes, such as Antley-Bixler syndrome and CHILD syndrome. The best characterized of these disorders is Smith-Lemli-Opitz syndrome, which is a disorder of the terminal step of cholesterol synthesis as described earlier.

Treatment of Inborn Errors of Metabolism

Most major advances in medical genetics over the past few decades have been in the areas of diagnostics and the understanding of the pathogenesis of genetic conditions. There is much to be said for advances like these. They provide invaluable insight into the central issues of these conditions, and their worth should not be downplayed. Still, in the realm of clinical medicine, patients are much more interested in treatments than diagnoses. In general, genetic therapies are lagging far behind genetic diagnoses. This idea will be covered in detail in Chapter 14, Genetic Therapeutics. As a group, advances in therapies for inborn errors of metabolism are far ahead of those for most other genetic conditions. This is largely due to the pathogenic nature of these disorders. Biochemical processes are ongoing and continuous, in contrast to, say, structural processes. Thus, IBEMs have a greater potential for therapy. In the following Clinical Correlation section, we will discuss the treatment of one such disorder, phenylketonuria, in detail.

Part 3: Clinical Correlation

Phenylketonuria (PKU) is an IBEM of phenylalanine metabolism. It is by far the best understood metabolic disorder in humans. Metabolic geneticists have had many decades of experience in dealing with patients with this disorder (Table 8-11). It is caused by a deficiency in the enzyme phenylalanine hydroxylase or one of the cofactor systems in this enzymatic reaction. The end result is impairment of the conversion of phenylalanine to tyrosine. With this metabolic block, there are multiple secondary metabolic abnormalities (Figure 8-3a-f).

Prior to newborn screening and effective therapies, children born with PKU had a severe phenotype (Figure 8-1). Many children died in the first few months of life. For those that survived, there were notable symptoms of mental retardation, seizures, microcephaly, an eczematous rash, hypopigmentation, musty smell to urine, discoordination, and autistic-like behaviors. Autopsy and imaging studies demonstrated severely disrupted myelination.

With the advent of public health programs in newborn screening, infants with PKU could be identified in the first few days of life. As such, therapies could be instituted prior to the onset of serious symptoms. The treatment of PKU is a classic example of restoring a normal phenotype without modification of a mutant genotype. The mainstay of treatment for persons with PKU is dietary modification. They are prescribed a semisynthetic diet, low in phenylalanine but adequate in other nutrients. They are provided just enough phenylalanine in this diet to allow for the needs of endogenous protein synthesis. It is notable how low this level actually is. The typical human diet (especially in the United States) has a marked excess of protein intake as compared to the actual metabolic needs. In fact, a patient with PKU can be maintained on a diet that has a minimum protein intake of about 1.5 g/kg/day. This diet is started as soon as the diagnosis is made, hopefully within the first 10 days of life. Patients are monitored regularly for phenylalanine and tyrosine levels. An interdisciplinary team of metabolic geneticists, nutritionists, and pediatricians follow these patients closely with the expectation of normal growth and neural development.

Table 8-11.	Major Events in the History of Phenyketonuria (PKU)

- 1934 – Dr. Asbjorn Fölling, a Norwegian physician, reports on two siblings with PKU. These children had severe cognitive deficits and a characteristic "musty" odor particularly appreciated in their urine. Phenylpyruvic acid was identified as the biochemical in the urine responsible for the odor. This was the first inborn error of metabolism to be described as associated with mental retardation.

- 1953 – Dietary therapy is developed for PKU. Therapy involves a metabolic formula deficient in phenylalanine. Effective therapy prevented early morbidity or developmental disabilities.

- 1963 – Development of the Guthrie test (bacterial inhibition assay). See Figure 8-2. This methodology was applied in the first mass screening of infants for PKU.

- 1973 – Launch of population screening for infants with PKU.

- 1990's – Identification of long-term issues in PKU treatment: adverse effects off of diet and the teratogenicity of untreated PKU.

- 2012 and beyond – All states in the US screen for PKU. Tremendous advances in therapeutic options make compliance with therapy significantly easier.

PKU was the first metabolic disorder that was successfully treated. As such there is a long history of experience and new discoveries along the path of treatment and intervention. Over time, many unexpected long-term sequelae have been identified. For instance, in the early days of PKU treatment, a presumption was made that therapy could be stopped after age five. This was based on the conclusion that most of the neurological abnormalities were due to aberrant myelin formation. Since the majority of myelination occurs in the first few years of life, it was assumed that therapy could stop after this window of time was complete. The short-term outcomes were impressive. Children that would have died or had severe neurological compromise survived and developed normally. Clearly, this was an amazing success story. Fortunately, a committed group of metabolic specialists banded together in what was known as the National Collaborative PKU study. Much of the effort on this project was unfunded volunteer work provided by specialists who simply wanted to know what the long-term outcomes of this never-before-seen entity (long-term normally developing persons with PKU) might look like. This collaborative identified several fascinating phenomena in this group.

First, although the treated children survived and had normal early neurodevelopment, over time a definite loss in IQ points was observed. Analysis of the study data demonstrated small, but definite, losses of IQ points for each year off of diet. This cognitive loss also was shown to be cumulative. The mechanism was shown not to be problems with myelin formation, but rather to problems with the transport of amino acids across the blood-brain barrier (BBB). Phenylalanine shares with other similar amino acids a common transport mechanism, called the large neutral amino acid transporter. In the case of PKU in which treatment is stopped in childhood, the devastating effects of dysmyelination are avoided. But, the extremely high circulating concentrations of phenylalanine compete with the other amino acids which share the same transport mechanism. The relative deficiency of transport of these other amino acids into the CNS results in problems with overall function, hence the loss in IQ. If PKU continues untreated, other findings are also seen in the adults. White matter changes are noted in the brain, and changes are seen in the cerebellum. These individuals demonstrate decreased performance on measures of attention, coordination, and information processing.

Another novel situation emerged with the successful treatment of children with PKU. As these children grew up as healthy, typically-developing young adults, the first group reached childbearing age in the early 1990s. As women with PKU but who as a group had not been treated since childhood began to have children of their own, another unexpected outcome was seen. Hyper-phenylalaninemia in the mothers was found to be teratogenic to the infants. Infants born to mothers with untreated PKU have essentially a 100% incidence of microcephaly and neurodevelopmental delays. The infants also often have dysmorphic features and congenital heart disease. Further work demonstrated that this adverse effect on the developing fetus could be avoided with reinstitution of the diet. In order to obtain maximum benefit, the diet must be rigid and begin prior to conception.

The logical conclusion from both of these later developing outcomes was straightforward: diet for life is now recommended. It is important to point out, that it is rather simple for us, the physicians, to recommend diet for life. But in practice, what this is asking of the patients is something quite involved. The metabolic formulas that they are asked to drink to provide nutrients without phenylalanine have an unpleasant taste. The newer formulas are significantly better than the early ones, which tasted surprisingly like quinine, but are nonetheless not great tasting. Also, the amount of protein that can be eaten is minimal. Meats are not allowed. Many vegetables, such as potatoes, are not "free foods" as they contain enough protein to be significant. Imagine having to count out 10 potato chips as your total allowance for lunch.

To help patients with compliance, several recent advances in therapy have emerged. As mentioned the newer formulas have a better taste. Sapropterin (trade name Kuvan) functions exactly like BH_4, the cofactor in the phenylalanine hydroxylase enzyme. The addition of sapropterin to the dietary therapy in PKU will further reduce blood phenylalanine levels and allow liberalization of the diet. Another addition to the therapy can be to supplement the large neutral amino acids. This will improve the ratio of phenylalanine to other amino acids that share the same BBB transporter. This also allows liberalization of diet. Phenylalanine ammonia lyase (PEG-PAL) converts phenylalanine to a nontoxic derivative. At this time, it is an investigational enzyme substitution therapy. Other therapeutic strategies are being explored. Enzyme replacement therapy (ERT) in theory should work. The major obstacle here is delivery of the enzyme to the appropriate site. ERT is currently not available for PKU. Also, without further advances in ERT, the risk to benefit ratio probably makes this therapeutic mode unlikely to be developed, given other more benign therapies. Placing a normal phenylalanine hydroxylase gene in place of the mutant gene in the patient (i.e., gene therapy) is a possible mode of therapy, but it is unlikely in the near future for both technical and ethical reasons.

In the end, what is the final outcome? Dietary treatment is clearly effective at ameliorating the severe effects of PKU. But early-treated children have mean IQ scores about one half a standard deviation lower than scores for their unaffected siblings and the corresponding population norms. Women with PKU can have normal children with early and rigorous therapy. Clearly, continued studies and advances in therapy are needed. Most importantly, the "PKU story" highlights the need for ongoing evaluation of patients with early identified metabolic disorders. Analogous to the National Collaborative PKU study, effective **Long term Follow-Up** programs are needed, especially given the rapid expansion of the recommended newborn screening panels (see Chapter 11 Genetic Testing and Screening).

■ Board-Format Practice Questions

1. In regards to inborn errors of metabolism:
   A. the original description was by Aborigines with a urine taste test.
   B. these are most commonly inherited as dominant disorders.
   C. disease can be caused by a deficiency of product upstream from the enzymatic block.
   D. disease can be caused by a surplus of metabolites downstream from the enzymatic block.
   E. deficiency of downstream product can cause disease.

2. A 10-day-old infant presents with poor feeding, vomiting, and lethargy. Sepsis (overwhelming bacterial infection in the blood) is suspected. A look at the prior history reveals normal pregnancy and delivery. The child was discharged after 48 hours of life. Over the next week, the baby became progressively more ill. If a genetic disease such as inborn errors of metabolism is suspected, which of the following is least informative?
   A. Family history of neonatal deaths.
   B. Family history of consanguinity.
   C. Infant's feeding/dietary history information.
   D. Any unusual odors.
   E. Chromosomal analysis.

3. Inborn errors of metabolism may have a plethora of presentations. Which one of the following is one such presentation?

   A. Overgrowth.
   B. Jaundice/high bilirubin levels.
   C. Tumor formation.
   D. Enlarged muscles.
   E. Enhanced intellectual functioning.

4. Inborn errors of metabolism:
   A. may cause structural congenital anomalies.
   B. have been described since the 16th century.
   C. because they are rare and have no effective therapies, are of limited clinical interest.
   D. early treatment and intervention almost guarantees no long-term problems.
   E. are distinct in their presentation from most other medical conditions.

5. In regards to phenylketonuria (PKU):
   A. with the advent of newborn screening, it is quite rare to see an untreated child in the United States.
   B. dietary therapy is effective and easy to implement.
   C. effective therapy prevents all complications of the disorder.
   D. high levels of phenylalanine in fathers with PKU results in birth defects in their infants (such as microcephaly and congenital heart disease).
   E. excess tyrosine leads to disorders of neurotransmitter concentrations.

Supplementary Readings

Clarke, Joe T. R. *A Clinical Guide to Inherited Metabolic Diseases.*

Hoffmann, Georg F., Johannes Zschocke, and William L. Nyhan. *Inherited Metabolic Diseases: A Clinical Approach.*

Nyhan, William L., and Pinar T. Ozand. *Atlas of Metabolic Diseases.*

Saudubray, Jean-Marie, Georges van den Berghe, and John H. Walter. *Inborn Metabolic Diseases: Diagnosis and Treatment.*

Scriver, Charles R., William S. Sly, Barton Childs, Arthur L. Beaudet, David Valle, Kenneth W. Kinzler, and Bert Vogelstein. *The Metabolic and Molecular Bases of Inherited Disease, 4 volumes.*

chapter

9 Family History and Pedigree Analysis

CHAPTER SUMMARY

Genetics is about family histories. Whether you are doing experimental breeding of mice or are exploring diversity in the human population, genetic traits are passed in family lineages. But when the focus is on a molecular or a developmental question, that relationship is easily taken for granted. On the other hand, pedigrees can be valuable when taking a broader view of gene expression, phenotypic variability, and patterns of transmission. Pedigrees can yield insights that single mating examples fail to provide. That is especially true for human genetics, where experimental matings typical of model organism studies cannot be performed.

Pedigrees are a simple way to summarize a lot of information about genetic relationships. One of the most famous pedigrees is that for hemophilia in the royal families of Europe (Figure 9-1). The most common form of this blood clotting condition is hemophilia A, a sex-linked trait associated with a defect in clotting factor VIII. Indeed, it was the first human genetic trait to be found to follow a sex-linked inheritance pattern. Other forms of hemophilia include hemophilia B affecting clotting factor IX, which is also sex-linked, and hemophilia C coding factor XI, which is autosomal. Although hemophilia A is more common, this type of trait heterogeneity can obviously complicate the genetic analysis of a pedigree if one carelessly ignores alternative explanations.

In the case of sex-linked hemophilia, genetics and history are clearly intertwined. A law in the Jewish Talmud, dating from about AD 600, implicitly recognizes the biological associations for this trait by allowing male children to be excused from ritual circumcision based upon having relatives with a bleeding disease. In the case of the descendants of Queen Victoria, hemophilia had serious consequences, at least indirectly, for the stability of the Russian royal family, the Romanovs, which ended with the death of Tsar Nicholas II and his family. His young son Alexei, a great-grandchild of Queen Victoria, suffered from hemophilia. The story of this family's isolation from the problems facing the Russian peasants and the powerful influence of the monk Rasputin form a sad tale of power, conflict, and human weakness. Alexei's medical condition gave Rasputin an influence in political activities that contributed to the overthrow of the Romanovs.

The Romanov family's execution generated famous rumors, including the supposed survival of the young sister, Anastasia, depicted in numerous books and movies. The story was finally resolved with establishment of the identities of family members taken from a hidden grave and confirmed using conclusive DNA evidence. In fact, the genetic study led to new information. The form of hemophilia seen in the European Royal families has generally been assumed to be the more common form, hemophilia A. But recent sequencing of the loci in preserved tissue samples from two members of the family, Alexei and his mother, the Russian Empress Alexandra, indicate that the locus was the less common sex-linked form, hemophilia B. Genetics and history are often linked in complex and interesting ways.

In this Chapter, we will begin by introducing some of the basic logic of representing genetic relationships in pedigrees. The Medical Genetics section will focus on actual cases and some of the difficulties encountered in evaluating the inheritance of often complex phenotypes. The general emphasis will be on the types of information that can be gained from a group of related individuals in contrast to our earlier focus on one mating or an individual alone.

Part 1: Background and Systems Integration

Pedigree Organization

In Chapter 6, we explored the genetic relationships among relatives by discussing basic Mendelian patterns of inheritance. Here we approach the analysis of gene transmission within families again, but in a slightly more formal way. Superficially, a **pedigree** is really nothing more than a series of Mendelian genetic crosses involving relatives. But we often find that seeing the patterns of expression in a pedigree can yield important clues about a genetic condition that the study of one isolated patient or family cannot.

Various approaches can provide information about patterns of inheritance. One of the first studies of this kind was

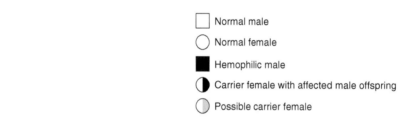

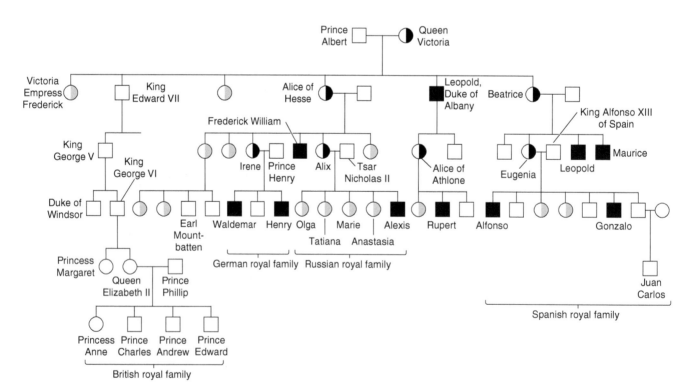

Figure 9-1. Well-publicized pedigree of hemophilia in the royal families of Europe.

done by George Darwin, the son of Charles Darwin, who explored the frequency of first cousin marriages in Great Britain. Indeed, George Darwin was the product of a first-cousin marriage between his father and his mother, Emma, a member of the Wedgwood china family. George Darwin's focus was on marriages between people with the same surname and yielded a frequency of 2.25% to 4.5%, with the British upper classes being at the high end of the range. Studies now utilize DNA markers, especially short tandem repeats (STRs) in the paternally-transmitted Y chromosome and hypervariable region mutations in the maternally-transmitted mtDNA.

Pedigrees are organized by generation. Symbols used to summarize information about the phenotypes and biological relationships are shown in Figure 9-2. Here is a useful hint: to begin to interpret an inheritance pattern, reverse the way you normally think about gene transmission. Rather than looking for the appearance of a trait among the progeny of a family, look from the progeny generation backward toward the parents. In other words, begin by looking at transmission patterns by moving your attention up the pedigree, not down it. If, for example, a child shows a dominant trait, then you expect one of the parents to show it. The other direction is not as certain. Just because a parent has a dominant trait does not mean that one of their few children will necessarily inherit it. Examples of this logic are explored in the next section.

The **proband** (or **propositus** [male], **proposita** [female]) is the first member in a family to be evaluated by the physician. If affected, that individual is the index case for the pedigree. Relatives may be first degree (parents, siblings, offspring of the proband), second degree (grandparents, grandchildren, uncles, aunts, nieces, nephews), or third degree (cousins, and so forth).

Finally, as with any analysis of human inheritance, pedigrees are susceptible to confusion by what we might call extramarital involvements. Even adoption is not always acknowledged publicly. Sensitivity to such issues is a natural and necessary element of all human genetic analyses. There can be a fine balance when issues of privacy and scientific accuracy are in play. Although pedigrees might only rarely include complications of this type, such possibilities should never be forgotten.

Basic Pedigree Analysis

One way to approach a pedigree is to ask a simple set of questions, since the number of common inheritance patterns is fairly small. To outline a logical approach, a few simplifying assumptions will be made. We will assume that the pedigree reflects the accurate biological relationships among genetically-related individuals and that the trait is a single-gene Mendelian characteristic, rather than a multiple-gene, or **polygenic**, predisposition.

First determine whether the trait is dominant or recessive. Dominance is easily recognized.

- If the trait is dominant, each affected child will have an affected parent. The lineage of the trait can be traced continuously up the pedigree (Figure 9-3).
- Furthermore, unaffected siblings will have only normal offspring.

But, if the trait commonly skips generations so that an affected child has phenotypically normal parents, then it does not fit the pattern of a dominant. The alternate hypothesis, recessive inheritance, is supported (Figure 9-4). To confirm recessive inheritance, note that if two affected individuals (both being recessive homozygotes) have offspring, all of the offspring will have the trait. Also be aware that recessive traits

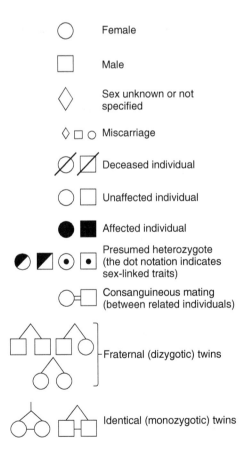

Figure 9-2. Symbols used in pedigree construction.

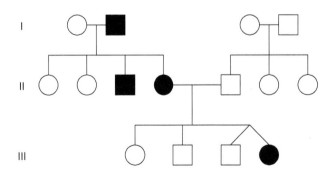

Figure 9-3. Sample pedigree for a simple dominant trait.

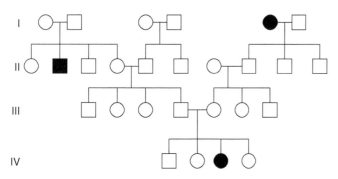

Figure 9-4. Representative pedigree showing an autosomal recessive trait. The appearance of affected offspring from normal parents is consistent with recessive inheritance. For offspring II-8 to -10, there is evidence the trait is autosomal, since a homozygous female for a sex-linked trait must pass it to all of her sons. Can you find another piece of evidence in support of autosomal linkage?

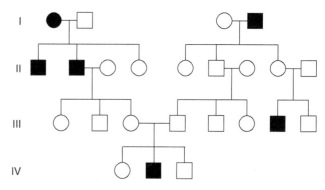

Figure 9-6. Representative pedigree for a sex-linked trait. Passage is never from father to a son, but an affected female has only affected sons. Here is a "test yourself" question: could the parents III-3 and III-4 be theoretically able to produce an affected daughter? The answer is "no." Why not?

may show up more often in pedigrees involving **consanguineous** marriages (matings between close relatives).

If a trait generally follows one of these common patterns but an occasional exception occurs, then consider additional factors like **incomplete penetrance** (Figure 9-5). A dominant trait that occasionally appears to skip a generation may simply be non-penetrant in an affected member of the family and thus undetectable by general visual assessment.

The next step is to determine linkage relationships (Figure 9-6). Is the trait or DNA marker sex-linked (i.e.,

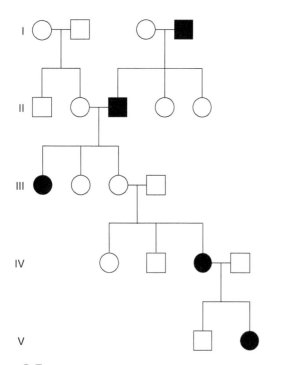

Figure 9-5. This pedigree is consistent with dominant inheritance, except for individual III-3, who apparently passes on the dominant trait but does not express it. This can be interpreted as an example of incomplete penetrance.

transmitted on an X chromosome or, more rarely, on a Y) or is it autosomal? For sex-linkage, we will limit our attention to the X chromosome. A good way to approach this question is to look for exceptions to the pattern expected for a sex-linked trait. If an exception to sex-linked transmission is found, the trait must be autosomal.

- Are there examples of both a father and a son expressing a dominant trait? Here the focus is on excluding sex-linkage by finding exceptions. The father only passes his X chromosome to his daughters. If a son inherits the trait from the father, it cannot be sex-linked (see, for example, Figure 9-5). Of course, one must be careful when a trait is common in the population or when both sides of the family carry it. In those cases a son and father might both be affected with a sex-linked condition, but the son inherited from the mother, not the father.
- For a recessive sex-linked trait, all sons of an affected (i.e., homozygous) mother will express the trait.
- When a sex-linked trait is recessive, it will appear most commonly, and perhaps exclusively, in the males of a pedigree. With only one X chromosome, a male will express a trait no matter whether it is dominant or recessive in females. But if the sex-linked trait is dominant, it might be expected to occur somewhat more frequently in females if a large number of individuals in a population are screened. This is simply because 2/3 of all X chromosomes are found in females.

Of course, there will be exceptions to these typical patterns. One must combine information about the pattern of inheritance with knowledge about the phenotype. If the trait is gender-specific, like female lactation, or is sex-influenced, like pyloric stenosis found more often in males or lupus erythematosis in females, then a simple analysis of affected genders in the pedigree alone can be misleading. Pedigree analysis is, after all, a kind of puzzle.

Sample Pedigree Evaluation: Applying the Rules

One reason to determine the mode of transmission and expression for a pedigree is to allow predictions about children who will be born into it. Once a trait has been characterized, it is possible to assign genotypes, or at least probabilities of a given genotype, to members of the pedigree and use that information to predict the trait's expression in the next generation.

Consider the pedigree in Figure 9-7. The first question is the type of expression, dominant or recessive. In this case, we hypothesize that the trait is recessive. The affected daughter in the second generation (II-7) shows the trait, but both parents are normal. Next, is the trait inherited autosomally or on the X chromosome? If the trait were sex-linked, the affected daughter would be homozygous and must have inherited the trait from both parents. With only one X chromosome, the father must express it, but he does not. Thus, we can conclude that the recessive trait is autosomally inherited.

Now knowing the manner of transmission, we can begin to assign genotypes to some individuals. For example, the first generation parents in the right-hand side of the pedigree (the female I-3 and male I-4) must both be heterozygous since they produce a homozygous recessive daughter. For convenience, let us assign the symbol *A* for the dominant and *a* for the recessive alleles (Figure 9-7b). On the

left-hand side, a phenotypically normal *AA* female I-1 and affected *aa* male I-2 have a phenotypically normal, thus heterozygous, daughter (II-3). In the absence of any conflicting evidence, we always assume that individuals, like male II-4, marrying into the pedigree are genetically normal for the trait. The mating that gives rise to male III-1 is, therefore, *Aa* × *AA*, and there is a ½ chance that male III-1 is heterozygous *Aa*.

Returning again to the right-hand side of the pedigree, let's consider the genotype of male II-5. In order for the child of interest (IV-1) to be homozygous for the *a* allele, the allele must be passed on by male II-5. What is his probability of his being heterozygous? The answer is 2/3. This number might initially surprise you (a common error is to say the probability is ½), but the logic is simple. Of the four possible outcomes of a mating between two heterozygous parents, one is eliminated by the pedigree; the male II-5 is not *aa* since he does not express the recessive trait. Thus, among the remaining three possible outcomes involving phenotypically normal offspring, two are *Aa* heterozygotes and the third is homozygous normal (*AA*). Then, if II-5 is heterozygous, there is a 0.5 chance of his passing the recessive allele to his daughter, III-2. For the yet-to-be-born child, IV-1, to show the recessive trait (a ¼ chance if both parents are heterozygotes), then all of these transmission events must have occurred. The overall probability requires applying the product rule.

The **product rule** applied to probabilities is simply that the likelihood of two or more events occurring together is the product of their individual probabilities. For example, the probability of flipping two nickels and getting a head both times is ½ (the probability of a head the first time) times ½ (the probability of getting a head the second time) = ¼. The other three outcomes are: head + tail; tail + tail; and tail + head. An assumption is, of course, that the events in question are independent.

Each member in a pedigree is the product of an independent fertilization event. The probability of inheriting the mutant *a* allele from a *Aa* heterozygote is, therefore, ½. The overall probability of a given outcome can be calculated by multiplying the probabilities of each required step leading to that hypothetical outcome. We can multiply the required steps in any order we wish, as long as all are included in the calculation. Ignoring the certainties (a probability of 1.0) and moving from generation II through IV, the calculation is ⅔ × ½ × ½ × ¼ = 1/24 of child IV-1 being *aa* and showing this recessive condition.

The analysis of a pedigree is, therefore, a combination of applying known information and calculating probabilities for elements that are unknown. By first determining the probable mode of transmission, one can convert individual phenotypes into genotypes. Then, breaking the pedigree down into individual families, one can predict the likelihood of specific transmission events. The overall assessment factors in these individual probabilities. Having a logical structure like this to work from allows you to approach even the most complex pedigree in an organized and confident manner.

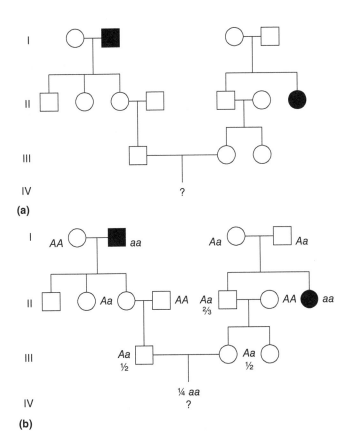

(a)

(b)

Figure 9-7. A pedigree to evaluate as a sample problem (see text).

Why pay money to have your family tree traced? Go into politics and your opponent will do it for you.

- Mark Twain

The Importance of the Family History

In a very real sense this is the most important chapter in this book. Most of you, the readers, will not be going into a career in medical genetics. Still, as we have stressed throughout the previous chapters, a working knowledge of medical genetics is a must for all current and future health care professionals. A detailed family history should be part of the medical record of each and every patient. This information is as critical to the chart as vital signs, examination findings and laboratory results. In addition, a carefully constructed and appropriately interpreted family history is an incredibly powerful diagnostic tool. Throughout this book we emphasize all of the amazing advances in molecular genetics. Exciting new tools are being developed continuously. And in the overall diagnostic yield (i.e., what will give you a tangible answer) the family history is equally effective as all of the available genetic testing options combined!

For centuries people interested in human genetic disorders have relied on the family history as an invaluable source of information. As technological advances have emerged at an amazing rate over the past few years, the question arises, "Is there still a role for the family history in the 'age of genomics'?" The answer is an emphatic "yes." Despite all of the advances in genetic technology, the family history still remains one of the most informative tools in a medical practice—of any type.

Traditional medical education about family history has been sorely underemphasized. All physicians should be skilled in obtaining and interpreting family history information. Every patient should have complete family history information as part of their medical record. This information should be systematically and periodically updated throughout the life course. It should then be incorporated into the overall medical plan. It can aid in diagnosis, treatment, and prevention of a host of illnesses.

The surgeon general, in cooperation with other agencies within the U.S. Department of Health and Human Services, launched a national public health campaign called the Surgeon General's Family History Initiative in November 2004. This initiative was developed to encourage all American families to learn more about their family health history. Every year since then, the surgeon general has declared Thanksgiving to be National Family History Day. Families are encouraged to discuss and record health problems that seem to run in their family as they are gathered together. The goals of this initiative are listed in Table 9-1.

Family Relationships

Pedigrees are simply graphic representations of members of a kindred and their relationship to each other. All health care providers should be comfortable in constructing and interpreting medical pedigrees. If the reader needs to review this process, it is reviewed in the first section of this chapter.

An important element in calculating risks for the transmission of a condition found in one family member for another is determining the degree of relationship of the person in question to the affected individual. In this context, relatives may be:

- First Degree: parents, siblings, offspring of the proband
- Second Degree: grandparents, grandchildren, uncles, aunts, nieces, nephews
- Third Degree: cousins, etc.

These (and other) degrees of relationships can be mathematically defined. Numbers such as the coefficient of relationship can be used to essentially describe the relative number of genes two individuals are expected to share based upon ancestry. The reader is referred back to Figures 6-27 and 6-28 for a quick review.

Obtaining a Family History in the Clinical Setting

At all levels, major health care organizations and authorities have come forth in support of the central role family health plays in the provision of clinical services. Besides the surgeon general's initiative, formal endorsements and resources have come from organizations like the American Medical

Table 9-1.	Goals of the United States Surgeon General's American Family Health Initiative

- Increase the public's awareness of the importance of family history in their own health
- Provide publically accessible tools to gather, understand, evaluate, and use family history information for lay individuals and health professionals
- Increase the awareness of health professionals about the importance of family history
- Increase the utilization of the family history by health care professionals and communicate this with their patients
- Increase genomics and health literacy
- Prepare both the American public and their health professionals for the coming era in which genomics will be an integral part of regular health care

Association and the American Academy of Family Practitioners. Current "standard of practice" recommendations are that *every patient,* in any practice setting should have family history as part of their medical record. It is recommended that a three generation pedigree should be obtained and periodically updated on all families in a medical practice. For pediatric patients, that would include the patient, their siblings, parents, aunts, uncles, cousins, and grandparents. For an adult it may also include the patient's children and grandchildren. Further generations should be included if the patient is aware of other relevant health history for more distant relatives. The typical type of information to be obtained in a family history is listed in Table 9-2.

Despite the resounding endorsements from major medical organizations, in reality the use of the family history in general medical practice falls far short of the published recommendations. Busy clinicians simply do not feel that they have sufficient time to obtain, organize, and analyze family history information. The solution requires innovative approaches to the family history that require the least amount of time of the practitioner. One of the best tools in this regard is to use a family history questionnaire. This form can be filled out in the waiting room at the time the patient is also filling out demographic intake information. The questionnaire can generate family history information from which a basic pedigree may be drawn by trained office staff. The completed pedigree can then be available on the chart as the practitioner enters the room along with the other important information typically provided like chief complaint, vital signs, and past medical history. At that point, all the physician needs to do is review the completed pedigree and apply the knowledge gained from training to interpret and act upon the information. Several good tools exist if the physician wants to use tools already developed. Most are readily available through internet sources. A few of the more well-known tools include:

- In association with the family history initiative discussed earlier, the surgeon general has created a computerized tool for obtaining a family's health history. It is written

Table 9-2. Typical Information To Be Obtained in a Three-Generation Pedigree

- Age or year of birth
- Age and cause of death (for those deceased)
- Ethnic background of each grandparent
- Relevant health information (*e.g.*, height, weight)
- Illnesses and age at diagnoses
- Information regarding prior genetic counseling and testing
- Information regarding pregnancies (stillbirths, infertility, spontaneous miscarriages, complications, prematurity)

to walk nonmedical persons through the process in an easy and fun context. It can be accessed at:
  ○ https://familyhistory.hhs.gov/fhh-web/home.action
- The American Medical Association also has tools for obtaining a family medical history. This site has separate forms for pediatric, adult, or prenatal patients. These can be accessed at:
  ○ http://www.ama-assn.org/ama/pub/physician-resources/medical-science/genetics-molecular-medicine/family-history.page
- The National Human Genome Research Institute also has several resources available at :
  ○ http://www.genome.gov/11510372

Families are indeed unique and complex. It is important that the person obtaining the family history information be aware of possible confounding issues. Certain family situations can lead to erroneous conclusions being drawn from the pedigree. For instance, it is estimated that 10% to 15% of people have **mis-assigned paternity**. That is, the person assumed to be the father is actually not the biological ancestor. Besides the obvious psychosocial implications of this information, it would of course obviate much of the information obtained in a pedigree were this information not revealed. This is also important in DNA testing, as will be discussed in a future chapter. By the nature of such testing, errantly-assigned paternity may be revealed unintentionally. Among other important considerations, this should be discussed during the informed consent process prior to obtaining the requisite samples.

Consanguinity is defined as the mating of two closely related individuals. The biological and genetic implications of this situation have been discussed in an earlier chapter. From the standpoint of obtaining a family history, there are several important points. Of course, there is the obvious stigma, and even legal ramifications, of such a union. For that reason, family members will often be hesitant to come forward with this information. Surprisingly, some individuals may not even be aware of a common ancestor and may actually identify this relationship through the process of obtaining the family history. Other potential sources of confusion include alternative relationships such as adoption, half-siblings, and persons with children via several different mates. Care must be taken to identify these relationships if at all possible in order to have the family history information accurately reflect the biological and genetic relationships within the family.

The issue of confidentiality is a crucial one in all aspects of clinical care. Because genetic conditions involve families and not just individuals, protecting confidentiality can require extraordinary efforts on the part of the practitioner. This is especially true for family practice physicians in which several members of the same family may receive their medical care from a single provider. Every effort must be made to keep each individual's information in strictest confidence. Such information should only be shared with other family members in the context of explicit and documented consent or when it affects the health of another person.

Interpreting the Family History

The recommended standard of practice, then, is to have an up-to-date three generational pedigree as part of every patient's medical record. Of course, this is just the first step. Simply having a pedigree on the chart does not by itself help in the care of the patient. The purpose of a book like this one is to prepare physicians to incorporate the principles of medical genetics into their daily practice. Thus, the practicing physician should be adept at interpreting the pedigree information for each patient. The pedigree should be scanned for relevant information. The practitioner should be comfortable in identifying what is significant in a family history. Every family will have medically notable conditions in some individuals. The trick is to identify when something is significant or not. Clearly, experience helps in this regard. The typical "red flags" that should alert the reviewer are by and large intuitive (Table 9-3). Factors such as the number of affected individuals, unusual presentations, and the degree of relationship should be considered. The practitioner should be alert to characteristics of the pattern of affected individuals. If it appears to be simple Mendelian inheritance (Chapter 6), then a monogenic etiology may be expected. If the pattern is clearly familial but does not follow a single gene pattern, a more complex explanation should be considered (Chapter 10). The Clinical Correlation section of this chapter provides an example of the way this might look in practice.

Responding to the Family History

Finally, it is not enough simply to obtain a family history and interpret it. The final step is to use the information to modify the patient's care. If the review of the pedigree identifies a significant family history, the practitioner should respond accordingly. In the event of a significant positive family history he or she should:

- Counsel the family—within their own comfort level for the particular condition
- Order specific indicated tests
- Identify at-risk family members
- Offer preventative strategies
- Utilize consultation as needed

Within the context of evidence-based medicine, the family history can actually be used to modify screening guidelines and recommended management protocols for many common disorders (Tables 9-4 and 9-5).

Table 9-4.	Conditions in Which Established Population Screening Guidelines Are Influenced by the Family History
Breast cancer	
Cardiomyopathy	
Colon cancer	
Coronary artery disease	
Diabetes	
Dyslipidemia	
Hearing impairment	
Hip dysplasia	
Hypertension	
Iron def anemia	
Liver cancer	
Osteoporosis	
Prostate cancer	
Thromboembolism	
Thyroid disease	
Visual impairment	

Data from Guttmacher AE: The Importance of Family History in Health. SACGHS. October 11, 2004. Available at: http://oba.od.nih.gov/oba/SACGHS/meetings/October2004/Guttmacher.pdf. Accessed August 28, 2012.

Table 9-5.	Conditions in Which Established Management Guidelines Are Influenced by the Family History
Breast cancer	
Colon cancer	
Coronary heart disease	
Developmental delay	
Diabetes	
Emphysema & COPD	
Heart failure	
Hypertension	
Pancreatitis	
Syncope	
Thromboembolism	
Thyroid cancer	
Urticaria	

Data from Guttmacher AE: The Importance of Family History in Health. SACGHS. October 11, 2004. Available at: http://oba.od.nih.gov/oba/SACGHS/meetings/October2004/Guttmacher.pdf. Accessed August 28, 2012.

Table 9-3.	Review of the Family History

"Red flags" in a family history
  Number of relatives affected
  Degree of relationship to proband
  Age of onset
  Least affected sex
  Related disorders

Positive family history
  Mendelian pattern
    Monogenic conditions
  Non-Mendelian pattern
    Complex disorder

Case 1

Within the context of regular medical practice, the family history can be used to modify care. For example, let's say that a new patient presents for "an office physical" to your practice. Your staff greets him at the reception desk and gives him the requisite forms to fill out. As part of this packet he is asked for demographic and insurance information. Another part of that packet collects information about his past medical history and other health care providers who have worked with him. Knowing what has been discussed in this chapter; your packet also has a printout of a family history tool, which he fills out. Your trained office staff takes the information from the packet and constructs a pedigree. When you enter the room, you note from his newly-constructed chart that the patient is a 52-year-old hispanic male who presents for a work physical. On the family history form he has checked "Yes" for a positive family history of diabetes, cancer, and heart disease. What intervention should you do based on this family history? If you are scratching your head, you are thinking "I don't have enough information"—and of course you are correct. So you flip the page and review the pedigree your staff has constructed for you. Look at Figure 9-8. Your patient is individual IV.1. In this pedigree, the family history does not look very remarkable, does it? There is only one person with cancer. This was pancreatic cancer at an advanced

age. Likewise, he only reports single occurrences of diabetes and heart disease with neither looking particularly remarkable.

But look at Figure 9-9. We think you would agree that this looks quite different from the first pedigree, and yet would have had the same "yes's" marked on the intake form. This pedigree is significant. There are multiple affected individuals with heart attacks and strokes. The ages of onset are quite early. In fact, upon further questioning, you are told that individual III-1, who died at 52 of a heart attack, actually had his first myocardial infarction at 38. Also note a 36-year-old first cousin (III-3), who is a female, died of a heart attack at 36! Finally, a quick review of the pedigree suggests autosomal dominant inheritance. In this case, your response is very different. Even though your patient is a healthy individual who simply came in for a physical exam, his family history screams at you: "do something." Here is your chance. You can actually be part of intervention before the problem, i.e., real prevention. What would you do next? At a minimum the easiest and least expensive step would simply be to gather more information. Asking for medical records (with signed releases) from the affected family members would be a great start. The rest of the answer is beyond the scope of this chapter. Look forward to Chapter 10 to get an idea of what your thought process might be in this scenario.

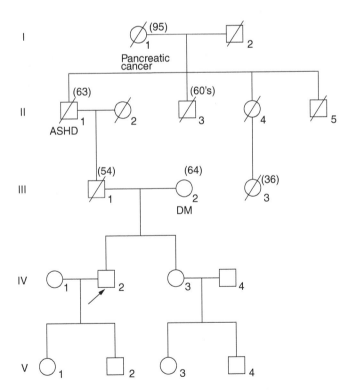

Figure 9-8. Possible pedigree from a new patient (IV-1) who presents for a work physical. On his intake form, the patient marked a positive family history of heart disease, diabetes, and cancer. (ASHD = atherosclerotic heart disease. DM = Diabetes mellitus)

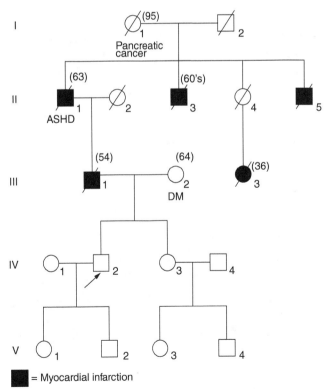

Figure 9-9. Second scenario of the new patient visit. Patient IV-1 has marked the same positive family history as in Figure 9-8. Notice the very different implications. (ASHD = atherosclerotic heart disease. DM = Diabetes mellitus)

Case 2

Consider the following case. You are a resident in orthopedic surgery. As part of your clinical rotations, you are assigned to an interdisciplinary cerebral palsy clinic. During the clinic you see a 20-year-old young man who has the diagnosis of "cerebral palsy." He has carried this diagnosis since early childhood. While looking through his chart, you notice that a family history is not part of his medical record. So you ask the simple question: "has anyone else in the family had cerebral palsy?" His mother is amazed by your question and answers, "yes." You then obtain a forma family history and construct the pedigree. The completed product looks like Figure 9-10a. Being the astute well-trained young doctor that you are, you look at this pedigree and quickly come to the conclusion that this looks like an X-linked recessive disorder.

Your knowledge of the diagnosis of cerebral palsy causes you to question the accuracy of the diagnosis. Ultimately, an MRI of the brain is obtained and the patient is found to have the findings of an olivopontocerebellar atrophy (Figure 9-10b). This is an actual case that we reported in 1989 as a rare case of an X-linked olivopontocerebellar atrophy. It highlights the power of simply asking the patient about his or her family.

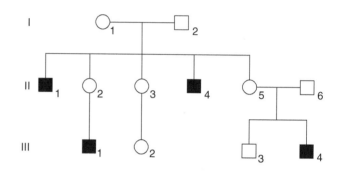

Figure 9-11. Pedigrees: sample board format questions. See answer section for explanation.

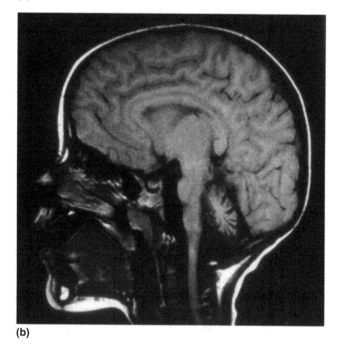

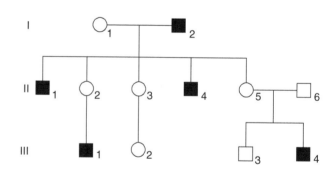

Figure 9-12. Pedigrees: sample board format questions. See answer section for explanation.

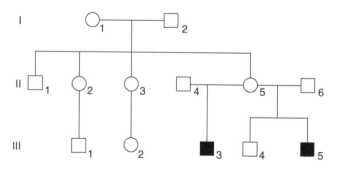

Figure 9-10. (a) Pedigree of a young adult (III-6) with the diagnosis of cerebral palsy. Note the affected uncle and cousin. (b) MRI of the brain of patient III-6.

Figure 9-13. Pedigrees: sample board format questions. See answer section for explanation.

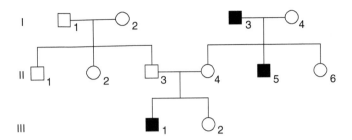

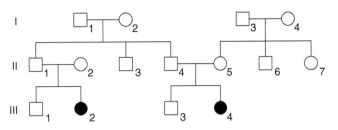

Figure 9-15. Pedigrees: sample board format questions. See answer section for explanation.

Figure 9-14. Pedigrees: sample board format questions. See answer section for explanation.

■ Board-Format Practice Questions

Questions 1–5 correspond to Figures 9-11–9-15, respectively. For each pedigree identify the most likely mode of inheritance. For some there may be more than one possible inheritance pattern. For test questions like these and on the board exams, you will be asked to select the *best* answer.

Multifactorial Inheritance and Gene × Environment Interactions

CHAPTER SUMMARY

The study of human inheritance often tends to focus on relatively simple traits. But as we explored in Chapter 2 and elsewhere, there is a broad avenue of molecular and developmental events that connect the DNA with a phenotype. When the work of Gregor Mendel was "rediscovered" in 1900, various researchers attempted to repeat and confirm his observations using a variety of plants and animals, including humans. Some studies supported the Mendelian genetic models. But many other cases were unsuccessful either because the organisms they chose had unusual genetic characteristics, like honeybee drones that are haploid, or because the traits they looked at did not have the simple phenotypic basis that we see in those studied by Mendel. Some people attribute these latter studies to bad luck in choosing an experimental system. But in fact they were setting the stage to explore a parallel, and very important, dimension of genetic complexity.

This is illustrated historically by the work of people like Francis Galton, a cousin to Charles Darwin, and Karl Pearson, one of the founders of modern statistics. A key trait they studied, human height (Figure 10-1), is now known to be influenced both by a number of genes segregating independently and by many environmental variables. The genotypes were not simple, so the application of Mendelian rules could not be detected. Galton's initial work actually predates the rediscovery of Mendel's papers by several decades, and indeed it was hotly debated whether quantitative traits have the same underlying genetic basis as seen in simpler Mendelian traits like flower color and seed shape. But far from being a dead end, work by pioneers like these led to the establishment of an important field of genetics, biometrical or quantitative genetics, based on the statistical analysis of genetic relationships.

Significant advances over the last couple of decades have seen the emergence of quantitative genetics as a field with important biomedical perspectives. It is leading to a deeper understanding of the way traits are influenced by quantitative trait loci (QTLs). This appreciation of the multilayered genetic underpinnings of normal phenotypic diversity and a large array of significant medical conditions reflects the continuing maturity of genetics as an explanatory science. In this chapter, we will discuss the basis of phenotype assessments and some of the ways this knowledge can be applied to benefit patients.

Part 1: Background and Systems Integration

Quantitative versus Qualitative Traits

Most of the phenotypes we have discussed to this point are relatively simple, in that they can be traced to mutations in one or a couple of genes and they generally follow predictable rules of transmission and expression. On the other hand, many important traits are influenced not by one gene, but by a battery of genes whose effects are over-shadowed by unknown environmental factors. In fact, if we analyze almost any trait in detail, we soon realize that all genes work within a complex network of biochemical interactions and environmental conditions. One only has to think back to phenomena like variable expressivity to see examples. But the fundamental inheritance mechanisms are the same.

How can one make genetic predictions about traits that are so complicated? The key, as usual, is to acknowledge that genetic

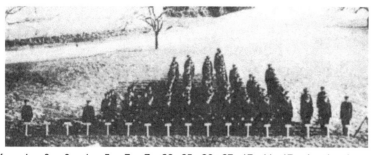

Figure 10-1. Human height was one of the earliest quantitative characters studied in detail. (a) Height distribution (inches) for 175 students in 1914 attending the Connecticut Agricultural College. (b) Graphical presentation of these student heights showing their close fit to a normal distribution. (a: Reprinted with permission from Albert and Blakeslee: Corn and Man. *Journal of Heredity.* 1914;5:51. Oxford University Press. b: Reprinted with permission from Brooker RJ: *Genetics: Analysis & Principles,* 3rd ed. New York: McGrawHill, 2008.)

Number of students	1	0	0	1	5	7	7	22	25	26	27	17	11	17	4	4	1
Height (inches)	58	59	60	61	62	63	64	65	66	67	68	69	70	71	72	73	74

(a)

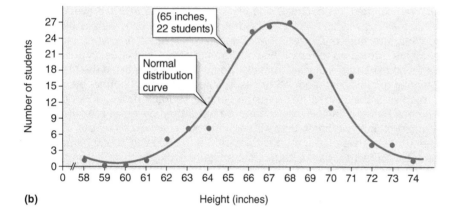

(b)

effects on human development are complex. But there are underlying patterns and relationships that allow us to work effectively with traits that might initially appear almost intractable.

The genetic boundary between "qualitative" and "quantitative" is blurred. But we can establish a context by defining a **qualitative trait** as one that can be categorized by a "quality" into two or more defined phenotypic groupings, like pigmented skin and albino. A **quantitative trait** is one that must be described by some quantity along a spectrum of expressions, like the range of skin pigmentation from dark to light.

This distinction is not simply descriptive. It distinguishes two completely different ways in which phenotypes must be analyzed. A qualitative trait, for example, distributes individuals into defined groups. When traits like this are analyzed statistically, one would present them in clear phenotypic categories (e.g., green versus yellow seeds) and use statistics like the chi square test to evaluate a fit between the observed proportions and a theoretical expectation. For a quantitative trait, on the other hand, the phenotypes are defined by their placement on some scale (e.g., height or degree of pigmentation). In this case, a comparison among groups is dependent on quantitative measurements like phenotypic averages and range of expression. The appropriate statistical tests are quite different. Groups are compared by t-tests, analyses of variance, or other approaches.

In the following sections we will discuss some of these statistical tests. But our goal will be larger. We will explore

the ways one can think about quantitative traits and their genotype × environment interactions. The objective is not just to document them mathematically, but instead to clarify the uncertainties behind complex information that patients and family members want to understand.

Quantitative Description of Phenotypic Distributions

One can visualize the array of phenotypes of a typical quantitative trait as a normal distribution. Such a distribution can be described using standard statistics. Even exceptions like threshold characters (Figure 10-2), in which a certain level of gene product must be reached before the trait is expressed phenotypically, can be interpreted in terms of an underlying distribution of developmental capacities.

The **mean** ($\bar{X}$) is the sum of all measurements (ΣX) divided by the number of individuals in the sample (N). But by itself, the mean overlooks an important element needed for prediction. It overlooks the variation seen among the individuals averaged in the sample. **Variance** (V) is a measure of this dispersal of the trait. More specifically, it is the average squared deviation of each data point from the mean.

$$\text{Variance} = \Sigma N_{i=1} (X_i - \bar{X})^2 / N - 1$$

The value $N - 1$ is called the **degrees of freedom** and is used to assess the strength of conclusion to be drawn in

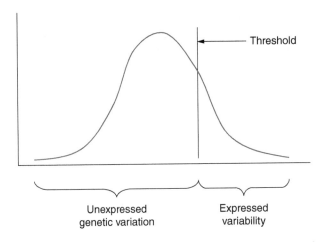

Figure 10-2. A normal distribution of biochemical product of gene activity can underlay a trait that is only expressed when a certain threshold amount is reached. Such traits may appear to be discrete, even though the underlying genetic mechanism is quantitative.

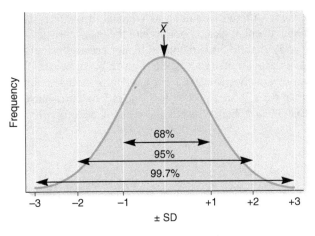

Figure 10-3. This rule is that the standard deviation will subdivide a normal distribution into predictable subgroups of the population. (Reprinted with permission from Brooker RJ: *Genetics: Analysis & Principles*, 3rd ed. New York: McGraw-Hill, 2008.)

many statistical tests. One can think about this measure by a simple thought experiment. Let's imagine gathering a group of data, such as child birth weights. The first child gives one measurement of weight, and so does the second child. So the average weight is calculated by adding the two weights and dividing by 2. But when assessing variance in weight, the first baby gives no indication about how much variability there is in such a measurement. The difference between baby 1 and baby 2, however, gives the first estimate of variation, the third baby gives a second estimate, and so forth. Thus, there are always one fewer estimates of trait variation than there are of trait mean.

$$\text{Standard deviation} = s.d. = s. = \sqrt{\text{variance}}$$

The square root of the variance is called the **standard deviation**, symbolized *s.d., s, or* δ. Similarly, the variance can be symbolized as V_x (i.e., the variance of *x*) or as s^2 or δ^2, since it is the square of the standard deviation. Generally, *s* and s^2 are used when referring to a measured characteristic of a specific sample, and δ and δ^2 are used when referring to the underlying theoretical population of data. You should always expect the mean and standard deviation (or variance) to be presented together in order to have a complete description of a quantitative trait's phenotypic expression.

One of the especially useful applications of the standard deviation is often called the "empirical rule." This rule is that the standard deviation will subdivide a normal distribution into predictable subgroups of the population (Figure 10-3), no matter what trait is being considered. Specifically, one standard deviation above and below the mean of a normal distribution will contain approximately 68% of the data points, while two standard deviations will contain about 95% and three standard deviations will contain 99.7%. For an example of its application, consider performance on a standard IQ test, on which the average score is 100 and the standard deviation is 15 IQ points. A typical population would be expected to have

68% of its members with an IQ score of 85 to 115 points. Half that number, 34%, would be expected to have an IQ between 100 (the mean) and 115. For more accurate evaluation of distribution differences, data are typically converted into units of standard deviation and compared to a table of standard normal deviations.

Polygenic Inheritance and Heritability

As the name suggests, "polygenic" refers to "many genes." The genetic basis of polygenic traits is now often found in the literature as quantitative trait loci or QTLs. Analytical techniques are making it possible to identify some of the loci that contribute most strongly to certain quantitative traits. But it is often enough just to measure the proportion of phenotypic variation that can be traced to segregating genetic differences among individuals, versus how much is due to environmental factors. It is the genetic component that is most influential in determining the trait's expression in the next generation.

Heritability is an important measure, but it is often misunderstood. One should not make the mistake of equating high heritability with high importance. It is a measure of the effect of segregating genetic variation, and critically important traits like those affecting survival or reproductive success (i.e., so-called "fitness traits") seldom tolerate high levels of variety. Directional selection to maximize an individual's survival and reproductive success has selected against less beneficial genetic variation that might have been present in the gene pool. For example, the heritability of IQ test scores in some populations is about 0.60, which means that about 60% of the phenotypic difference among individuals can be explained by genetic allele difference. On the other hand, the heritability for an important fitness trait like egg production in chickens or *Drosophila* is estimated to be only about 0.21 and 0.18, respectively. Thus, heritability simply measures the proportion of phenotypic variation that can be explained by genetic differences among individuals, it is not a statement about the biological importance of the characteristic.

Heritability is symbolized h², not because there is such a thing as its square root (there is no "h"), but because it is the ratio of two variances (s²). For this part of the discussion, however, we will follow the style that uses V to represent variance. Specifically, heritability is the ratio of the proportion of all phenotypic variance (V_P) that can be explained by genetic segregation (V_G), i.e., to genetic differences among members of the sample. V_P in turn has various components, the two most important being genetic segregation and environmental effects (V_E) (Figure 10-4). Thus, for practical purposes,

$$h^2 = V_G/(V_G + V_E)$$

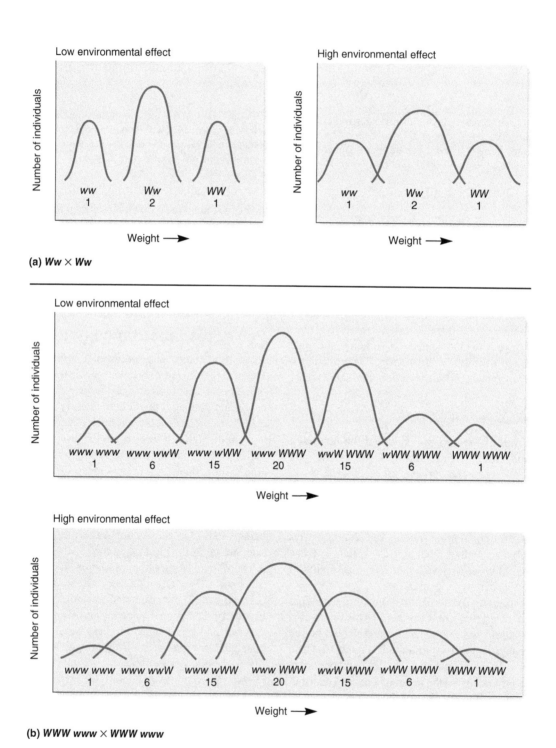

Figure 10-4. An example (using weight as a sample trait) of the effect of the number of alleles and environmental variation on quantitative genetic distributions. (Reprinted with permission from Brooker RJ: *Genetics: Analysis & Principles*, 3rd ed. New York: McGraw-Hill, 2008.)

There is one other aspect of heritability that is critically important to remember. Heritability is a measure of the proportion of phenotypic variation that can be accounted for by genetic differences among members of the sample. But we know that gene pools vary from one time to another and from one population to another. For that reason, heritability is valid only in making predictions about genetic makeup or responses to selection for the population in which it is measured. It cannot validly be generalized from one population to another. Ignoring this simple population genetic fact led to many inaccurate and destructive statements about the genetic differences among races in traits like IQ, since comparisons often generalized heritabilities in unfounded ways.

Genotype × Environment Interactions

Environmental differences can be as important as genetic differences in phenotypic expression. Indeed, the same genotype can be expressed in quite different ways as a relevant environmental factor changes. This type of relationship is called a genotype × environment (G × E) interaction.

A classic example of a G × E interaction is the temperature-sensitive activity of melanin production in Siamese kittens. The enzyme is catalytically more active in cooler conditions, so more pigment is synthesized in the tips of the ears and the paws. Temperature, nutritional components, light wavelength and intensity, and even internal conditions like age and sex can influence the expression of a given genotype.

Genetic Heterogeneity

We pointed out earlier how a single genotype can result in different phenotypes because of environmental influences. The opposite can also be true. The same phenotype can be traceable to genetically different backgrounds. **Genetic heterogeneity** refers to the situation in which a condition or disease could be traced to different underlying genotypes. Different genes or different alleles of a single gene might be involved in each case analyzed. Thus, tools like microarrays or DNA sequencing that uncover the individual makeup of each case are important aides to accurate diagnosis. Given the developmental complexity of even the simplest anatomical structure, cases of genetic heterogeneity should become even more commonly recognized.

One example of genetic heterogeneity is found in the condition retinitis pigmentosa (RP). This is a collection of literally dozens of genes or gene regions at which mutations affect photoreceptor structure or longevity in the eye. This is **locus heterogeneity**. Some mutations are, not surprisingly, more common than others. About 10% of the RP cases, for example, can be traced to mutations in the rhodopsin gene on chromosome 3.

A related situation is found in **allelic heterogeneity**. In these situations, different alleles have distinctly different phenotypic consequences. In fact, in some instances the conditions were thought to be linked but genetically unrelated until

sequencing and other molecular techniques uncovered their relationship. There are a growing number of examples of this phenomenon. One is associated with different mutations in the gene coding for β-globin. One mutation causes sickle cell disease while others result in various forms of β-thalassemia.

Concordance in Twins

Twins provide a special opportunity to explore the repeatability of genetic expression. Monozygotic (MZ) or identical twins share the same genotype and largely the same developmental environment. Dizygotic (DZ) or fraternal twins are probably as similar as are monozygotic twins in their shared developmental environment, but they differ genetically as much as any other typical sibling pair. By measuring the degree of phenotypic agreement, **concordance**, between monozygotic versus dizygotic twins, it is, therefore, possible to estimate the genetic influence on a trait. Some examples are shown in Table 10-1.

It is important to note that although monozygotic twins start off as genetically identical, things can change quickly. Once the twinning event has occurred and the two zygotes resume/continue their development, divergences can occur. Postconception mutations can and often do occur. Since these are largely random events, what occurs in one MZ twin is not what will happen in the other. Thus, even though they started off as genetically identical, there are likely to be multiple genetic differences in the twins by delivery. As was discussed in Chapter 7 (Mutations) many of these genetic differences may affect no observable phenotypic change—and thus the twins still appear "identical." However, on occasion one twin may acquire a mutation that does result in a phenotypic change that is present in one MZ twin but not the other (Figure 10-5). The twins are thus said to be **discordant** for that trait.

Table 10-1.	Trait Concordances in Monozygotic (MZ) and Dizygotic (DZ) Twins		
Trait	MZ Concordance	DZ Concordance	h²*
Manic-depressive psychosis	67	5	~ 1.0
Bronchial asthma	47	24	0.71
Hypertension	25	7	0.62
Rheumatic fever	20	6	0.55
Cancer, at any site	16	13	0.15
Death from acute infection	8	9	0

*Note that heritability is not a direct calculation from the MZ and DZ concordance values, so consider its magnitude independently from the other data; data for all comparisons other than cancer and death from acute infection are highly significant (Based on Cavalli-Sforza and Bodmer, 1971, *The Genetics of Human Populations*, Freeman and Co., San Francisco.)

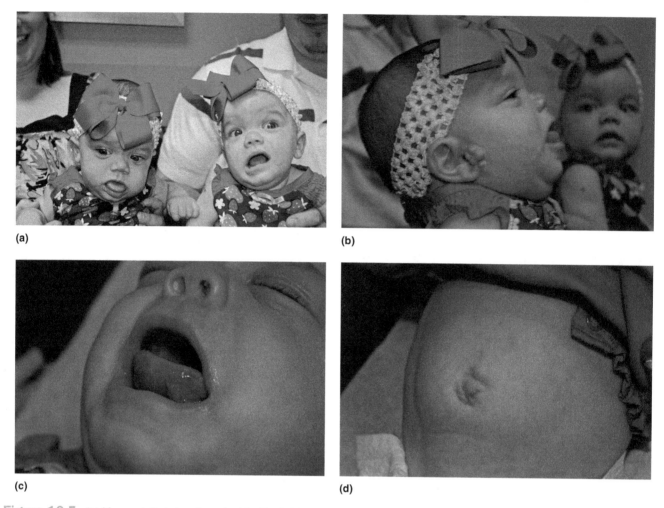

Figure 10-5. (a) Monozygotic twins discordant for Beckwith Wiedemann syndrome (macrosomia, macroglossia, omphalocoele). Note the difference in the phenotype of the twins. (b, c, d) Twin A showing features of Beckwith-Wiedeman syndrome—(b) Preuricular ear tags, (c) Macroglossia, and (d) Ompahlocoele (repaired).

A caveat in twin studies is that it is sometimes difficult to distinguish monozygotic from dizygotic pairs. Tests like DNA fingerprinting may be needed to establish the degree of genetic similarity. In addition, monozygotic twins share the same genotype, but they also share many potentially important environmental conditions like nutritional level and cases of infectious disease. Comparing identical twins raised together with the rare examples of identical twins raised apart might provide a partial answer. But when adopted independently, identical twins are often raised in families with similar environments, such as city living versus rural, education level of the adoptive parents, or number of other children in the household. Twin data are, therefore, informative but not without limitation.

It is also useful to keep in mind that one can use other examples of shared genotype to quantify the genetic influence on a trait, or its **recurrence risk**. Recurrence risk is related to the degree of shared genotype expected among relatives. For a condition traceable to a single gene, the recurrence risk for siblings is 0.50 and it decreases by half for each step of separation in the pedigree (e.g., aunt – nephew = 0.25; first cousins = 0.125).

Part 2: Medical Genetics

Thus far we have discussed cytogenetic abnormalities (Chapter 5) and single gene disorders (Chapter 6) as major categories of etiologies of human genetic disorders. These inheritance modes would best be characterized as uni-factorial. That is, a single key genetic change is responsible for the majority of the phenotype. Historically, these conditions were the first described and are among the best understood genetic conditions. However, these conditions are also relatively rare when all human medical disorders are considered. In general, the more common diseases tend to have more complex

Table 10-2.	Common Medical Disorders With a Proven Genetic Basis
Allergies/asthma	
Autoimmune disorders	
Atherosclerosis	
Cancer	
Diabetes	
Epilepsy	
Hypertension	
Infertility and pregnancy loss	
Longevity and aging	
Major affective disorders/schizophrenia	
Obesity	
Outcome from head trauma	

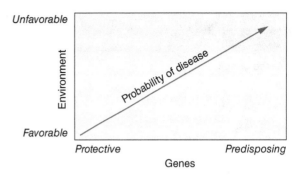

Figure 10-6. Graphic representation of the concept of cumulative liabilities in multifactorial inheritance. As the number of adverse genetic and environmental factors accumulate, the chances of disease expression likewise increases.

modes of inheritance. Still, they will have significant genetic contributions to explain their occurrence (Table 10-2). In the first part of this chapter the concepts of gene-environment interactions were explained. Here we will discuss the applications of these concepts in clinical practice.

Multifactorial Inheritance

"Multifactorial" as the name implies means "many factors." This simply means that both genetic and environmental factors have significant contributions to the phenotype. It is important to note that in a literal sense, all medical conditions are "multifactorial." It is hard to imagine any condition that does not have some degree of genetic basis to it and some degree of environmental modification of the phenotype as well (i.e., the Mendelian and chromosomal disorders as discussed can/do have environmental influences that can modify the phenotype somewhat). By convention the simplest model or mechanism is designated for a given condition to give the most accurate predictions of outcomes (recurrence risk/familial pattern/transmission mode). Thus, Mendelian disorders and chromosomal disorders are not conventionally classified as having "multifactorial inheritance."

So, then, what constitutes multifactorial inheritance? The major features include:

1. Genetic variability exists yet *no uni-factorial mechanism* can be identified to explain the transmission pattern.

2. Family studies indicate an increased risk for relatives to be affected.

3. Environmental factors may exert a significant influence on the phenotype.

Conditions that exhibit multifactorial inheritance usually involve complicated pathophysiologic or morphogenetic processes. This means that the search for an etiology becomes

significantly more complicated. The search is not for "the gene" responsible for the condition. Rather, the pattern that best describes what is observed may involve multiple different genes interacting with more than one environmental factor. As described in the first part of this chapter, the expression of multifactorial traits involves a biologic **threshold**. The concept is that every individual has a set of **liabilities** toward a given condition. These liabilities are both the genetic and environmental factors. Each individual has their own unique combination of protective or predisposing genes and favorable or unfavorable environmental influences (Figure 10-6). For any given person, an increasing number of liabilities push that person toward the biologic threshold. When the cumulative contributions of all genetic and environmental liabilities exceed a certain threshold, the capacity of the organism to buffer against the liabilities is overcome, and the trait is observed (Figure 10-2).

As multifactorial traits are observed in families, several general characteristics are observed in their transmission. The basic principles of inheritance exhibited by multifactorial traits include:

1. The condition does not segregate through the family in a recognizable Mendelian (single gene) or other uni-factorial manner.

2. The recurrence risk of the condition is increased in relatives as compared to its occurrence in the general population.

3. There is a nonlinear decrease in the recurrence risks with an increasing distance of relationship. In general, recurrence risks are higher in first or second degree relatives. Once the distance of relationship becomes greater than third degree, the risk has fallen back to the general population baseline risk.

4. There is an increased risk with an increasing number of affected individuals.

5. Within the spectrum of variably expressed conditions, there is an increased risk seen with an increased severity of the disorder seen in the affected individuals.

Table 10-3.	Multifactorial Conditions Reported With a Significant Sex Bias
Increased in Males	
Condition	Increase (M:F)
Pyloric stenosis	5.0
Legg-Perthes	5.2
Hirschprung	3.7
Talipes equinovarus	2.0
Cleft lip + palate	1.6
Increased in Females	
Condition	Increase (F:M)
Idiopathic scoliosis	6.6
Cong. hip dysplasia	3.3
Anencephaly	1.6
Spina bifida	1.2
Cleft palate	1.4

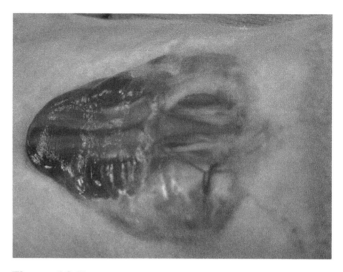

Figure 10-7. Lower back of an infant with an inferior neural tube defect (i.e., spina bifida/meningomyelocoele).

Table 10-4.	Empiric Recurrence Risks for Neural Defects (NTD)
Familial Risk Factor	**Risk for a Subsequent Affected Child (%)**
One child with NTD	5
Two children with NTD	10
Three children with NTD	21
Parent with NTD	4

6. Many multifactorial traits show a sex bias (i.e., they occur more often in one sex than the other) (Table 10-3). Interestingly, an increased recurrence risk is noted if the affected person(s) is of the less commonly affected sex.

For most multifactorial traits we do not know enough about the genetic and environmental factors involved to be of practical use in the clinical setting. For most, then, etiologic-specific counseling is not possible, and this is often confusing and frustrating to patients. However, there is still helpful information that can be provided. If a multifactorial condition is common enough to gather reasonable population data, empiric recurrence risk data may be available and provided to the family. **Empiric risk** counseling is the application of observational population data when little is known about underlying factors. The recurrence risk for a particular family is based upon what has been observed in other, similar families. It involves identifying recurrences in defined subpopulations that are condition and situation specific.

Neural tube defects (NTDs), for example, are congenital malformations of the embryonic neural tube. Failure of the neural tube to close properly will lead to anomalies of the brain and/or spinal cord and the surrounding bony structures (Figure 10-7). There is a range of expression depending upon where/how much of the neural tube fails to close. They are relatively common birth defects, occurring in about 1 to 2 per 1000 births. Neural tube defects exhibit multifactorial inheritance. Because they occur commonly enough, empiric risk data have been obtainable (Table 10-4). Such data are applicable in the clinic setting. Such a scenario might happen something like this: a young couple is seen in which their child was born with a neural tube defect. The pregnancy was uncomplicated. A careful review of the family history reveals no other known family member with a neural tube defect as far back as anyone can remember. Examination of the child does not demonstrate anything else wrong with the child other than the NTD. The couple now wants to know "what are their chances of having another child with an NTD?" In referring to the data in Table 10-4, it can be determined that the answer to their question is 5%. Although this may seem quite simple, there is still a lot of useful information embedded within. As per the discussion above, several deductions based on the multifactorial model can be made. First, the 5% risk clearly does not suggest a Mendelian (single gene) disorder. Second, this risk can be compared to the baseline (population) risk. That is, the recurrence risk is "only" 5% (and for the family that means a 95% chance that a subsequent child will *not* have an NTD). Still, a 5% recurrence risk as compared to a general population incidence of 1/1000 represents a 50-fold increase.

Depending on the amount of data available, even more information can be discerned from empiric data. Cleft lip and cleft palate are among the most common structural congenital anomalies seen in humans (Figure 10-8). Orofacial cleft occurs in 1 to 2 per 1000 live births. About half of the patients born with a cleft have cleft in conjunction with other structural anomalies (i.e., "complex" clefts). The other patients just have a cleft; that is isolated or nonsyndromic clefts. The occurrence of isolated clefts can be explained by a multifactorial model as described earlier. Although intense research continues around defining the etiology of clefts, much is still

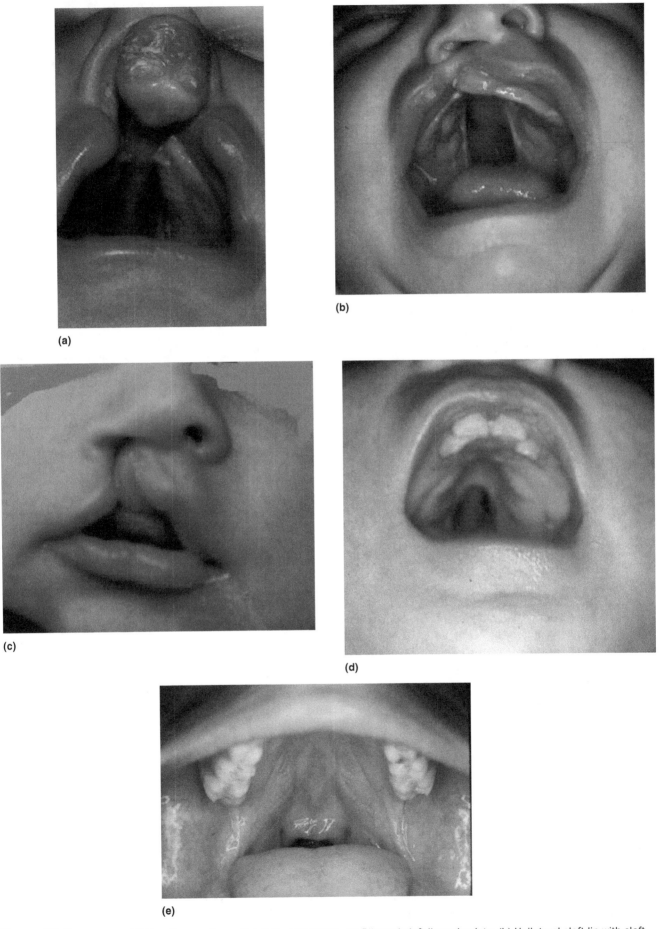

Figure 10-8 Patients exhibiting the spectrum of cleft lip and palate. (a) Bilateral cleft lip and palate. (b) Unilateral cleft lip with cleft palate. (c) Unilateral cleft lip with alveolar notching. (d) Cleft palate. (e) Submucous (occult) cleft palate.

Table 10-5.	Recurrence Risk Data for Cleft Lip With/Without Cleft Palate
Population baseline incidence	0.1%
Recurrence risk by degree of relationship to affected person	
First degree	4%
Second Degree	0.7%
Third degree	0.3%
Recurrence risk by nature of relationship to affected person	
Sibling	4%
Child	4.3%
Recurrence risk by number of affected relatives	
1 affected first degree relative	4%
2 affected first degree relatives	10%
[3 or more affected first or second degree relatives should raise the question of a unifactorial disorder]	
Recurrence risk by severity	
Unilateral cleft lip	2.5%
Unilateral cleft lip and palate	4.1%
Bilateral cleft lip	5.6%
Recurrence risk considering sex bias	
Affected male, risk of affected sister	2.8%
Affected female, risk of affected sister	4.4%

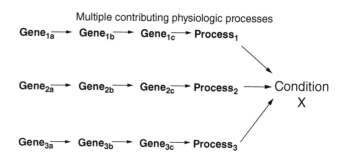

Figure 10-9. Diagram of multiple physiologic processes each with multiple contributing genes for a hypothetical disorder (condition X) that exhibits multifactorial inheritance.

not known. In general genetic testing for nonsyndromic clefts is not readily available. As such, when a patient with a nonsyndromic cleft is seen, genetic counseling is provided using empiric data. Because clefting is a relatively common condition, and because multiple large population surveys have been published, extensive empiric data exist (Table 10-5). The data in this table are regularly used when counseling with families of children with clefts. The data in this table highlight the major features of multifactorial inheritance (relationship to baseline incidence, relationship to affected individual, number of affected persons, severity of expression, and sex bias).

A Better Understanding of Multifactorial Inheritance

Currently, for NTDs and many other conditions, this type of information is still the only clinically available recurrence risk information that can be given to families. In fact, this is what is routinely used in clinics on a regular basis. While it is helpful to have such information available to share with families, it is not ideal. It should be noted that by the very nature of the information, it is a population *average*. In reality, the 5% recurrence risk quoted for the hypothetical couple above is actually not their actual recurrence risk but rather an average risk for a group of couples with similar circumstances.

The individual risk for a given couple could be quite low (as it often is) or sometimes could be significantly increased. However, in the absence of etiologic specific information it cannot be determined which is true for a specific case.

Clearly what is needed is a better understanding of the underlying genetic and environmental factors that contribute to the expression of any given multifactorial trait. The more that is discovered about the factors that are involved, the better (more specific and more accurate) are the predictions that can be made. As mentioned previously most multifactorial conditions involve complex, interacting physiologic processes. Typically each of these processes will have multiple components to them—each separately genetically regulated. Figure 10-9 shows how this might look. Thus, by earlier ways of thinking, the question might have been asked: "what gene causes condition X?" In hindsight, the reason for this was simply oversimplified view of multifactorial inheritance that was prevailing at the time. A quick look at the figure shows that the more accurate question would be: "which of the several possible genes is at work in a particular family with condition X?"

A good example of this can be seen in how our understanding of diabetes and the genetics underlying it have changed over time. Diabetes mellitus (DM) is a metabolic disorder characterized by carbohydrate intolerance (high serum blood glucose levels). There are several types of diabetes classified by the purported physiologic mechanism. The most common type is type II occurring in almost 10% of all adults in the United States. The primary pathogenic change in type II DM is insulin resistance. The inheritance pattern of type II DM is best described as multifactorial. In the 1980s, ambitious researchers set out to find "the gene" that causes type II DM. Despite valiant efforts, little progress was made. Early studies identified **candidate genes** based upon the understanding of the condition's physiology. It thus was logical to suspect that mutations in genes like the insulin receptor or the insulin gene itself might be responsible for type II DM. As these possibilities were explored, it became quickly evident that what might be a very logical assumption was in fact wrong. In fact, most of the candidate genes that researchers have deduced have proven to not be significant (Table 10-6).

Over the past 30 years, much headway has been made in understanding the etiology of type II DM. Using powerful

Table 10-6.	Candidate Genes for Type II Diabetes Mellitus

Genes now excluded as major contributors to type II diabetes
Insulin receptor
Insulin gene
Insulin-like growth factor II [IGF 2]
Glucose transport genes [Glut]

Genes now shown to be significant contributors to the occurrence of type II diabetes

Gene	Gene Function
KCNJ11	Islet cell potassium channel
SUR1 (ABCC8)	Sulfonyl urea receptor
TCF7L2	Regulates proglucagon gene expression
IGF2BP2	IGF2 receptor binding protein
ID1	Major control of beta cell formation and differentiation
Connexin 32/ Connexin34	Gap junction proteins
FTO	Fat mass and weight influence
FAT/CD36 antigen	Fatty acid metabolism
NR4A1/ NR4A3	Growth factors
Tomosyn-2	Inhibitor of insulin secretion
HMGA1	Decreases insulin receptor production

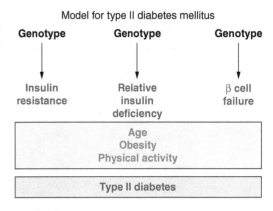

Figure 10-10. Influences on the occurrence of type II diabetes mellitus. Three major physiologic processes interface with environmental factors.

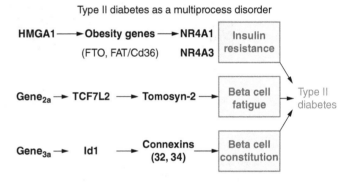

Figure 10-11. Diagram of multiple physiologic processes each with multiple contributing genes for type II diabetes mellitus as an illustrative multifactorial disorder.

genome scanning techniques, many major genetic factors that predispose to type II DM have been identified (Table 10-6). It is fascinating to look at this list and realize that discovering these linkages would probably never have happened without whole genome analysis. Logic simply would not have led researchers to the answers. Once these factors are identified, they can then be linked to the primary physiologic processes involved. For our example of type II DM, the major physiologic processes involved appear to be resistance to:

1. insulin stimulation (not mediated by the insulin receptor),

2. beta cell constitution and mass, and

3. beta cell fatigue.

The beta cells are the cells in the pancreas that make and secrete insulin. Of course these genetic predispositions must interact with environmental modifiers. Over the decades, the environmental risk factors for diabetes have not changed. Obesity, decreased physical activity, and age are clear modifiers of the genetic background. The relationship of all of these factors to the overall occurrence of type II DM can be visualized as in Figures 10-10 and 10-11. The final step then is to apply this knowledge in the clinical realm. Genetic testing would need to be performed to identify which gene(s) were contributory for a given factor. Recurrence risk counseling could then be given as etiologic specific information. Therapies would be designed to address the specific pathogenic mechanism that

was disrupted. For diabetes and many of the other so-called common disorders, that end point is within sight.

Polygenic (Oligogenic) Inheritance

Polygenic inheritance, as the name implies, means "many genes." But environmental influences are also important in determining the final phenotype. Although many geneticists use the terms 'multifactorial' and 'polygenic' interchangeably, here we want to focus on the genetic component. The concept of polygenic inheritance is that there are multiple genes that individually contribute to the phenotype in a cumulative manner. The additive effect of the overall genetic contribution then determines a relative "size" or degree of expression. Traditionally, polygenic inheritance has been used to describe the expression of quantitative traits (e.g., height, weight, head circumference, blood pressure, and so forth). Clinical observations of polygenic traits usually identify mathematical relationships of the traits within families. Height, for example, is one of the best understood polygenic traits. Simple observations of people quickly identify the heritable nature of height. It is intuitive that taller people tend to have taller children (Figure 10-12). In the event of one tall parent and one short parent, the children usually end up somewhere in between.

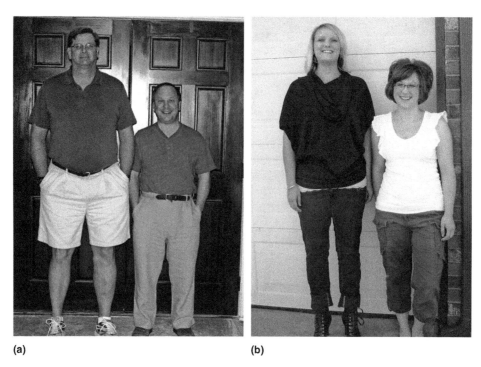

(a)   **(b)**

Figure 10-12. (a) Two adult men, fathers of one daughter each. (b) It shouldn't be hard to guess which daughter goes with which father.

Multiple large **auxologic** studies scanning many decades have identified several important features of the inheritance of height. First, there is a clear sexual dimorphism. Simply, males tend to be taller than females. Within families with the same parents, the male children as a rule are taller than the female children. Second, the primary determinant of a child's height is the heights of the parents. The heights of other, more distant, relatives have little influence or predictability on the height of a given child. Clinically this relationship can be represented by the formulas below:

Height (cm) of male child
$$= \frac{\text{Height of father (cm) + Height of mother (cm) + 13 cm}}{2}$$

Height (cm) of female child
$$= \frac{\text{Height of father (cm) + Height of mother (cm) − 13 cm}}{2}$$

Albeit simple, these two formulas provide an accurate estimate of final adult height of a child given the parental heights. The expected height then is simply an average of the parent's height with an adjustment for the sex of the child. The first question that usually follows is: "so then how come all male siblings of the same parents aren't the same height?" The answer is simply that this number is a calculated *mean* height of the children. The rest of the equation is a standard deviation of 5 cm around this mean.

Let's apply this then. Assume a mother that is 5′4″ tall (162.5 cm) and a father that is 6′1″ tall (185.4 cm). Using the formula mentioned earlier, the target height (expected mean) of their male children would be 180.5 cm. If 1 SD is 5 cm,

then 95% (mean + 2 SDs) of their male children would be predicted to be between 170.5 cm and 190.5 cm. This information has great clinical utility. When children are seen for a short stature evaluation, there are two major and complementary questions that need to be answered:

1. What is the target height of the child (i.e., how tall do we think they *should* be when growth is complete), and

2. What is the predicted height (i.e., how tall do we think they *will* be when growth is complete).

Comparison of these two answers allow the determination of which patient has "normal" versus pathologic short stature.

Similar relationships also exist for other quantitative traits in people. Intelligence as estimated by IQ testing is another such example. The relationship of a child's IQ is also close to an average of the parents' IQs. Notably, however, the sexual dimorphism observed for height does not apply to IQ (i.e., females have predicted IQs that are the same as their male full siblings).

Early thinking on polygenic inheritance envisioned numerous genes (maybe in the hundreds) each with a small additive effect to the phenotype. The final expression then would be the cumulative "score" of all of the pluses and minuses toward the phenotype. That is, a person with 80 positive height genes and 20 negative height genes would be expected to be above of above average height. Current evidence suggests a slightly different situation. For most polygenic conditions, there are actually a small number (maybe 3-5) major gene influences that account for the majority of the phenotype. Just a few genes segregating

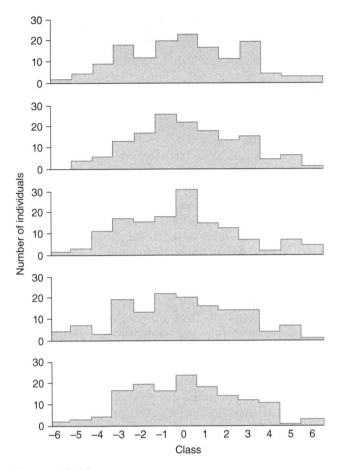

Figure 10-13. Phenotypic distributions produced in a representative quantitative trait in which only two segregating genes account for 90% of the genetic effect. (Reprinted with permission from Thoday JM and Thompson JN: The number of segregating genes implied by continuous variation. *Genetica.* 1976;46:335-344.)

Table 10-7.	Examples of Reported Genes in Which Mutations Produce an Increased Susceptibility to Environmental Factors
Gene	**Increased Susceptibility**
Factor V Leiden mutation	Blood clots with oral contraceptives, smoking
GSTM1 (glutathione transferase, class mu 1)	Lung cancer and smoking
EPHX1 (epoxide hydrolase)	Alcoholic cirrhosis, fetal hydantoin syndrome
NRAMP1 (natural resistance-associated macrophage protein 1)	Tuberculosis infections
CCR5 (C-C chemokine receptor 5)	HIV infections
APOE (apolipoprotein E)	Alzheimer disease, outcome in head trauma

independently can generate a statistically normal distribution of the trait (Figure 10-13). The remainder of the phenotype (and a smoother distribution) can be accounted for by environmental buffering and the relatively smaller contributions of any number of other "minor" modifying genetic changes.

Genetic Susceptibility to Environmental Factors

A particularly important aspect of gene-environment interactions is the concept of genetic susceptibility. **Genetic susceptibility** refers to genetic changes that an individual possesses that alter his or her response to specific environmental exposures. Understanding how a person's genome influences their response to the environment has tremendous implications for

targeted treatments and, even more importantly, prevention. Table 10-7 lists just a few examples of known genetic susceptibilities. In reviewing this list, we hope you are impressed by how significant these susceptibilities can be.

Let's use the first one on the list, factor V Leiden, to highlight this concept. A single nucleotide polymorphism in the factor V clotting gene called the Leiden mutation occurs in about 7% of the general population. This particular mutation makes factor V more resistant to degradation—so it hangs around longer than usual. The consequence of this is an increased tendency to form pathologic blood clots. Persons who are heterozygous for the Leiden mutation have significantly increased risks for spontaneous thrombi, abnormal clotting in association with precipitating events such as surgery or trauma and even with oral contraceptive use. In fact, some estimates suggest that this mutation potentially accounts for 40% of all pathologic thrombi. Since the Leiden mutation occurs in 7% of the general population, it is easy to extrapolate that about 0.1% of the population will be homozygous for the mutation. Homozygotes for the Leiden mutation have an order of magnitude greater increased risk of thrombi. Consider, then, what the risk might be in a middle-aged woman, who is homozygous for the factor V Leiden mutation and who also smokes and then starts oral contraceptives! The hope is that this type of knowledge can be used in preventative strategies utilizing genetic screening to identify genetic susceptibilities, identify and avoid high risk exposures, and prevent morbidity and mortality.

Part 3: Clinical Correlation

In Chapter 3 teratogens were briefly introduced. Here is a good place to look at these in a little more detail. **Teratogens** are environmental exposures that a woman may encounter during pregnancy and that can adversely affect fetal development. In the not-so-distant past, the prevailing understanding was that the womb was an almost impervious barrier that protected the developing baby safely inside the mother. Beginning in the 1960s, the science of teratology emerged and quickly expanded. It is now understood that the fetus is not protected from many environmental exposures that the mother may encounter. Table 10-8 lists just a few of the more important human teratogens. As a group, teratogens are extremely important as they represent one cause of congenital anomalies (birth defects) that are completely preventable.

Exposure to alcohol (ethanol) may easily be the most common teratogenic exposure in our society. It is amazing that fetal alcohol syndrome (FAS) was not medically defined until the mid-1970s. Since that time, a tremendous body of literature has emerged on the effects of fetal exposure to alcohol in the womb. As it turns out, there is a wide range of outcomes in fetal exposures to alcohol. At the severe end of the spectrum is FAS. The features of FAS include characteristic facial changes (most notably smooth philtrum, thin upper lip, and short palpebral fissures), microcephaly, decreased linear growth, and several types of structural anomalies (Figure 3-31). Children with FAS also have cognitive and behavioral problems. However, not all children exposed to significant amounts of alcohol in the womb will turn out to have FAS. In fact, what is observed in children with significant *in utero* alcohol exposures is that about one third will have FAS, one third will have neurodevelopmental and behavioral problems that can be attributed to the exposure, and one third will have no apparent effects of the exposure. Taken as a whole, these can be referred to as the *spectrum of alcohol-related birth defects*.

Salient to the theme of this chapter (gene-environment interactions), research suggests that the explanation for the wide range of outcomes after *in utero* alcohol exposure is indeed genetic susceptibility. Differences in both the fetal and maternal genome seem to affect the final outcome. Some of these genetic differences have been shown to be genetic changes that influence the metabolism and elimination of alcohol. For now, it is simply not predictable as to which fetus will have which outcome. By far, the most important point to take from this is: there currently is no known safe amount of alcohol exposure for a given fetus. It is sobering to know that there are still medical practitioners who will "prescribe" alcohol for pregnant women to "calm their nerves" or who tell women it is permissible to drink after the first trimester of pregnancy has passed. It is critical for all health care professionals to understand the appropriate stance on this issue. The only recommendation that should be made *is the complete avoidance of alcohol throughout pregnancy for all women*. It is also important to stress that most pregnancies in the United States are not identified until 6 to 8 weeks of gestation. If steps are going to be taken to avoid such exposures, education and public health measures are needed to reach all women of childbearing age. The importance of this cannot be overstated. It has been estimated that one-third of all neurodevelopmental and neurobehavioral disabilities could be eliminated by simply avoiding fetal exposures to alcohol!

Although much remains to be learned about the actual genetic changes that alter susceptibility of the fetus to alcohol, there are other examples for which more detailed information exists. For example, fetal hydantoin syndrome (FHS) is another teratogenic syndrome analogous to FAS. FHS is seen in children exposed to the anticonvulsant medication hydantoin or its derivatives during gestation. Children with FHS have characteristic craniofacial features, growth disturbance, neurodevelopmental delays, limb anomalies, nail hypoplasia, and hirsutism (Figure 10-14). Similar to what has been observed in FAS, not every child exposed to hydantoin

Table 10-8.	Major Human Teratogens
Ethanol (fetal alcohol syndrome)	
Antiepileptic medications (fetal hydantoin syndrome)	
Infections ("ToRCH" infections)	
Cigarettes/other nicotine containing products	
Toluene (inhalants)	
Substances of abuse	
Prescribed medications	
Other the counter medications, vitamins, herbals, and "naturals"	
Chemotherapy drugs	
Maternal medical conditions (e.g., diabetes, phenylketonuria)	

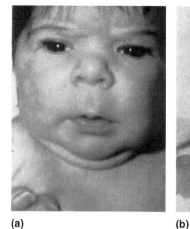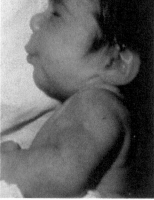

(a)   **(b)**

Figure 10-14. Infant with fetal hydantoin syndrome. (Reprinted with permission from Buehler BA, Bick D, Delimont D: Prenatal prediction of risk of the fetal hydantoin syndrome. *N Engl J Med.* 1993 Nov 25;329(22):1660-1661.)

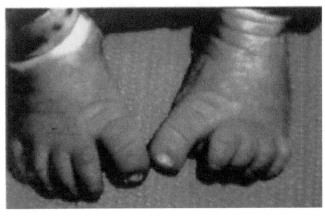

(c)

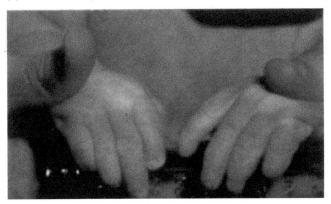

(d)

Figure 10-14. *(Continued)*

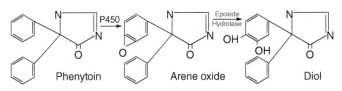

Figure 10-15. First two metabolic steps in the degradation of phenytoin. (© Dilantin).

derivatives during gestation will have FHS; in fact only about one-third will. In trying to sort out the question: "why do only some of the children with this exposure have FHS?" researchers focused on the metabolism of the drug (Figure 10-15). Ultimately, the genetic susceptibility of FHS was shown to be due to mutations in the gene for the enzyme epoxide hydrolase (the second step in the drug's metabolism). With almost 100% predictability, it can be determined which children will have FHS when exposed to hydantoins in the womb—those with defects in epoxide hydrolase. Thus for FHS, the susceptibility to the teratogenicity of the drug can be demonstrated to be an autosomal recessive condition that operates at the fetal level. This exciting discovery was reported in 1990 and was one of the first examples where the molecular basis of the susceptibility to an environmental exposure was proven.

■ Board-Format Practice Questions

1. Suppose that a condition, *blueism*, occurs commonly in a population of individuals. After careful genetic analysis of hundreds of people in the population, you discover three different genes that are located on three different chromosomes (*blueism* 1, *blueism* 2, and *blueism* 3). A mutation in any one of these genes can cause this condition. From this information you can conclude that:
   A. *blueism* exhibits multifactorial inheritance.
   B. *blueism* exhibits polygenic inheritance.
   C. there are marked environmental influences on *blueism*.
   D. there is no environmental influence on *blueism*.
   E. *blueism* exhibits genetic heterogeneity.
2. Which of the following is true about conditions that show a multifactorial inheritance pattern?
   A. The recurrence risk is lower if more than one family member is affected.
   B. If the expression of the disease in the proband is more severe, the recurrence risk is lower.
   C. The recurrence risk is higher if the proband is of the less commonly affected sex.

   D. The recurrence risk for the disease is quite high even in remotely related relatives.
   E. Environmental influences are not important.
3. Assume that nose size is inherited in a polygenic manner. Based on this you would predict that:
   A. at least 50 different genes contribute to the size of the nose.
   B. a person with a big nose who mates with a person with a small nose would most likely have children with normal sized noses.
   C. there would be a high threshold effect for persons with few liabilities for a large nose.
   D. a survey of the population would likely show a bimodal curve with most persons having either a large or a small nose.
   E. women would tend to have smaller noses than men.
4. Pyloric stenosis (PS) is a condition that is associated with hypertrophy (enlargement) of the muscle of the pyloris (outlet of the stomach). Infants with PS usually have severe vomiting beginning around 2 to 6 months of life. PS is inherited in a multifactorial manner. It is more

common in boys. A couple's first born child (a male) was born with PS. It began when he was 2 months old. They come to you with questions about recurrence risk. Correct information to give them would include:

A. their recurrence risk would be lower if the first (affected) child had been a female.
B. if the PS had been less severe (onset at 6 months), the recurrence risk would be lower.
C. if there are any other affected relatives, the risk would be lower.
D. the recurrence risk is about 20% to 25%.

E. the inheritance of pyloric stenosis could also be called monogenic.

5. In regards to *in utero* alcohol exposure:

A. it is an uncommon occurrence.
B. it has no real clinical importance.
C. all children exposed to alcohol in the womb will have FAS.
D. the best medical recommendation is the complete avoidance of alcohol for all stages of pregnancy.
E. there are no genetic effects on the impact of such exposures.

chapter 11

Genetic Testing and Screening

CHAPTER SUMMARY

It is probably obvious that for most subjects the quality of understanding is limited by the quality of information. If our information is faulty, so is our understanding. Conversely, as we learn more, our understanding of processes and events will improve. The advent of shared databases, the internet, and other communication tools has given us unprecedented insight into unfolding events around the world. Similarly, advances in molecular, biochemical, and other diagnostic technologies are changing the limits of genetic testing and screening. But we must put this into an historical perspective. Molecular insights have set the foundation for recent changes in the relatively short history of technological advancement. Not long ago, resources like personalized DNA databases and targeted genetic testing were hardly even imaginable. But today, the only certain prediction about the future of individualized genomic data is that information will increase.

When considering available genetic tests, one quite reasonable question is: "why not just get the most detailed information first? Do a DNA sequence." This is, after all, the age of genomics (Figure 11-1). DNA sequencing is being applied to identify genetic variation among individuals, within population groups, and in hundreds of species throughout the animal and plant worlds. But sequencing can be comparatively expensive and time consuming. In addition, it can give more information than is really necessary to answer most clinical questions. Indeed, sometimes the mass of information can actually bury the key result.

In this chapter we will explore some of the growing array of genetic tests that are currently available, although we must recognize that this field will advance rapidly as new techniques are discovered and applied. This creates a continuing challenge for physicians and genetic counselors. But that is not bad. A growing battery of analytical tools and data sources—in other words, the "information challenge"—is good news for the medical profession and for patients. Still, it means that all of us need to stay up-to-date on new advances. This chapter will focus on some of the practical aspects of testing and evaluating genetic conditions in patients. What are some of the tools available to analyze a patient's condition? What principles guide screening and interpretation? Not surprisingly, the topic of this chapter will probably change almost daily in the world of the practicing clinician.

But behind this advance in technology hides an age-old question. What does it all mean? It is not uncommon for the results of a DNA screen to report "finding of unknown clinical significance." The warning should be clear. More information does not necessarily make you smarter.

Part 1: Background and Systems Integration

Linkage Disequilibrium

Segregation patterns were discussed in Chapter 5 on Cytogenetics. There we saw that, if two genes are on different chromosomes or are more than 50 map units apart on the same chromosome, they will assort independently. In the Mendelian cross of $A\ a\ B\ b \times a\ a\ b\ b$, for example, the four segregating types from the dihybrid parent will each have an expected frequency of ¼: AB, Ab, aB, and ab. But if the two genes are

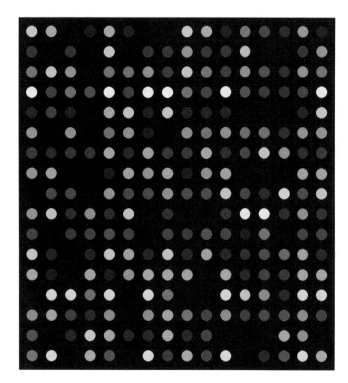

Figure 11-1. A small portion of a large DNA microarray or "gene chip." Each of the colored spots shows binding of fluorescently-labeled cDNA made from the RNA isolated from a tissue sample. Spot color indicates the amount of binding and thus the relative amount of RNA in the original sample.

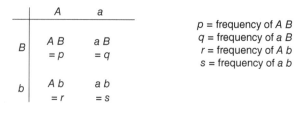

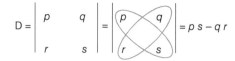

Figure 11-2. Linkage disequilibrium is measured by the gametic determinant, D, which quantifies the deviation from random association (or linkage *equilibrium*) between pairs of alleles. It is the determinant of a matrix composed of the four ways in which alleles of two genes can be linked. The product of the two *cis* linkages, p and s, should equal the product of the two *trans* linkages, q and r, unless there is some nonrandom association among alleles.

located closely together on the same chromosome, there will be a tendency for the linked alleles to be inherited together, so the four types will deviate from expected equilibrium values. Depending upon the arrangement of alleles in the dihybrid parent, two of these four combinations (say, *AB* and *ab*) will occur more often than expected by chance.

When we generalize from this familiar Mendelian mating to view the behavior of genes in the population, the same basic expectation still holds. Alleles combine as a function of their frequency in the mating. In a population, however, the frequencies of the *A* and *a* alleles (and of the *B* and *b* alleles) are generally very different. Still, the alleles are predicted to assort as a function of their individual frequencies, an application of the product rule of probability. But if there is some association between these two genes in the population, such as being closely linked together on the same chromosome, allele combinations will not be at random (i.e., they will not be at equilibrium). In other words, there will be **linkage disequilibrium**.

Linkage disequilibrium is generally expressed in terms of the expectations from matrix algebra as shown in Figure 11-2. The determinant of a matrix (D) is the difference between the products of the two *cis* and two *trans* associations of gametes, $(A\,B \times a\,b) - (A\,b \times a\,B)$. Thus, D is formally the "gametic determinant," the determinant of a matrix composed of the four combinations of alleles at two loci. In the context of genetics, it is the difference between the *cis* and *trans* linkages

in the population sample and is simply a measure of association. If there is no preferred association between the two variables, they are "dis-associated" and the *cis* arrangements have the same frequency as the *trans* arrangements. In that case the value of D is zero. But if alleles at the *A* and *B* loci are linked, either in *cis* or in *trans*, the value of D is significantly positive or negative, depending on whether the *cis* or the *trans* linkages are favored. This idea is applied broadly in measuring the association between segregating DNA markers and traits of genetic interest.

As with most metrics, however, there are caveats. For example, there can be statistical association without functional association if, for example, the population has recently gone through a bottleneck and recombination has not yet had time to achieve linkage equilibrium. In addition, a functional association among alleles is usually strong evidence of linkage between those genes, but related genetic functions showing linkage disequilibrium need not always be linked chromosomally. They may simply be linked by function.

Types of Genetic Tests

The ability to detect diagnostically relevant markers in the human genome depends on several layers of information. Some important landmarks in the history of genetic testing are shown in Table 11-1. There is no question that new techniques will continue to improve the quality of diagnosis. Available techniques differ in their cost, their ease of availability, and their ability to resolve specific underlying genetic conditions. No one technique is appropriate for all situations. Furthermore, knowing the genetic source of a condition is only the first step of the process. Treatment options, if any, are a separate question.

At one end of the spectrum of genetic connections, a karyotype allows us to identify large-scale changes in

Table 11-1.	Timeline Noting Important Milestones in Genetic Testing
1953	Double helix structure of DNA identified
1956	Human chromosome modal count established at 46
1959	Down syndrome is the first genetic disorder with genetic test to identify the etiology
1970	*in situ* hybridization
1970s	Chromosome banding techniques developed
1973	Recombinant DNA technology, restriction endonucleases
1975	Maternal serum screening for fetal anomalies
1985	Polymerase chain reaction (PCR)
1987	Fluorescent *in situ* hybridization (FISH)
1992	Comparative genomic hybridization (CGH)
1997	Isolating fetal DNA in maternal blood
2001	Human genomic sequencing
2004	Identification of large scale polymorphisms (CNVs) in the human genome
2006	Direct to consumer marketing of whole genome SNP analysis
2007	Next generation sequencing

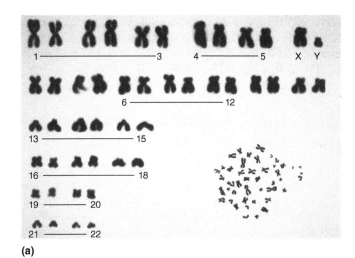

(a)

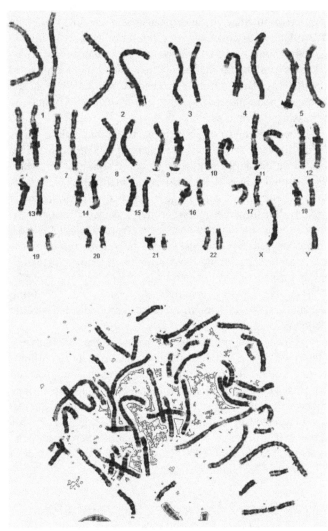

(b)

chromosome number and structure. Some examples of this were discussed in Chapter 5. Using high resolution karyotype images of prometaphase chromosomes, which are incompletely condensed, about 800 to 1000 chromosomal bands can be detected (Figure 11-3). Thus, each band contains on average about 25 genes. Changes in chromosome structure that involve losses or duplications of big sections can be diagnosed this way, as of course can any change in whole chromosome number.

In the next several sections, we will explore some widely-applied techniques that give higher-resolution information about a patient's genome. There is no question that these approaches will change rapidly as existing techniques are refined and new ones are designed and implemented.

Fluorescent *in situ* Hybridization (FISH)

Any cloned locus can be mapped to its position on a metaphase chromosome by fluorescent *in situ* hybridization (FISH). A sample of cells arrested in the process of division is placed on a microscope slide, and the chromosomes are fixed and the DNA is carefully denatured while still retaining its fundamental chromosome organization. A labeled probe prepared from a cloned DNA fragment is then placed on the slide and incubated to allow hybridization to occur on the chromosome *in situ*. After removing un-hybridized probe, the chromosome can be viewed under UV light with a microscope so that fluorescent regions and chromosome banding landmarks can be

Figure 11-3. (a) Low resolution karyotype. Random spread in lower right corner. No banding pattern seen. (b) Prometaphase (high resolution) karyotype. Lower panel is a random spread. The upper panel shows the chromosomes arranged by size and number (karyotype). Note the extended banding; this is about a 600-band study. (a: and b: Reprinted with permission, Dr. Warren G. Sanger, University of Nebraska Medical Center.)

correlated (Figure 5-24). The resolution of this technique, however, is only as good as the resolution of karyotype bands. Standard DNA cloned fragments of about 100 kb each for use as FISH probes are available from many genetic resource centers worldwide as bacterial artificial chromosomes (BACs).

Single Nucleotide Polymorphism (SNP) Analysis

A growing application of linkage disequilibrium associated with genome sequencing is found in single nucleotide polymorphism (SNP) analysis. SNPs (typically pronounced "snips") are single nucleotide differences that fit the definition of polymorphism, i.e., in which the most common form is found at a frequency of less than 99% in a population. One of the leaders in SNP discovery is The SNP Consortium (TSC), a group of pharmaceutical companies and the U.K. Wellcome Trust that has discovered over 1.8 million SNPs in the human genome. Some of the laboratories are now characterizing representative SNPs for their allele frequencies in several world populations. There are an estimated 10 million SNPs in the human genome and the objective is to develop a SNP database for association studies.

The importance of SNPs is mainly in their role as DNA locus markers. While it is true that some SNPs can be the basis of a mutant phenotype in a coding region, others serve as neutral landmarks for association mapping. This allows their cosegregation with a trait of interest to be followed in order to localize the trait's genetic placement. In that way, they are used for applications ranging from mapping the most important genetic components for a polygenic trait to allowing comparisons among DNA samples in forensic or parental investigations. As targeted sequencing efficiency expands, SNP markers can help in individual decisions like identifying the medications that might be most appropriate for specific genotypes.

A related approach is the basis of the International HapMap Project, an international project to identify chromosomal regions. It would be prohibitively expensive to screen all 10 million SNPs to map a trait, so the HapMap Project focuses on linked groups, or haplotypes. Each haplotype can be represented by a unique SNP, called a **tag SNP**, so the number that needs to be tracked to map a given target gene is reduced to about 500,000. This will be discussed further in Chapter 15 (Population Genetics).

Array-Based Comparative Genomic Hybridization (aCGH)

The **comparative genomic hybridization** (CGH) is a technique to measure DNA changes in DNA copy number. It is applied, for example, in screening tumor cells for deletions, duplications, and aneuploidy with high efficiency. For array-based CGH, control DNA is labeled with one fluorescent dye (yellow), and the test DNA is labeled in a contrasting way (red). The two samples are mixed, yielding an orange spot on the microarray for each section in which the control and test samples are the same genomic concentration. But if the genomic region in the test sample differs from the control, the microarray spot will fluoresce differently. Red indicates a duplication, and thus a relative excess of red label from the test sample, while a yellow fluorescent spot indicates a deletion in the test DNA and thus a relative excess of yellow label from the control sample. In general this technique gives specific genome map information and can detect any change larger than 50 kb or so, although some applications of the technique can have a resolution of 100 bp or less.

Gene Sequencing Strategies

Techniques for determining the DNA sequence of a gene first developed in the early 1970s, and the chain-termination method developed by Frederick Sanger soon became the preferred approach. **Dideoxy sequencing** (or **Sanger sequencing**) uses a modified DNA replication reaction in which a proportion of a given dideoxyribonucleotide (ddNTP; Figure 11-4) is added to the mix. As the name suggests, a dideoxyribonucleotide is missing two oxygens ("di"-"deoxy"; –H instead of –OH at both the 2′ and the 3′ positions) in comparison to the deoxyribonucleotides of normal DNA, which is missing a hydroxyl group at only the 2′ position. The replication enzyme responsible for extending the new DNA chain requires a 3′–OH for addition of a new nucleotide. When it encounters the 3′–H of a dideoxyribonucleotide instead, chain elongation stops. Four complementary sequencing reactions are set up, each with a portion of one of the dideoxynucleotides (ddATP, ddTTP, ddCTP, or ddGTP) included in the reaction (Figure 11-5). Fragment lengths are compared by running these four reactions side-by-side so the nucleotide that caused termination can be determined for each size of fragment. The resulting list is the sequence of nucleotides making up the complementary (newly synthesized) strand.

Modifications of this approach use radioactively-tagged nucleotides or a fluorescently-labeled primer which support automation of the sequencing process. Dye-terminator sequencing, for example, involves four separate fluorescent dyes, one for each ddNTP. The resulting strands pass along thin capillary tubes past a laser fluorescence detector that

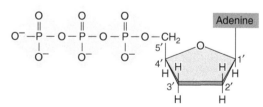

2′, 3′-Dideoxyadenosine triphosphate

Figure 11-4. A dideoxynucleotide, ddATP. The 3′ group is missing an oxygen molecule, so DNA polymerase cannot attach a new nucleotide to this position. Chain elongation stops. (Reprinted with permission from Brooker RJ: *Genetics: Analysis and Principles,* 3rd ed. New York: McGraw-Hill, 2008.)

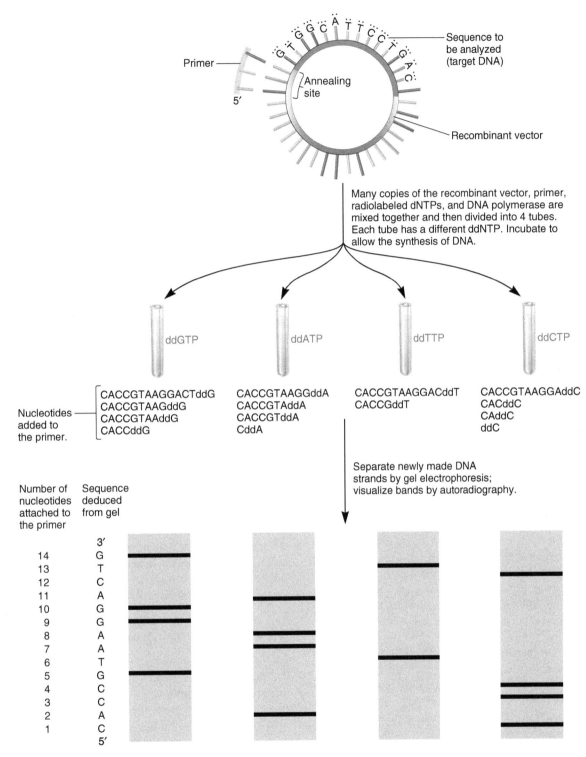

Figure 11-5. An example of DNA sequencing by the dideoxy method of Sanger. Beginning with a single-stranded DNA template, reactions are carried out with a primer, the four dNTPs, and polymerase. In each of four reactions, however, a small proportion of one of the dideoxynucleotides (ddNTPs) is included. When one of these is incorporated into the growing strand, chain elongation stops. The lengths of all strands ending in a given ddNTP can be read by their migration distances on a gel. Comparing across all four kinds of gels, one can read the termination nucleotides and deduce the sequence. (Reprinted with permission from Brooker RJ: *Genetics: Analysis and Principles*, 3rd ed. New York: McGraw-Hill, 2008.)

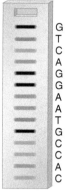

(a) Automated sequencing gel

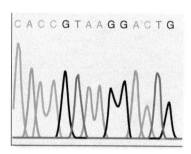

(b) Output from automated sequencing

Figure 11-6. Automated sequencing is based on reading the nucleotide incorporated into each terminal (ddNTP) position by its fluorescence. As each length of fragment is passed along a capillary tube, a fluorescence detector reads and records its wavelength. This readout is complementary to the original template DNA being sequenced. (Reprinted with permission from Brooker RJ: *Genetics: Analysis and Principles*, 3rd ed. New York: McGraw-Hill, 2008.)

determines the incorporated ddNTP by its emitted wavelength (Figure 11-6). A common limitation of automated sequencing is the length of fragments, up to about 1000 bases, that can be processed efficiently. This limitation is due, at least in part, to the reduced ability to distinguish long fragments that differ by only one nucleotide at a time. Techniques that sequence individual DNA molecules are also being developed.

High-Throughput Sequencing

The application of advanced genetic screening for patient diagnoses and research requires rapid and inexpensive sequencing technologies. This is an area of medical genetics that is expected to continue to grow rapidly. One avenue of development is high-throughput technologies in which thousands, or even millions, of sequences are processed at the same time.

One early example of a high-throughput approach is massively parallel signature sequencing (MPSS), a bead-based system. Although it was only performed by the original company, Lynx Therapeutics, before becoming obsolete, many of its properties are found in the "next-gen" outputs of later sequencing systems. These yield hundreds of thousands of short DNA sequences for cDNAs or PCR products.

Next Gen Sequencing

One of the first "next generation," or next gen, systems was Polony sequencing used to sequence a complete *Escherichia coli* genome in 2005 with high accuracy at a significantly reduced cost. It applied a multiplex sequencing approach to read millions of immobilized DNA strands at a fraction of the cost of more traditional Sanger dideoxy sequencing.

A sequencing-by-synthesis process is called **pyrosequencing**. Prepared single-stranded DNA fragments 300

to 800 bp long are attached to beads in a water-in-oil emulsion before being amplified by PCR. Each bead is then placed in a tiny well on a fiber-optic chip. After adding the sequencing reactants, the four DNA nucleotides are added in a fixed order to all wells of the plate. Each time the appropriate nucleotide is added to the growing strand, it generates a light signal that is recorded by a camera. 454 pyrosequencing depends on large-scale parallel sequencing that can yield about 500 Mb of data per 10-hour run. In 2006, 454 Life Sciences, a biotechnology company that specializes in this high-throughput approach, reported sequencing the first million base pairs from the Neanderthal genome, and in 2007 its Project Head Jim reported the completion of the first sequence from an individual, James Watson, codiscoverer of DNA structure.

In contrast to pyrosequencing, Illumina sequencing extends the DNA only one nucleotide at a time. It uses reversible dye-terminators and four types of fluorescently-labeled ddNTPs that are incorporated and photographed, before the dye and terminal 3′ blocker are removed and the next cycle is initiated. In 2010, the full Neanderthal genome was published using a combination of 454 and Illumina sequencing technologies.

Whole Exome Sequencing

As you remember, the exon is the portion of the DNA sequence that codes for the mature mRNA molecule, i.e., the part of a gene that codes for a protein. This accounts for most but not all of the genes in the human genome. Using microarrays to capture DNA segments that match a defined set of coding exons, sequencing focuses on the coding portion of the genome. This can be called "exome capture." When applied clinically, however, it is important to keep in mind that the functional defect may be not actually be in an exon, but instead may be upstream, in an intron, or may be in a gene that does not code for a protein. In these cases, this technique will miss the DNA site of the problem.

RNA or Transcriptome Sequencing

RNA sequencing focuses on a more limited target, specifically the expressed RNAs present in the tissue at a given time. For that reason, it is especially valuable for the study of diseases like cancer. This supports the development of a whole new field of study, transcriptomics, which explores the results of gene regulation rather than the larger picture of genome content.

Although there are different technical systems to accomplish RNA sequencing, they often target mRNA with its 3′polyadenylated (poly-A) tail to separate coding from noncoding mRNA (only coding mRNA has a poly-A tail). This can be done using magnetic beads with poly-T oligonucleotides attached. After reverse transcription, the resulting cDNA can be sequenced by a choice of the techniques described here.

A side benefit of this approach is the "flow-through," i.e., the RNA without a poly-A tail. The large ribosomal RNA fraction can also be removed, using probe hybridization. The resulting fraction is a rich resource for noncoding RNA gene discovery.

Genome-Wide Association Studies (GWAS)

Studies of gene associations date back to the beginning of experimental genetics. After all, even classical gene mapping is done by measuring associations. But the power of computer analyses applied to very large datasets has brought this approach to a new level of sophistication. Genome-wide association study (GWAS) focuses on how a trait of interest appears in combination with genetic markers like SNPs spread among all the chromosomes. In contrast to more targeted linkage studies, GWAS simply looks for connections. It is, in effect, an approach that combines linkage disequilibrium associations with the high resolution markers provided by SNPs.

Associations have already been identified for more than a hundred human diseases and phenotypic characters. But the strength of the GWAS approach is also its weakness. It simply looks for associations. Associations can lead to the discovery of a causal connection between a marker and a trait, but not all associations are functional. A rum and cola drink can be intoxicating. So can bourbon and cola. But that does not mean that cola is the intoxicating element, even though it is superficially the common factor. The large numbers of tests that are performed lend themselves to accidental or false-positive associations that can be misleading.

Other Approaches

Other techniques being developed include sequencing individual molecules as they pass through nanopores, sequencing with microchips, and microfluidic sequencing in which thermal cycle amplification and electrophoretic separation of fragments are done on a small glass wafer. The creativity of these DNA technologies will undoubtedly have a growing influence on diagnostic approaches and upon our knowledge of normal genetic control of development in complex biological systems.

Genetic Screening

Genetic screening is the search in a defined population for individuals with:

1. a particular disorder

2. a predisposition to a disease

3. changes that may lead to a disease in their descendants, or

4. changes that can produce other variants not known to be associated with disease.

A **genetic test** is done with the directed purpose of achieving a diagnosis, i.e., is a problem present or not. Screening is performed to measure a person's result against a population-based standard to try and define who is at higher risk for a condition. Diagnostic testing is then offered to, or performed on, persons for whom screening shows they are at higher risk. Often, the laboratory procedures for screening and testing are exactly the same—such as in tandem mass spectrometry used in newborn screening—but the definitions of "normal" are different. Likewise, the reason for performing the study in the first place is different.

Genetic screening should be designed to maximize both **sensitivity** and **specificity**. A perfect screen would have 100% sensitivity and specificity. As a quick review, the sensitivity of a diagnostic test refers to how well the technique identifies the presence of a condition. If the test shows the presence of the condition in 19 out of the 20 times it occurs, the test's sensitivity is 95%. Those individuals correctly flagged by the screening would be termed "true positives." Those missed by the screen would "false negatives."

A test's specificity, on the other hand, refers to those instances when the condition is "detected," but is actually absent. These errors are called "false positives," and 100% specificity refers to having no false positives. Of course those correctly identified as not having the condition would be the "true negatives." All types of screening should then be designed to maximize the detection of the targeted condition (true positives) and minimize the false positives. While in theory this sounds straightforward, in practice this may not be easy to do. Many factors such as cost, limits in methodology, and sample procurement may limit these parameters in a given screen.

Traditionally, genetic screening has been based on several key principles.

1. The condition must be sufficiently frequent in the screened population for associations to be identified statistically.

2. The condition should be serious or fatal without intervention.

3. But, the condition should also be treatable or preventable.

4. An effective follow-up program should be feasible.

5. The required screening and management must be cost effective.

6. Specimens must be easy to collect.

7. Analysis of the results must lend itself to mass screening and be simple, reliable, and reproducible.

While these are certainly the classically defined principles, in practice they do not always apply well. For instance, the changes in newborn screening over the last decade have significantly affected this list. There are conditions now identified in newborns that meet criteria #2, but not #3.

Non-ketotic hyperglycinemia is one such example. For such conditions we have moved from screening because we can treat, to screening because we can test. The logic in the latter situation would be that treatments may be found in previously "untreatable" conditions if the cases can be identified early.

A similar situation exists with maternal serum analyte screening for chromosomal aneuploidy. Trisomy 18 is fatal with or without intervention and is neither treatable nor preventable in a way that increases survivability.

Part 2: Medical Genetics

Genetic Testing

The completion of the Human Genome Project (HGP) has spurred many remarkable advances in human genetics. Undoubtedly, one of the most significant spin offs has been the advancement in genetic diagnostic testing. The last decade has seen a veritable explosion of new technologies that can be directly applied in the clinical realm. In Chapter 1, a timeline of technological events and milestones in medical genetics was presented. The overall "newness" of medical genetics itself is apparent. Even more impressive are the specific advances in diagnostic testing.

It is amazing to see that it was not until 1956 that the chromosome modal number of 46 was firmly established for humans. Shortly after that, in 1959, the chromosomal imbalance of trisomy 21 was identified, making this the first condition that had a specific genetic abnormality that could be used in the diagnosis of the condition (i.e., Down syndrome). After that, chromosomal analysis remained the mainstay of clinical genetic testing for the next several decades. Cytogenetic techniques (such as extended banding methods) improved over this time, but relatively few "new" testing modalities were available. Beginning about the mid-1980s things began to change. Advances in molecular techniques were refined and then applied in clinical diagnostics. Since 2001, with the completion of the Human Genome Project, further advances have been developed at a staggering pace. New technologies are introduced into the clinics, only to become outdated in a couple of years. The last decade has seen numerous diagnostic modalities come and go almost before their full utility has become known. Table 11-1 provides a timeline for some of the major advances in genetic diagnostics over the past 60 years.

Discussions on **genetic testing** should probably start with the question: "what is a genetic test?" In the strictest sense, a genetic test would be defined as a diagnostic investigation that involves the analysis of DNA. This could include chromosomal analysis, linkage studies, *in situ* hybridization, or gene sequencing. In the broader sense, genetic testing could include non-DNA based tests for genetic disorders such as performing enzyme analysis or measuring metabolites for an inborn error of metabolism. Thus, there are numerous "types" of genetic tests.

In the first section of this chapter, the major categories of types of genetic tests are discussed in light of the technology involved. Another way to organize thinking about genetic tests would be by indication, i.e., by the reason for which they are performed. In general the methodologies are the same,

with the difference being the "Why?" *Diagnostic testing* is performed to identify a specific genetic cause (etiology) of a medical condition. *Carrier testing* is used to identify a person who is unaffected with a particular condition, but who may harbor a genetic change that can be heritable. *Prenatal testing* involves identifying genetic changes in the unborn fetus. This type of testing of course requires obtaining fetal cells. This can be accomplished via several mechanisms including chorionic villus sampling, amniocentesis, cordocentesis, and even isolating fetal cells or naked fetal DNA from the maternal circulation. It is also now possible to do *preimplantation testing*. This involves performing the test on cells from a developing embryo prior to implantation during assisted reproduction. The amazing part of this technology is that cells can be removed from the developing embryo during the pluripotent stage of development without apparent disruption of normal embryonic development.

Sometimes genetic testing may be performed in an asymptomatic individual who is at risk for developing a disorder in the future. This has been termed *predictive* or *presymptomatic testing*. Again, the methodologies are much the same as for any other genetic indication. However, the ethical issues involved in this type of testing can be quite complex—especially if testing for conditions that may develop later in the patient's life and for which there is no effective treatment or prevention. As frequently demonstrated by the entertainment industry, genetic testing may be used in forensic investigation. *Forensic testing*, then is the application of genetic testing technologies applied in the investigation of criminal or legal matters.

Advances in Genetic Testing

The application of new genetic technology to clinical medicine typically has not lagged far behind the original development of the techniques. As new methods are developed in research laboratories, there is a strong impetus to translate these into clinically applicable (diagnostic) tests.

Cytogenetics

Cytogenetic studies became readily available in the 1970s. Early karyotypes displayed chromosomes in the metaphase stage of cell replication. These chromosomes were tightly packed and did not display many (if any) discernible bands (Figure 11-3a). At this level of resolution the only changes that could be identified were changes in whole chromosome

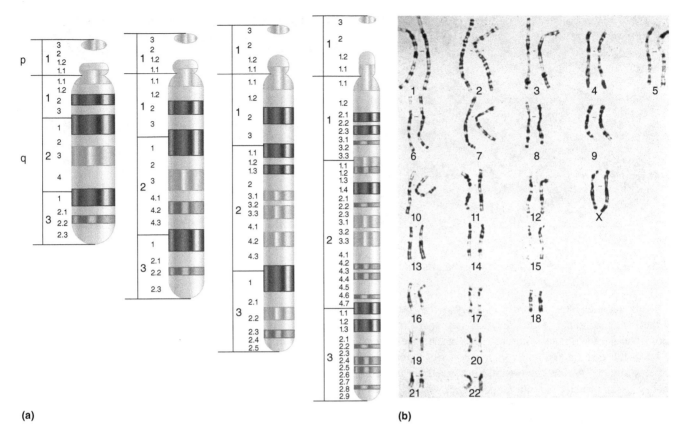

Figure 11-7. (a) Schematic demonstrating the increasing levels of resolution seen with increased banding of chromosomes. (b) High resolution (prometaphase) karyotype showing resolution at about 750 observable bands. (b: Reproduced with permission of Warren G. Sanger, PhD, University of Nebraska Medical Center, Omaha, Nebraska.)

number (aneuploidy) or large duplications/deletions. Over the past four decades, improvements in cytogenetic techniques have produced studies that are much less compact and display a much larger number of identifiable bands (Figure 11-7a). At the time of this writing, the accepted standard for a clinical karyotype is a prometaphase study that exhibits 650 to 700 bands (Figure 11-7b). At this level of resolution, 1 band corresponds to approximately 4 to 5 Mb of nucleotides. Thus, at the level of what the eye can see by the microscope, changes involving a handful of genes can be seen. While chromosome studies are still a major tool in the geneticist's tool box, the overall utility is decreasing as newer techniques are introduced.

Fluorescent *in situ* hybridization

Fluorescent *in situ* hybridization (FISH) as described in the first section of this chapter utilizes fluorescent probes attached to known segments of DNA to identify submicroscopic changes in the chromosomes (Figure 5-24). In the 1980s FISH detectable chromosome changes were reported in association with well-described genetic syndromes, which previously had no definable etiology. Using this technology, genetic confirmation of a clinically suspected condition was possible for several such conditions.

Williams syndrome is characterized by short stature, infantile hypercalcemia, cognitive deficits, congenital heart malformations other vascular anomalies, and a distinctive personality type described as loquaciousness (a "cocktail personality"). Patients with Williams syndrome have a distinct facial appearance: small upturned nose, long philtrum (length between the nose and upper lip), wide mouth, full lips, small chin, and puffiness around the eyes). For those patients with Williams syndrome that have blue or green eyes, a "starburst" (stellate) pattern can be seen in the iris (Figure 11-8). As with most genetic syndromes, the features can vary greatly from person to person, from striking to barely noticeable.

Prior to the advent of FISH testing, the diagnosis of Williams syndrome was made solely on clinical criteria. For many cases the clinical parameters were unambiguous and a clinical diagnosis could be made with certainty. In the more subtle cases, it was often difficult to settle on a diagnosis with any degree of confidence. This often led to many robust discussions among geneticists for these patients: did they have Williams syndrome or something else? Ultimately a FISH detectable deletion of chromosome 7q11.23 was discovered in patients with Williams syndrome (Figure 11-9). This particular deletion has been shown to be present in over 95% of patients with Williams syndrome. At the time of its development, the FISH test was indeed exciting and revolutionary. Finally there was a molecular test that could confirm or rule out the diagnosis. This was very satisfying to clinicians and patients/their families alike.

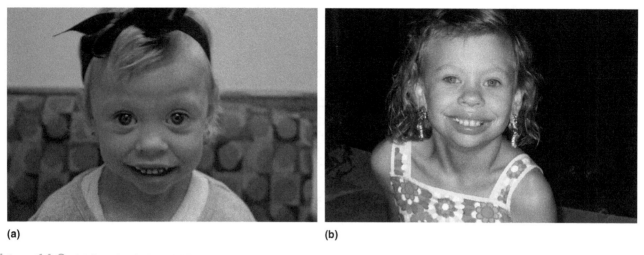

(a)   **(b)**

Figure 11-8. (a) Preschool girl with Williams syndrome at the time of diagnosis. (b) Same young lady, school age.

Another interesting part of this story is the insight that further understanding of this deletion has provided to the pathogenesis of Williams syndrome. One of the genes known to be in the deleted Williams syndrome "critical region" is the elastin gene. As the name would imply, elastin is a connective tissue protein with elastic properties. The deletion in Williams syndrome typically involves only one copy of the region. Thus, patients with Williams syndrome will have haplo-insufficiency of the genes—and their products–in this region. Many of the physical and cardiovascular changes in Williams syndrome can be attributed to having only half of the normal amount of elastin in their tissues. As mentioned, there are several other syndromes besides Williams syndrome that can also have diagnostic confirmation by such "single locus FISH" testing. The identification of these conditions has led to the designation of a new category of conditions: **micro-duplication/micro-deletion syndromes** (Table 11-2).

Over the past two decades, FISH technology has been used in many other different types of clinical diagnostics. Probe panels that have whole chromosome coverage can be used for **chromosome painting** (Figure 5-26a). This type of technology is particularly helpful in identifying unknown segments of abnormal chromosomes, such as **marker chromosomes**. In addition, different colored probes corresponding to different chromosomal regions can be applied as a **multi-color FISH** study (Figure 11-10b).

One practical advantage of FISH studies over conventional chromosome testing is that FISH testing can be done on nondividing (interphase stage) cells. In the interphase cell, the DNA of the chromosomes is "uncoiled." That is, the DNA has not been compacted into discrete visible chromosome structures. In this form, the chromosomes cannot be visualized, and thus the study is non-interpretable. To obtain a usable karyotype, living cells need to be obtained and then cultured. Any cell capable of dividing can be used. The most common cell type used is white blood cells (neutrophils), because they are relatively easy to obtain, and they readily divide with a little prompting in the laboratory. Other cell types used for clinical studies include fibroblasts obtained from a skin biopsy or amniocytes obtained during amniocentesis for prenatal studies.

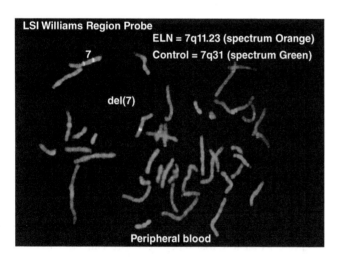

Figure 11-9. Single locus FISH test demonstrating a 7q11.23 deletion seen in patients with Williams syndrome. Note the absence of the orange probe on one of the chromosome 7's (Courtesy Dr. Warren G. Sanger, University of Nebraska Medical Center.)

Table 11-2.	Microdeletion Syndromes That Can Be Diagnosed Utilizing Single Locus FISH (Fluorescent *in situ* Hybridization)
Alagille syndrome	deletion 20p11.2
Angelman syndrome	deletion 15q11q13
DiGeorge/Velo-cardio-facial	deletion 22q11.2
Langer-Gideon syndrome	deletion 8q24.11
Miller-Dieker syndrome	deletion 17p13.3
Prader-Willi syndrome	deletion 15q11q13
Smith-Magenis syndrome	deletion 17p11.2
Williams syndrome	deletion 7q11.23

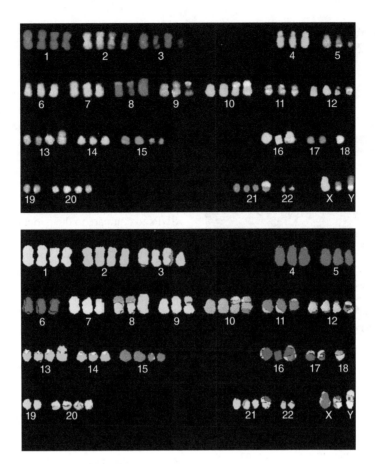

Figure 11-10. Multi-color FISH study. (Reprinted with permission from MacLeod RAF, Nagel S, Kaufmann M, et al: Multicolor-FISH analysis of a natural killer cell line (NK-92). *Leukemia Research.* 2002 Nov;26(11):1027-1033.)

The cultured cells are then allowed to grow and further divide. In the middle of the cell division, the cells are treated with a compound called colchicine, which interferes with the formation of microtubules and thus of the spindle fibers in cell division. This then halts the cells while in the midst of mitosis at the time of metaphase or prometaphase. At these stages the chromosomes are discrete and readily visualized, so they can be analyzed for structural changes. Typically cytogenetic results could be available within 72 hours using this process. However, there are clinical situations in which knowing the modal number of chromosomes earlier than that can be extremely helpful. Examples of such situations would include prenatal diagnosis, or a child born with a disorder of sexual differentiation, or a child with a suspected chromosome aneuploidy (such as trisomy 13) in which critical case management issues hinge on knowing the karyotype information. The nature of FISH technology does not require dividing cells, and thus can allow for more rapid diagnoses in such situations (Figure 11-11).

The next major advancement in genetic testing technology became available in the late 1990s with the advent of the **subtelomeric FISH** panel. Because of their biology, the telomeric regions of the chromosomes undergo a great deal of rearranging. As such, these are regions of the chromosomes that have a high chance of generating imbalances. This panel was developed as a set of 41 FISH probes hybridizing to the subtelomeric regions of each chromosome (Figure 11-12). One side note: there are 41 rather than 46 probes, because

the five acrocentric chromosomes (13, 14, 15, 21, and 22) do not have a "p" arm. The use of the subtelomeric FISH panel in clinical diagnostics was revolutionary. One example is in the genetic evaluation of mental retardation (MR). The **diagnostic yield** (rate of identifying a positive result) for subtelomeric FISH was shown to be 7.5% for severe to profound MR and 0.5% for mild to moderate cases. While to many these numbers may not seem all that impressive, this was a major leap in testing yields for clinical geneticists. Prior to subtelomeric FISH testing, the chromosome test was the major diagnostic tool. Down syndrome at an incidence of 1 in 800 live births was the most commonly identified cause of

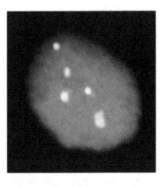

Figure 11-11. Interphase FISH on an amniocentesis specimen. This study demonstrates the prenatal identification of trisomy 13.

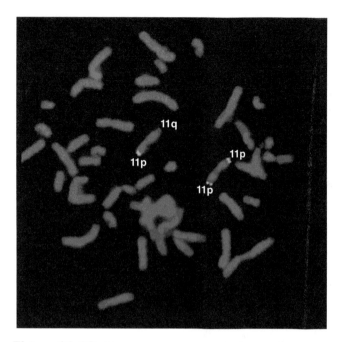

Figure 11-12. Metaphase spread hybridized with the subtelomeric probe for 11p (green) and 11q (red). (Reprinted with permission from Clarkson B, Pavenski K, Dupuis L, et al: Detecting Rearrangements in Children Using Subtelomeric FISH and SKY. *American Journal of Medical Genetics,* 2002, 107:267-274.)

mental retardation. Further advances in technology have now made subtelomeric FISH obsolete.

Chromosomal microarray

A **microarray** is large numbers of molecules distributed in a very small space—often arranged as rows of embedded wells on a microscope slide. **Chromosomal microarray** (CMA) refers to the application of microarray technology to accomplish whole genome scanning utilizing any one of a number of different platforms. This testing modality will identify microduplications or micro-deletions in the patient's genome.

In Chapter 5 we introduced the technique of **array comparative genomic hybridization** (aCGH). This technique utilizes slides with hundreds of thousands of tiny wells imbedded with probes composed of short segments of known DNA sequences (Figure 5-28). The patient's DNA is hybridized to these probes coupled with fluorescent markers (i.e., FISH probes), which are read by automated color detecting lasers. The pace at which aCGH technology has advanced over the past 10 years is staggering. The original aCGH chip that was available for clinical use had about 400 DNA probes that were obtained from DNA constructs called **bacterial artificial chromosomes** (BACs). Over the past 10 years aCGH platforms have mostly transitioned to oligonucleotide derived probes, which has allowed the addition of many more probes. At the time of this writing, the standard aCGH oligonucleotide chip used in the clinical setting has between 180,000 and 205,000 probes! With this technology, there is now clinically available high resolution whole genome analysis in a single

technology. The resolution of this current platform is coverage of the genome at around 1 Mb intervals. To put this in perspective, one of the larger known human genes, *dystrophin*, is about 1.8 Mb in size, so a standard oligonucleotide array will have two or more probes within the dystrophin gene! It is worth noting that the probes used in such studies are not evenly distributed across the genome. Certain regions have a higher density of coverage due either to more knowledge of, or interest in, certain regions. Further refinements and different approaches to aCGH are constantly being developed.

Another CMA platform uses SNPs as the standards for comparisons. "SNP chips" utilize literally millions of known SNPs to compare to the patients genome. In general the information that is garnered from SNP analysis is comparable to that obtained from aCGH chips. However, SNP chips have the added advantage of providing information such as identifying areas of uniparental disomy (see Chapter 12) and runs of homozygosity by descent (common regions of the genome due to consanguinity).

The results of CMA studies report the identification of changes in "copy numbers." In the normal situation, there should be two copies of every probe (with the exception of X-linked genes in males). The results of CMA studies, then, report **copy number variants** (CNVs)—that is deviations from the normal (modal) number of copies expected at a genetic locus that are found with the patient. When a CNV is identified in a patient, the next step is to determine its significance. At present, the rapid advances in testing technology have outpaced clinical understanding. Currently for many identified CNVs the significance is simply not known. Given the knowledge base and collective experience of laboratory geneticists, an identified CNV will be classified and reported by the laboratory as either benign (known not to be disease causing), pathogenic (known to be disease causing), or of unknown clinical significance.

The clinical impact of chromosomal microarray studies cannot be overstated. The application of CMA studies has tremendously increased the ability to identify specific genetic diagnoses. In fact, current clinical guidelines list CMA as a "first tier" diagnostic test for the work-up of multiple congenital anomalies, cognitive deficits, and autism. It is extremely gratifying for geneticists (and for the patients and their families) to be able to identify a cause of their problems after decades of searching. It is interesting to note, however, that the increase in diagnostic yield has not been in direct proportion to the number of probes added. For instance, the diagnostic yield noted in mental retardation using aCGH has increased from about 5% with the 400 panel probe chip to 15% with the 180,000 chip.

Not surprisingly, introducing a test that scans the genome in 180,000 places has produced many unexpected results, beyond the straightforward diagnostics. While CGH studies now provide diagnostic answers in previously undiagnosable cases, they also identify CNVs for which little to no clinical information exists. These findings have been designated "copy number variants of unknown clinical significance." Identifying such changes during the course of a diagnostic evaluation can be difficult both for the family and the clinician. But, as noted earlier, the increase in the number of probes has not led to an equivalent increase in diagnostic yield. For instance, the jump from a 44,000 chip probe to an 180,000 chip probe increased the yield of true diagnostics by only about 3%.

An interesting phenomenon associated with the application of CMA diagnostics has been the identification of new "syndromes without names." Traditionally, genetic syndromes have been associated with an eponymic designation (e.g., Down syndrome, Turner syndrome, and so forth). In the early days of medical genetics, syndromes were described clinically and then paired with a name of a person critical in the description of the condition. Later, an associated genotype might be identified. So, for example, in 1866 John Langdon Down made the key description of the syndrome to which his name is forever linked. Later, in 1959, cytogenetic analysis identified the genotypic correlation—trisomy of chromosome 21—with the syndrome.

With the introduction of whole genome analysis (such as CMA studies), individuals have now been identified with specific chromosomal changes in which the order of these events has been reversed. That is, in these cases, the genotypic abnormality is identified *before* any clinical description of the conditions has been made. By default, the condition is actually known by its genetic description. For example microdeletions of chromosome 1q21.1 have been identified in a large number of patients with neurodevelopmental and neurobehavioral problems. This condition shows a large range of variability and may also involve structural congenital anomalies (Figure 11-13). The identification of this CNV has preceded any phenotypic description, and thus has no associated eponym. The condition is simply referred to as the "1q21.1 microdeletion syndrome." It is fascinating to note that many families find this unsettling. They would like to know: "what is the "name" of the condition that the patient has?"

Finally as exciting and revolutionary as these advances in testing are, their long-term utility is in question. Just as subtelomeric FISH panels came and went in a matter of a few years, it is likely that newer developments in genetic testing technology may make them obsolete in an equally short period of time. We fear that, even at the time of the publication, what we have written here may be in need of updating. But for future patients, that advance in knowledge is a wonderful thing.

Determination of nucleotide sequences

Another approach to genetic testing involves determining the actual nucleotide(s) present within a specific gene. Early clinical tests used **restriction endonucleases** that could identify specific polymorphisms at targeted nucleotide positions of specific genes. While accurate, this methodology was limited in which genes and specific polymorphisms could be tested. **DNA sequencing** utilizes a variety of methods to identify the order and type (A, G, T, or C) of the nucleotide bases for a specific

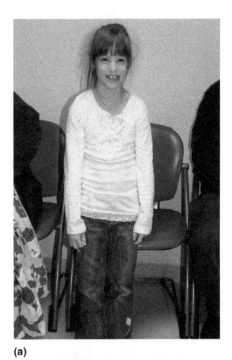

(a)

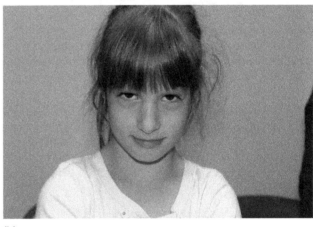

(b)

Figure 11-13. Patient with 1q21.1 deletion. The child has mild developmental delays and neurobehavioral problems.

gene (Figure 11-14). Advances in sequencing technology eventually allowed clinicians to request sequencing of entire genes. As with most new technologies, early gene sequencing studies took a long time and cost a considerable amount of money. Continued improvements included the development of newer sequencing techniques that utilize methods to analyze numerous sequences at once for study. This greatly increased the speed of sequencing from **linear sequencing** (starting at the beginning of one gene and sequencing it from start to finish). **High throughput sequencing** was developed using this principle and was significantly faster than linear sequencing because of advances in automation and multi-sample processing. Although this process involved longer runs of sequencing, it still required performing each sequence just once. High

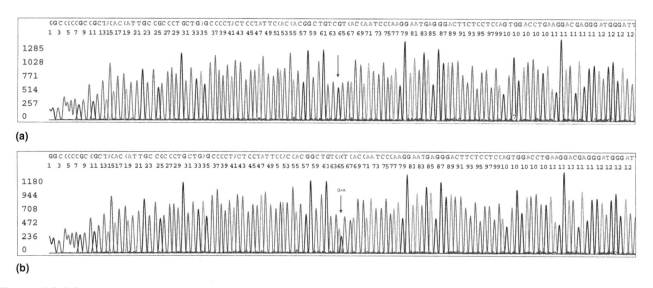

(a)

(b)

Figure 11-14. Sanger method of DNA sequencing. This particular test is sequencing of exon 4 of the transthyretin (TTR) gene. Mutations in this region have been associated with hereditary amyloidosis. (a) Normal sequencing results. (b) Note the mutation (G > A change) at position 64 in this read out. (Courtesy of Dr. Charles Sailey, Arkansas Children's Hospital.)

throughput sequencing can be used to identify mutations in specific genes known to be associated with a specific disorder that is suspected in a particular patient (Figure 11-15).

The most recent advancement has been the advent of **massively parallel sequencing** often referred to as **Next Gen sequencing.** There are multiple clinical applications of next gen sequencing now available to clinicians. Currently there are two major types of studies. **Whole exome sequencing** provides genomic information on all of the known coding regions (exomes) of the human genome. Whole exome sequencing is accomplished by "exome capture," which pulls a defined set of matching coding exons from within the full

genomic DNA using microarrays and then sequencing the identified sequences. Since exomic sequences account for only about 1% to 2% of the entire human genome, this allows for much less data to handle than whole genome sequencing. Since the exons are the coding portions of the genomic material, the majority of truly pathologic mutations are predicted to occur in these sequencings. A small number of pathologic mutations in the noncoding regions may cause disease by changing splice sites or altering gene regulation, but these would represent a small fraction of known disease causing polymorphisms. **Whole genome sequencing**, then, is simply sequencing all 3 billion bp in the human genome.

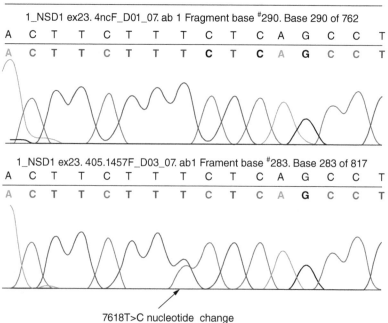

Figure 11-15. Diagram demonstrating a single nucleotide polymorphism (mutation) in the NSD1 gene associated with Sotos syndrome. (Courtesy of Dr. Darrel Waggoner, University of Chicago.)

It is hard to over-express just how amazing these advances have been. In the late 1970s using the chemical degradation sequencing methods developed by Maxam and Gilbert, gene sequencing could proceed at a pace of 1.5 kb (1500 bp) of DNA per person-work year. At the time of this writing, genomic DNA can be sequenced at the rate of 3 Gb of DNA per person-work year. Because of the rapid pace at which this science is advancing, it is highly likely that this number will already be out of date by the time of publication! The Human Genome Project, which was completed in 2001, took over 12 years and $15 billion to sequence the human genome. Many advances in techniques actually happened in the midst of the project that helped speed it to completion. Toward the end of the project, it was possible to sequence the 3 billion bp of the human genome in 3 years for about $4 billion. Using current technology, it can be achieved in 1 month for around $25,000. At the time of this writing, there are several commercial laboratories that offer clinical (fee for service) whole genomic testing. Currently whole exome sequencing can be obtained for $7000 to $9000. Likewise, whole genome sequencing can be ordered for around $20,000. If you are not astounded by this information, you have watched way too many sci-fi movies in your lifetime!

Of course technology is not going to stand still. Already predictions are being made for further advances that should produce sequencing rates of 60 Gb per hour in the next 2 to 3 years at a cost of around $1000, and being completed from start to finish in a couple of hours. As was already highlighted earlier in the discussions on CGH, the "brute force" genetics that happen in the laboratory have to be interpretable before bringing the techniques into the clinical realm. As mentioned in Chapter 7 (Mutations), it is predicted that all people have about 30,000 identifiable polymorphisms in their genome. Thus, if one were to perform whole genome sequencing on an individual, the test would be expected to identify 30,000 positive results. Just think what that laboratory report would look like! Obviously a simple reporting of all identifiable polymorphisms would not be useful for anyone. The real key for introducing whole genome sequencing into the clinical setting is going to lie in its interpretation. Information is going to have to be culled, sorted, and prioritized into some meaningful, useful format. This has led several prominent geneticists to speak of the "one thousand dollar genome with the million dollar interpretation"!

Practical Issues in Genetic Testing

As exciting as the advances in genetic testing may be, the excitement must be tempered with an understanding of many practical issues involved with such rapid developments. Many of the issues include cost factors, ethical considerations, and pragmatic details of actually getting the test done. There is also the reality that there is no treatment for most of the diagnosable conditions: there is currently no way to correct a genetic defect. A full discussion of these issues would require more space than we can include in this book. The ethical issues alone could fill a few volumes. However, we should mention several of the more pressing issues in genetic testing.

The first consideration is simply "should the test be done?" The old adage that "just because you have a hammer doesn't mean you hit everything with it" applies to genetic testing. While the science may be exciting, it is always crucial that the best interest of the patient be the paramount factor in making decisions regarding their care. When ordering a genetic test, several important factors should be considered. It is imperative that the patient be provided true **informed consent** in this process. While this is true of all medical testing, the highly sensitive and personal nature of genetic testing makes this even more critical. Prior to ordering any genetic tests, the patient should be informed of key pieces of information including what will the test tell them/not tell them. Also the utility of the test should be reviewed. For some conditions having a genetic diagnosis may not be the right choice. Particular consideration should be given for conditions that are done for predictive/pre-symptomatic reasons (i.e., testing to see if the patient will develop the condition in the future). This can be especially intense if the condition is a later onset progressive condition for which there is no prevention or treatment. Figure 11-16 depicts a continuum of testing utility from high utility to potentially harmful.

The spectrum of utility in genetic testing

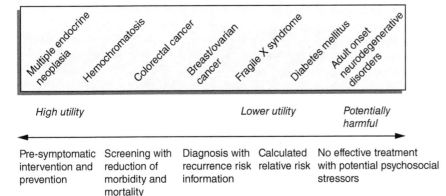

High utility		Lower utility		Potentially harmful
Pre-symptomatic intervention and prevention	Screening with reduction of morbidity and mortality	Diagnosis with recurrence risk information	Calculated relative risk	No effective treatment with potential psychosocial stressors

Figure 11-16. Spectrum of utility of genetic testing from high to potentially harmful to the patient.

There are many more key elements in a complete informed consent for genetic testing. The most common reason that patients will decline testing is over fear of **genetic discrimination**. The concern is: "can my genetic information be used against me?" Questions are raised about how this information might affect aspects of their life, such as confidentiality, insurability, or employment. The past several years have seen great improvements in protecting patients' rights in regards to genetic testing. A landmark piece of legislation was passed in 2008. The **Genetic Information Non-Discrimination Act** (GINA) provides key safeguards for patients undergoing genetic testing. Important aspects of this bill include protection against loss of health insurance and employment discrimination. While this bill has been a tremendous source of protection and comfort for patients considering genetic testing, it is still not all-encompassing. For instance life insurance (as compared to health insurance) is not a protected element. This information should be fully discussed with patients prior to having genetic testing. Table 11-3 provides a list of some of the key elements that should be part of a fully executed informed consent. Another important piece of legislation that will be helpful in assuring that patients have access to genetic testing is the **Affordable Care Act**. The legislation as constructed mandates that as of 2011 children cannot be discriminated against by insurance as having a "preexisting condition," and in 2014 this will apply to everyone. Thus, someone diagnosed with a genetic condition at age 2 years, 12 years, or 25 years will not be refused insurance coverage.

Patients should also be informed of what the potential costs and nonmonetary investments of testing might be. This should be reviewed in light of what the potential benefits are and the balance between the two (i.e., the cost: benefit ratio). Costs of the test, of course, include the actual fee for performing the test. For some genetic tests the cost can be relatively modest (less than $200), but for others it may be several thousands of dollars. It is important to note that the "cost" of the test for the patient includes much more than just the dollar amount of the bill. Other costs to the patient include lost time from work or school, anxiety over the testing, and even physical discomfort if the test requires an invasive procedure

such as a spinal tap or sedation for the procedure. Another very real concern is third-party coverage of the tests. At all levels, governments, agencies, and corporations are trying to reduce health care costs by any means feasible. Genetic tests are particularly vulnerable in this environment as they are poorly understood and constantly changing. As such, many third-party payers have taken the stance that "new" is synonymous with "investigational." Unfortunately a great deal of time and effort is often required on the part of the patient and the ordering health care provider to determine whether third-party payers will or will not cover a particular test. Hopefully help in the form of additional legislation will be forthcoming. One can only hope.

Another important aspect to be discussed with patients undergoing genetic testing is the **diagnostic yield of the test.** That is, if the test is performed, what is the chance that it will actually give an answer? While all of the technological advances we have described are indeed exciting, it is important to recognize that they still do not always give an answer. Not by a long shot. Currently, diagnostic yields are reported by diagnostic categories. Such categories include conditions such as multiple congenital anomalies, cognitive impairments (mental retardation, learning disabilities), cerebral palsy, or autism. Table 11-4 lists the most recently reported yields in the diagnosis of some of these major categories now as compared to 30 years ago. Again, it is exciting to note the impressive gains, but you must also recognize how much is still unknown. Once more, we emphasize the need to discuss this aspect of testing with the patient before proceeding. In the light of the fact that an answer is often not found, the patients should be informed of options for extraction and storage of DNA for future use. This option can be particularly important for family members if the patient being tested is critically ill and potentially may not survive to have testing done in the future when more advances are anticipated.

The approach to genetic testing can be quite simple, such as testing a patient for sickle cell anemia in which only one mutation in a single gene is known to cause the condition. Conversely the differential diagnosis may be quite broad and include testing options for several quite different etiologies. In general, the "shotgun" approach of ordering many tests at one time is discouraged. A stepwise (tiered) approach is preferable. For most major diagnostic categories, national guidelines have been developed outlining such suggested approaches for

Table 11-3.	Important Elements of Informed Consent in Genetic Testing

Nature of the test

Purpose of the test

Effectiveness of the test

Limitations of the test

Implications of taking the test including medical risks and benefits

Future uses of sample and genetic information

Meaning of test results and the plans for delivering them

Who will have access to the samples and the genetic information?

Right to confidentiality

Table 11-4.	Reported Diagnostic Yields for Selected Conditions	
	1970s(%)	**2012(%)**
Single anomalies	20	25-30
MCA/syndromes	20	30-50
Mild mental retardation	10-15	30-40
Severe mental retardation	40-50	80
Autism	6-8	30

each. A significant question arises as to how any one practitioner can be aware of all the possible diagnostic genetic tests (which number in the thousands) and published testing algorithms out there? Fortunately, online (internet based) resources exist to help. One such resource is a federally funded site that acts as an information clearing house for genetic testing. This is a wonderful continually-updated resource for this type of information. We encourage you to add http:\genetests.org to your Favorites on the web browser.

One final topic about genetic testing is worth mentioning here. In recent years, several commercial companies have begun to market a variety of different genetic tests directly to individuals, bypassing the patient's health care provider. Some of the more popular types offered in this manner include paternity, lineage/ethnicity/genealogy, and nutrigenomic testing. This so-called "direct to consumer marketing" has certainly raised a lot of concerns and prompted robust debate on both sides. Issues debated in this arena include voiced concerns over the paternalism of medical establishment *versus* unchecked recklessness for capitalism. Some of the key questions in this dialogue include:

1. How will privacy be handled?

2. What constitutes a "medical test"?

3. Who should regulate all of this?

4. How will informed consent be assured?

5. Who will guarantee the value of such information?

It will be fascinating to watch how this all plays out over the next many years!

Genetic Screening

Genetic screening as noted in the first section of this chapter is not the same as testing. In general the methodology is the same. The difference is in the "Why." Testing is a diagnostic endeavor to identify the cause of a person's disease or disorder. Screening is the search in a population for "healthy" persons who possess a genotype which:

1. is associated with a predisposition to a disease

2. may lead to a disease in their descendants, or

3. produce other variants not known to be associated with disease.

Genetic screening can be conducted at many different levels. One way to look at the different types of screening is by the timing of screening (i.e., at what point in an individual's life cycle is the screening accomplished). Table 11-5 lists several types of screening grouped by the timing that the screening is typically performed. Another way to look at screening is by the type of person(s) to be screened. **Individual screening** involves checking single persons for a specific condition. The person is being evaluated not because of a symptom or problem, but rather because of their relative *potential* for

Table 11-5.	Timing and Types of Screening

Preconception screening
  Nutritional/folic acid review
  Teratogen assessment
  Ethnic specific carrier screening

Pregnancy
  Advanced maternal age identification
  Combined first trimester screening
  Second trimester maternal serum screening for fetal disorders ("quad screen")
  Integrated screening (first and second trimester screening)
  Parental cystic fibrosis carrier screening

Newborn
  Genetic/metabolic panel (Table 11.7)

Adult
  Family History assessment/pedigree analysis (see Chapter 9)
  Pre-symptomatic screening for adult onset disorders

having a problem. Examples of individual screening include lead screening in a pediatric patient, heterozygote (carrier) testing of the parents of a child with cystic fibrosis, or likewise testing the mothers of boys with fragile-X syndrome.

Alternatively, **selected population screening** can be used to screen certain subgroups of the population for conditions known to occur at a higher frequency in that group. One such selection criterion is screening based upon ethnicity. Certain ethnic groups are at such a high risk for a particular condition that selected screening is warranted (with the condition occurring at a low frequency in general population). Table 11-6 lists some of the better known ethnic-associated conditions for which selected population screening might be appropriate. One group that bears further mention is persons of Eastern European descent (Ashkenazi Jewish population). This specific ethnic group is known to have a higher frequency

Table 11-6.	Selected Genetic Conditions That Occur at an Increased Frequency in Specific Ethnic Subgroups of the General Population
Ethnic Group	**Genetic Conditions**
Eastern European (Ashkenazi) Jewish	Multiple conditions (see Table 11.7)
African	Sickle cell
African, Mediterranean	Hemoglobinopathies
French Canadian	Tay-Sachs disease, several others
Native Alaskans	Congenital adrenal hyperplasia
Acadian/Cajun	Usher syndrome type III, several others
Northern European	Cystic fibrosis
Irish	Neural tube defects

Table 11-7.	Conditions With a High Carrier Frequency Rate in Eastern European (Ashkenazi) Jews
Condition	**Carrier Frequency**
Gaucher disease Type 1	(1:15)
Tay-Sachs disease	(1:29)
Familial dysautonomia (Riley-Day syndrome)	(1:30)
Canavan disease	(1:40)
von Gierke disease (GSD 1A)	(1:60)
Fanconi anemia Type C	(1:90)
Niemann-Pick Type A	(1:100)
Mucolipidosis IV	
Crohn disease	
Torsion dystonia (DYT1)	
Nonsyndromic hearing loss (Connexin 26/30)	
Breast and ovarian cancer due to BRCA 1 and 2	
Hemophilia C (Factor XI deficiency)	
Familial Mediterranean fever	
Bloom syndrome	

of carriers of several monogenic disorders (Table 11-7). As noted previously in Chapter 9 (Family History and Pedigree Analysis), health care providers should have family history information—including ethnicity—as part of every patient's medical record. If a patient reports Ashkenazi Jewish ancestry, the health care provider should be aware of the potential disorders that are associated with it and provide targeted screening upon request. This is particularly crucial to ascertain prior to pregnancy as some of the screening methodologies are much more complicated during pregnancy. In general, however, persons of Ashkenzi Jewish descent are well aware of these risk factors, and as a community are well organized and proactive in supporting their community in such efforts.

The broadest approach to genetic screening of course would be that of **general population screening.** This type of screening involves testing entire unselected populations for specific conditions that might be present in any individual person. In deciding which conditions are right for whole population screening, all of the basic principles of population screening discussed in the first section of this chapter should be carefully considered. The prototype for population screening is the practice of newborn screening in the United States and many other developed countries. The premise of newborn screening is to identify infants with specific disorders that, if detected, can be treated early with the resulting prevention of death or disability. Newborn screening began in the United States in the 1970s. Since that time it has evolved

and expanded into one of the most successful efforts in all of public health endeavors. From the early beginnings of the program where states tested for a handful of disorders, the majority of states now screen for most of the 29 conditions suggested by the American College of Medical Genetics and Genomics Recommended Core Screening Panel (Table 11-8). As technology advances and a better understanding of other conditions evolves, this core panel should continue to expand. In fact, quite recently, severe combined immune deficiency (SCID) and critical cyanotic congenital heart disease (CCHD) have been added to the recommended panel. Several other

Table 11-8.	Recommended Uniform Newborn Screening Panel
3-Methylcrotonyl-CoA carboxylase deficiency (3MCC)	
3-Hydroxy-3-methyglutaric aciduria	
Argininosuccinic aciduria (ASA)	
Biotinidase deficiency	
Carnitine uptake defect/carnitine transport defect	
Citrullinemia, type I	
Congenital adrenal hyperplasia (CAH)	
Congenital hypothyroidism	
*Critical Congenital Heart Disease (CCHD)**	
Cystic fibrosis (CF)	
Galactosemia	
Glutaric acidemia type I	
Hearing loss	
Holocarboxylase synthase deficiency	
Homocystinuria	
Isovaleric acidemia	
β-Ketothiolase deficiency	
Long-chain L-3 hydroxyacyl-CoA dehydrogenase deficiency (LCHAD)	
Maple syrup urine disease (MSUD)	
Medium-chain acyl-CoA dehydrogenase deficiency (MCAD)	
Methylmalonic acidemia (methylmalonyl-CoA mutase and cobalamin disorders)	
Phenylketonuria	
Primary congenital hypothyroidism	
Propionic academia	
S,S disease (Sickle cell anemia); S, βeta-thalassemia; S,C disease	
*Severe combined immunodeficiences (SCID)**	
Trifunctional protein deficiency	
Tyrosinemia, type I	
Very long-chain acyl-CoA dehydrogenase deficiency (VLCAD)	

*Italicized conditions have just been added to the recommended panel (2012).

conditions are currently under consideration and likely will be added to the recommended panel in the near future.

As would be easily predicted, genetic screening is wrought with controversy. While the proponents of screening point to the great success of preventing disease and disabilities, many thoughtful individuals have raised several real concerns that warrant strong consideration in the implementation of such programs. Some of the more pressing issues in genetic screening include:

- Mandated screening—for almost all states in the United States, newborn screening is legislatively mandated. The thought behind mandated screening is taking the best interest of the infant as a priority at a time when they cannot advocate for themselves. However, most states do have an "opt out" option for parental declaration of conflicting religious or moral objections.
- Right not to know—tied to the issue of mandated screening is the basic principle of personal liberties. What if I don't want to know such results?
- Confidentiality—who has access to this information, and can it be shared without my permission?

- Genetic discrimination—similar to the discussions on genetic testing, the issue of confidentiality is paramount in screening. Since this information can be part of a legislated mandate, is the law putting me at risk of having my genetic information used against me? Of course, all of these issues are interrelated, as confidentiality also comes into play here.
- Use/disposal of specimens—many researchers recognize the potential wealth of information that could be available from population screening efforts. They are of the opinion that such specimens should be made available for research "for the better good of all." However, those already concerned over the mandated procurement of specimens see further use and distribution of the samples as proceeding down that very "slippery slope" of loss of personal freedoms.

Obviously the short musings above do little justice to the incredibly complex and deeply emotional issues discussed. Ethical and legal discussions of such topics could fill libraries. For now, we just mention these so the reader is aware of some of the major talking points in this arena.

Part 3: Clinical Correlation

Kabuki syndrome (also known as Niikawa-Kuroki syndrome) was described by two Japanese physicians in 1981. The disorder received its name from a characteristic set of facial features that include long palpebral fissures, a broad and depressed nasal tip, large prominent earlobes and eversion of the lower eyelids (Figure 11-17). The appearance was said to be reminiscent of the makeup of the actors of Kabuki, a traditional Japanese theatrical form. Kabuki syndrome was originally known as Kabuki makeup syndrome, but the term "makeup" has been dropped as it was considered offensive by some families.

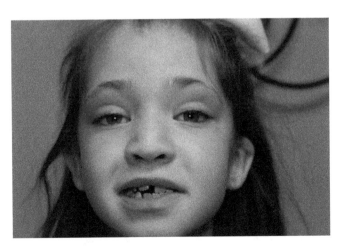

Figure 11-17. Young girl with Kabuki syndrome. Characteristic facial appearance that has been likened to the masks worn by Japanese Kabuki performers. This patient has a known MLL2 gene mutation.

Besides the characteristic facial changes, patients with Kabuki syndrome may have a variety of other signs and symptoms including cognitive deficits, postnatal slow growth, orofacial clefting, congenital heart malformations, scoliosis and other skeletal changes, shortened fifth fingers, and persistence of the fetal digital pad prominences.

Since its original description, the etiology of Kabuki syndrome was unknown. Most cases were typically isolated (nonfamilial). A few familial cases were described suggesting a genetic etiology. Standard genetic testing like chromosome studies and microarray studies failed to identify a specific etiology. For quite a long period of time, then, the diagnosis was made solely on clinical parameters without any confirmatory testing available. Often this was adequate, but given the highly variable nature of this condition, many cases presented a significant diagnostic dilemma.

In 2010 a research group used the technique of exome sequencing, as described earlier, in a small cohort of patients with Kabuki syndrome. Using this powerful technique, they were able to identify a gene, the MLL2 gene, in chromosome region 12q12 to 12q14 as the cause of Kabuki syndrome in about three-fourths of the patients tested. Besides identifying this gene as being a cause of Kabuki syndrome, the testing showed that all cases were due to a heterozygous mutation, establishing this as an autosomal dominant condition. Subsequent studies have now confirmed the suspected genetic heterogeneity of this condition. Several patients with Kabuki syndrome who did not have MLL2 mutations were subsequently shown to have mutations in the KDM6A gene on chromosome Xp11.3 by a combination of chromosome, microarray, and sequencing techniques.

■ Board-Format Practice Questions

1. Condition A is appropriate for population screening. Condition B is not. What possible reasons could explain this?
   A. Condition A is a much rarer disorder than condition B.
   B. Condition B is easy to screen; A is not.
   C. Condition B is a serious condition; Condition A is not very clinically problematic.
   D. There is no effective treatment for condition B; there is for A.
   E. The screening tests for conditions A and B are both very expensive.

2. Genetic screening:
   A. can identify at risk individuals.
   B. is highly cost ineffective.
   C. is politically incorrect to target specific ethnic groups in screening.
   D. is unlikely to affect general medical practices.
   E. is usually limited to DNA testing.

3. Performing which of the following would be considered genetic screening rather than genetic testing?
   A. Selected biochemical studies on a newborn for a suspected metabolic disorder.
   B. Serum markers in pregnant women to identify fetuses with chromosome disorders.

C. DNA tests on an individual for an adult onset genetic disorder.
   D. Neurologic examinations on people with tremors.
   E. A sweat test on a child with pneumonia to see if he/she has cystic fibrosis.

4. What is the difference between genetic testing and genetic screening?
   A. The types of methodology used in each.
   B. The costs of doing one or the other.
   C. The reason for doing one or the other.
   D. The laboratories that do one or the other.
   E. The age of the patient.

5. About how many conditions are infants tested for by newborn screening in most states in the United States?
   A. 5
   B. 10
   C. 30
   D. 75
   E. 150

12

Atypical Modes of Inheritance

CHAPTER SUMMARY

For there even to be a chapter titled "Atypical Inheritance" in a book that focuses on human genetics, we are actually highlighting an important fact. On one hand, in spite of our developmental and functional complexity, the number of genetic rules is surprisingly small. The mechanisms of inheritance are generally so direct that most examples are "typical." But that is not always the case. The path from an inherited DNA sequence to an expressed phenotype can sometimes be a convoluted and complex one. Most of the time this complexity is seen in the way genetic processes and their products interact with each other and with the environment. But not always.

A couple of examples will illustrate how our normal assumptions can lead to surprises. After fertilization, the regular nuclear divisions of mitosis yield a population of genetically identical cells that differentiate into the tissues of the adult. True? Yes, but not necessarily. Somatic mutation or other genetic events can yield genetic mosaics (Figure 12-1) in which subpopulations of cells within the individual differ from each other. But in other situations the genome itself does not change. Only the ability of the genes to function is affected. This is called **genetic imprinting** and is a normal phenomenon. It is similar to inactivation of one X chromosome in females in that some portions of the chromosome are turned off.

One example is a type of dwarfism in mice caused by imprinting of the insulin-like growth factor 2 (*Igf2*) gene. Let *Igf2*+ represent the normal allele and *Igf2*− represent the dwarf allele. Normally imprinting results in the inactivation of the *Igf2* allele the offspring inherits from the mother. If a heterozygous offspring (*Igf2*+/Igf2−) inherits the normal allele from the father, it will be average sized. But, if it inherits the normal allele from the mother, the normal allele will be inactivated (*Igf2*+/Igf2−) and the offspring will be dwarf. Sometimes the genome is not even involved. *Drosophila* can inherit carbon dioxide sensitivity from their mother due to a rhabdovirus passed cytoplasmically just like the maternally inherited mitochondria.

The more we learn about the genome, the more we realize how diverse the body's information pathways can be. Influences on development go well beyond the traditional role of genes controlling the synthesis of enzymes and structural proteins. Some special cases have been mentioned in other contexts. Here we will look at a sample of these mechanisms to explore their medical significance in a more applied fashion.

Part 1: Background and Systems Integration

Mosaicism

It is common to assume that cells within the same individual share the same genotype. But that is not necessarily the case. **Mosaicism** refers to the situation in which different cells within the same organism have different genotypes.

Given the lower rate of genetic repair found in somatic cells compared to the germline, it is likely that all individuals are mosaics for some genetic differences. The earlier in development a somatic mutation occurs, the larger the number of cells that carry and potentially show it. Usually this is not noticed,

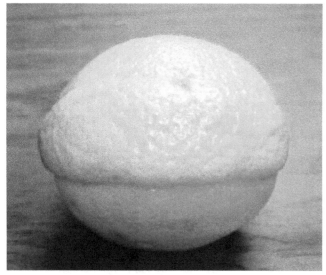

(a)

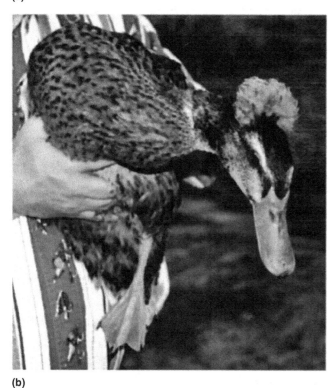

(b)

Figure 12-1. Mosaicism can occur in any multicellular speci-men. Specific mutations may cause phenotypic differences that correlate with the distribution the affected cells. (a) Segmental mosaicism in an orange showing hypertrophy (overgrowth) of one section. (b) Clonal mosaicism seen in the feathers of a duck. The small patch of abnormal feathers on the head is actually a collec-tion of abdominal feathers.

because the mutated genes are either inactive in the affected tissue or the pathogenic defect can be covered by normal cells nearby. So, an individual can be genetically, but not pheno-typically, mosaic. However, depending upon the nature of a particular mutation, the level of mosaicism and the distribution

of the cells carrying the mutation, phenotypic differences may be observed.

X-chromosome inactivation in females represents a unique mechanism of mosaicism. As a means for dosage compensation in mammals, one of the two female X chromo-somes is inactivated very early in embryogenesis, resulting in **functional mosaicism** for any X-linked heterozygous gene. Although inactivation is random most of the time with about half the cells inactivated for each allele, there can be **skewed inactivation** toward one chromosome so that one allele is phe-notypically expressed more often than the other. This is usu-ally a signal that there is a deleterious X-linked mutation: the cells preferentially inactivate the X with the mutation. Another example of genetic mosaicism is seen in most cancers, in which the tumor is genetically different from the normal cells around it.

Uniparental Disomy

In the usual situation, an individual typically inherits one copy of each chromosome from each parent. As the name suggests, **uniparental disomy** ("one parent-both bodies"—UPD) is an exceptional condition in which both copies of a given gene, gene region, or chromosome originate from the same parent. In the case of isodisomy, both alleles are the same, while in heterodisomy the alleles differ from each other but originate from the same parent (Figure 12-2). Several mechanisms have been proposed to explain this phenomenon. Most proposed mechanisms involve a genetic error with a second error that by chance corrects the first error. For example, consider events affecting a trisomic individual. Two of the chromosomes come from one parent and the third comes from the other parent. But if the latter copy is subsequently lost, the result will be a return to normal disomy, but with both copies originating from the same parent. The reverse situation would be an initial monosomic conception with a second division error resulting in a subsequent gain of two chromosomes from the original. Yet a third possible mechanism has been termed **gamete**

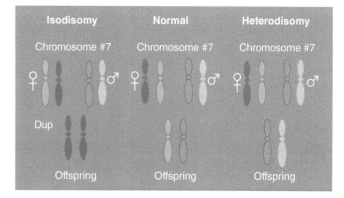

Figure 12-2. Schematic demonstrating UPD. The normal segregation pattern is in the middle. The panel on the left shows maternal isodisomy. The panel on the right shows paternal heterodisomy.

complementation. In this situation, two abnormal gametes with reciprocal errors (one missing a chromosome with the other having two copies of the same one) correct each other at conception.

Imprinting

Imprinting was discussed briefly in Chapter 5 (Cytogenetics). This parent-of-origin epigenetic phenomenon is reintroduced here to put it into context with other examples of atypical gene expression. Before transmission, genes can be marked by differential methylation or histone alterations that affect their later levels of gene expression. These epigenetic changes are maintained throughout all somatic cells and are only erased when germline cells for the next generation are formed. Low levels of gene expression generally result from methylated alleles, while higher gene expression is generally found for alleles that are unmethylated. But methylation does not always mean inactivation; the effect depends on the gene. For loci that undergo imprinting, therefore, the phenotype of the offspring is determined both by the specific allele(s) it inherits and by which parent transmitted each one. The result is essentially **monoallelic** expression for the gene. Since some genes are imprinted in the parental female and others in the male, it is necessary that the imprinting be erased and then re-established each generation.

In mammals only a small proportion of genes (perhaps only 1% or less) undergo imprinting. In humans thus far fewer than 100 imprinted genes have been identified, with most working during the embryonic and placental phases of development. Because of these imprinted genes, naturally occurring cases of **parthenogenesis** cannot occur in humans.

To explore the phenomenon experimentally, a mouse embryo series was produced that carried small chromosomal regions from either the mother alone or the father alone. This series of **UPDs**, explored in more detail in the next section, was used to define an imprinting map. Many chromosome sections were found to contain several imprinted genes. In fact, about 80% of the known imprinted genes are located in clusters, called imprinted domains, suggesting that they might be regulated as a group.

It is important to note that imprinting is a *normal* phenomenon. For the approximately 80 human genes known to be imprinted, monoallelic expression is what is expected for that locus. As with most features in biological systems, any deviation (over or under expression) from the expected norm usually results in an abnormal phenotype. Figure 12-3 depicts a hypothetical imprinted gene and several possible scenarios of how specific genetic changes can alter the normal level of gene expression. Knowing that imprinting is a normal occurrence, it is interesting to speculate why such a mechanism is needed. Possible reasons that have been suggested include regulation of placentation, avoidance of parthenogenesis, providing flexibility during development, playing a role in the immunological escape of the fetus, and "dominance modification."

Other Types of Gene × Gene Interactions

In Chapter 6, we described genetic heterogeneity, in which a large number of different gene mutations can give rise to the same phenotype. One example was retinitis pigmentosa, a phenotype that can be produced by defects in a range of contributing gene processes. One of these is actually **digenic inheritance**, i.e., the condition is produced when mutations occur together in two different genes.

A classic example of digenic inheritance is comb shape in roosters (Figure 12-4). Here the rose comb (*R–*) is dominant to *rr* and the pea comb (*P–*) is dominant to *pp*. *R* and *P* are co-dominant and produce a walnut comb. The double recessive (*rrpp*) yields a single comb. In these examples, the phenotype produced by the combined action of the two genes is not simply predictable from knowing the effect of each gene alone.

Phenotypes can usually be explained in terms of simple diploid genotypes. But occasionally it is necessary to postulate the involvement of a third allele, i.e., to postulate **triallelic inheritance**. Although it is generally difficult to identify these situations, some estimates put them at less than 10% of the known cases. In those few instances, however, traditional Mendelian risk estimates used by genetic counselors may not be completely accurate.

By using the term **multi-locus inheritance** we mean that the observed phenotype is influenced by genes at more than one locus. This should not come as a surprise to the reader at this point. We have already discussed several examples of multi-locus inheritance. In Chapter 10 (Multifactorial Inheritance and Gene × Environment Interactions) we discussed polygenic inheritance. Clearly polygenic inheritance falls within the definition of "multi-locus" as it represents the cumulative (often additive) effects of multiple loci on a quantitative trait. Likewise the digenic and triallelic inheritance patterns described earlier are also examples of multiple loci influencing a specific phenotype.

Another example of multi-loci interactions is that of **modifier genes**. A study of modifier genes reflects more a specific perspective than a unique type of gene interaction. Modifier genes are simply genes that influence the expression of other genes. Generally the context refers to the variable expression of the gene or mutation of primary interest. Modifier genes are loci of secondary importance or more minor effect that influence the degree of severity of the primary gene.

An example from *Drosophila* will illustrate the phenomenon. The fly's wings are supported by longitudinal and cross veins that stabilize it during flight (Figure 12-5a). A number of mutations have been isolated that either reduce the length of the vein or increase the amount of venation formed on the wing (Figure 12-5b, c). But as for other quantifiable traits like this, all sampled populations carry genes that either lengthen or shorten a vein gap or that add to or remove extra venation. In other words, all natural populations appear to be segregating for alleles that modify the expression of the mutations that

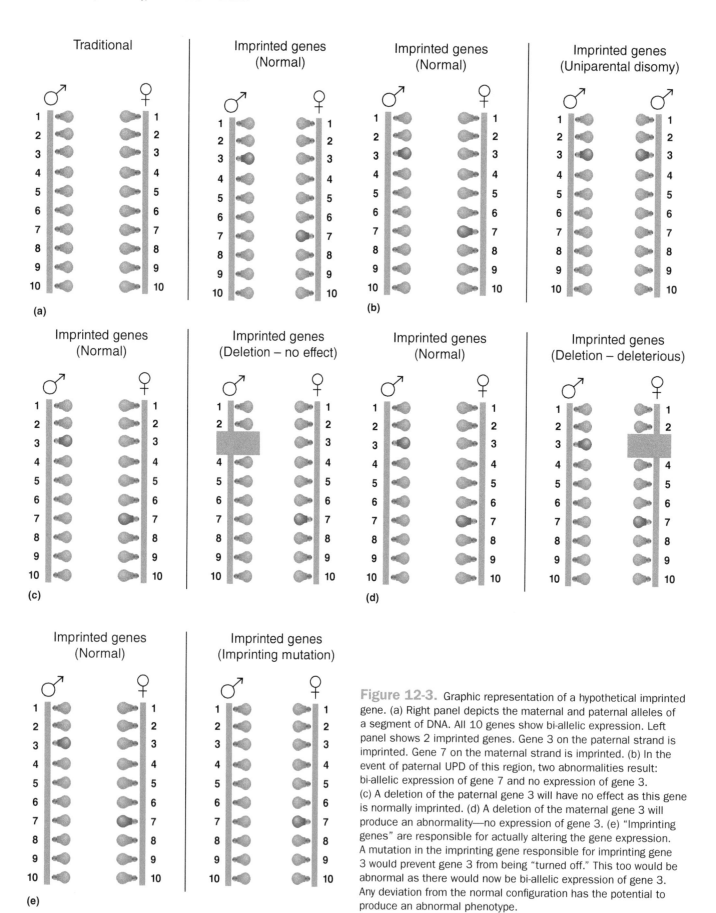

Figure 12-3. Graphic representation of a hypothetical imprinted gene. (a) Right panel depicts the maternal and paternal alleles of a segment of DNA. All 10 genes show bi-allelic expression. Left panel shows 2 imprinted genes. Gene 3 on the paternal strand is imprinted. Gene 7 on the maternal strand is imprinted. (b) In the event of paternal UPD of this region, two abnormalities result: bi-allelic expression of gene 7 and no expression of gene 3. (c) A deletion of the paternal gene 3 will have no effect as this gene is normally imprinted. (d) A deletion of the maternal gene 3 will produce an abnormality—no expression of gene 3. (e) "Imprinting genes" are responsible for actually altering the gene expression. A mutation in the imprinting gene responsible for imprinting gene 3 would prevent gene 3 from being "turned off." This too would be abnormal as there would now be bi-allelic expression of gene 3. Any deviation from the normal configuration has the potential to produce an abnormal phenotype.

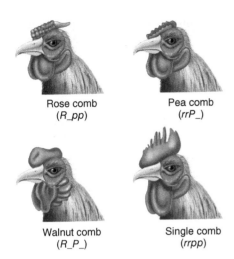

Rose comb
(R_pp)

Pea comb
(rrP_)

Walnut comb
(R_P_)

Single comb
(rrpp)

Figure 12-4. The comb appearance in a rooster depends on two genes, rose (R) and pea (P). Different combinations of dominant and recessive genotypes at these two loci determine four common comb types. (Reprinted with permission from Brooker RJ: *Genetics: Analysis & Principles*, 3rd ed. New York: McGraw-Hill, 2008.)

affect *Drosophila* wing vein length. This may not seem very surprising until you step back and consider: in a normal fly the veins extend all the way to the edge of the wing, and they have done so for millions of years. Why would all tested populations of *Drosophila* carry modifiers of a trait that has not varied for thousands of generations?

The answer is subtle, but important. Just because we detect a gene's action by the way it modifies something we choose to measure does not mean we are looking at the actual role of that modifier gene in development. For *Drosophila* wing vein lengths, the modifier genes are not there to influence the expression of a shortened vein. In nature the veins are never short. Instead, the modifier genes appear to be part of a developmental buffering system for wing blade organization. The lesson from this example is that a phenotypic association does not always indicate the primary functional relationship between a gene and its role in development.

Opposite (Anti-Sense) Transcripts

The traditional understanding of the process of transcription in humans is that the coding strand of DNA is copied as messenger RNA. In this process, one strand, the **coding strand**, is read in a 3′ to 5′ direction. However, anywhere along the genome either strand has the potential to act as the template. In other words some genes run one direction, some the other. In a few remarkable cases, at one locus, the same segment of double-stranded DNA contains genetic information on both strands. The products of such a "double read" have been termed opposite (or anti-sense) transcripts. It is important to note, however, that in either situation the RNA polymerase still transcribes the DNA strand in its 3′ to 5′ direction. Natural antisense transcripts (NATs) have been identified from most eukaryotes, including humans, and the RNAs generated include both protein-coding and noncoding examples.

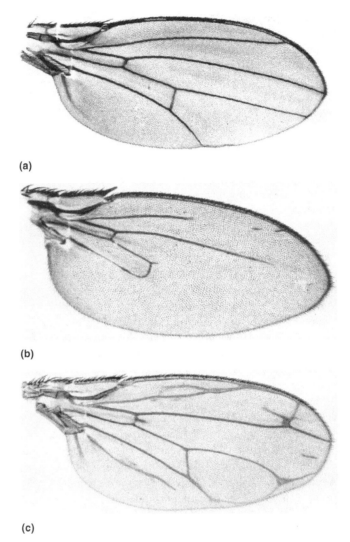

(a)

(b)

(c)

Figure 12-5. *Drosophila* wings provide a model system for studying major genes and quantitative variation affecting expression. (a) Normal wing. (b) *Veinlet* mutation reduces venation. (c) *Plexus* increases wing vein fragments. Polygenic modifiers of *veinlet* and of *plexus* expression can make the mutant wings indistinguishable from the normal.

Transposable Elements

Transposable elements ("jumping genes") are mobile segments of genetic material that are present in all eukaryotes. They are nonrandomly distributed throughout the genome. By a series of mechanisms, they can move themselves or a copy from one chromosomal locus to another. In the process of moving about, they may increase (or decrease) the amount of DNA in the genome of the cell. If such changes occur in gamete precursor cells, the change is potentially heritable. Potentially one-third of the entire human genome is made up of repetitive sequences that represent degenerate copies of transposable elements.

Transposable elements (also called **transposons**) are classified by the type and size of nucleic acids involved and the mechanism of movement. Class I transposons (**retrotransposons**) transcribe DNA into RNA and then utilize reverse transcriptase to remake a DNA copy of the RNA to insert into a new location. There are several different types of retrotransposons. The types and characteristics vary among species. In humans, two types should be mentioned. **Long interspersed elements** (LINEs or L1) are found in large numbers in most eukaryotic genomes. They are transcribed to an RNA using an RNA polymerase II promoter that is within the LINE itself. **Short interspersed elements** (SINEs) are shorter DNA segments. SINEs do not have their own reverse transcriptase enzyme and rely on other mobile elements to move about. The most common SINEs in humans and other primates are called Alu sequences. Class II transposons consist of only DNA that moves directly from locus to locus. Class III transposons are also known as **miniature inverted-repeats transposable elements** or MITEs.

The major clinical implications of transposons are that they act as mechanisms for the spontaneous generation of mutations (i.e., they are **mutagens**). This then represents a "natural" source of genetic variation. In migratory populations, such as *Drosophila*, there is a well-described phenomenon of hybrid dysgenesis. When two different strains of *Drosophila* meet, intermingle, and mate, the spontaneous mutation rate increases phenomenally. This sudden increase in mutation rate has been shown to be due to a transposable element in the flies known as a P element.

The most common mechanism of transposon generated mutations is insertional mutagenesis. The movement of the element into a normal gene may simply disrupt the gene. Alternatively, the element may exert its influence on nearby genes by affecting the promoter or enhancer.

Genetic Anticipation

Anticipation as a genetic term refers to a phenotype of a condition that becomes more severe (phenotypically worse) as it passes from one generation to the next. As clinicians have observed families through time, **genetic anticipation** has often been postulated. Until relatively recently there have been significant disagreements as to whether or not genetic anticipation was an actual phenomenon. Skeptics held the opinion that what was being observed was simply a bias of ascertainment: when a genetic condition was diagnosed in a single family member, it then became easier to identify the condition in subsequent (or previous) generations. Thus, the condition would appear to be getting worse through the generations, although it actually was not.

The debate was ultimately resolved when genetic anticipation was identified in association-specific genetic markers—expanding trinucleotide repeats. Trinucleotide repeats, also known as **microsatellites**, can cause disease by expanding the number of repeated copies at a locus. An individual with a low number of repeated units is typically normal, but the number of repeats has the potential to change each generation. If the size of the repeat increases, it can ultimately disrupt gene function by a variety of mechanisms to the point where the individual becomes symptomatic.

Epigenetics

Epigenetic inheritance is the transmission of information from a cell or multicellular organism to its descendants without that information being encoded in the nucleotide sequence of the genes. It occurs through interactions among developmental processes above the level of primary gene action. Epigenetic variation does not follow the rules of Mendelian inheritance, is often the result of changed gene expression, and may be reversible. It may be somatically inherited, but it is not transmitted through meiosis.

All of these examples show how much information potential the genome contains beyond its traditionally-recognized role in gene regulation and protein coding. The interpretation of genetic causality must, therefore, always be done with an open mind. Most patients may fit into well-understood patterns of inheritance and expression. But one should always be open to the significance of the unexpected or the complex.

Part 2: Medical Genetics

The mechanisms of "atypical inheritance" described in the first section of this chapter are fascinating indeed. Simply knowing that such mechanisms exist is worthwhile just for their intellectual curiosity. However, the importance for the health care professional is that all of these mechanisms have "real life" clinical applicability. For this section of the chapter, we will not describe mechanisms again. Instead we will provide clinical examples of each and discuss how they might appear in patient encounters.

Mosaicism

Somatic mosaicism

Mosaicism can become clinically recognizable depending upon the nature of the mutation and what cells harbor the mutation. Somatic mutations can occur in the embryo very early after conception. If so, a large number of cells may be "affected" and clinical features may be recognized that reflect the distribution of the cells harboring the mutation. Marfan syndrome is a connective tissue disorder characterized by exceptionally long limbs and digits, hyper-flexible joints, fragile stretchy skin, ocular abnormalities, and cardiac abnormalities such as dissecting aortic aneurysms and valvular prolapse. Most cases of Marfan syndrome have been shown to be due to mutations in a connective tissue protein called *fibrillin*. The young lady shown in Figure 12-6 has a distinct body asymmetry. From a clinical standpoint, her doctors felt that she had the features of Marfan syndrome on one side of her body and not the other (i.e., she had "hemi-Marfan syndrome"). Skin

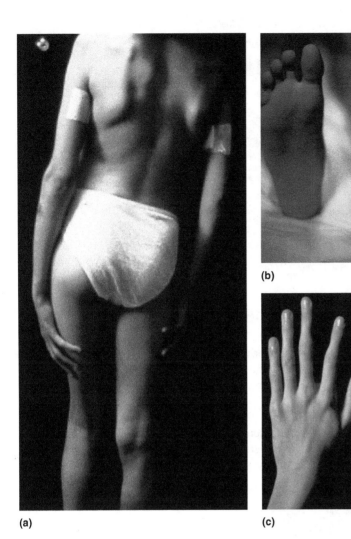

(b)

(a)

(c)

Figure 12-6. Adolescent female with clinical features of Marfan syndrome on the left side of her body. (a) Note the hip tilt due to leg length discrepancy. (b, c) Note excessive length of left hand and foot. (Reprinted with permission from *Am J Hum Genet.* 1990;46:661-671.)

biopsies performed on each side of her body confirmed that one side of her body had deficient *fibrillin*, while the other side had normal amounts (Figure 12-7). The explanation for this would be somatic mosaicism with a *fibrillin* mutation in the cells of the left side of her body. Of course somatic mutations can occur at any point in embryogenesis throughout all of postnatal life. Small clonal patches of cells harboring a mutation might be completely asymptomatic or evident as something as subtle as a freckle.

Gonadal mosaicism

Somatic mosaicism localized to the germ cells (gonadal mosaicism) has special implications as germ cell mutations are potentially heritable. If the mutation is only in the germ cells, there will likely be no physical manifestations in the parents as the germ cells are not performing a specific "function" for the body other than reproduction. However, such a mutation may produce problems in the next generation. For example, osteogenesis imperfecta (OI) is an autosomal dominant skeletal disorder characterized by the tendency to have fractures easily. Like most conditions there is a marked variability ranging from a severe form that is lethal at birth to milder forms that are associated with the tendency to have

a fracture with only mild trauma. Figure 12-8a, b shows two siblings with a moderately severe form of OI. Both children had over 20 fractures each simply as a result of the birthing process. As noted in Figure 12-8c, these are the only two children to this couple. Neither parent has OI. Given this information, one would be tempted to predict that in this family OI was an autosomal recessive disorder. However, molecular testing revealed that this was not the situation. Most cases of osteogenesis imperfecta are caused by abnormalities in type I collagen. Type I collagen is a multimeric protein composed of two alpha-1 polypeptide chains (COL1A1) and one alpha-2 chain (COL1A2). Mutation testing in these two siblings showed that each one of them carried an identical mutation of only one copy of their COL1A1 gene! Since only one allele of the COL1A1 gene had a mutation, this means that for these children the disorder was autosomal dominant (COL1A1 is on chromosome 17).

So then, what is the explanation for both children having an identical mutation? The odds of two spontaneous identical mutations are astronomically small. The answer then is in the title of this section—**gonadal mosaicism**. One of the parents has this mutation in some of their germ cells. Because the mutation is not present in other tissues, the parent is unaffected.

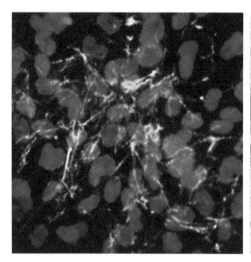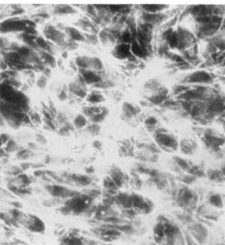

Figure 12-7. Two panels of immunohistochemical staining of the protein *fibrillin* from skin biopsies on the left and right side of the patient in Fig. 12-6. Almost complete absence of *fibrillin* is seen in the panel from the left side of the patient which corresponds with this patient's clinical picture of "hemi-Marfan syndrome."

Gonadal mosaicism can be present in either parent, but in this particular family, genetic analysis of individual sperm confirmed that it was the father who harbored the same mutation that was found in his children. Additional testing demonstrated that this mutation was present in about 40% of his sperm. Thus, a plausible presumption of autosomal recessive inheritance would be wrong. For this family it is an autosomal dominant condition. As such the recurrence risk for future children would not be 25%, but actually 40%, reflective of the degree of mosaicism in the father's spermatozoa.

Uniparental Disomy

As noted earlier, UPD is a unique situation in which an individual has inherited both copies of an allele or chromosome from one parent, rather than the typical situation of receiving one copy from each parent. The first question that might arise could be: "so what? What harm could there be in inheriting both copies from the same parent?" As it turns out, there are several fascinating consequences of such events. Take for example cystic fibrosis (CF) (Figure 4-21). Cystic fibrosis is an autosomal recessive disorder caused by mutations

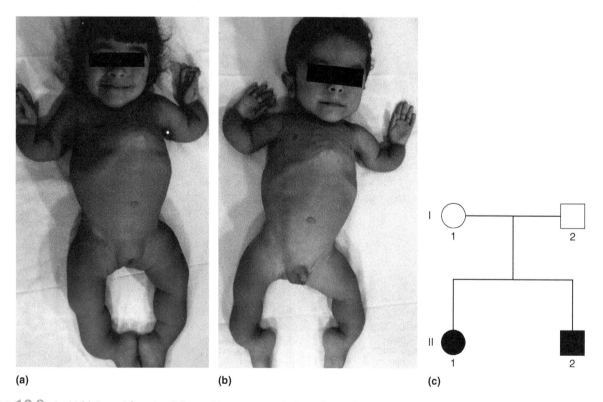

Figure 12-8. (a, b) Male and female siblings with osteogenesis imperfecta. Both children have multiple abnormally healed fractures. (c) Pedigree of this family. Initial inspection might suggest autosomal recessive inheritance. See text for explanation.

in a gene called CFTR—a membrane transporter of chloride ions. Once DNA testing became available, children could be tested to identify the particular mutations causing their disorder. Likewise their parents can be tested to identify which parent is carrying which mutation–information that can be useful for others in the family as they try and ascertain their particular risks. As families were tested, an interesting observation was sometimes encountered. A child with CF would be tested, and two identical mutations would be identified on their two alleles. When the parents were tested, one parent would be identified as having one of the two mutations, but the other would have no identifiable mutation. Further studies were conducted to verify paternity and to rule out new mutations. Ultimately, these studies identified UPD as the explanation! Figure 12-2 provides a schematic demonstrating UPD. Population studies have suggested that maternal UPD may be present in 1 in 500 children with CF. (Note that in order for the child to be affected with CF, that there would have to be uniparental *isodisomy*). A very important aspect of this occurrence would be in recurrence risk counseling. In the typical situation of autosomal recessive inheritance, the recurrence risk for a couple who has had a child with CF would be 25%. In the event of UPD, the same rare abnormal event would have to happen a second time making recurrence essentially zero.

Imprinting

As noted earlier, fewer than 100 human genes are currently known to be imprinted. Specifically then, for this handful of alleles, the normal situation is for monoallelic expression. Disruption of the normal imprinting pattern can result in an abnormal phenotype. Several fascinating human disorders are now known to occur as a result of abnormal imprinting. We encourage you to review the section above on imprinting and to understand Figure 12-3 completely before reading any further.

The first described and probably best understood "imprinting disorders" are Prader-Willi syndrome (PWS) and Angelman syndrome. Prader-Willi syndrome (Figure 12-9) is characterized by hypotonia, cognitive deficits, typical facial changes, obesity, and small hands and feet. Patients with PWS exhibit many features and behaviors that are due to

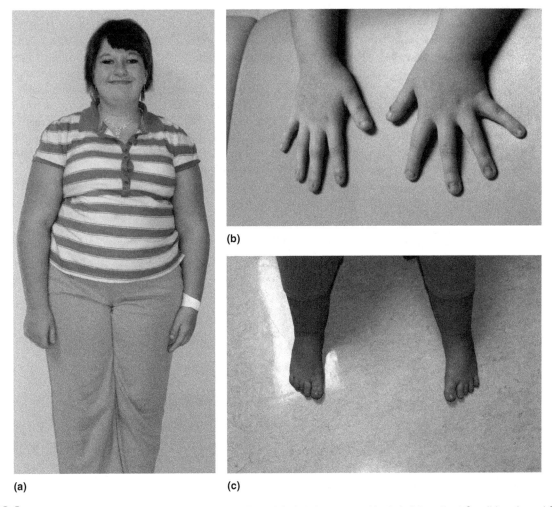

(a) (b) (c)

Figure 12-9. Young woman with Prader-Willi syndrome (a) Typical facial changes and body habitus. (b,c) Small hands and feet.

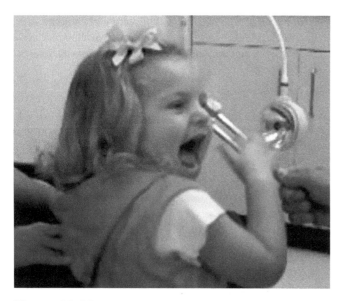

Figure 12-10. Young girl with Angelman syndrome showing a positive "tuning fork sign".

hypothalamic dysfunction (poor satiety control, hyperefficient metabolic rate, hypogonadotrophic hypogonadism). Patients with Angelman syndrome also have a characteristic appearance (Figure 12-10) that is distinctly different from that of PWS. These patients often have seizures and an abnormal gait that is somewhat spastic/hypertonic in nature. In addition they often show "happy" behavior under circumstances not expected to evoke a happy response.

High resolution cytogenetic studies and cytogenetic microarrays have shown that a specific deletion of chromosome region 15p11-13 is found in 70% to 80% of patients with either disorder (Figure 12-11). The obvious question

arising from this observation, of course, is how can the same deletion produce two very different phenotypes? Investigations revealed a parent-of-origin answer. For those patients in which the deletion was on the paternally inherited chromosome 15, the phenotype was PWS. Conversely, if it was the maternally inherited chromosome 15 with the deletion, the phenotype was Angelman syndrome. Further studies have shown that for the 20% of patients with PWS who do not have a chromosome 15 deletion, maternal UPD of chromosome 15 is present. If one considers these two observations, a quick conclusion becomes apparent. The common theme is that PWS occurs if the paternal component of this region of chromosome 15 is missing—either because it is deleted or because the person has inherited both copies of chromosome 15 from the mother. Ultimately these differences have been shown to be due to imprinted genes in this region.

As noted earlier, imprinted genes are often found in clusters called **imprinting domains**, which likely have linked functions of the genes in the region. Clearly this region of chromosome 15 is such a region with several known imprinted genes. Two of these genes are particularly notable. The small nuclear ribonucleoprotein polypeptide N (*SNRPN*) gene seems to be highly associated with PWS and the ubiquitin protein ligase E3A (*UBE3A*) gene with Angelman syndrome.

The genetic etiology of Angelman syndrome is slightly more complicated than PWS. Like PWS, around 70% of patients with Angelman syndrome will have a 15q11-13 deletion, which will be of *maternal* origin. However, only about 5% of patients with Angelman syndrome will have UPD. But as predicted, when this is the case, it will be paternal uniparental disomy. The remaining cases of Angelman syndrome are largely due to mutations in the imprinted gene *UBE3A*.

Besides these two conditions, there are several other human disorders that are known to be due to disorders of

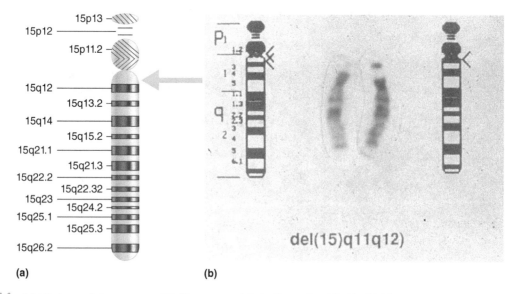

(a) (b)

Figure 12-11. (a) Idiogram of chromosome 15. The arrow points to the region 15q11. (b) Idiograms and photomicrographs of two different chromosome 15s demonstrating a 15q11 deletion.

Table 12-1.	Disorders Caused by Abnormalities of Imprinting

Albright hereditary osteodystrophy/McCune-Albright syndrome

Beckwith-Wiedemann syndrome/Russel-Silver syndrome

Familial nonchromaffin paraganglioma

Maternal/paternal uniparental disomy 14 syndromes

Transient neonatal diabetes mellitus

imprinting. A list of some of these is in Table 12-1. It is interesting to note that many of these are **inverse disorders** like Prader-Willi and Angelman syndromes. While the conditions listed are largely recognizable syndromes and conditions, it is likely that imprinting errors play a role in more complex conditions. Studies have suggested a role of imprinting defects in conditions like Alzheimer disease, autism, schizophrenia, and even some cancers.

More Examples of Gene-Gene Interactions

The traditional definition of **compound heterozygosity** is the presence of two different mutant alleles at a particular gene locus, one on each allele of the pair (Figure 12-12). In a monogenic, autosomal recessive disorder, it simply means that each allele carries its own unique mutation. This is in fact quite common given the degree of genetic heterogeneity typically present in human genetic disorders.

With better access to molecular diagnostic information, more complex mechanisms of inheritance have been identified. **Digenic inheritance** as noted before occurs when mutations occur at two different loci. For example, most states in the United States currently perform newborn screening for hearing loss. Newborn hearing loss is relatively common, occurring in about 1 newborn per 1000 births. If a congenital hearing loss is identified, a genetic evaluation to identify the cause is indicated. The two most common causes of hearing loss identified in infants are teratogenic (congenital

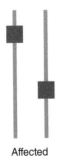

Figure 12-12. Graphic representation of compound heterozygosity for a simple autosomal recessive disorder at a single locus.

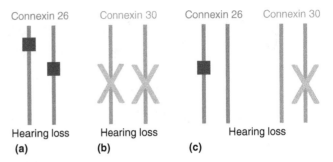

Figure 12-13. Compound heterozygosity at two different loci in hereditary hearing loss. (a) Autosomal recessive hearing loss due to mutations in the gene connexin 26. (b) Autosomal recessive hearing loss due to deletions in the gene connexin 30. (c) Compound heterozygosity for a connexin 26 mutation and a connexin 30 deletion also produces hearing loss. This could be termed "digenic" inheritance.

cytomegalovirus) and mutations in a gene called connexin 26 or *GJB2*. Connexin 26 is one of the so-called "gap junction proteins" that allows for rapid ion transport that circumvents osmosis by directly connecting the cytoplasmic regions of contacting cells. This gene is located on chromosome 13. In fact, connexin 26 mutations account for almost 15% of all hearing loss in newborns.

Typically infant hearing loss due to connexin 26 mutations is inherited as a straightforward autosomal recessive condition (Figure 12-13a). Given the high frequency of connexin 26 related hearing loss, it is not surprising that the carrier frequency of connexin 26 mutations is relatively high at about 1 in 30 individuals of Northern European descent. Connexin 30 is another gap junction protein. It also lies on chromosome 13 just upstream and close to connexin 26. About 1 in 100,000 people in the general population carry a connexin 30 gene deletion. Given the low carrier frequency it is rare, but occasionally there is an individual who is homozygous for this deletion (Figure 12-13b). These individuals, then, also have an autosomal recessive hearing loss. When genetic testing for the genes became available, an interesting phenomenon was noted. A significant number of newborn were seen in which only a single connexin 26 mutation was identified. Early assumptions were that this was simply chance and unlikely to be the cause of the hearing loss. However, this occurrence was soon recognized as occurring significantly more often than could be predicted by chance and carrier frequency.

Ultimately it was shown that 20% of connexin 26 heterozygotes with neurosensory hearing loss also have a connexin 30 deletion (Figure 12-13c). This compound heterozygosity at two different loci is thus the cause of the hearing loss. The inheritance can be described as digenic inheritance.

Bardet-Biedel syndrome (BBS) is a recognizable condition with the key clinical features being mental retardation, pigmentary retinopathy, polydactyly and other digital abnormalities, central obesity, and hypogenitalism (Figure 12-14). As originally described, BBS was felt to be an autosomal recessive disorder. Research into the genetics of BBS has

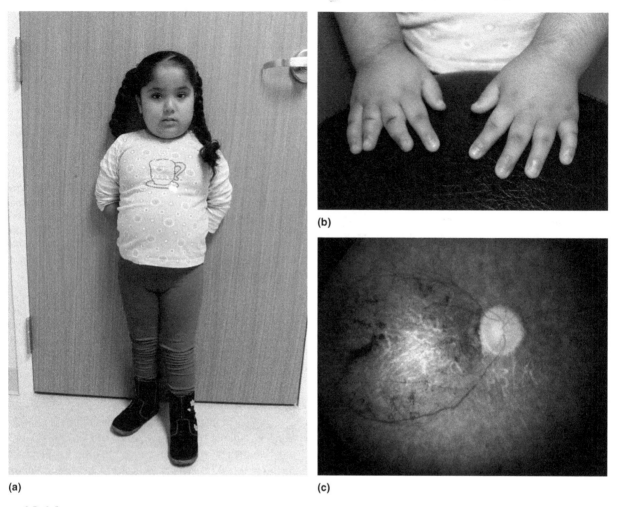

(a)

(b)

(c)

Figure 12-14. Young girl with Bardet-Biedel syndrome. This child has cognitive deficits, short stature, mild obesity, and pigmentary retinal abnormalities.

revealed genetic heterogeneity with at least 15 genes thus far described that are associated with this condition. The majority of cases of BBS typically show simple autosomal recessive inheritance due to mutations in the BBS 1 gene

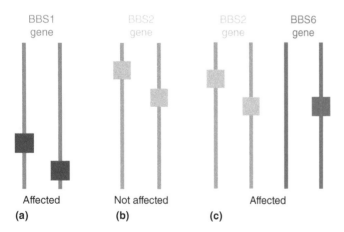

Figure 12-15. Compound heterozygosity involving 3 alleles at 2 different loci for Bardet-Biedel syndrome. This could be termed "triallelic inheritance." See text for detailed descriptions.

(Figure 12-15a). Notably, mutations on both alleles of the BBS 2 gene do not cause any apparent disease (Figure 12-15b). However, patients who are homozygous for BBS2 mutations who also harbor a single BBS6 mutation will be affected with Bardet-Biedel syndrome (Figure 12-15c). This type of compound heterozygosity involving three alleles at two different loci has been termed "triallelic" inheritance.

Multi-locus Inheritance

Multi-locus inheritance as defined in the first section of this chapter means that the observed phenotype is influenced by genes at more than one locus. For many of the most common human medical conditions (if not all) this is the case. The examples above of digenic and triallelic inheritance patterns clearly meet this definition.

Modifier genes are simply genes that influence the expression of other genes. Usually these are genes that have small quantitative effects on the level of expression of another gene. One might appropriately ask: "isn't this what was defined as polygenic inheritance?" In many ways this is correct. The distinction here is subtle, and maybe not always

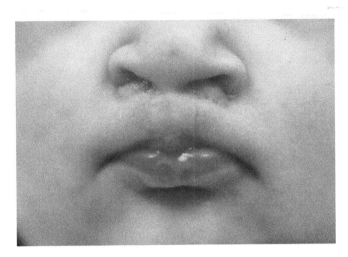

Figure 12-16. Van der Woude syndrome. The child has a repaired cleft lip and palate. Note the paired lower lip pits.

completely delineated. One can model polygenic inheritance as having multiple genes each more or less equally influencing a single quantitative trait. Modifiers genes, on the other hand, exert influence on a major gene's effects. Take the example of van der Woude syndrome. Van der Woude syndrome is an autosomal dominant condition caused by mutations in IRF6 on chromosome 1q32. The major phenotypic feature that can be tracked through a family is that of bilateral lower lip pits (Figure 12-16). Cleft lip and/or cleft palate are variably expressed in association with the lip pits (Figure 12-17). It is obviously the same gene with the same mutation within a family, so why then do only some have clefting? Linkage studies have identified a locus at 17p11.2 that contains a gene (yet to be identified) that influences the expression of clefts in patients with van der Woude syndrome.

Multi-locus interactions are particularly notable in cancer. It is now known that all cancers are genetic (the reader is reminded

that this is not synonymous with heritable, since mutations can occur in somatic tissue alone). The current understanding of the etiologic pathogenesis of cancer is a model of sequentially accumulated mutations (Figure 12-18). That is, multiple genes are involved in neoplasia initiation and progression. All evidence points to the clonal nature of cancers. This means that all of the daughter cancerous cells share a common origin from a cell line that has accumulated mutations in all of the genes necessary to change the growth characteristics of the cells from benign to malignant.

Opposite (Anti-Sense) Transcripts

The use of a section of DNA for more than one transcript is not uncommon in viruses, in which compaction of information is at a premium. But when only a tiny percent of the whole human genome is actually used to code for all of the required protein products, it seemed improbable for portions to overlap in coding function. Improbable, i.e., until it was discovered. In reality, the generation of products is a function of their usefulness, not some probability of their spatial distribution. Current estimates suggest there are at least 1600 such transcript pairs scattered across the human genome.

Interleukin-14 (*ILI4*) is one such example in humans. Two distinctly different transcripts are created from the opposite strands of the *ILI4* gene: *IL14α* and *IL14β*. Another example is the *Lit1* gene in Beckwith-Wiedeman syndrome (see the clinical correlation in Part 3 of this chapter). Abnormal processing of natural antisense transcripts has been implicated in diverse group of human conditions, such as cancer, Alzheimer disease, and hemoglobinopathies.

Transposable Elements

As noted in Part 1 of this chapter, transposable elements (transposons) are migratory segments of the genome. There are several different types of transposons that differ by their size, nucleic acid type, and the mechanism of movement. The major clinical implication of transposons lies in their mutagenic potential. In some situations, this is actually a normal and desired effect. Transposons play a key role in the generation of antibodies in a normal immune response. In the processes of recombination and "somatic hypermutation" that are necessary to generate a wide diversity of antibodies, the presence of a natural source of "shuffling the deck" is advantageous. Transposons have also been shown to play a role in the origin and perpetuation of several genetic disorders. In Chapter 7 (Mutations) it was noted that some loci have a higher than average mutation rate. For many of these "mutation hotspots," the higher mutation rate has been shown to be related to the presence of nearby or internal transposons. A list of a few of these is provided in Table 12-2. Transposons are implicated in the pathogenesis of cancer and aging. It is interesting to note that the HIV-1 virus and other similar human retroviruses demonstrate replication patterns that are strikingly similar to retrotransposons.

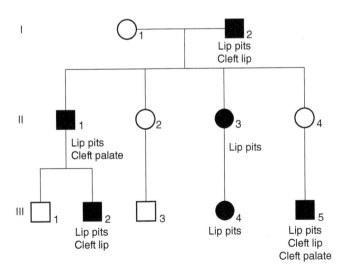

Figure 12-17. Pedigree of a family with van der Woude syndrome.

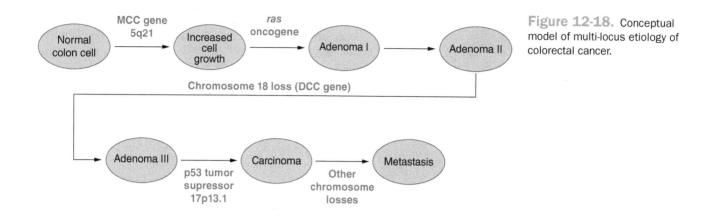

Figure 12-18. Conceptual model of multi-locus etiology of colorectal cancer.

Table 12-2.	Disorders Shown to Be Related to Transposon Generated Mutations

Acute intermittent porphyria (hydroxymethylbilane synthase gene)

Duchenne muscular dystrophy (dystrophin gene)

Familial adenomatosis polyposis (APC gene)

Hemophilia A (factor VIII gene)

Hemophilia B (factor IX gene)

X-linked severe combined immunodeficiency (IL-2 receptor gene)

Genetic Anticipation

Genetic **anticipation** is defined as the apparent worsening of a disorder with subsequent generations. For decades the issue was debated. Was anticipation real or simply a bias of ascertainment? If it were real, what possible mechanism could explain it? The issue was finally resolved with the identification of the underlying pathogenesis of fragile X syndrome. (Before the genetic basis of fragile X syndrome was discovered, the associated phenotype had been described as "Martin-Bell" syndrome.) Fragile X syndrome is now known to be an X-linked condition associated with mental retardation and autistic like behaviors. Boys with fragile X have mildly dysmorphic facies (somewhat thin and elongated with large ears), macrocephaly, hypotonia, joint laxity, and postpubertal macroorchidism (Figure 4-27). In the mid-1970s several laboratories were studying families with X-linked mental retardation. As part of these studies, a marker was found in some families. In these families, a "fragile site" could be expressed on the X chromosome at location Xq28 if the cells were cultured in folate-deficient media (Figure 12-19).

Using this marker, investigators were able to look at this subgroup of families with X-linked mental retardation separately. In doing so, they identified a novel inheritance in these families. The transmission of fragile X syndrome within families showed X-linked semi-dominant inheritance with anticipation—but only when transmitted through the mother. This unique pattern was designated the "Sherman paradox" named after Stephanie Sherman who described it. Figure 4-28 shows a hypothetical pedigree of a family with fragile X syndrome. In this drawing, all of the mentioned features can be seen. The condition is X-linked; hence no male-to-male transmission is seen. The condition is semi-dominant with partial (milder) expression in females. The observed anticipation is represented by the statistical recurrence risks. Note the increasing recurrence risk with each generation—but only if transmission is maternal. Herein was the first objective evidence of genetic anticipation!

Further research ultimately identified a fascinating mechanism of pathogenesis in fragile X syndrome. The condition was shown to be due to an "expanding gene." Specifically, the normal gene, designated *FMR1*, was found at a locus that was better defined as Xq27.3. A series of trinucleotide (CGG)

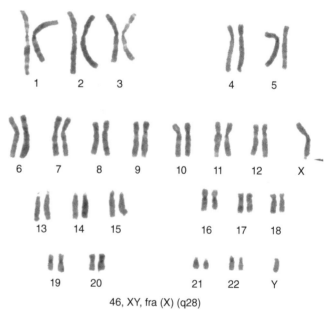

Figure 12-19. Karyotype showing the "fragile site" on the X chromosome at location Xq28.

Table 12-3.	Correlation of Trinucleotide Repeat Number and Phenotype in Fragile X Syndrome	
Clinical Status	**CGG Repeat Number**	
Normal	6-46	
Transmitting male	52-200	
Carrier female	52-200	
Affected males	>200	
Affected females	>200	

repeats was identified in the 5′ untranslated region of the gene. Normal individuals typically have 35 to 40 CGG repeats in this region. Fragile X syndrome is now known to be caused expansion of the CGG repeat number in the *FMR1* gene. When the number of repeats exceeds 200, abnormal methylation occurs with resulting suppression of *FMR1* transcription and decreased production of the normal protein. The normal protein product of this gene is designated the fragile X mental retardation protein (FMRP). This protein is found in most tissues, but has its highest concentrations within the brain and testicles. The protein is critical in the formation and organization of synapses. Thus, fragile X syndrome is ultimately caused by deficiency of the FMRP. Additional studies have shown that the clinical spectrum of problems seen in families with fragile X syndrome correlate with the number of repeats, which expand as the mutation is transmitted to the next generation (Table 12-3). Thus, the argument could be definitively settled. Genetic anticipation is a real phenomenon, and a specific mechanism that can explain how it can occur had been discovered. Current technology then allows for ready diagnosis of fragile X syndrome. Using any one of several techniques, the number of trinucleotide repeats can be quantified to establish or rule out the diagnosis (Figure 12-20).

Myotonic dystrophy (Figure 12-21) is a muscle disease characterized by myotonia (the inability to relax muscles adequately after a sustained contraction). Affected individuals may show a variety of other medical complications including cataracts, heart arrhythmias, hypogonadism, and male pattern baldness. Clinicians had long suspected that myotonic dystrophy showed genetic anticipation. Thus, shortly after the discovery of the expanding trinucleotide repeats in fragile X syndrome, a similar mechanism was discovered in myotonic dystrophy. In a similar fashion, myotonic dystrophy was shown to have genetic anticipation due to an expanding trinucleotide repeat. There are, however, several significant differences. The trinucleotide repeat in fragile X syndrome is CGG, but in myotonic dystrophy it is CTG. The location of the repeats in fragile X is the 5′ untranslated region. In myotonic dystrophy, it is in the 3′ untranslated region of the gene dystrophia myotonica protein kinase (DMPK). In fragile X syndrome, the repeat only enlarges as it passes through maternal meiosis. In myotonic dystrophy the repeat can enlarge as

it is transmitted by either sex; however, the expansion tends to be larger as it is transmitted by mothers.

Since the discovery of the trinucleotide expansions in fragile X syndrome and myotonic dystrophy, several more **trinucleotide repeat disorders** have been described (Table 12-4). Interestingly, most of these conditions are neuromotor disorders. As with fragile X and myotonic dystrophy, these disorders differ in the trinucleotide repeat, its size and stability, where in the gene it is located, and whether or not the repeat is translated or transcribed (Figure 12-22). Categories have been established to group the conditions that have similar properties of the repeats. Category I includes conditions due to repeats affecting the coding region of the gene. Two well-known examples are Huntington disease and the spinocerebellar ataxias (due to CAG repeats). Category II expansions are also found in the exons of genes but tend to be phenotypically diverse and generally small. Category III expansions tend to be the largest and are located outside the protein-coding region of a gene. Fragile X and myotonic dystrophy are included in this third group.

While we will discuss pathogenesis in more detail in Chapter 16, it is worth brief discussion here. The specific question is: "how do expanding trinucleotide repeats cause disease?" To date at least three mechanisms have been identified:

1. Loss of function. As already described before, fragile X syndrome is caused by a loss of functional protein due to abnormal methylation. Friedreich ataxia, the only known trinucleotide repeat disorder that shows autosomal recessive inheritance (not surprisingly) also is due to protein insufficiency.

2. Gain of function. In some conditions, the mechanism of disease is not a deficiency of a protein product, but rather a direct toxicity from excess metabolites, which inhibit other enzyme and/or regulatory systems. Huntington disease is one such example. Normally the enzyme GAPDH binds to stretches of glutamine. Excess glutamine (>760 CAG repeats) will inhibit the enzyme, which results in cumulative cell death. As is the case in Huntington disease, most of these conditions show an adult onset degenerative phenotype.

3. Dominant negative effect. Sometimes the trinucleotide change results in an abnormal product that interferes with its normal physiological function. This is the proposed mechanism in myotonic dystrophy.

One way of looking at these three mechanisms is to consider a race. Always remember that the normal physiological state is balance. Think about two people in racing lanes with *the goal being to run at the same pace*. A loss of function mutation would make one racer run slower than the other. A gain of function mutation would make one run faster than the other. A dominant negative effect would be if one had a leg injury that caused them to weave out of their lane and run into the second runner disabling both of them.

Normal female

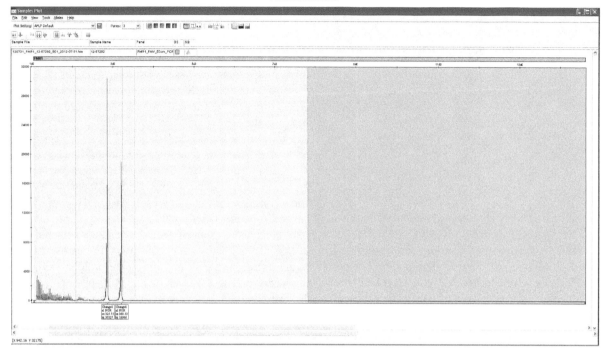

(a)

Normal male

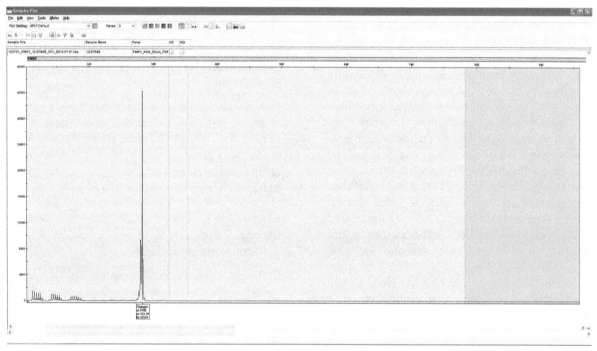

(b)

Figure 12-20. Molecular testing for the trinucleotide repeats in fragile X syndrome. Shown are 3 chromatograms depicting repeat number. (a) Normal female. Note the two peaks, one for each X chromosome. (b) Normal male. One peak, one X chromosome. (c) Male with full expansion. This individual has over 200 CGG repeats noted by the large displaced peak. (Chromatograms courtesy of Dr. Jennifer Wei, Ambry Genetics.)

12-56893 full mutation

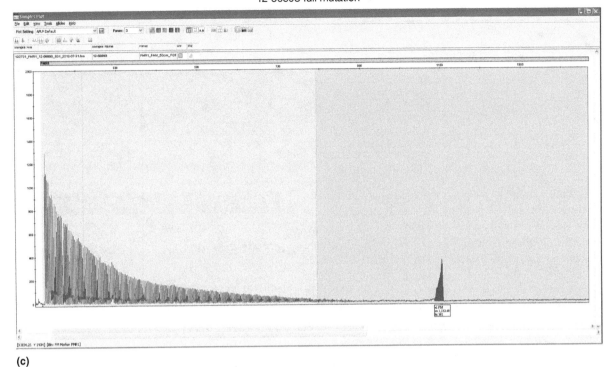

(c)

Figure 12-20. (Continued)

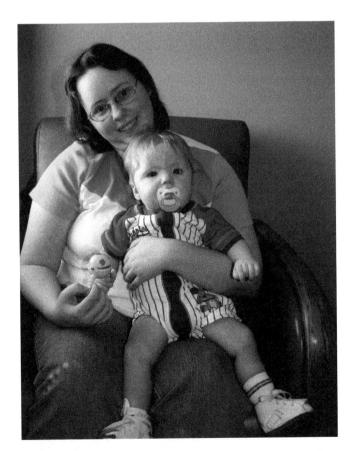

Figure 12-21. Mother and child with myotonic dystrophy. The mother is more mildly affected having only mild myotonia. Note the hypotonia in the child.

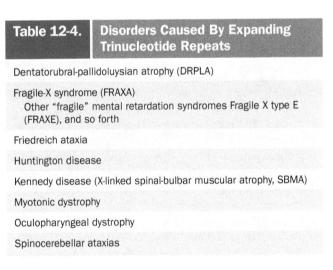

Table 12-4.	Disorders Caused By Expanding Trinucleotide Repeats
Dentatorubral-pallidoluysian atrophy (DRPLA)	
Fragile-X syndrome (FRAXA) Other "fragile" mental retardation syndromes Fragile X type E (FRAXE), and so forth	
Friedreich ataxia	
Huntington disease	
Kennedy disease (X-linked spinal-bulbar muscular atrophy, SBMA)	
Myotonic dystrophy	
Oculopharyngeal dystrophy	
Spinocerebellar ataxias	

Epigenetics

A very important and rapidly emerging field of genetics concerns epigenetics. One of the many reasons that humans have a relatively small number of genes compared with much simpler organisms is the fact that we can do a lot more with the genes we have. As discussed in earlier chapters, this would include mechanisms such as multiply cleaved transcripts or posttranslational modification of proteins. Another mechanism of getting varied responses from a single specific genetic code is epigenetic modification.

Epigenetic mechanisms are those that can change gene expression without modifying the code itself. While the reader

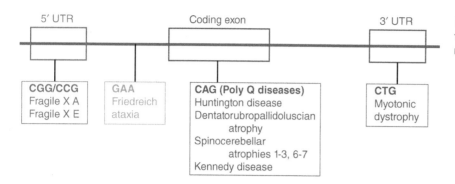

Figure 12-22 Schematic showing the different types of trinucleotide abnormalities that may be seen in different disorders.

may not have specifically recognized it as such, epigenetic mechanisms have already been introduced in earlier parts of this book and were discussed under different topic headings. The inactivation of an X-chromosome in Lyonization is one such example. Changes in methylation as discussed earlier in this chapter in the role of imprinting genes is another. Other examples of epigenetic mechanisms are listed in Table 12-5. It is beyond the scope of this text to discuss this very complex and expansive topic in detail. The greatest importance in understanding the concept of epigenetic mechanisms lies in their therapeutic potential. The fact that many human diseases, including cancer, have an epigenetic etiology has encouraged the development of new therapeutic options

Table 12-5.	**Types of Epigenetic Mechanisms**
Chromatin modifications
DNA methylation
Histone modification
RNA-associated silencing
Imprinting X-inactivation

that might be termed "epigenetic therapies." Many agents have been discovered that alter methylation patterns on DNA or the modification of histones, and several of these agents are currently being tested in clinical trials.

Part 3: Clinical Correlation

Beckwith-Wiedemann syndrome (BWS) is a recognizable multiple anomaly syndrome (Figure 12-23 a-c). It is characterized by macrosomia (large body size), macroglossia (large tongue), and omphalocoele. Other features include visceromegaly (enlarged internal organs)—especially the kidneys and pancreas—often severe neonatal hypoglycemia, abnormal earlobe creases, posterior helical pits, and an increased risk of embryonal tumors (Wilms tumor, hepatoblastoma, neuroblastoma, rhabdomyosarcoma). Clinical observations noted a clear familial nature to BWS without a Mendelian inheritance pattern. Other notable observations included an association of discordance of the phenotype in monozygotic twins (Figure 10-5) and an increased presence of BWS after certain types of *in vitro* fertilization methods.

Ultimately, molecular genetic studies of BWS identified an extremely complex inheritance pattern. The different mechanisms involved here tie together much of what has been discussed in this chapter. If after reading this clinical correlation, you understand it well, you have it down!

In short, the majority of cases of BWS are due to problems with genes within the locus 11p15. Of the identified cases:

1. For BWS 50% to 60% of cases are due to a problem with a gene in this region called *Lit1*. In the normal situation *Lit1* is an imprinted gene. The maternal allele is usually methylated and thus "turned off." The paternal allele is normally expressed. An error that causes

loss of the methylation (hypo-methylation) of *Lit1* (the normally imprinted maternal allele is thus activated) will result in increased *Lit1* expression and a person with BWS. It is also interesting to note that the gene *Lit1* has within its coding sequence a gene that has an opposite transcript. The gene *KCNQ1* is a gene that codes for a potassium channel protein. Its coding sequence is read in the opposite direction of *Lit1*. Thus, an alternative name for *Lit1* is *KCNQ1OT1* (KCNQ1 opposite transcript)!

2. In contrast, 2% to 7% of all BWS cases are due to a problem with a gene called *H19* in this same region. In the normal situation *H19* is an imprinted gene. The paternal allele is usually methylated and thus "turned off." The maternal allele is normally expressed. An error that causes gain of methylation (hyper-methylation) of *H19* (the normally non-imprinted maternal allele is turned off) will result in decreased *H19* expression. Decreased *H19* expression leads to increased *IgF2* expression (another gene in this region that is a growth factor) and likewise a person affected with BWS.

3. For BWS 10% to 20% of cases are due to paternal uniparental disomy of the 11p15 region.

4. For BWS 5% to 10% of cases have an identifiable mutation in *CDKN1C* (another imprinted gene in this region).

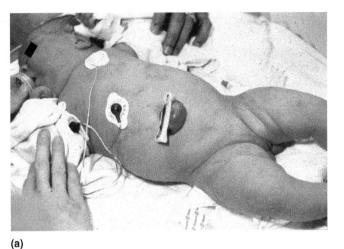
(a)

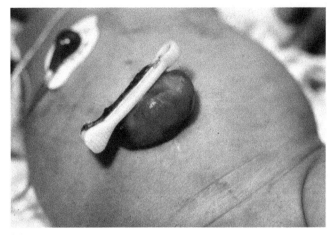
(b)

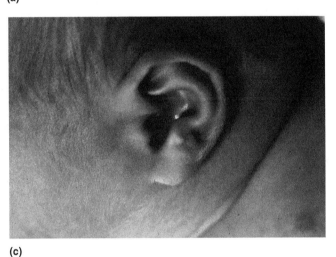
(c)

Figure 12-23. (a) Newborn female with Beckwith-Wiedemann syndrome. (b) Close-up view of the child's omphalocoele. (c) Abnormal helical pits.

5. Finally, about 1% of patients with BWS will have a chromosome 11 rearrangement of the region 11p15 such as a maternal translocation or inversion or a paternal duplication.

Thus, when a patient is born with Beckwith-Wiedeman syndrome, any of these five etiologies are possible. From the information mentioned, it would seem obvious that the implications for things such as recurrence risks differ greatly depending on the cause. Therefore, targeted genetic testing must but performed—usually in a tiered (stepwise) set of tests. When an etiology is defined, this very complicated information needs to be communicated to the family in an understandable and usable manner. This is not an easy task—one that benefits from the skills and training of a genetic counselor.

■ Board-Format Practice Questions

1. Suppose that there is an important growth factor during fetal development (GF). Like most polypeptide hormones it has a receptor (GFR). It appears that during fetal life only the paternal GF gene is active and only the maternal GFR gene is active. Mutations that cause both copies of either gene to become active typically result in fetal overgrowth. This is an example of:
   A. Uniparental disomy.
   B. Genomic imprinting.
   C. Unstable DNA.
   D. Genetic anticipation.
   E. Partial expression.
2. In regards to imprinting, which of the following statements is most likely true?
   A. Imprinting represents a pathologic mechanism of gene expression.
   B. Imprinting changes the DNA code.
   C. Imprinting is erased during meiosis.
   D. The most common mechanism of imprinting is by DNA glycosylation.
   E. All human gene loci are normally imprinted.

3. In regards to X-inactivation:
   A. Males will usually have one Barr body in their cells.
   B. Because it is random and thus there is almost always a distribution of very close to a 50:50 proportion of one or the other X being inactivated.
   C. A structurally abnormal X chromosome is preferentially inactivated, leaving the normal X active.
   D. It is permanent in germ cells
   E. Its clonal distribution suggests that it occurs late in embryonic development.
4. Which part of the Sherman paradox can be explained by the phenomenon of expanding trinucleotide repeats?
   A. X-linked inheritance.
   B. Semi-dominant pattern of transmission.
   C. Genetic anticipation.
   D. Females being more severely affected than males.
   E. Mosaicism.

5. Which of the mechanisms below is an epigenetic mechanism?
   A. X-autosome chromosome translocation.
   B. Genomic imprinting.
   C. Microsatellites.
   D. Spontaneous mutation.
   E. Expanding trinucleotide repeats.
6. Which is a mechanism whereby expanding trinucleotide repeats could cause disease (i.e., pathogenesis)?
   A. Dominant negative effect.
   B. Insertional mutations.
   C. X-inactivation.
   D. Reverse (opposite) transcription.
   E. Modifier genes.

chapter 13

Disorders of Organelles

CHAPTER SUMMARY

The functions of cell organelles like the nucleus and mitochondria are critical to the processes on which life depends. But that does not mean they are easy to study. From a general biology course you probably learned facts like a nucleus controls the growth and reproduction of a cell and ribosomes are the sites of protein synthesis (Figure 13-1). But for a moment, take a step back and ask a more basic question, "How do we know these things?" Just seeing the microscopic structures inside a cell is hard enough. How can we know the way they actually work? For medical genetics, the next question is then obvious. What are the medical effects of a genetic change in the structure or activity of a cell organelle? Can that knowledge lead to appropriate treatment?

Asking how we learn things about a structure as tiny as a cell organelle leads us to an important insight about the way science, including medical science, progresses. The real champion is how human ingenuity can figure out a process, especially a small, elusive one hidden somewhere in the complexity of the body—or of a cell. Let's step back in history to remind ourselves of both the limitations and the scientific revolutions that have been spurred by experimentation at the level of a cell. Then we will look at one specific example of discovering the role of a cell organelle.

Imagine yourself in the early 16th century. If you were a physician, not a common profession at the time, you would work with a limited and even misleading view of how the body functions. The prevailing explanation of life is a mystical one. But changes are underway. The publication of *De humani corporis fabrica* in 1543 by Andreas Vesalius helped introduce to science an emphasis on personal observation rather than a dependence on accepted authority. It replaced the authoritative position held by the studies that Galen published about 1300 years earlier. William Harvey's *De motu cordis* (1628) traced the flow of blood to and from the heart and led to a mechanistic, rather than a mystical, explanation of nutrient and oxygen transport. The invention of optics for magnification, which began as a novel entertainment, opened biologists to the microscopic realm.

Robert Hooke described the cellular structure of bark in *Micrographia* (1665)–". . . these pores, or cells, were not very deep, but consisted of a great many little Boxes, separated out of one continued long pore, by certain Diaphragms . . . ." This was the first use of the word "cells" to describe biological structure, because the images reminded him of the spartan cells in which monks slept. Thus, a previously unknown dimension was being opened to view. It was Matthias Schleiden and Theodor Schwann (1838 and 1839, respectively) who formalized the theory that all living material is composed of cells. The light microscope revealed basic elements of cell organization and tissue differences. But it was not until just after the Second World War that the electron microscope began to resolve ultrastructure sufficiently to see the internal organization of cells in detail.

Seeing cell organelles in sharp resolution is not the same as understanding their function. Indeed, a nondividing nucleus is not a very imposing image. Looking at it unveils little about how it works. Imagine for a moment you are a researcher interested in the function of an organelle like the nucleus. How can you correlate a microscopic cell particle with a defined function? Joachim Hämmerling explored this question experimentally, but not in the 16th century, or even the 18th. His experimental demonstration that the nucleus controls the growth and regeneration of eukaryotic cells was done as recently as the 1940s and early 1950s. This is an area of biological research that clearly illustrates in a powerful way the creative insight of good science. It also reminds us how important experimental organisms are in uncovering information that is valuable to medicine and other applied fields. We can learn things by taking advantage of the special characteristics of a model organism, where the same question would be difficult if not impossible to answer using human cells or tissue.

Hämmerling took advantage of the very large cell size of marine algae of the genus *Acetabularia* (Figure 13-2). An inch-long *Acetabularia* cell is composed of a cap and a stalk. A rhizoid or rootlet contains the nucleus. Such a large cell can be surgically dissected and its parts can be transferred or fused together. For example, when Hämmerling cut a cell into these three sections, the cap died and the rhizoid with its nucleus regenerated a new stalk and cap. Surprisingly, the stalk by itself initially regenerated a cap, but then when the new cap was removed, the stalk was not able to continue regenerating. It died. Something in the stalk allowed it to regenerate for a brief time, but the root containing the nucleus could do so repeatedly. We now understand that the temporary ability of the isolated stalk to regenerate is due to mRNA in the stalk. But mRNA cannot be replaced if the nucleus is missing. To confirm the nuclear role in a separate experiment, Hämmerling grafted the stalk from a fringed *A. crenulata* onto the rhizoid of the smooth-capped *Acetabularia mediterranea*. The regenerated cap took on characteristics associated with the nucleus, not the stem. With experiments like these, Hämmerling confirmed the functional role of this nuclear organelle.

The story of the growth of microscopy shows how advances in technology can open new vistas for biomedical discovery and for applications to benefit patients. We have seen this more recently in the case of microarrays and personalized medical treatment options. The questions may be old. What is always "new" is the creative way a researcher can devise to approach them. Being receptive to new tools and remaining open-minded to new explanations will always define the foundations for success at the frontiers of biomedical knowledge.

In this chapter, we focus on the microscopic basis of cell function and some of the medical consequences of abnormalities in selected key cell organelles. To illustrate these, we have chosen to put some microscopic images of normal and abnormal cells together for direct comparison. This means that references to figures may tend to jump back and forth a bit between sections. But we think the resulting image comparisons will be more meaningful this way.

Part 1: Background and Systems Integration

The cell has two domains, the nuclear and the cytoplasmic. The cytoplasm is composed of the fluid component (the cytosol) and the formed elements (organelles other than the nucleus) (Figure 13-3). The functions of these two domains are intricately interconnected. The nucleus and most of a cell's other organelles, are bounded by membranes, although the composition and specific roles of the membrane will differ from one organelle to another. Transitory interconnection of membranes throughout the cell insures a high degree of molecular communication among cell components. Other non-membrane organelles, like ribosomes and the cytoskeleton,

interact directly with molecules and formed elements in the cytoplasm. Not surprisingly, then, defects in organelle structure and function can have extensive consequences for all levels of biological activity.

All are critical for cell function, but because of their role in energy metabolism the mitochondria are among the most important for medical genetics. We will first review briefly some major types of microscopy, because this guides what can be visualized about cell and organelle organization. We will then explore both normal and defective organelle functions, with primary emphasis on the mitochondria.

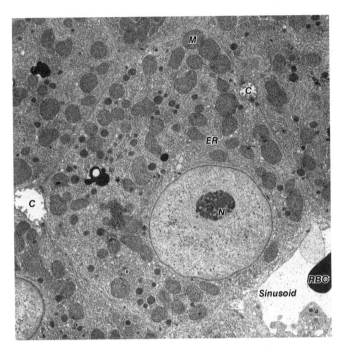

Figure 13-1. Electron microscopy opens cell ultrastructure to a world of detail that could not be imagined by early researchers. But seeing structure does not always explain function. (Reprinted with permission from Cheville, N., *Ultrastructural Pathology*, Iowa State University Press, Ames, IA. p 2, 1994.)

Types of Microscopy

Cells are tiny. But it is a mistake to think that the more magnification, the better. One must choose a magnification that makes sense for the question being asked. Electron microscopy can provide fine resolution of the internal structures in a cell, but often the most useful diagnostic information will come from a less magnified view. To prepare material for different types of light or electron microscopy, the tissue must be stabilized and stained. Structures are fixed with chemicals like formaldehyde for light microscopy or glutaraldehyde for electron microscopy. Water is then removed so the tissue can be embedded in a non-aqueous medium like paraffin or plastic. From this block, thin sections are cut and stained. The choice of stain will control what aspects of the complex cell structure will be enhanced. Other techniques allow surfaces of large structures and even internal activities in living cells to be studied in detail.

Light microscopy can resolve tissue organization up to a little more than 1000 × with an oil immersion lens. There are three main types of light microscopy that allow different kinds of cell structure to be visualized. Bright field microscopy depends on staining cell components with dyes that are acidophilic (mostly proteins) or basophilic (primarily nucleic acids and certain sugars) (Figure 13-4). Osmium tetroxide covalently bonds to lipids. Some staining protocols involve double staining, such as defining the nucleus with one stain and counterstaining the cytoplasm with another. Other common stains, like Wright's used for white blood cells, are a mixture of different stains (i.e., polychrome stains).

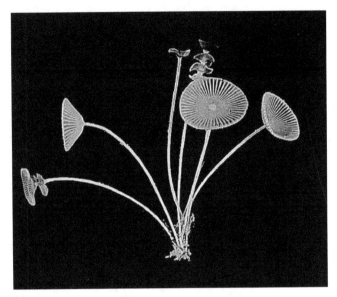

(a)

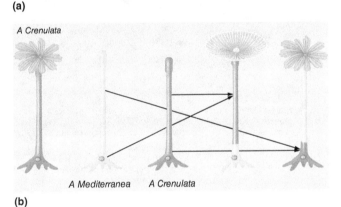

(b)

Figure 13-2. Each *Acetabularia* is a single cell. (a) With a nucleus near the rootlet and with an umbrella that regenerates when foraged upon. The species *Acetabularia mediterranea* and *A. crenulata* differ in the shape of the umbrella at the top of each cell. (b) By removing and transplanting the cap, stalk, and nucleus containing rootlet, J. Hämmerling confirmed that genetic control of growth and regeneration resided in the nucleus.
(a: Reproduced with permission from Wolfgang Sterrer, originally appearing in Sterrer W. Marine Fauna and Flora of Bermuda. New York: John Wiley & Sons, 1986.)

A second type of light microscopy is phase contrast, a powerful tool to visualize living cells. This approach depends on the way light changes its speed when passing through structures that have different refractive indices. Phase contrast optics causes these structures to appear lighter or darker in the field of view. While imaging living cells, phase contrast can give detailed information about cell responses to stimuli (Figure 13-5). Nomarski differential interference can even produce detailed three-dimensional images. These are compared in Figure 13-6.

A third approach to light microscopy uses fluorescent stains that have a high affinity to certain types of cellular molecules. This is a very powerful technique, because one can

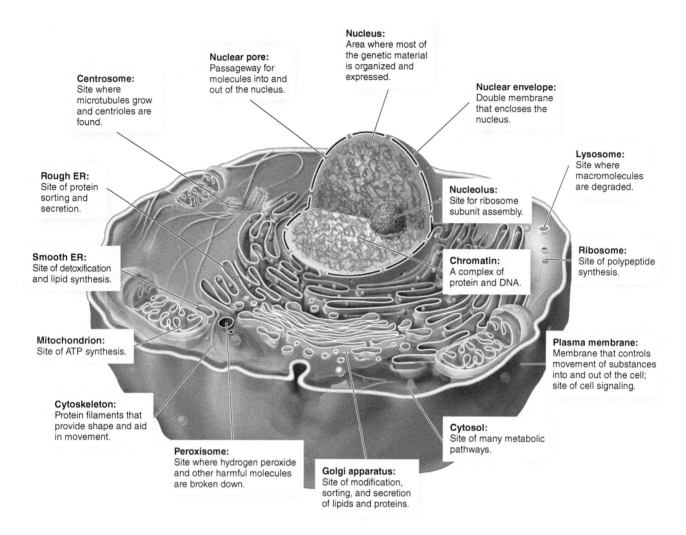

Figure 13-3. An overview of the functions associated with primary organelles in an animal cell. (Reprinted with permission from Brooker et al., *Biology*, 2nd ed, New York: McGraw-Hill, p 70, 2011.)

couple fluorescent materials to a large array of antibodies for almost any cellular molecule. Materials can be multiply-stained to visualize the physical relationships among molecules that are close together in the cell (Figure 13-7).

There are two fundamental types of electron microscopy, transmission electron microscopy (TEM) and scanning electron microscopy (SEM). TEM requires very thin sections (on the order of 40-90 nm) prepared from tissue embedded in a resin block and stained with heavy metals like osmium tetroxide or uranyl acetate. Combining these with immunological agents can target specific cell activities like the movement of a molecule through a membrane as seen in Figure 13-8. TEM magnification is related to the available energy for the electron beam, with powers up to 10,000,000 × now possible.

For SEM, a very thin coating of gold-palladium or other metal is applied via a plasma to the surface of a dry structure. A focused electron beam produces reflected or emitted electrons that are captured by a detector and projected as an image on a monitor. Although initially used to explore surface structures, internal organization can also be imaged after breaking or fracturing a section of tissue. In Figure 13-9, for example, freeze-fracturing of the double membrane surrounding the nucleus clearly shows the nuclear pores and inner membrane.

An Overview of Cell Membranes

Membranes are composed of phospholipids and a range of protein and other organic molecule components (Figure 13-10). Artificial phospholipid membranes can form spontaneously, even in a test tube, because of the interaction between their hydrophilic region and the ubiquitous water environment surrounding them both inside and outside the cell. The hydrophobic fatty acid tails create a boundary between the two watery layers. While some cellular components can be anchored in a membrane, the lipid bilayer structure is somewhat fluid allowing molecules like protein receptors to move within it. Molecular interactions with water define many of the membrane's cellular processes.

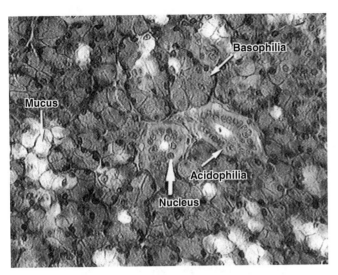

Figure 13-4. Stains help explain biochemical differences among cells and their organelles. Here hematoxylin, that behaves like a basic dye, colors the DNA of the nucleus and the RNA of the cytoplasmic ribosomes purple, but eosin, an acidic dye, colors the cytoplasmic proteins pink. These two types of staining are called basophilia and acidophilia, respectively. The neutral carbohydrates do not stain. (Courtesy of Paul Bell and Barbara Safiejko-Mroczka, Histology course web site, University of Oklahoma.)

About half the molecular mass of a membrane is protein and half is lipid, although this will differ from one kind of membrane to another. A membrane protein is, however, much larger than a phospholipid, so the number of lipid molecules in a typical membrane outnumbers the proteins by 50 × or more. The diverse functions associated with different membranes are mainly a function of their protein component.

The plasma membrane that surrounds the cell serves as the communication interface with the environment, creating the intracellular domain and the surrounding extracellular environment. It is a very complex structure, with some specialized domains carrying out functions like regulating secretion or nutrient uptake. Lateral sides of a cell form a range of connections with adjacent cells that can influence intercellular interaction. Desmosomes and tight junctions anchor adjacent cells together, and gap junctions form molecular communication channels between adjacent cytosols. The extracellular matrix (ECM) serves animal cells in somewhat the same way as the cell wall in plants. Its primary components are glycoproteins, like collagen, which alone makes up about half the protein in a human body. Surface adaptations like cilia, flagella, and microvilli also play key roles in cell function. Microvilli are tiny fingerlike processes that increase the absorptive surface of an exposed membrane on cells like those lining the digestive tract. Cilia and flagella use dynein, one of the so-called "motor molecules" to move cells like sperm through the body or move materials like mucus past cells lining the respiratory tract to trap and eliminate dust and other particles.

A key characteristic of a biological membrane is its selective permeability. Because of its phospholipid component, lipids and lipid-soluble materials can generally pass through easily. Water and some small water-soluble molecules tend to diffuse beside the protein elements distributed in the membrane. In such cases, a specialized transport protein is not necessary. But many larger molecules and charged ions have very low permeability and require a membrane transport mechanism. In facilitated transport, a specialized protein creates a passage through which the targeted molecule can move passively. Active transport, on the other hand, requires energy from adenosine triphosphate (ATP) to generate protein shape

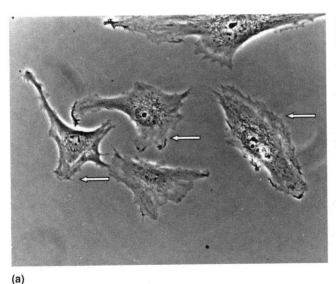

(a)

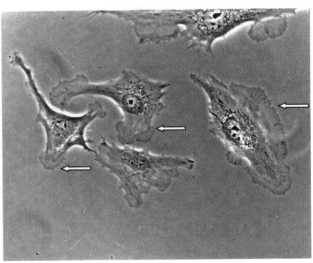

(b)

Figure 13-5. Phase contrast of living cells can allow observation of cell behavior and measurements of a response to chemical exposure. Here, the effect of neomycin on motility of human glioma cells in culture is compared: (a), before introduction of neomycin into the cell environment; (b), 2 minutes after exposure to neomycin. (Courtesy of Barbara Safiejko-Mroczka, University of Oklahoma.)

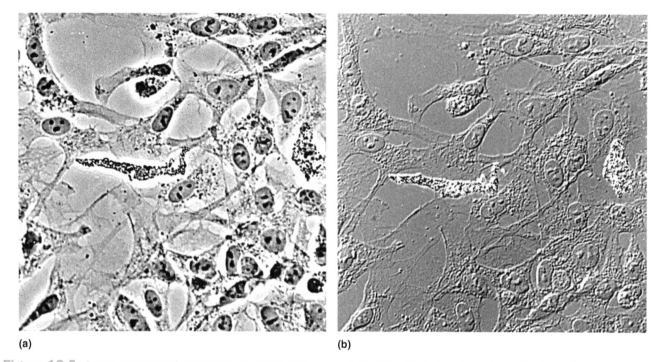

(a)   (b)

Figure 13-6. Phase contrast (left) and Nomarski (right) of the same field of fibroblasts in culture shows the three-dimensional capability of Nomarski. The cultured neural crest cells in these fields are alive. (Reprinted with permission from Junqueira, L., and J. Carneiro, *Basic Histology*. New York: McGraw-Hill, p 4, Fig. 1-3 b and c, 2003.)

changes that move a targeted molecule across the membrane, often against the passive movement of diffusion. Many of the variations seen in cell membrane activity are, therefore, due to differences in the presence of facilitated transport and active transport channels.

Because of its central role in life processes, heritable defects of the cell membrane are not common. Most defects associated with the plasma membrane are the result of toxins, trauma, or other disease influences. Among congenital disorders, however, we can identify examples of the

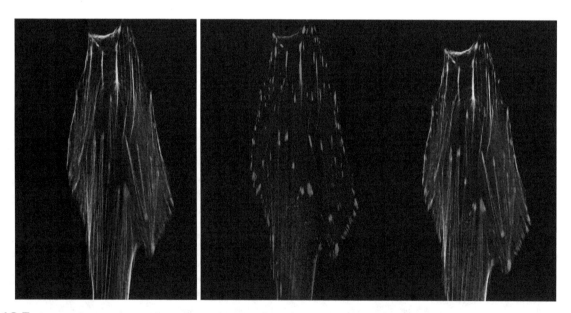

Figure 13-7. Immunofluorescence with multiple stains. The same human gingival fibroblast labeled using Bodipy conjugated phallacidin to reveal filamentous actin (left), and with anti-vinculin antibody and rhodamine conjugated secondary antibody to label vinculin present in focal contacts (center). The right-hand figure shows double-labeling of the F-actin and vinculin distributions in the same cell. (Courtesy of Barbara Safiejko-Mroczka, University of Oklahoma.)

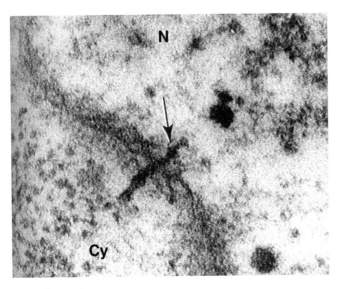

Figure 13-8. Molecule movement through the nuclear envelope, believed to be the passage of a ribosomal subunit through a nuclear pore (Cy, cytoplasm; N, nucleus). (Reprinted with permission from Stevens, B., and H. Swift. *J. Cell Biol.* 31:72, 1966.)

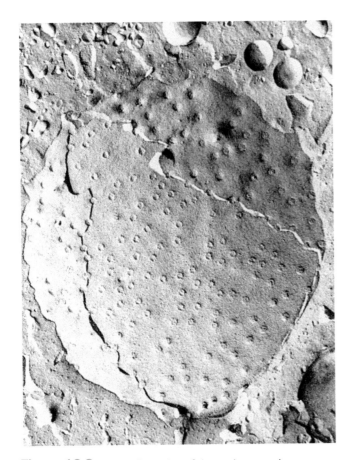

Figure 13-9. Freeze-fracturing of the nuclear membrane enables us to view the inner membrane and the nuclear pores that connect the cytosol with the nuclear region. (Reprinted with permission from Junqueira, L., and J. Carneiro, *Basic Histology.* New York: McGraw-Hill, p 56, Figure 3-7, 2003.)

inadequate number or even total absence of a specific membrane receptor, changes in cell adhesiveness, abnormalities in cell-to-cell communication, and the presence of exceptional proteins.

Mitochondria

As organelles, mitochondria are special. They have DNA and their replication is independent of the nucleus. They also have a key role in energy transformation—ATP synthesis—that makes them indispensible for life. These roles give mitochondria an especially important place in a survey of cell organelles.

Although a small amount of ATP synthesis occurs in the cytoplasm, most occurs in mitochondria (Figure 13-11). ATP carries a high energy phosphate bond (often symbolized ~P). When that phosphate is removed leaving adenosine diphosphate (ADP) (ATP $\rightarrow$ ADP + ~P), the high energy phosphate can transfer energy to other molecules and reactions. So it is not surprising that disorders of the mitochondria have their largest impact in tissues like the brain and muscles that have the greatest demand for energy through synthesis and use of ATP.

There are two functional domains in each mitochondrion, one in the fluid internal matrix and one embedded in the folded internal membrane, the cristae. Glucose digestion in the cell cytoplasm yields a small net gain of two ATP molecules plus two molecules of pyruvate, which enter the mitochondrion as acetyl-CoA (Figures 13-12 and 13-13). There, enzymatic breakdown by the **Krebs** (or **citric acid**) **cycle** (Figure 13-14) occurs in the mitochondrial matrix.

Finally, sequential oxidation-reduction reactions by the cytochromes of oxidative phosphorylation (OXPHOS; also called the electron transport chain; Figure 13-15) produce most of the cell's ATP yield. But the fact that mitochondria have their own DNA is what makes them stand out for medical geneticists as a special case of organelle biology. Key principles of mitochondrial inheritance are summarized in Table 13-1.

The human mitochondrial DNA (mtDNA) genome is present in about 5 to 10 copies per mitochondrion, with up to 1000 or so mitochondria per cell depending on the energy expenditure of each type of tissue. In fact in some cells like a frog egg the vast majority of the DNA in the cell is mtDNA, not nuclear DNA. In most mammalian tissues, however, about 1% of the cellular DNA is mtDNA. The human mitochondrial genome is a circular molecule of 16,569 bp and does not contain introns. Its use of the genetic code differs slightly from that of a nucleus. The UGA triplet codes for tryptophan instead of serving as a "stop codon," and AGA and AGG serve as stop codons instead of coding for the amino acid arginine. AUA and AUU sometimes serve as start codons, in place of AUG.

Species differ widely in the number of genes encoded in their mtDNA genome. The human mitochondrial genome codes for only 13 of the 80 or so proteins needed to control

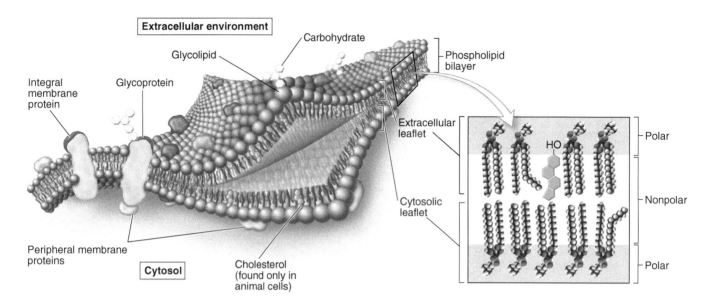

Figure 13-10. The fluid-mosaic model of membrane structure is based on the way membrane phospholipids, with both a hydrophobic and a hydrophilic region, will spontaneously form a bilayer in which proteins and other macromolecules can float. (Reprinted with permission from Brooker et al., *Biology*, 2nd ed, New York: McGraw-Hill, p 98, 2011.)

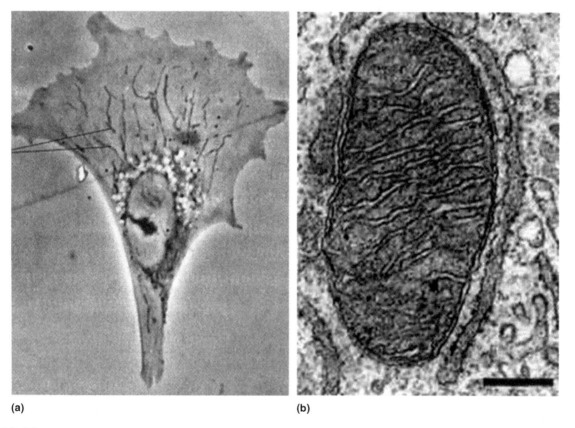

(a)   (b)

Figure 13-11. (a) Mitochondria in a cell, seen as dark elongated bodies. (b) An electron micrograph of a mitochondrion, showing the inner folded membrane (cristae). (Reprinted with permission from Karp, G., *Cell and Molecular Biology: Concepts and Experiments*, 3rd ed, Wiley, p 184, 2002.)

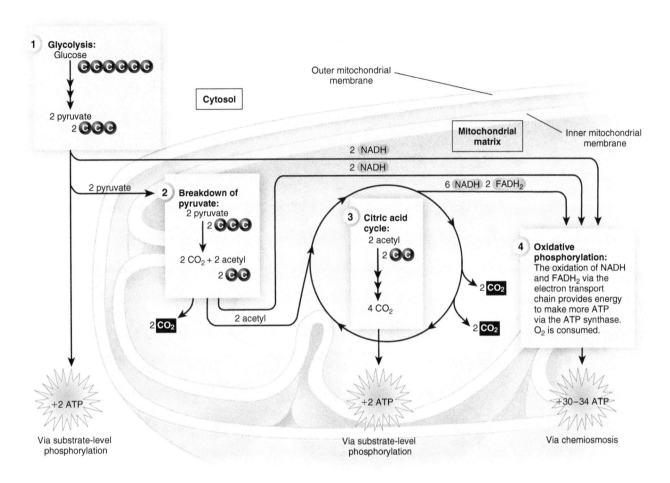

Figure 13-12. A summary of the metabolism of glucose in: (1) the cytoplasm, and in the mitochondria by (2) pyruvate breakdown, (3) the Krebs or citric acid cycle, and (4) oxidative phosphorylation (OXPHOS). (Reprinted with permission from Brooker et al., *Biology*, 2nd ed, New York: McGraw-Hill, p 138, 2011.)

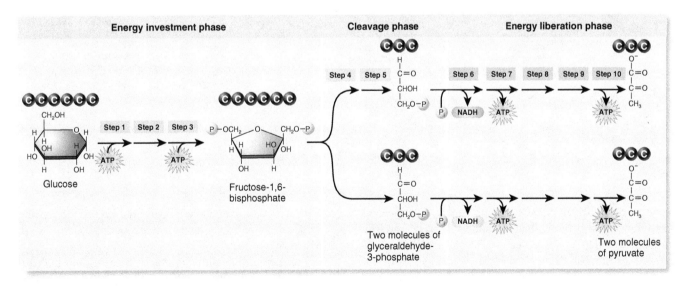

Figure 13-13. Glycolysis in the cytoplasm yields two molecules of pyruvate for each glucose molecule. (Reprinted with permission from Brooker et al., *Biology*, 2nd ed, New York: McGraw-Hill, p 139, 2011.)

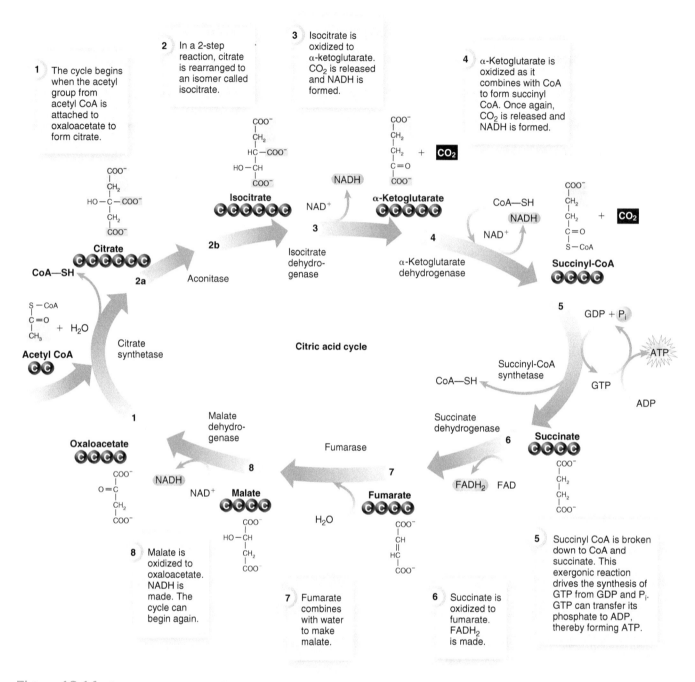

Figure 13-14. One carbon is removed from pyruvate when it enters the mitochondrion as acetyl CoA. In the Krebs or citric acid, cycle the remaining two carbons are removed as CO_2 and energy is passed to ATP and to carrier molecules that transfer it to the electron transport chain. (Reprinted with permission from Brooker et al., *Biology*, 2nd ed, New York: McGraw-Hill, p 143, 2011.)

the process of OXPHOS. The rest are coded in the nucleus and follow normal Mendelian genetic inheritance patterns. In contrast, mtDNA is passed from females to all their offspring. The mtDNA from the sperm is generally lost by the 2- to 4-cell stage. So, just because a disorder can be traced to a mitochondrial function does not mean it is going to follow maternal transmission rules. One needs to understand the specific genetic origin of each trait to determine its transmission pattern. In other words, it is important to distinguish

clearly between a mitochondrial disorder and mitochondrial inheritance. Some examples of mitochondrial conditions are shown in Figure 13-16.

One special phenomenon that affects cellular makeup is **replicative segregation**. This is a phenomenon that largely depends on chance (Figure 13-17). If there is just one type of mtDNA sequence in a cell, it is **homoplasmic** ("homo" = same; "plasmic" referring to the cytoplasm makeup). But mutations occur in mitochondria. If a cell

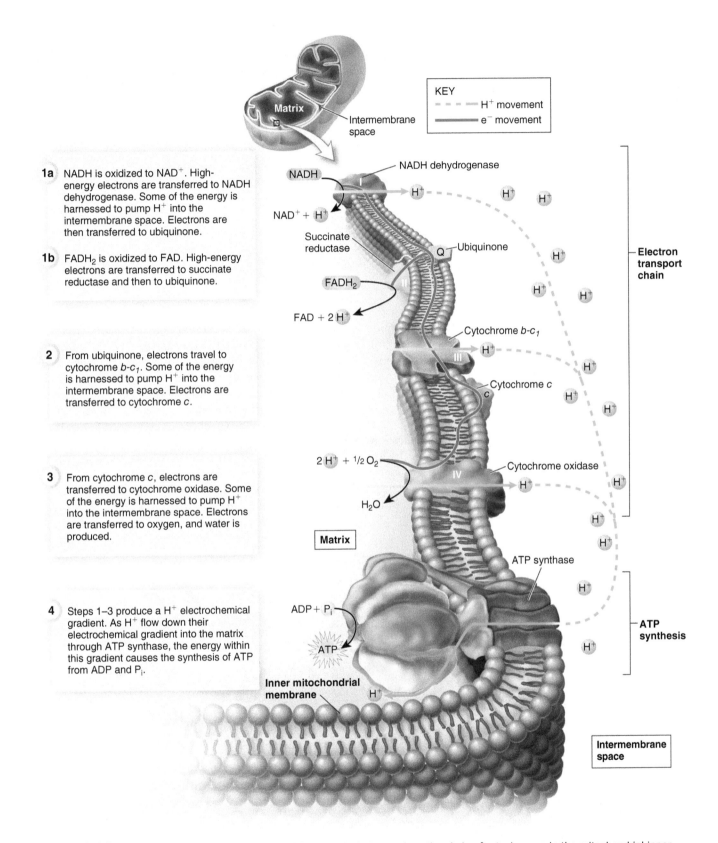

KEY
— — — H^+ movement
——— e^- movement

1a NADH is oxidized to NAD^+. High-energy electrons are transferred to NADH dehydrogenase. Some of the energy is harnessed to pump H^+ into the intermembrane space. Electrons are then transferred to ubiquinone.

1b $FADH_2$ is oxidized to FAD. High-energy electrons are transferred to succinate reductase and then to ubiquinone.

2 From ubiquinone, electrons travel to cytochrome b-c_1. Some of the energy is harnessed to pump H^+ into the intermembrane space. Electrons are transferred to cytochrome c.

3 From cytochrome c, electrons are transferred to cytochrome oxidase. Some of the energy is harnessed to pump H^+ into the intermembrane space. Electrons are transferred to oxygen, and water is produced.

4 Steps 1–3 produce a H^+ electrochemical gradient. As H^+ flow down their electrochemical gradient into the matrix through ATP synthase, the energy within this gradient causes the synthesis of ATP from ADP and P_i.

Labels in figure: Matrix; Intermembrane space; NADH dehydrogenase; NADH; $NAD^+ + H^+$; H^+; Succinate reductase; $FADH_2$; $FAD + 2 H^+$; Q—Ubiquinone; Cytochrome b-c_1; Cytochrome c; $2 H^+ + 1/2 O_2$; H_2O; Cytochrome oxidase; Matrix; ATP synthase; $ADP + P_i$; ATP; Inner mitochondrial membrane; H^+; Intermembrane space; Electron transport chain; ATP synthesis

Figure 13-15. Oxidative phosphorylation, or OXPHOS, passes electrons along the chain of cytochromes in the mitochondrial inner membrane, the cristae. The final product is ATP synthesis with water as a byproduct. (Reprinted with permission from Brooker et al., *Biology*, 2nd ed, New York: McGraw-Hill, p 144, 2011.)

Table 13-1.	Basic Principles Associated With Mitochondrial Inheritance
Semiautonomous inheritance	mtDNA is inherited cytoplasmically and is distributed to daughter cells with the cell divides
Maternal inheritance	transmitted independently of the nucleus and therefore does not follow Mendelian ratios
Replicative segregation	if more than one type of mtDNA is present in a cell, they can be partitioned by drift and can eventually lead back to a single type per cell
"Bottleneck" phenomenon	number of mtDNA copies per mitochondrion decreases, yielding a restriction that reduces mtDNA diversity
Threshold expression of phenotype	once the nature and effect of a mutation exceeds the cell's need for energy, expression of the mutation begins
High mutation rate	mutation rate is higher than for nuclear genes
Genotype/phenotype correlation	mtDNA mutations are highly polymorphic and there is not a clear association between a specific mutation and a given phenotype
Accumulation of mutations	somatic and mtDNA mutations accumulate as a person ages

has more than one mtDNA sequence, it is **heteroplasmic**. But the organelles are not regularly distributed at each cell division, so over time the daughter cells will change proportions, showing replicative drift, and can even return to homoplasmy.

The DNA outside the nucleus is under separate replication control. Mitochondria divide independently of the nucleus. It should, therefore, be no surprise that replication processes differ between the nucleus and this organelle. An important example is error correction. Mutation rate is much higher—perhaps even 10-fold or more higher—in mitochondria than in nuclear DNA. One possible explanation is that

a mutation in a mitochondrion does not necessarily affect the function of the cell that contains it. It is functionally masked because there are so many nonmutant mitochondria to compensate for it. Selection against the new mutation may be zero. In addition, mtDNA does not have the histone associations that might mediate mutagenic effects. There is, therefore, a much lower selection pressure to favor efficient mtDNA repair enzymes.

Bottlenecks can affect mtDNA representation. A bottleneck is simply a reduction in number that leads to random sampling variation. In this case, the number of mtDNA molecules in oogonia is reduced to only about 1 to 30 copies.

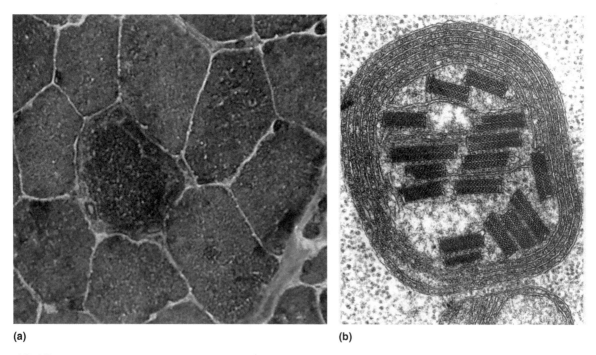

(a)   (b)

Figure 13-16. Abnormal mitochondria showing: (a) ragged red fibers, and (b) and crystalline inclusions in the mitochondrial matrix.
(a: From Donald R. Johns in Karp, G., 2002, *Cell and Molecular Biology: Concepts and Experiments*, 3rd ed, Wiley, p 213, Figure 1; b: From Morgan-Hughes, J., and D. Landon, Engel, A., and C. Franzini-Armstrong, eds *Mycology*, 2nd ed, McGraw-Hill, 1994.)

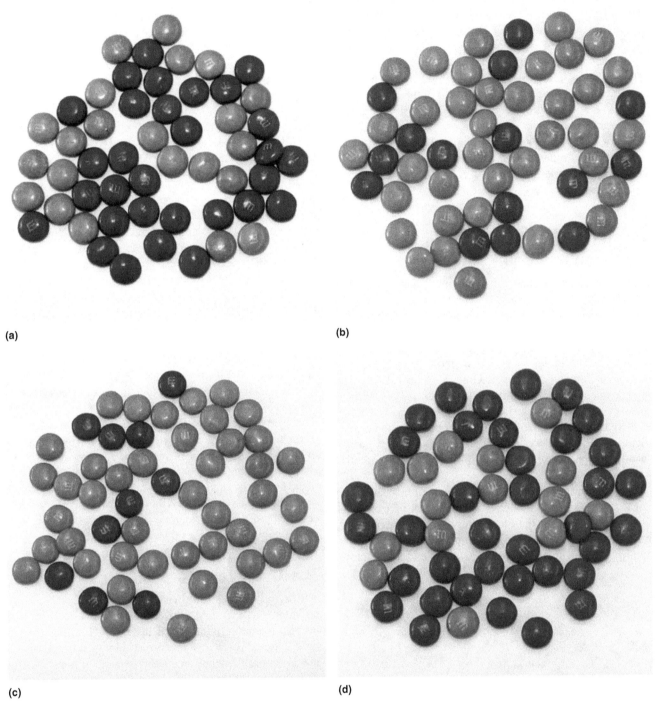

(a)

(b)

(c)

(d)

Figure 13-17. The consequences of random sampling during replicative segregation of mitochondria is illustrated here by random samples of red and green chocolate candy pieces. Although drawn from the same pool of candy pieces, the random samples held different proportions each time.

During oogenesis, the number increases again by about 100 ×. After fertilization, there is rapid nuclear DNA replication, but the number of mitochondria and mtDNA molecules does not change a lot. It is mainly affected by tissue specialization that reflects functional demands. In Chapter 15 we will return to this idea of bottlenecks and sampling error in a different context, the population.

In scientific applications, just as in our daily activity, a bottleneck means the same thing. It is a restriction. In biology, it is generally a restriction in numbers of individuals or component parts. Although a phenomenon like a genetic bottleneck may seem like a rare special case, it is not. It is just one of the many factors that commonly affect expression of inherited diseases. As a whole, we can view the influences on a biological trait as a threshold phenomenon. In earlier discussions, we explored variation in penetrance and expressivity. Below a threshold level, the trait is unexpressed, but above a threshold of contributing conditions it is exposed and changes the phenotype. Factors like the specific nature of the mutation, the proportion of the mtDNA that carries the mutation, and the relative dependence of the affected tissue on ATP and the processes of OXPHOS will determine a mutation's phenotypic expression. We have seen that a change in a critical enzyme can change phenotypes a lot, but mutations in other steps might be masked. If that can be true of an enzyme, it can also be true for an organelle like a mitochondrion.

Molecular Traffic of the Endoplasmic Reticulum and Golgi Complex

Much of the molecular synthesis occurring in a cell is associated with an extensive membrane network called the endoplasmic reticulum (ER). Rough endoplasmic reticulum (RER; Figure 13-18) refers to the portion of this membrane that has attached ribosomes giving it a rough appearance in an electron micrograph. The proteins that are synthesized there can be transported along the RER to the Golgi complex (also called the Golgi apparatus or Golgi body), where they are further processed and then packaged into vesicles for transport within the cytoplasm or out of the cell. The smooth endoplasmic reticulum (SER), on the other hand, lacks attached ribosomes. It is primarily associated with detoxification and the synthesis of steroid hormones.

In addition to housing the cell's synthetic biochemistry, the ER can engage in some kinds of quality control over protein secretion. To leave the ER, recently-synthesized proteins must be correctly folded or, if they are subunits of a more complex protein, they may need to be assembled. Abnor-

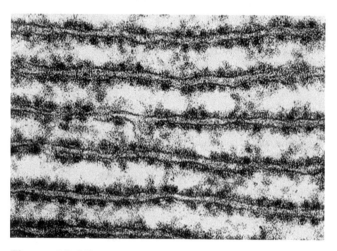

Figure 13-18. Endoplasmic reticulum with attached ribosomes is called rough endoplasmic reticulum (RER). (Reprinted with permission from Cheville, N., *Ultrastructural Pathology*, Iowa State University Press, Ames, IA, p 23, 1994.)

mally-folded proteins and other defective molecules can be destroyed. Chaperone proteins help facilitate this process by anchoring abnormal proteins in the lumen of the ER from which they are transported back to the cytosol and digested. But this recycling also means that defects in these processes can lead to the abnormal retention of proteins, leading to serious ER storage diseases.

Endosomes, Lysosomes, and Other Membrane-Bounded Vesicles

Endosomes are membrane-bounded organelles that isolate materials that are newly-ingested into the cell (endocytosis). But there are many other similar vesicles carrying out a range of functions, such as sequestering various cell products or isolating chemical reactions in the cytoplasm. Lysosomes, for example, are the principal location of cellular digestion. Indeed, this is one way the cell can safely produce and use materials like proteolytic enzymes that would otherwise be fatal to a cell's survival. A large number of lysosomal enzymes have been identified, and pathologies of the lysosomes involve releasing these enzymes into the cell or into extracellular spaces. Lysosomal storage diseases occur when they fail to digest properly (Figure 13-19).

Peroxisomes typically contain one or more enzymes that remove hydrogen atoms from targeted molecules and produce hydrogen peroxide (H_2O_2) in an oxidation reaction with oxygen. An important aspect of this reaction is the breakdown of fatty acids, in which β-oxidation shortens the fatty acid chains to yield acetyl CoA used in various biosynthetic reactions. One key example is the synthesis of plasmalogens, the most abundant type of phospholipid in the myelin of nerve cells. Not surprisingly, peroxisomal abnormalities are often associated with nervous system disorders.

The Cytoskeleton

The cytoskeleton is a dynamic system of microtubules and filaments that are involved in cell shape, cell division, internal transport, and movement (Figure 13-20). There are three types of protein filaments in animal cells. Actin filaments (microfilaments) make the reversible transition from globular monomers to a filamentous two-strand polymer and thereby effect rapid changes in cell shape and movement. The microtubules, on the other hand, are more rigid hollow cylinders composed of the protein tubulin. They direct transport of materials, including organelles, within the cell. Finally, intermediate filaments are made up of a large, diverse group of proteins that can create a mesh-like network that gives mechanical strength to the cell. An example is the interconnected filaments that strengthen the elongated cellular structure of neurons.

Along this dynamic system of protein corridors, accessory proteins assist in assembly and disassembly of cytoskeletal components. Accessory proteins include the motor proteins, which use energy from ATP to change shape and move

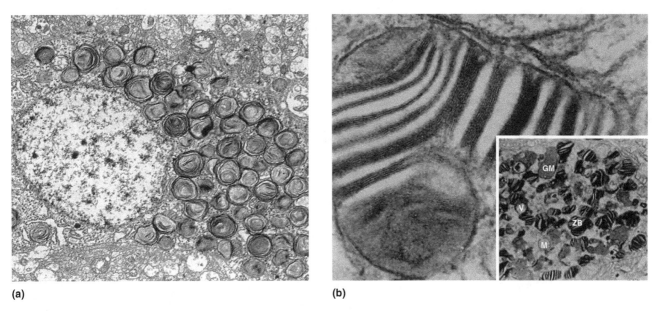

(a)   (b)

Figure 13-19. (a) Gangliosidosis is a lysosomal storage disorder, Tay Sachs. (b) Zebra bodies, Hurler syndrome. (a: From Karp, G., 2002, *Cell and Molecular Biology: Concepts and Experiments*, 3rd ed, Wiley, p 315; b: From Cheville, N., *Ultrastructural Pathology*, Iowa State University Press, Ames, p 154, 1994.)

(or "walk") along the filament pathways to transport organelles or other cell components to which they are attached. An important example of the cytoskeleton with specialized function is the mitotic spindle that moves chromosomes during cell division.

Cilia, Flagella, and Cell Surface Specializations

The cell surface is quite complex. Many functional proteins such as ion channels, gap junction proteins and receptors are distributed across the surface of cell membranes. Cilia and flagella are other specialized elements of the cell surface.

Their structures are similar; both are composed of microtubules and the motor protein dynein (Figure 13-21). They also share many of the same genes that code for proteins common to both. In both, the core is composed of nine microtubules composed of a doublet fused together and with two single microtubules in the center. Pairs of dynein arms are attached to each microtubule doublet. When activated, these dynein arms "walk" up the adjacent microtubule causing the tubules to slide past each other in much the same way as actin and myosin filaments slide past each other in muscle contraction. But in the case of cilia and flagella, the tubules are connected at points along their length so the sliding actually causes the structure to bend. While they are quite similar, there are some distinct differences between cilia and flagella. Flagella are

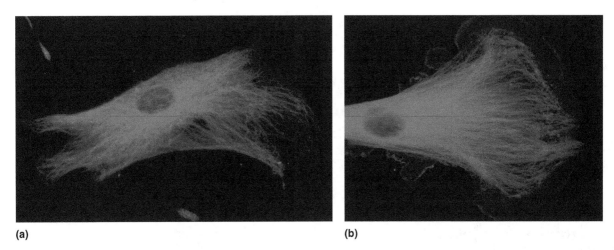

(a)   (b)

Figure 13-20. Cell cytoskeleton shown as tubulin distribution in human fibroblasts labeled with anti-tubulin antibody and rhodamine conjugated secondary antibody. Left, untreated; right, treated with neomycin to induce formation of protrusions. (Courtesy of Barbara Safiejko-Mroczka, University of Oklahoma.)

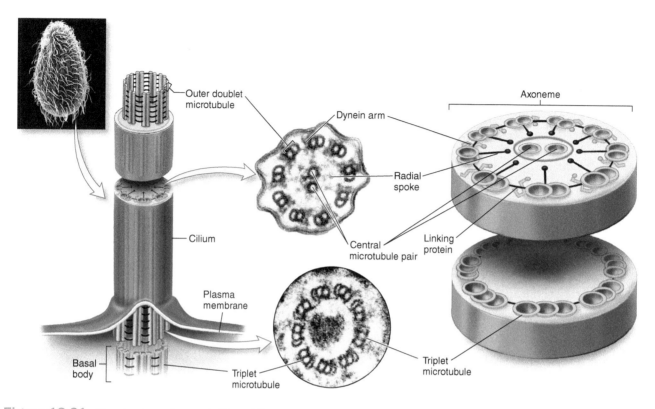

Figure 13-21. The structure of normal cilia and flagella. (Reprinted with permission from Brooker et al., *Biology*, 2nd ed, New York: McGraw-Hill, p 77, 2011.)

longer than cilia and typically beat with a whiplike motion (the Latin word for flagellum actually means 'whip'). Cilia are shorter and more numerous on a cell surface. Their movement is described as being more of a coordinated, rhythmic wavelike movement. The movement of cilia is in two parts with power and recovery phases that have been likened to the breast stroke in swimming.

Flagella primarily function in cell motility. However, they may also function as sensory organs—being responsive to chemicals and temperature. In humans, the best known examples of flagella are the tails of sperm. Abnormalities of this structure (Figure 13-22) can lead to infertility from nonmotile sperm.

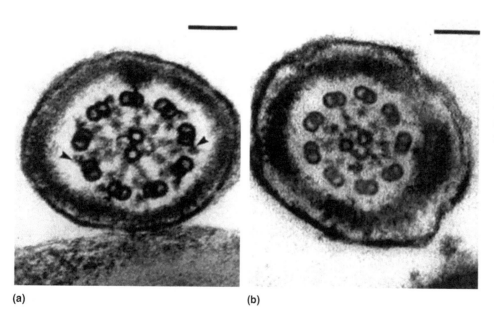

(a)   (b)

Figure 13-22. Defect of inner dynein arms. The loss of inner dynein arms is the ultrastuctural alteration that is most often seen (original magnification × 85,000). (Reproduced, with permission, from Theegarten D, Ebsen M. *Diagnostic Pathology*, 6:115 doi:10.1186/1746-1596-6-115, 2011.)

There are two types of cilia: immotile (primary) and motile. The immotile cilia are primarily sensory in function and can be found on the surfaces of almost every cell. They serve as essentially cellular "antennae" to send and receive chemical signals. They are very important in cell-cell recognition and other critical interactions among cells. Motile cilia exist to move liquids across cell surfaces. They are typically found in the fallopian tubes and the respiratory epithelium.

The Nucleus and Centrioles

The focus of this chapter is on cell organelles that play a central role in certain heritable medical conditions. It may seem we have overlooked one of the most important of these, the nucleus. Along with the centrioles that generate the spindle for nuclear division, the nuclear region of a cell is clearly of critical importance for cell function. But for a moment, let's look at the overall organelle, rather than the information coded within its chromosomes. Why do changes in the structure of this organelle not appear as a common source of medical problems? Although the answer may seem obvious, it is still worth highlighting. It is true that the nucleus controls the growth and reproduction of a cell. It, therefore, follows that, if the essential structure of the nucleus is abnormal, the cell will not be able to carry out its most fundamental role and will probably die.

This also illustrates a more general fact about genetic research. Genetics can identify the role of a gene by seeing the abnormalities that occur when the gene mutates. But a mutation affecting the ability of a cell to divide or to transcribe its encoded information cannot survive long. There is no phenotype to trace. The loss of such a valuable experimental approach helps us appreciate the ingenuity that researchers have brought to bear on questions about the function of the nucleus and other cell organelles. Extrapolating from mutations to understanding the normal function of a gene is what gives genetics its power as an experimental approach. But when the mutation causes the loss of the cell, that asset disappears. In spite of that limitation, the ingenuity of researchers is now drawing upon other approaches.

Nuclear size and shape give hints about its level of activity. A nucleus that is large, lightly staining, and with an enlarged nucleolus is probably transcriptionally active. A large basophilic nucleus may have an elevated DNA level, but a small one may be less active with transcription down-regulated. Certain cells like lymphocytes may have irregular nuclei normally. However, unusual nuclear shapes are often found in cells of malignant tumors.

In this overview of cell ultrastructure, we have limited our attention to some of the main organelles that are involved in human genetic disease. In the next section, we will discuss examples of how abnormalities in organelle structure and function can explain some heritable conditions.

Part 2: Medical Genetics

Introduction

The function and importance of subcellular organelles has been detailed in the first section of this chapter. As with most other chapters in this book, the Medical Genetics correlate is what happens when things go wrong. Each organelle has a specific set of functions. When those functions are impaired, there are usually clinical consequences. One of the most fascinating aspects of these correlations has been the discovery of what is seen clinically in these situations. Often, the outcomes are quite unexpected. If one were to try and predict the outcomes based on knowledge of structure and function, you would often be wrong. For instance, as discussed below, no one would ever have predicted that mutations in the laminin proteins of the nuclear membrane would be associated with progeria (premature aging syndromes). Conversely, in this era of genomics, the typical scenario is to start with the disorder and then search the entire genome rather than think about the condition and go check out logical candidates.

In this section we will discuss mitochondrial disorders in detail, as these represent an important group, both numerically and in treatment potential. For the rest of the organelles to be discussed, we will focus mainly on the known disease entities associated with dysfunction of each type.

Mitochondria

It is extremely important to discuss mitochondrial disorders. Collectively they are actually quite common. The range of symptoms associated with these conditions encompasses just about every symptom group described, i.e., they are in the differential diagnosis of almost any human malady. Still, they are commonly underdiagnosed. If the clinician does not consider them, they will simply be overlooked. Besides the relatively common occurrence of these conditions, there is also treatment potential for many.

The key to understanding mitochondrial disorders is to consider their primary role as generators of biologic energy. Mitochondria exist to facilitate aerobic energy generation through OXPHOS. The reliance on OXPHOS for energy varies during developmental stages and among tissues. During embryonic development, the blastocyst stage is a time of increased oxygen consumption associated with increased numbers of mitochondria and mtDNA. For the rest of the first half of gestation there is low oxygen tension with a major reliance on glycolysis: i.e., OXPHOS is not heavily utilized. From the last half of gestation through the first 10 years post-natally, OXPHOS activity rises with a gradual decrease to adult levels by about 20 years of age.

OXPHOS gene expression in different tissues varies with changes in mtDNA levels, nuclear OXPHOS genetic activity, nuclear-cytoplasmic interactions, and environmental influences. Mitochondrial density is related to the overall number of mitochondria per cell as well as the number of mtDNA copies per mitochondrion. These factors vary greatly among tissues. Those tissues that have functions that have higher energy needs tend to have more mitochondria. In humans, the mtDNA content is highest in the brain, eyes, muscle, liver, kidney, and heart (in decreasing order) with the overall involvement of these organs reflecting this fact (i.e., CNS dysfunction is the most common presenting problem in mitochondrial disorders).

The pathophysiology of mitochondrial dysfunction is complex and involves interactions with multiple other physiological systems. Mitochondrial disorders include multiple conditions that share in common structural and functional differences in the mitochondria. This includes defects in aerobic cell metabolism, the electron transport chain, the Krebs's cycle or any of several combinations of these. In general, mitochondrial damage results in decreased mitochondrial activity (including superoxide dismutase) plus the inability to regenerate proteins. This results in the generation of metabolic by-products including free radicals that in turn will damage proteins (structural and enzymatic) and the mtDNA itself. This leads to further elevation of anaerobic by-products with further decline in mitochondrial functions.

Mitochondrial inheritance has been discussed in detail in the first section of this chapter. If you are not quite clear on the details, you are encouraged to go back and review this. Of paramount importance is that clear distinction needs to be made between **mitochondrial disorders** and **mitochondrial inheritance.** The term "mitochondrial *disorder*" refers to recognizable clinical disorders that are due to dysfunction of the mitochondria. It is important to remember that the mtDNA only codes for 13 of the large number of proteins needed for normal mitochondrial metabolic functioning. Thus the vast majority of mitochondrial proteins are encoded in the *nuclear* genome. It then follows that many mitochondrial disorders are inherited as Mendelian traits (see Clinical Correlation section). Mitochondrial *inheritance*, then, refers to pattern of transmission seen in those mitochondrial disorders in which the causative mutation is located in the mtDNA. For these conditions, the unique pattern of mitochondrial inheritance as described earlier (maternal transmission) holds. As of the time of this writing, mutations in 13 mitochondrial genes and 228 nuclear genes have been reported in association with human medical disorders.

The complex requisite interaction between the mitochondrial genome and the nuclear genome cannot be overstated. For the mitochondria to work appropriately, both genomes have to be working correctly and be carefully synchronized. Because both genomes may code for proteins involved in the same pathway(s), certain disorders of mitochondrial function can be inherited as either classic Mendelian or

mitochondrial inheritance. For instance, diabetes insipidus, diabetes mellitus, optic atrophy, and deafness (DIDMOAD) is a well-described entity. It has long been recognized that the primary pathophysiology of this condition involves mitochondrial physiology. It is now known that DIDMOAD can be caused by mutations in the mitochondrial genome or by mutations in an autosomal gene at chromosome locus 4p16. Obviously the familial implications of these two are markedly different. Thus, when a patient is diagnosed with DIDMOAD, careful identification of the underlying genetic etiology is critical. One cannot simply infer an inheritance mode based solely on the clinical impressions.

The clinical characteristics of mitochondrial disorders are tied to their roles in energy metabolism. Typically they are progressive in nature. They exhibit high intra- and interfamilial variability. The overall phenotype depends on multiple factors such as the level of heteroplasmy, the distribution of heteroplasmy (i.e., among which cells, tissues and organs), other modifier genes (including those in the nuclear genome), the timing of the life cycle (the level of heteroplasmy can change over the life of an individual), and the specific biologic threshold of a particular function.

As noted earlier, mitochondrial disorders have a myriad of presentations. They can present as almost anything and at any time in a person's life. Simply, if you do not think about them you will miss them. Mitochondrial disorders often present in childhood. Table 13-2 lists the most common presenting symptoms and the time in childhood when they usually present. In pediatric intensive care units, children are often seen with "multisystem failure." The commonly considered causes of this are infectious and toxic etiologies. However, many of these children actually have mitochondrial disorders—often undiagnosed. The presentations of mitochondrial disorders are somewhat different in adults than in children. The most common presenting symptoms in adulthood are listed in Table 13-3. Another important consideration of mitochondria in adult health is their role as contributing factors to other primary pathologic conditions. Changes in mtDNA have been shown to contribute to a number of late onset processes such as Alzheimer disease, Parkinsonism, and multiple sclerosis. The accumulation of mitochondrial mutations undoubtedly plays a large part in the "normal" aging process. Presbycusis (age associated hearing loss) is particularly tied to mitochondrial dysfunction. It is

Table 13-2. Childhood Presentations of Mitochondrial Disorders

Neuromuscular symptoms (44%)

Non-neuromuscular symptoms (56%)
  Liver, heart, kidney, GI, endocrine, hematologic, dermatologic

Age of Onset:
  Neonatal (<1 month): 36%
  Infantile (1-24 months): 44%
  Childhood (>24 months): 20%

Table 13-3.	Adult Presentations of Mitochondrial Disorders
Ataxia	
Deafness	
Diabetes	
Myopathies	
Neuropathy	
Vision loss	
Monoallelic	
Triallelic	
Uniparental disomy	

also important to note that there are a few presenting findings that are strongly associated with mitochondria disorders. The finding of "ragged red fibers" on a muscle biopsy (Figure 13-16) is essentially pathognomonic for mitochondrial disorders. Likewise, in any patient with chronic progressive external ophthalmoplegia (CPEO) mitochondrial disease should be considered.

Several mitochondrial "syndromes" have been described. These are a small number of specific disorders that have been described where mitochondrial mutations are either inherited or occur early enough in development to dominate most cells. These disorders characteristically affect muscle and nervous tissue, particularly the optic tracks. One such example is Leber hereditary optic neuropathy (LHON) shown in Figure 13-23. Patients with LHON exhibit a progressive optic nerve atrophy beginning early in adulthood. The condition has been reported with at least 18 different mutations in the mitochondrial genome. Table 13-4 lists several more examples of mitochondrial syndromes. In reality, the description of mitochondrial syndromes represents an artificial distinction clinically. Such descriptions reflected the functional limitation of knowledge and technology (for testing). It is now known that there are multiple phenotypes associated with same mutation and multiple mutations associated with the same phenotype. Thus the best practice these days is to describe the phenotype carefully and then pair it with the specific genetic abnormality identified (genotype) in a particular patient or family.

At the present time, advances in genetic testing technology (see Chapter 11) have greatly increased the ability to diagnose mitochondrial diseases. It is relatively easy and not extremely costly these days to sequence the entire mitochondrial genome. Testing for nuclear gene abnormalities is significantly more expensive and time consuming. Undoubtedly, this will get much better as NextGen sequencing is developed as a clinical testing modality. For now, the diagnostic approach to mitochondrial disorders is best accomplished as an algorithmic approach using the family history, clinical symptoms, and the medical history to direct the type and order of tests.

Molecular Traffic of the Endoplasmic Reticulum and Golgi Complex

The ER has a variety of different functions. Its functions can differ depending on the individual type, function, and needs of a given cell. The ER can even adapt with time in response to cell needs. One of its primary functions is in facilitating protein folding and transport. It plays a major role in post-translational protein modification including glycosylation and disulfide bond formation. The Golgi complex processes and packages proteins from the ER.

Several conditions have been found to be due to disorders of the ER/Golgi complex functions. In the Clinical Correlation section of Chapter 2, congenital disorders of glycosylation are discussed in detail. As noted earlier, the process of glycosylation occurs in the ER. Some disorders of myelination (Charcot-Marie-Tooth disease, Pelizaeus-Merzbacher disease, the vanishing white matter syndrome, and spastic paraplegia type 17) are due to ER dysfunction. Other ER problems include the skeletal dysplasia pseudoachondroplasia which is an ER storage disorder, some endocrinopathies (congenital hypothyroid goiter, diabetes insipidus), familial hypercholesterolemia, and congenital lipodystrophy 2. One disorder attributed to problems of the Golgi complex is the I-cell storage disorder (the abnormal enzyme phosphotransferase is a Golgi enzyme). Also Golgi dysfunction has been implicated in Alzheimer disease pathophysiology.

Endosomes, Lysosomes, and Other Membrane-Bounded Vesicles

Membrane bound vesicles serve multiple functions. They are involved in endocytosis and other protein transport, storage of multiple compounds, and complex enzymatic processes. Endosomes are endocytic vacuoles that transport molecules to the lysosomes. Niemann Pick C is caused by abnormal endocytic transport of lipids, particularly cholesterol.

Lysosomes are vesicles that contain enzymes that are acid hydrolases. They function to clear compounds from the cell. In general the enzyme functions of the lysozymes are much less specific than those involved in the synthesis of biochemicals. They essentially function in the intracellular "digestion" of macromolecules. In addition, in many organisms, lysosomes can be involved in programmed cell death. Disorders in lysosomal function lead to **lysosomal storage disorders** (LSDs). Because lysozymes work in clearing compounds from the cells, the end result of lysozyme dysfunction is the progressive accumulation of these compounds within the lysozymes. Over time the continued accumulation of compounds that should be cleared leads to engulfed lysozymes. As the lysozymes continue to enlarge they disrupt all aspects of cell function.

Pompe disease is a lysosomal storage due to deficiency of the enzyme acid maltase (acid alpha-glucosidase). This enzyme nonspecifically degrades glycogen in the lysosomes to clear this compound from the cells. Because glycogen is found abundantly in the muscles, glycogen accumulates rapidly in these cells (Figure 13-24). Progressive accumulation of glycogen in

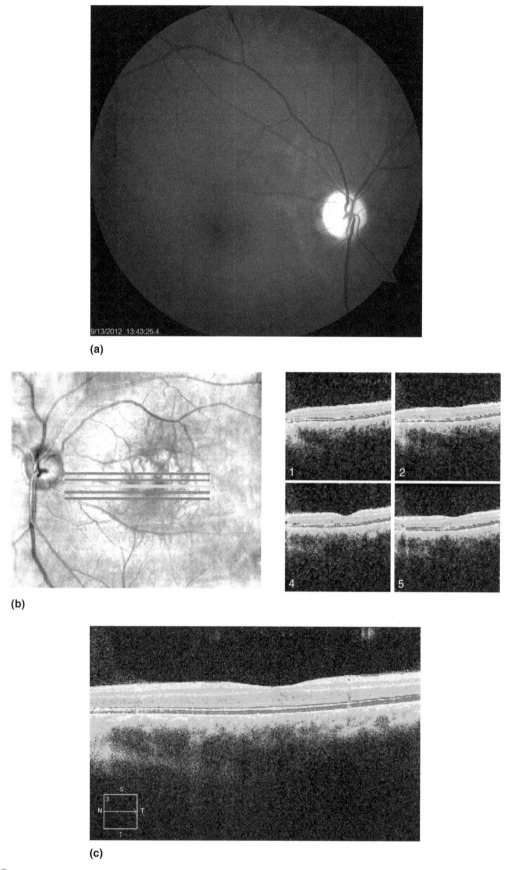

Figure 13-23. Retinal photograph of Leber hereditary optic neuropathy (LHON). The retina in this patient demonstrates central retinal vessel vascular tortuosity and optic atrophy.

Table 13-4.	Examples of Mitochondrial "Syndromes"	
Name	**Symptoms**	**Associated Mutations**
Kearns-Sayre syndrome	Ophthalmoplegia Cardiomyopathy Pigmentary retinopathy Myopathy with ragged red fibers	Various mitochondrial deletions
LHON (Leber hereditary optic neuropathy)	Optic atrophy Onset early adulthood	18 different mitochondrial mutations
MELAS	**M**itochondrial myopathy **E**ncephalopathy **L**actic **a**cidosis **S**trokelike episodes Symptoms in infancy	At least 10 different mitochondrial mutations
MERRF	**M**yoclonic **e**pilepsy **R**agged **r**ed **f**ibers	At least 6 different mitochondrial mutations
NARP	**N**europathy **A**taxia **R**etinitis **p**igmentosa	Mutations in gene encoding subunit 6 of mitochondrial H(+)-ATPase

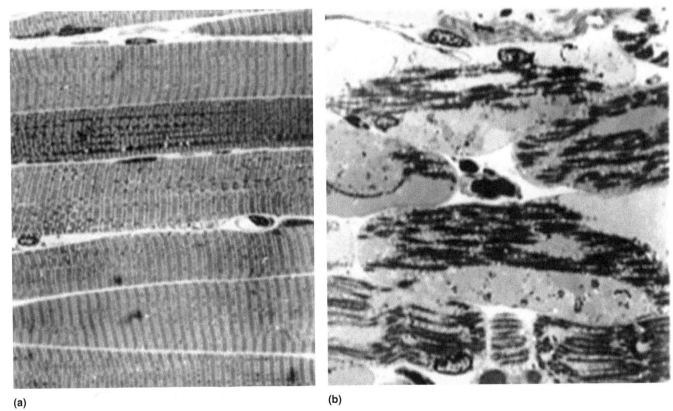

(a)　　　　　　　　　　　　　　　　　　(b)

Figure 13-24. (a) Normal muscles fibers in microscopic section. (b) Muscle biopsy of a child with Pompe disease. Note the massively congested lysosomes, which are full of glycogen, and the distorted normal architecture of the muscle fibers. (Reproduced, with permission, from Amalfitano A, Bengur AR, Morse RP, Majure JM, Case LE, Veerling DL, Mackey J, Kishnani P, Smith W, McVie-Wylie A, Sullivan JA, Hoganson GE, Phillips JA 3rd, Schaefer GB, Charrow J, Ware RE, Bossen EH, Chen YT. Recombinant human acid alpha-glucosidase enzyme therapy for infantile glycogen storage disease type II: results of a phase I/II clinical trial. *Genet Med.* 2001 Mar-Apr;3(2):132-138.)

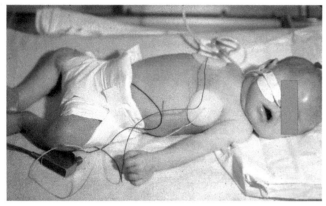

(a)

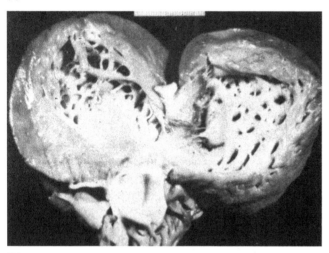

(b)

Figure 13-25. (a) Severely hypotonic infant with Pompe disease (also known as glycogen storage disease type II). (b) Postmortem picture of a heart in a patient with Pompe disease showing a severe cardiomyopathy secondary to massive stores of glycogen.

the muscles leads to muscle deterioration and weakness and a hypertrophic cardiomyopathy (Figure 13-25). Without treatment, infants with classic (complete) Pompe disease usually die in the first year of life. There are many types of lysosomal storage disorders which share in common the mechanism of lysosomal congestion, but differ by the accumulated chemicals and the clinical features of the condition. Table 13-5 provides a list of some of the known lysosomal storage disorders.

Significant interest in the lysosomal storage disorders has emerged over the past several years due to their therapeutic potential. As mentioned before, these are progressive disorders that have the potential for reversal of symptoms. Over the years many strategies have been tried that involve multiple ways to replace/insert normal enzyme into the patient to reverse the lysosomal storage. Currently two treatment modalities (Figure 13-26) are being used to treat these conditions: tissue transplantation or direct infusion of bioengineered enzyme (**enzyme replacement therapy** or ERT). Because treatment is most effective the earlier it is started, it has been suggested that

Table 13-5.	Examples of Lysosomal Disorders

Hydrolase deficiencies
   Glycogen storage disease type II–Pompe disease
   Glycoproteinoses—Mannosidosis
   Mucopolysaccharidosis–Hurler syndrome, Hunter syndrome
   (Total of 7 types with multiple subtypes)
   Neutral lipid storage–Wolman disease (cholesterol ester storage disease, CESD)
   Pycnodysostosis—Cathepsin K deficiency
   Sphingolipidoses—Niemann-Pick types A and B

Lysosomal transport disorders
   Cystinosis
   Sialic acid storage

newborn screening for LSDs should be strongly considered. This will be discussed in more detail in Chapter 14.

Peroxisomes are amazingly complex organelles. To date over 70 enzymatic functions have been identified in the peroxisomes. Some of their known major functions include β-oxidation of very long and long chain fatty acids, peroxide-based respiration, plasmalogen and bile acid synthesis, and glyoxylate transamination. There are two categories of peroxisomal disorders. Type 1 disorders involve multiple enzymes. These are typically disorders of the formation and assembly of the organelles themselves. Type 1 peroxisomal disorders include Zellweger syndrome, neonatal adrenoleukodystrophy, infantile Refsum disease, and rhizomelic chondrodysplasia punctata. Type 1 peroxisomal disorders are typically severe conditions that affect overall brain function. Type 2 disorders are those in which a single enzymatic function of the peroxisome is affected. Examples

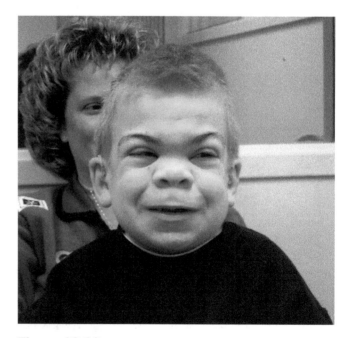

Figure 13-26. Adolescent male with mucopolysaccharide storage disorder type II (Hunter syndrome). Hunter syndrome is X-linked. He is also pictured with his affected brother in Fig. 8-10.

of these conditions include X-linked adrenoleukodystrophy (ABCD1 gene), Pseudo-Zellweger syndrome (PMP70 gene), Adult Refsum disease (phytanic acid oxidase), and hyperoxaluria (alanine-glyoxylate aminotransferase).

The Cytoskeleton

Early thoughts on cellular organization were that the cytoplasm was an amorphous collection of fluid bound by the cell membrane and separated from the nucleus by its own membrane. It is now known that the cytoplasm is not merely a buffered solution of free floating enzymes and other biochemicals, but rather it contains a series of complex structural (filamentous) proteins that exist for cellular architectural support and organization. The collective term given to these filaments is the "cytoskeleton." The proteins of the cytoskeleton come in several varieties, which include actin microfilaments (6 nm), intermediate filaments (10 nm), and the microtubules (23 nm). The intermediate filaments are composed of several important subunits including vimentin, keratins, and lamins.

Actins are microfilament proteins of the cytoskeleton. They are highly conserved across species and are one of the most prevalent proteins in cells. They have several functions including cell support, cell mobility, and molecular trafficking. Mutations in actin have been shown to cause a congenital myopathy known as nemaline myopathy. Filamins are cytoskeletal proteins that interact with actin as a basic anchoring protein. Several filamin A disorders have been described including frontometaphyseal dysplasia, Melnick Needles syndrome, otopalataldigital syndromes 1 and 2, and periventricular heterotopia.

The protein dystrophin is a component of the sub-sarcolemmal cytoskeleton. It is coded for by one of the largest known human genes (almost 2 Mb). The dystrophin gene is located at Xp21. The dystrophin protein acts as a biological "shock absorber" during muscle cell contraction. Abnormalities of this protein result in unrestrained contraction, which ultimately leads to disruption of the cellular membrane and muscle cell loss (Figure 13-27). The dystrophinopathies are a group of related disorders due to abnormalities of dystrophin. The phenotype of Duchenne muscular dystrophy (DMD) is most often associated with complete dystrophin dysfunction. DMD is an X-linked recessive disorder that, therefore, primarily affects boys. The typical presentation is that of a normal young boy who begins to develop difficulties walking at around 4 to 5 years old. Around this same time, hypertrophy of the calves is noted. Thereafter, progressive muscle wasting/weakness are noted. Most commonly young men with DMD die in young adulthood (Figure 13-28).

Epidermolysis bullosa refers to a group of skin disorders characterized by blistering of the skin associated with minimal pressure, friction or trauma. The disorder is genetically heterogeneous. Most commonly, it shows autosomal dominant inheritance; a few types show autosomal recessive inheritance. The common pathophysiology of these conditions is shearing

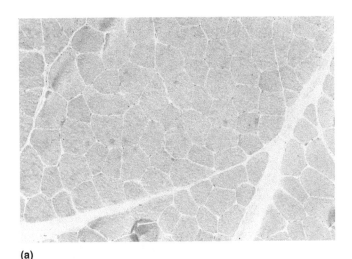

(a)

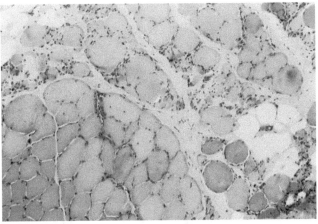

(b)

Figure 13-27. (a) Histopathologic picture of normal muscle. (b) Slide of dystrophic muscle. Note irregular fiber size and staining and the multiple central nuclei.

within the epidermal cells. Epidermolysis bullosa simplex (EBS) is an autosomal dominant disorder that has a blister pattern affecting mainly the hands and feet (Figure 13-29). EBS is caused by mutations in the cytoskeletal keratins, keratin-5 or keratin-14 gene.

Other disorders reported in association with mutations of cytoskeletal proteins include hepatic cirrhosis, chronic pancreatitis, pulmonary fibrosis, red blood cell membrane disorders (elliptocytosis and spherocytosis), and hearing loss. Disorders of the cytoskeleton have also been implicated in the pathogenesis of neurodegeneration, heart failure, and cancer (invasion).

The Nucleus and Centrioles

As with the cytoskeleton, mutations that lead to abnormal proteins involved in the nuclear membrane and centriole have been associated with recognized human disorders. The **nuclear lamina** is a dense collection of intermediate filaments and membrane associated proteins on the inner portion of the nuclear membrane. It has many important

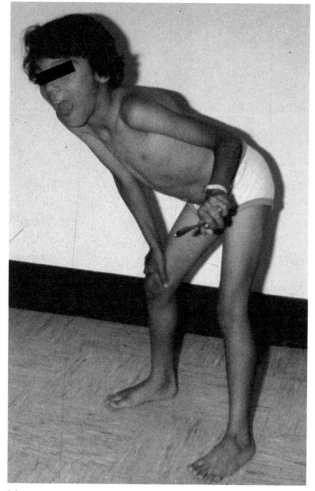

(a)

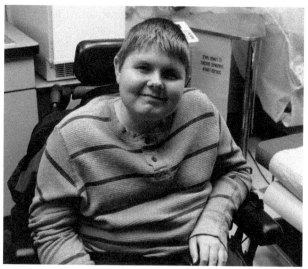

(b)

Figure 13-28. (a) Young man with Duchenne muscular dystrophy demonstrating a positive "Gower sign." When asked to pick up a reflex hammer off of the floor, he cannot straighten back up without pushing off of his legs. This is a sign of proximal muscle weakness. (b) Adolescent male with more advanced Duchenne muscular dystrophy. He is now non-ambulatory due to advanced muscle deterioration.

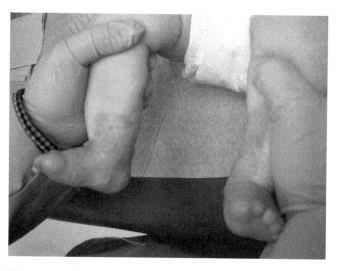

Figure 13-29. Lower extremities of an infant with epidermolysis bullosa. These patients have recurrent generalized blistering especially in pressure prone areas. The blistering typically does not scar. Dermatopathology shows cleavage within basal keratinocytes.

roles including providing mechanical support to the membrane, regulating DNA replication and cell division, chromatin organization, and anchoring the nuclear pore complexes embedded in the nuclear envelope. Lamins are filamentous proteins of the nuclear lamina. Currently three lamin protein genes (LMNA, LMNB2, LMNB1) have been associated with 13 known disorders, including 11 discrete phenotypes caused by LMNA mutations such as Hutchinson-Gilford progeria (Figure 13-30), Emery-Dreifuss muscular dystrophy, mandibuloacral dysplasia, generalized lipodystrophy, and restrictive dermopathy.

The centriole is a relatively small, tubular organelle located in the cytoplasm close to the nucleus. Its primary role appears to be involved in the nuclear division. The centriole is a self-replicating organelle. The hydrolethalus syndrome is a severe multiple anomaly syndrome. As the name implies, the outcome is very poor. Seventy percent of cases are still born; the remaining infants die shortly after birth. The condition is associated with a long list of congenital anomalies. The most common include complex central nervous system malformations, atrioventricular canals, polydactyly, stenosis of the airway, and abnormal pulmonary lobulations. Hydrolethalus syndrome is known to be caused by mutations in a gene designated HYLS-1. The protein product of this gene is a core centriolar protein that links the core centriole architecture to cilia.

Cilia, Flagella, and Cell Surface Specializations

There are two major types of cilia found on the surfaces of human cells. Immotile (primary) cilia have a primarily sensory function and occur on almost every cell type. Motile cilia are found on specialized cells that have specific needs for motility. They are found in high concentrations on

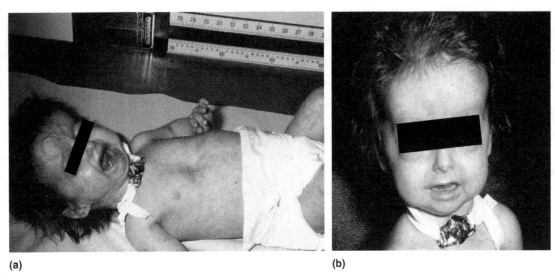

(a) (b)

Figure 13-30. Young child with Hutchinson-Gilford progeria. Note the appearance of premature aging.

the cells of the lining of respiratory tract, middle ear, and fallopian tubes.

Immotile (primary) cilia

Since primary cilia are found on most cell types, abnormalities of these structures have been associated with a large variety of clinical problems. Reported disorders associated with disrupted primary ciliary function include hepatic cystic disease, polycystic kidney disease (Figure 13-31), retinal dystrophies, ocular colobomas, infertility, polydactyly, and brain malformations (Figure 13-32). In the past few years, several well-described conditions have been shown to

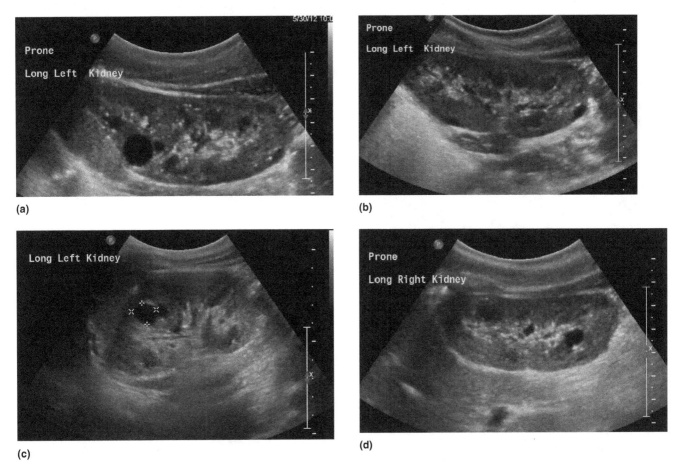

(a) (b) (c) (d)

Figure 13-31. Renal ultrasounds showing multiple cysts in both kidneys. This child has autosomal recessive polycystic kidney disease.

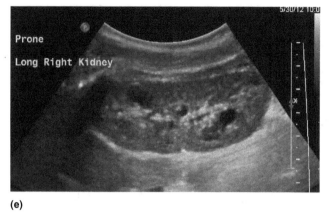

(e)

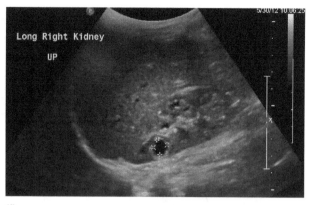

(f)

Figure 13-31. *(Continued)*

be disorders of the cilia. Collectively they have been called "ciliopathy syndromes." Table 13-6 lists some of these disorders. These conditions have in common abnormalities of the primary cilia and multiple congenital anomalies that include varying combinations of the anomalies noted above, plus other unique findings. Bardet-Biedel syndrome described in Chapter 12 (Figure 12-14) is a well-known disorder of the primary cilia.

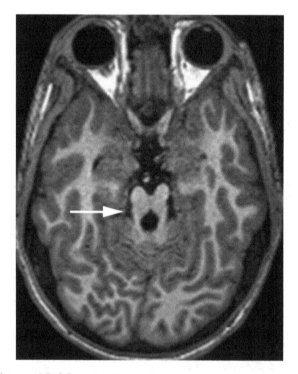

Figure 13-32. Axial T1 brain image showing the "molar tooth sign," a very characteristic brain malformation seen with Joubert syndrome. Joubert syndrome is a known "ciliopathy" disorder.
(Reprinted with permission from Macferran KM, Buchmann RF, Ramakrishnaiah R, Griebel ML, Sanger WG, Saronwala A, Schaefer GB. Pontine tegmental cap dysplasia with a 2q13 microdeletion involving the NPHP1 gene: insights into malformations of the mid-hindbrain. *Semin Pediatr Neurol.* 2010 Mar; 17(1):69-74.)

Motile cilia and flagella

Motile cilia and flagella are structurally very similar. In fact, flagella are essentially very long motile cilia. The majority of genes that code for both types of these structures are the same. Motile cilia are important for regional cell motility and for movement of fluids across the cell surface. Flagella serve a primary function in locomotion. Disorders of motile cilia and flagella, reflect their known distribution in cells (epithelium of the respiratory tract, middle ear, and the fallopian tubes as well as the tails of sperm).

A primary disorder of flagella has been described. In cases of male infertility, spermatic analysis is a first round assessment. Morphologically abnormal sperm termed "stump tail" or "short tail" sperm have been described. These sperm are described as having short, thick, and irregular flagella. On electron microscopic examination they are noted to have findings of dysplasia of the fibrous sheath. The primary problem ultimately appears to be dysplastic development of the axonemal and periaxonemal cytoskeleton of the spermatic flagella. Genetic studies in individuals with this anomaly have identified mutations in several

Table 13-6.	Examples of Ciliopathies: Disorders of Primary (Immotile) Cilia
Biedel-Bardet syndrome	
Cerebellar vermis hypoplasia or aplasia, oligophrenia, congenital ataxia, ocular coloboma, and hepatic fibrosis (COACH) syndrome	
Joubert syndrome	
Meckel-Gruber syndrome	
Nephronopthisis	
Oral-facial-digital syndromes I, VI	
Polycystic kidney disorders	
Senior-Lokien syndrome	

related genes. The A-kinase anchor proteins (AKAPs) are found in the fibrous sheaths of sperm. Their function is to direct protein kinase A activity by anchoring the enzyme close to its substrates. Several patients with short tail spermatic abnormalities have been reported with abnormalities of these genes. Reported mutations include partial deletions in the Akap3 (12p13) and Akap4 (Xp11.22) genes and complete deletions of Akap4.

Because of the shared structural identity of motile cilia and flagella, mutations in the genes that code for any of their common structural proteins may affect both of these structures.

Kartagener syndrome (also called primary ciliary dyskinesia or PCD) is a well-described entity. The primary manifestations of PCD are **situs abnormalities**, chronic respiratory problems, and infertility. It is easy to understand these symptoms in light of

ciliary and flagellar dysfunction. An interesting observation is that only 50% of patients with Kartagener syndrome will have situs abnormalities. The explanation for this appears to be that the correct placement of organs depends in part on the directional beating of cilia. If ciliary motion is impaired, the organs can essential "fall" randomly in either direction. Thus by chance, they will fall into the normal position about half the time. The other half of the time they will fall in the opposite (abnormal) direction. The condition shows marked genetic heterogeneity. To date at least 16 loci have been associated with the disorder. All of the associated genes share in common a primary function of the ciliary/flagellar mechanism. These include abnormalities of some of the key structural proteins (dyneins), components of the radial spokes, assembly of the units, and stabilizers of the assembled structures.

Part 3: Clinical Correlation

As noted earlier, certain clinical signs and symptoms are strongly associated with mitochondrial dysfunction. The presence of such findings provides the clinician with important clues as to the possible origin of a patient's disease. In the early 1990s several families were reported with problems that clearly appeared to be mitochondrial in origin. Affected individuals had progressive external ophthalmoplegia (inability to move the globe of the eye), myopathy with ragged red fibers seen on biopsy (Figure 13-16), and neurosensory hearing loss: there is a failure in the tissues of high energy requirement causing a combination of muscle, sight, and hearing problems. For medical geneticists this pattern of problems screams of mitochondrial dysfunction. Review of the pedigrees, however, showed vertical transmission with several instances of male-to-male transmission suggestive of autosomal dominant inheritance. However, additional investigation into these families revealed mutations in the mitochondrial genome (usually large scale and often multiple deletions) in the affected individuals. The other fascinating observation in these individuals was that each of them had *different* mitochondrial mutations! Ultimately it has been shown that all of this information can be explained by a novel

genetic mechanism. These disorders are now known to be due to mutations of nuclear-encoded proteins that disrupt the integrity of the mitochondrial genome. To phrase this another way, the mutations in the nuclear genes affect the normal replication of the mitochondrial DNA. What is observed in the families then is a Mendelian pattern of transmission of randomly generated mitochondrial mutations.

These families highlight a very important biological fact. Having the different proteins in a single organelle encoded by two or more independent genomes requires a high level of coordination. In this light, a new class of genes has been described that are involved in this process. **Regulators of organelle gene expression (ROGEs)** are nuclear genes that—as the name implies–regulate the mitochondrial genes. This regulation of mitochondrial gene expression usually occurs via posttranscriptional mechanisms (transcript maturation and translation). ROGEs have been shown to have multiple mechanisms of influence on the mitochondrial genome. Examples of some of these include influences on mitochondrial formation, level of OXPHOS activity, balance between aerobic and anaerobic metabolism, and the removal of dysfunctional mitochondria.

■ Board-Format Practice Questions

1. Which of the following is a characteristic of mitochondrial inheritance?
   A. Male-to-male transmission.
   B. Replicative segregation.
   C. Expression in homozygotes.
   D. A spontaneous mutation rate lower than that of nuclear genes.
   E. Bottlenose phenomenon.
2. A patient (20-year-old woman) presents to your clinic wanting to be tested for a mitochondrial disorder.

She tells you that her bother has been diagnosed with a mitochondrial disorder. You would tell her which of the following?
   A. Because her brother is affected, and the condition is mitochondrial, she could not be affected.
   B. Since she does not have any symptoms now as a young adult, she could not be affected.
   C. If she has the same condition as her brother, she should be affected to the same degree as he is.

D. The most helpful information would be to know the particular mutation that is present in her brother.

E. She should not have any children and should have a sterilization procedure soon.

3. You are evaluating a child with multisystem problems. As you ponder ordering some diagnostic tests, you could appropriately decide which of the following?

A. Because the child has chronic respiratory problems you should test for peroxisomal disorders.

B. Perform a renal biopsy.

C. Because the child is showing severe premature aging, you should do testing for genes coding for the nuclear membrane proteins.

D. You can safely assume the condition is autosomal dominant and counsel as such—avoiding doing any tests.

E. Because multiple organ systems are involved, testing won't be able to give you an answer, so you should not do any tests.

4. You see a patient in the newborn nursery. The child has multiple congenital anomalies. As part of a thorough evaluation you discover that the child has polydactyly, polycystic kidneys, retinitis pigmentosa, and a "molar tooth sign" on the brain MRI. Given this pattern of anomalies, you would conclude that the primary pathogenesis of this child's problems is likely due to abnormalities of:

A. Primary cilia.

B. Mitochondria.

C. Peroxisomes.

D. Lysosomes.

E. Endosomes.

5. You see a new patient who is a 2-month-old boy. He is seeing you because his brother has Hunter syndrome (an X-linked lysosomal storage disorder). On your exam he has no dysmorphic features and is exhibiting normal growth and development. His parents have multiple questions. Which of the following would be a correct statement to share with them?

A. Since Hunter syndrome is X-linked and he is not a female, he will not have it.

B. Since he looks normal at this point, he probably does not have Hunter syndrome.

C. Since he had newborn screening and that was normal, he could not have Hunter syndrome.

D. Enzyme replacement therapy is now available for Hunter syndrome. Early confirmation of his status would be important.

E. Lysosomal transplantation should be performed soon on this child.

chapter 14. Genetic Therapeutics

C H A P T E R   S U M M A R Y

By this point in the book, we feel sure you as readers have appreciated the heavy emphasis on diagnostics. In fact, the mainstay of clinical genetics is still in identifying the etiology and pathogenesis of specific disorders. However, as the practice of clinical genetics has progressed, so have advances in therapies. There are now several available modalities of genetic treatments. Up until recently, however, most treatments provided by medical geneticists primarily involved counseling and case management. The treatment of inborn errors of metabolism (IEM) dates back to the mid-1960s. These treatments have involved dietary adjustments, specialized formulas, and vitamin/cofactor supplementation. More recently tissue transplantation and enzyme replacement therapies have become available. New treatment modalities have been developed for non-metabolic disorders. Bioengineered pharmaceuticals are now commonplace. Other treatment options like personalized medicine strategies, tissue cloning, gene correction, and true gene therapy all sit poised for transition out of clinical trials and into standard medical care. In the first section of this chapter we will discuss the mechanisms of the different modes of genetic therapies. In the second section we will discuss the clinical application of these therapies.

Part 1: Background and Systems Integration

What are Genetic Therapies?

In the broadest sense, genetic therapies can include any treatment or medical intervention for genetic disorders. Alternatively, it can include a treatment that uses a genetically based technology regardless of the disease etiology. Thus, one could propose that an aortic replacement surgery for a patient with Marfan syndrome could be classified as a "genetic therapy." Likewise, a monoclonal antibody treatment for cancer or multiple sclerosis might be considered a "genetic therapy." A narrower definition of "gene therapy" would be only those treatments in which there is actual manipulation of the patient's DNA to produce a therapeutic response. For the purposes of this chapter, we will shoot for somewhere in between.

Conventional "Therapies"

The discipline of clinical genetics began to emerge in the 1960s. The role of the clinical geneticist was primarily diagnostic back then. Genetic testing at that point was largely limited to low resolution (400 band) G-banded chromosome studies and a handful of metabolic tests. Likewise, no molecular therapies existed then. The **clinical geneticist** functioned primarily as a diagnostician. Beyond diagnostics, the geneticist had a limited number of modalities in which to "treat" the patient. Over time, the type of roles that a geneticist performs has greatly expanded. Currently the majority of clinical geneticists work in a primarily academic environment. Still there are increasing numbers of clinical geneticists in private practice or working as members of single-specialty teams like a large pediatric practice in which they do some pediatrics, but manage the genetic patients for the group.

Case management

This has always been a key role of the geneticist. Patients with genetic disorders often have conditions that are rarely encountered by other health care professionals. As such, the question of: "what do we do for them?" is an often asked query. The clinical geneticist in collaboration with the patient's primary care physician and other ancillary health care providers plays a key role in assuring that their patients receive the requisite screening, surveillance, and ancillary medical services that are unique and specific to their diagnosis. Examples of such management would include assuring that all patients with Down syndrome have an echocardiogram at the time of diagnosis, or that patients with Beckwith-Wiedemann syndrome have periodic tumor surveillance (serum alpha-fetoprotein levels and renal ultrasounds).

Genetic counseling

This is an independent discipline. A **genetic counselor** is a health care professional trained in the science of genetics and the social sciences of psychology and counseling. They are accomplished in working with families throughout their experience with the clinical genetics team. Genetic counselors are particularly adept in explaining the complex concepts of genetics to nonmedical persons. They also excel in crisis intervention, resource identification, and coordination of services. Training in genetic counseling is a 2 or 3 year specialized master's degree. Genetic counselors are certified by the National Board of Genetic Counseling. At the present time, genetic counselors can be separately licensed in only a handful of states in the United States. Genetic counselors may work with pregnant couples and cancer patients. Others provide supportive care in managing pediatric and adult medicine patients and in genetics laboratories.

Interdisciplinary specialty teams

Many patients with genetic disorders will have multiple and complex needs. The range of specialists needed to optimize outcomes can be staggering. It would be nearly impossible for a family to make independent visits to all of these specialists. Besides the practical issues of making multiple medical visits, coordination among specialists can be extremely cumbersome. A successful solution to this problem is the formation of interdisciplinary teams. Interdisciplinary specialty teams assemble a selected group of specialists needed to provide optimal care for a specific disorder. One advantage of such teams is of course the fact that the patient can obtain "one stop shopping", i.e., all of the necessary specialists under one roof. One especially important advantage is the coordination of care. Not only are all of the specialists in one place, but they can talk directly to one another rather than trying to communicate by letters, emails, or phone conversations. The list of possible specialty teams in theory is as long as the list of known disorders. Table 14-1 lists some of the most common interdisciplinary clinics in which clinical geneticists and genetic counselors participate.

The final conventional therapy to mention is that of the *treatment of inborn errors of metabolism*. If you would like a review of these disorders, Chapter 8 covers the physiology of them in some detail. Although the treatment of most genetic conditions remains limited, therapy for IEMs began in earnest in the 1960s and has continued to progress. Multiple novel approaches for the treatment of metabolic disorders have been developed. Table 14-2 provides a summary of some of the major types of approaches. Critical partners in these therapies

Table 14-1.	Examples of Interdisciplinary Clinics Involving Medical Genetics/Genetic Counseling

Autism

Cancer genetics

Connective tissue disorders

Disorders of sexual differentiation (DSDs)

Down syndrome

Endogenetics/growth disorders

Fetal alcohol syndrome

Metabolic disorders

Neurogenetics

Neuromuscular

Neurosensory genetics
   Hereditary hearing loss
   Ocular/retinal genetics

Orofacial clefts/craniofacial

Perinatal management

Table 14-2.	Possible Treatment Modalities for Inborn Errors of Metabolism

Dietary modification
   Avoidance of offending substance
   Galactosemia
   Restriction of intake of specific dietary elements
   Phenylketonuria
   Distribution of calories
   Glycogen storage disorders

Enzyme replacement therapies
   Gaucher, Fabry, Pompe

Cofactor replacement
   Biotinidase

Detoxifying agents
   Hyper-ammonemias

Bone marrow transplantation
   Some storage disorders

Gene therapy

ADA deficiency (SCIDS)

Combination therapy

are dieticians with special expertise in metabolic disorders (**metabolic dieticians**).

Biopharmaceuticals

The term **biopharmaceuticals** in general refers to medicines developed using various biotechnologies. If the technique

Table 14-3.	Examples of Genetically Engineered Drugs

Alpha-interferon

Azidothymidine (AZT)

Enzyme replacement therapies for inborn errors of metabolism
  Acid alpha-glucosidase (Pompe disease)
  Alpha-galactosidase A (Fabry disease)
  Alpha-L iduronidase (Hurler syndrome)
  Arylsulfatase B (Maroteaux-Lamy syndrome)
  Glucocerebrosidase (Gaucher disease)
  Iduronate-2-sulfatase (Hunter syndrome)
  Tissue-nonspecific isozyme of alkaline phosphatase (hypophosphatasia)

Erythropoietin

Factor VIII (hemophilia A)

Hepatitis B vaccine

Human growth hormone (hGH)

Human insulin

Tissue plasminogen activator (TPA)

Table 14-4.	Requirements for Gene Therapy

Gene expression sufficiently understood

Gene transfer into target cells possible

Pathogenesis of disorder sufficiently understood

Recombinant gene technology

Relevant gene cloned

Relevant gene identified

Sufficient and appropriate expression of the gene at the appropriate time

Sufficient and appropriate expression of the gene for the appropriate length of time

Target cell(s) known

utilized involves manipulation of nucleic acids (DNA or RNA), these may commonly be referred to as "genetically engineered drugs." Such medicines may be proteins, nucleic acids, or even microbes. They can be used for therapeutic or *in vivo* diagnostic purposes. Often the generation of these drugs requires some sort of biologic system to manufacture the compound from the assembled genetic template. These would include such different methods as biological secretions (such as milk), cultured cells (such as Chinese hamster ovaries), or selected gene activation in human cells. A few examples of such drugs are given in Table 14-3. This list provides only a representative sample of an ever increasing number of such drugs.

Gene Therapy

The concept of genetic correction was discussed in Chapter 7 in the Clinical Correlation section. In that section we discussed a new class of drug that has the potential for therapy for genetic disorders that are nonsense mutation mediated. The mechanism of action is that it allows ribosomes to read past premature stop codons. For details, you may want to refer back to that section. This investigational new drug is currently in clinical trials. If studies do eventually demonstrate that this is an effective therapy it would be truly amazing. The medication is taken orally as a tasteless powder that can be dissolved in liquids such as water or milk. Clearly this is the first of what is likely to become many related drugs that share in common a mechanism of correcting genetic errors. However, just because a mutation is corrected, it does not necessarily mean that the problem is fixed. This is covered more in the second section of this chapter.

Genetic correction as described before could represent one form of "gene therapy." In a more narrow definition, true gene therapy could mean the treatment of a disorder by the introduction of a genetic element. While the concept of introducing genes into host systems seems rather straightforward, the mechanics are far from simple. The basic requirements for effective gene therapy are listed in Table 14-4. In general, three basic types of information need to be available. The nature of the mutation involved, the type of function that the gene in question performs (i.e., pathogenesis), and an effective method of gene transfer must be understood. An understanding of the mutation would include knowledge of site of the mutation, the nature of the amino acid change(s), and the expression pattern (dominant versus recessive, and so forth). Most importantly, the pathogenesis of the condition should be well understood. For instance a mutation in a gene that affects a developmental embryonic process would not be a good candidate for gene therapy. For example correcting a mutation in a gene that controls limb bud growth would not be helpful in a child already born with a malformed or missing arm. Correcting the gene after the fact would be of no help. In contrast, correcting the abnormality in a gene that controls an ongoing process would have the potential to effect a true cure. Thus, correcting a mutation in a gene that codes for an enzymatic protein would have the potential of producing a normal enzyme which from that time forward could perform the normal biological function for the patient.

Cloning

There are very few words that invoke a more guttural response from society than the term "cloning." This is unfortunate—and largely a function of misinformation and misunderstanding. The lay public generally perceives cloning as the duplication of a genetically identical human. This of course is replete with all sorts of ethical and social implications. However, cloning in a literal sense refers to the process of making a genetically identical copy of *something*, not necessarily an entire organism.

Cloning has proved to be a very effective strategy in a variety of different settings. For example, cloning is used routinely in agriculture today. Plants grown from cuttings are literally clones of the parent plant. Also, livestock produced by splitting embryos at the 4-cell stage that can be grown into a separate embryo will improve the overall yield for a herd. Such applications can even be used to re-establish colonies of endangered or extinct species.

Cloning can occur at many different levels. Cloning of a specific DNA segment can be used to obtain material for further study. The resulting cloned (copied) collections of DNA molecules are maintained in clone libraries. A second type of cloning exploits the natural process of cell division to make many copies of an entire cell. The genetic makeup of these cloned cells, called a cell line, is identical to the original cell. Cloning may also occur at the tissue or organ level. Such efforts have tremendous potential for medical treatments as described in the following section. And of course, yet another type of cloning produces complete, genetically identical organisms such as Dolly the famous Scottish sheep.

Personalized Medicine

In the Clinical Correlation section of Chapter 1 we introduced the concept of personalized medicine. We defined personalized medicine as the application of genomic and molecular data to an individual's health care. The general principles of personalized medicine are to tailor the delivery of health care, facilitate the discovery and clinical testing of new products, and to help determine a person's predisposition to a particular disease or condition. Personalized medicine develops not only the tools to help providers deliver the care that works best "on average," but at the same time develop a new class of tools for identifying and employing the best care for each individual patient. In a very real sense, personalized medicine is the ultimate "genetic therapy."

Part 2: Medical Genetics

Clinical genetics is a relatively new discipline in medicine. Specialists exclusively practicing as geneticists began to appear in the 1960s. Slowly, the number of practicing clinical geneticists has risen to a little over 1000 by 2007. But this still only represents 0.18% of all practicing physicians in the United States. For much of the past five decades, the majority of the work done by genetic physicians has focused on diagnostics. Geneticists are skilled in the evaluation of individuals and families in an attempt to identify the etiology of a particular condition or set of symptoms. The identification of an etiology is a critical piece of the health care of an individual. For many people, simply knowing "why" is important for their own piece of mind and for dealing with the particulars of the condition. Knowing the cause can also help the family in many other ways such as identifying co-morbid conditions, defining prognosis, and for recurrence risk counseling.

In the realm of clinical genetics, therapeutics has always tended to lag behind diagnostics. Still, the role of the physician has traditionally focused not just on diagnostics, but on treatments. There are many reasons for this discrepancy. In Chapter 11 we discussed the amazing and rapid advances in genetic testing and screening. These advances continue to increase diagnostic yields and the amount of information that can be given to families. For the foreseeable future, clinical geneticists will continue to play a major role in the discovery of the causes of disease spurred by the ever-increasing number of powerful molecular tools that are constantly being introduced. In this section we will highlight the second aspect—therapeutics. The past 10 years has seen a dramatic rise in the number of therapeutic options that the geneticist has to work with. While the therapies employed by the geneticist may not be as tangible as the removal of an inflamed appendix, these are treatments all the same.

It is important to note that geneticists are not the only physicians who utilize genetic therapies. Oncologists, for example, have used genetic therapies for decades. Genotype information is routinely used to direct specific therapies, and DNA/RNA based tools are being increasingly used. With the continued advancements of genetic technologies, all health care providers will be using "genetic therapies" in the not so distant future (and in fact, the future may be now).

Conventional "Therapies"

Case management

The past decade has seen a great emphasis placed on establishing the **Family Centered Medical Home**. Primary care physicians are trained to function as the center of a medical system of care where the medical home where all of the patient's information and care resides. In this regards, the medical genetics team can function as a **Medical Home Neighbor**, a professional partner of the medical home who works in collaboration to assure comprehensive and patient centered services. Many of the patients that the geneticist cares for have complex problems and require access to a plethora of specialists and services. Coordination of care is the key issue. Geneticists are not here to assume care, but to bring to the medical home expertise and information about genetic disorders that will complement the work being done in the primary care setting.

Genetic counseling

The mainstay of genetic therapies from the beginning has been to provide genetic counseling. Genetic counseling is the complex process of providing critical information about genetic conditions to a family in a process that is understandable, relevant, and sensitive. Medical geneticists work in collaboration with genetic counselors to provide this information. As with most medical practices, there are differences in the division of labor from practice to practice. Regardless of who does what part, the key element is that families get the information they need in a format that is both understandable and useful. A major challenge of genetic counseling is in the explanation of difficult concepts. Genetics is not typically a day-to-day conversation for most people. Of course, patients vary greatly in their level of understanding. In addition, the acute stress of the situation may cloud interpretation and retention. Also, as has been discussed throughout the last 13 chapters, current technology can be quite complicated.

Consider this scenario: You have a patient who is a 7-year-old boy who you have just diagnosed with fragile X syndrome (Figure 4-27). In order to inform the family of the type of inheritance that is seen in fragile X, you would want to tell the family: "your child has fragile X syndrome, which is an X-linked semi-dominant trait that shows genetic anticipation due to an expanding trinucleotide repeat in the FMR-1 gene." Presumably you, the reader, took a little while to grasp these concepts as you worked you way through Chapter 12. Think then about how you might explain the above information to the child's mother who has no medical background, did not finish high school, and, because she is a carrier of a fragile X expansion, has an IQ of 75 herself!

Often, genetic diagnoses are made and discussed under extremely stressful conditions. For example, there are few situations that are more intense than the discovery of an unanticipated congenital anomaly in the delivery room. The birth of a child with congenital anomalies represents a loss of the perceived "normal" child. Parents in these situations will experience the typical stages of grieving. Likewise simply having a child with special needs adds another level of pressure to the already difficult task of raising a child. Persons with Special Health Care Needs (SHCN) present added stresses to parenting in many ways including financial, loss of insurance, time off work (multiple specialists), fear or jealousy of siblings, need for respite, and the unfortunate discomfort associated with public curiosity and meddling. In addition, the diagnosis of a genetic disorder in a family often exacerbates pre-existing conflicts and tension. The current divorce rate in the United States is a little over 50%. For families with special needs children the estimates are 85%! It is here that the genetic counselor or other psychosocial ancillary care person can be useful. Working with families in these situations and helping them maneuver the complex process of dealing with often overwhelming circumstances is why the discipline exists.

Interdisciplinary services

Think for a moment about the example of a child born with a cleft lip and palate (Figure 10-8). An initial assumption would be that child with a cleft would need a surgeon to repair the cleft, and that would pretty much take care of the situation. In reality, there are multiple possible medical complications and extenuating conditions of oro-facial clefting. Current health care standards now recommend that all children with

Table 14-5.	List of Specialties on a Cleft Lip and Palate Team

Primary team members

Audiology

Dentistry (pediatric and adult)

Clinical genetics

Genetic counseling

Otolaryngology

Orthodontics

Plastic surgery

Speech pathology

Accessible specialists

Behavioral psychology

Neuropsychology

Ophthalmology

Oral maxillofacial surgery

Prosthodontics

clefts, be evaluated and have their care coordinated through a cleft team. The ideal team that provides care for children with clefts is comprised at least 14 different specialists! A list of specialists that might participate in a cleft lip and palate team is provided in Table 14-5. Granted, not every child will need to see every specialist on every visit. Still, in order to achieve optimal outcomes, children with clefts and other craniofacial malformations need access to such a team. Just imagine what it would mean for the family if they had to make visits to all of these specialists independently. Interdisciplinary services, such as a cleft team, epitomize family-centered services. Not only are all of the specialists under one roof at one time–"one stop shopping"–but communication is optimized. The team can make coordinated treatment plans and recommendations that will optimize the outcomes for each patient. As noted in the first section of this chapter, many different types of interdisciplinary teams exist. Table 14-1 lists some of the more common types of teams in which participation by the clinical geneticist is particularly helpful.

Treatment of inborn errors of metabolism

The earliest true treatments for genetic disorders were those for metabolic disorders. The development of a modified formula low in phenylalanine that was effective in treatment of phenylketonuria (PKU) was reported by Professor Horst Bickel around 1955 (see Table 8-11). This therapy prevented the mental retardation and high likelihood of death in infants with untreated PKU. Since that time the treatment of PKU has become quite sophisticated (refer to the Clinical Correlation Section of Chapter 8). The treatment of PKU stands as the premier example of successful treatment of inborn errors of metabolism. Multiple, often combined, therapies are now available for many metabolic disorders. Primary treatment options include dietary modifications, cofactor replacement, administration of detoxifying agents, enzyme replacement therapies, and tissue transplantation (see Clinical Correlation section).

Biopharmaceuticals

The first mass produced pharmaceutical manufactured using genetic engineering was human insulin produced from altered *Escherichia coli* bacteria in 1982. Over the last 30 years many such drugs have been developed (Table 14-3). The development of these drugs has greatly enhanced medical treatment for many disorders. Currently the vast majority of persons treated with insulin now use a form made by genetic engineering rather than extraction from bovine or porcine sources–as was the case into the 1970s.

One particularly fascinating story in this regards is that of growth hormone therapy. Human growth hormone deficiency (GHD) was discovered in the 1920s. Shortly thereafter, attempts to treat GHD began. Early strategies used growth hormone (GH) extracted from cattle–as was the case with insulin. In the 1950s the first treatments with GH extracted from human (cadaver) pituitary began. In 1960, the federal government established the National Pituitary Agency to centralize and administer the distribution of pituitary-source GH. The need for such an agency was that this source of GH was quite limited and needed to be rationed and prioritized for dissemination—only the most severe GHD children could be treated. The use of human pituitary GH extracts was halted in 1985 when several children receiving this therapy were found to have a lethal neurodegenerative disorder known as Creutzfeldt-Jakob disease. (Creutzfeldt-Jakob disease is part of a family of disorders known as transmissible spongiform encephalopathies. One such condition that you may be familiar with is the so called "mad cow disease.") Fortunately, at around the same time that CJD was reported in these patients, genetically engineered human growth hormone (hGH) was in the final stages of development. Currently there are several companies that now make hGH by genetic engineering techniques. This technology has resulted in an adequate, uninterrupted supply of GH for all persons needing the drug. Also, the risk of biological contamination—as in the pituitary source GH—has been eliminated.

The story of the development of genetically engineered hGH is a fascinating one. There are many intriguing facets of this story if you find yourself inclined to search for more information. Likewise, there are other examples of other conditions in which treatment has been revolutionized by the development of similar therapies. It is, however, important to point out that things are not always as simple as they first appear. While genetically engineered drugs are wonderfully exciting and helpful, their development has not been without complications. Several important issues have emerged that are clinically relevant in their use.

Cost is a significant issue in the use of genetically engineered drugs. The research and development (R&D) costs of bringing these drugs can be staggering. In the case of human insulin, these costs can be shared across a large population–with almost 10% of the US population developing diabetes mellitus sometime in their life. Thus most people with diabetes can take engineered human insulin at a very affordable cost. However, this is not the case with other, less common disorders. Take for instance the example above of hGH. Currently an annualized cost of treatment is around $20,000-40 000 per year depending on the age and size of the patient. For conditions that are even less common the costs can be staggering. Current annualized cost estimates for the treatment of some of the lysosomal storage disorders are: Gaucher disease (~ $150,000 per year), Fabry disease (~ $250,000 per year), or Hunter syndrome (~ $500,000 per year). As one might imagine, payment for drugs this expensive is a very difficult problem to deal with. Some of the more critical issues along these lines include:

1. Who will pay for the drug?

2. Life-time maximum payments (ceilings) even if there is payment coverage.

3. When does the treatment become standard therapy instead of investigational?

4. Is there such a thing as a cost:benefit ratio that can be objectively applied?

Other problems that have been encountered with such therapies have included problems with the product development and manufacturing. There are also fiscal considerations from the manufacturer's side. What if the drug is not fiscally sound, i.e., what if it is not worth making? If the decision is made to stop production, what about the patients who were dependent on the pharmaceutical? On the other end of the spectrum, there are potential problems with expanded use/abuse. Going back to our example of hGH, there have been significant issues raised regarding its potential uses. Originally hGH was used solely for treating patients with complete growth hormone deficiency (GHD). Over time, with abundant supplies, its use has been expanded to partial GHD. In addition, the use of hGH has been expanded to a variety of other conditions (Table 14-6). Note the last indication listed in Table 14-6. The FDA has now approved

Table 14-6.	Licensed Indications for the Use of Human Growth Hormone Therapy
Growth hormone deficiency (complete and partial)	
Turner syndrome/SHOX gene mutations	
Chronic renal failure	
Prader-Willi syndrome	
Intrauterine growth retardation (without catch-up growth by age 2 years)	
Normal variant (idiopathic) SS	

the use of hGH therapy for normal variant short stature! A very long, intense ethical discussion can ensue over the pros and cons of treating "normally short" children. It is beyond the scope of this chapter to do so. However, you are encouraged to simply ponder what potential issues such a usage of hGH raises. Yet another possibility is the abuse of hGH as a performance enhancing drug. Many recent stories about high profile athletes and "doping" charges highlight the potential for abuse of such therapies.

The final conclusion of all of this is simple. Genetically engineered pharmaceuticals are truly amazing in their potential to treat human disease. They often present the first method ever developed for treating certain complex and rare disorders. Still, caution has to be maintained. While the science may be straightforward, the practical application (getting the drug to the patient) may be fraught with many unanticipated complications.

Gene Therapy

The first thing that comes to mind for most people when genetic treatments are discussed is the term "gene therapy." **Gene therapy** may be defined in several different ways. Narrowly defined gene therapy could mean using DNA as a pharmacologic agent. Alternatively, one could define it as those therapies in which genes (more specifically runs of nucleic acids) are transported into a patient's body to effect a therapeutic outcome. The greatest hurdle in implementing gene therapy is the difficulty in transferring the normal gene sequence into a living organism without disrupting normal biological functions. Simply put, how do you get the correct gene into the correct place without producing unwanted problems? Many different techniques for gene transfer have been tried. Some of the more commonly employed strategies include viral vectors, plasmids, chemical methods, and antisense oligonucleotide strands.

One of the early success stories in human gene therapy was the treatment of severe combined immunodeficiency (SCIDS) in the 1990s. SCIDS as the name implies is an immunodeficiency disorder with symptoms in early childhood. The disorder is an autosomal recessive disorder caused by mutations in the gene adenosine deaminase (ADA). Inactivity of this enzyme renders white blood cells incapable of carrying out normal immunologic responses. The approach to treating SCIDS with gene therapy involved taking a bacterium carrying a plasmid that had the normal human ADA gene incorporated in it. The cloned ADA gene was transferred from the bacterium to an inactivated retrovirus. Bone marrow from the patient with SCIDS was then harvested and infected with the retrovirus, thus transferring a functional copy of the ADA gene into the T cells. The genetically altered T cells were then transplanted back into the patient (Figure 14-1). Using this approach, patients with SCIDS were effectively "cured" of their disease. As these patients have been followed, limitations in this treatment modality have been noted including a low level of the retroviral transduction (<1%) and difficulty in maintaining transformed cells in the periphery. Unanticipated "side effects" like an increased risk of developing cancer also complicate such therapies.

There is thus a balance between optimism and realism that must be communicated to patients and to the public at large. The potential of gene therapy literally to cure human disease cannot be overstated. However, as noted earlier, there are practical and technical issues that continue to impede the translation of preclinical studies into effective clinical protocols. There are also critical issues of safety and regulation. When discussing gene therapy as a possible treatment option for patients, the clinician must be honest about the practical reality of gene therapy.

Despite these limitations the science of gene therapy continues to advance. In recent years, gene therapy has emerged as a truly independent discipline. There are now even

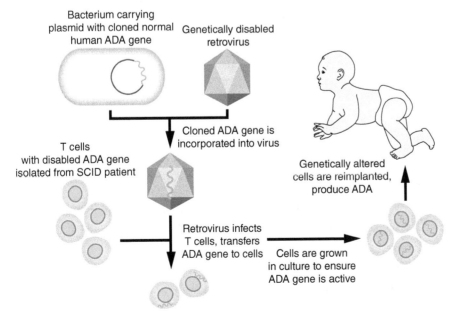

Figure 14-1. Schematic of gene therapy trials for severe combined immunodeficiency (SCID). (From Klug WS, Cummings MR, Spencer CA, et al: *Concepts of Genetics*, 10th ed. Benjamin Cummings, 2011.)

Table 14-7.	Clinical Trials with Gene Therapy
Adenosine deaminase deficiency	
AIDS/HIV	
Cancer	
Coronary artery disease	
Cystic fibrosis	
Duchenne muscular dystophy	
Growth hormone deficiency	
Hemoglobinopathies	
Hemophilia B	
Hypercholesterolemia	
Inborn errors of metabolism (multiple)	
Parkinson disease	

clinicians who work solely within this field. In fact, many clinical trials with gene therapy are currently underway (Table 14-7).

Cloning

As we noted earlier, people react emotionally to the term "cloning." Just the overall consideration of making a duplicate of one's self reaches down to some of the most basic edicts of humanity. Unfortunately, these initial reactions have greatly limited the public from an accurate understanding of the concept. **Cloning** simply means making an identical copy of something. It is important to emphasize that cloning in the medical arena can occur at any of several different levels—cells, tissues, organs, or organisms. The tremendous ethical concerns that are typically raised are usually focused on the latter. These concerns have likewise overshadowed the tremendous potential that cloning has for the treatment of human disease. At the level of cells, tissues, and organs, the potential benefits are staggering—and largely noncontroversial. Some specific examples might include:

1. Cloning of an individual's neuronal cells could generate therapies for problems like spinal cord injuries or neurodegenerative conditions (including potentially even normal aging).

2. Cloning of organs for auto-transplantation. For instance a person with 80% to 90% of total body surface area burns will be in need of large amounts of tissue for grafting. Using cloning techniques from the small amounts of non-affected skin could generate adequate supplies of the patient's own skin (which would also alleviate issues with graft rejection). In conditions such as hepatic or renal failure, cloning an entire replacement organ from an individual's own cells would again alleviate graft issues and also eliminate the need for cadaver-source donors.

3. Cloning of a specific anatomic structure would aid in reconstructive options for problems such as injury or

congenital anomalies. For instance, cloning of an entire ear appears to be a reasonable expectation in the near future.

In a very real sense, all of these examples would fit our definition of "genetic therapies." Also, while these may seem somewhat dramatic and maybe a little too amazing to be true, they are none-the-less on the horizon. Despite the limitless potential that such interventions promise, the huge ethical issues associated with the cloning of individuals has largely overshadowed such promise in the eyes of the public. Deep concerns exist over the moral and ethical questions of cloning people—and even other animals. While final resolution on such issues will need careful consideration and discussions among all interested disciplines (ethics, politics, religion, law), certain principles are straightforward enough to discuss here.

One of the most misunderstood concepts of the cloning of individuals is the idea of making an exact duplicate of one's self. It is critical to recognize that our genetic code is not the sole determinant of who we are as individuals. As individuals we are products of not only our genetic make-up, but of environmental influences, experience and chance as well. One only has to think about the practical example of monozygotic (MZ) twins. Almost everyone has had the chance to know a set of siblings who are monozygous twins. Simple observation will quickly highlight the fact that those two persons, while similar, are not exactly the same. Simply put, although they are genetically identical they are not developmentally identical. Even the concept of being genetically identical is an oversimplification. While monozygotic twins start off genetically identical, genetic differences likely happen throughout gestation (see Chapter 7, Mutation).

Because of the rate of spontaneous mutations, MZ twins will almost certainly have several acquired genetic difference even by the time of birth. Likewise, MZ twins do not even share an identical *in utero* environment. Twins differ in their position in the womb and in blood flow in the womb. Clinical geneticists have long observed the not infrequent occurrence of discordant phenotypes in MZ twins (we refer you to similar discussions in Chapter 10 on "Concordance" and to Figure 10-5).

At the present time, the bulk of international law and consensus is on the side of extreme caution. A legal moratorium currently exists in the United States on the cloning of individual humans. Before this would ever become a sanctioned practice, many ethical and legal issues will have to be resolved. Several practical issues will have to be ironed out as well. For instance, the famous sheep Dolly (Figure 14-2) was conceived by a nuclear transplantation of the nucleus from a donor cell of an adult sheep. Thus even at the time of birth, Dolly possessed a mature genome and actually died a premature aging death. Thus, it is clear that careful oversight is needed in this realm. However, such caution should not stymie efforts for less controversial interventions that could greatly benefit our patients.

Personalized Medicine

The concept of personalized medicine was introduced in the Clinical Correlation section of Chapter 1 of this book.

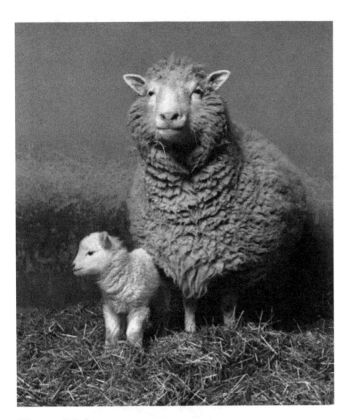

Figure 14-2. Dolly, the famous sheep (right) that was 'conceived' by nuclear transplantation producing a literal clone of the donor. (Courtesy of the Roslin Institute, The University of Edinburgh.)

Personalized medicine may be defined as health care targeted to the inherent biology and physiology of an individual leading to improvements in their medical care. Simply, this is medicine tailored to the individual with direction coming from the person's own unique situation. As we have emphasized a number of times, a large contributor to individual diversity is one's own genomic constitution. Thus, the ultimate "genetic therapy" is that in which knowledge of an individual's genome directs their medical care. Personalized medicine can occur at several levels. In its simplest form it may be using the person's family history information to identify specific risks that warrant testing, screening or interventions hopefully to prevent disease. In Chapter 9 we emphasized the importance of having family history information on every patient. The well-trained modern health care professional should have a working knowledge of genetics to be able to review and accurately respond to a patient's family history. Even in this era of modern genetic diagnostics, the family history remains equally effective in identifying and diagnosing conditions in a family. This is indeed personalized medicine at its classic best!

Using any number of the remarkable molecular tools discussed in Chapter 11, personalized medicine can now be taken to the molecular level. The next 10 years will see the era of molecular-based personalized medicine ushered in. Currently there are just a few logistical hurdles, such as reimbursement and regulation, that need to be addressed. However, there is no question that direct clinical utility of such science will occur in the very near future (Table 1-5).

Part 3: Clinical Correlation

One of the many areas in which exciting advances have been made in genetic therapeutics is in the treatment of the lysosomal storage disorders. The lysosomal storage disorders (LSDs) are a group of conditions that share a common pathogenic mechanism. All of these conditions are problems with enzymatic catabolic processes (see Chapter 8). The different LSDs are characterized by which biochemical accumulates abnormally within the cells (see Chapter 13). The progressive accumulation of substances within the lysosomes eventually disrupts cell function. As such, the typical LSD patient has a normal phenotype at birth. Over time, an abnormal phenotype emerges that is characterized by the type and degree of accumulation of abnormally stored compounds.

Hurler syndrome is an example of a lysosomal storage disorder. It was described in 1919 by a German physician, Dr. Gertrude Hurler. It is caused by a deficiency of an enzyme called alpha-L-iduronidase. As with most inborn errors of metabolism, it is inherited as an autosomal recessive trait. The enzyme alpha-L-iduronidase cleaves the alpha-L-iduronic acid residues off of the glycosaminoglycans (GAGs) dermatan sulfate and heparan sulfate. Another term for GAGs is "mucopolysaccharides." Thus Hurler syndrome and other related conditions are collectively referred to as the "mucopolysaccharide storage disorders" (MPSs). Hurler syndrome has been designated type I MPS.

Infants with Hurler syndrome are phenotypically normal at birth. Growth and development usually proceed normally for the first couple of years of life. Early symptoms may include repeated ear infections and enlarged tonsils. Eventually, the abnormal accumulation of GAGs will lead to other phenotypic changes. Accumulation of the GAGs in the bones will lead to a pattern of changes known as dysostosis multiplex. This can include an enlarged skull with shallow orbits. The cranial bone is thick and the cranial sutures may initially be widened, but eventually close prematurely. The ribs are narrow where they attach to the vertebrae and widen as they approach the sternum—sometimes described as being "oar-shaped." The clavicles are short, thickened, and have irregular margins. The vertebral bodies show a hook-shaped configuration of vertebral bodies. The pelvis is malformed with small femoral heads and flaring of the iliac wings. The long bones have diaphyseal splaying and the epiphyses are dysplastic. The phalangeal bones are widened and tapered—described as being "bullet-shaped" (Figure 14-3 a-c). Progressive accumulation of GAGs in other tissues leads to hepato-splenomegaly, clouded cornea, the development of hernias, and a progressive coarsening

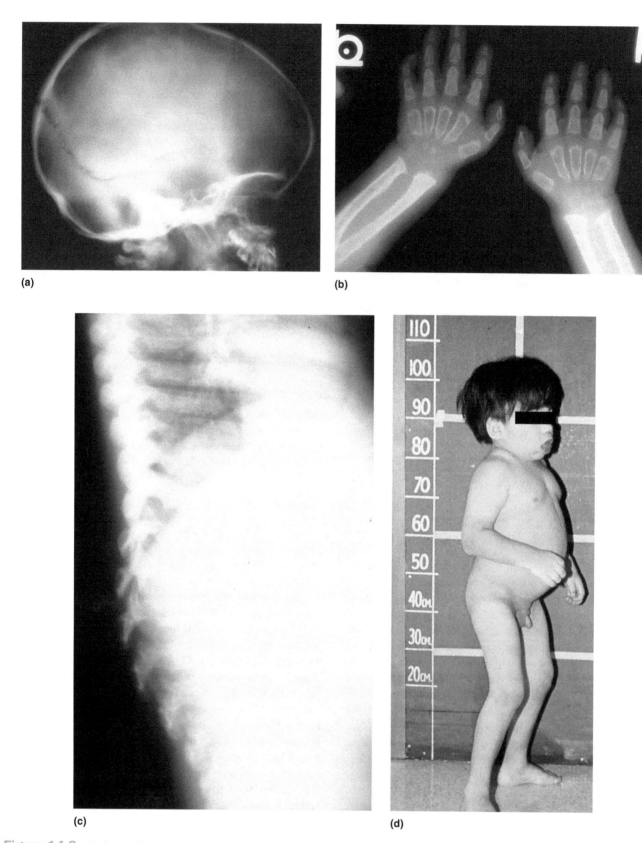

(a)

(b)

(c)

(d)

Figure 14-3. Hurler syndrome. (a-c) X-rays demonstrating dysostosis multiplex (see text for details). (d) Young male with Hurler syndrome prior to the advent of therapeutic options. This patient has advanced signs and symptoms of his disease.

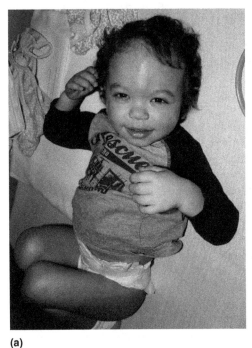
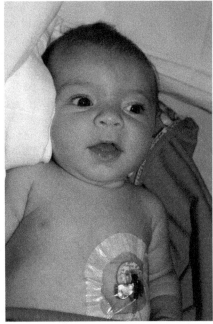

(a)   (b)

Figure 14-4. Siblings with Hurler syndrome (mucopolysaccharidosis type I). (a) A 2½-year-old male post stem cell transplantation. He is doing well and is developmentally normal. (b) The younger female sibling of the boy in (a), diagnosed *in utero* also having Hurler syndrome, with confirmation at birth. She has been on enzyme replacement therapy since the first few weeks of life, and is posttransplantation herself. She has neither physical stigmata nor imaging changes seen in untreated mucopolysaccharide storage disorders.

of facial features (Figure 14-3d). The most serious complication is a progressive neurodegeneration due to abnormal storage of GAGs in the central nervous system. The natural history of Hurler syndrome is neurologic regression and worsening behaviors with an early demise typically in the teenage years.

Early attempts (1960s and 1970s) at treating Hurler syndrome included the surgical placement of pregnancy membranes (i.e., amnion) into the abdomen of these patients. This treatment actually provided some relief—albeit temporary—from the progression of the disorder. Over the past several years, modern approaches to the treatment of Hurler syndrome have emerged (Figure 14-4). Genetically engineered enzyme replacement therapy became available in 2003. Patients treated with this modality receive intravenous infusions every 1 to 2 weeks of the manufactured human enzyme. Thus far the treatment seems to be effective in reducing the accumulation of the GAGs in peripheral tissues. One significant barrier to effective therapy is the delivery of the enzyme across the blood brain barrier. Current clinical trials are under-

way looking at the effectiveness of intrathecal administration of the drug.

Another method of correcting the enzymatic defect is tissue transplantation. Several centers in the United States and Europe offer stem cell transplantation as another method of providing the missing enzyme for Hurler syndrome and other LSDs. Transplantation has the advantage of being a "permanent" method of providing enzyme, but it carries with it the high risk of transplantation and the long-term issues of immune suppression. As with enzyme infusion, the problem with enzyme transfer across the blood-brain barrier remains a complicated issue.

Until the above therapies were developed, the "treatment" of children with Hurler syndrome was largely supportive. The condition was invariably progressive, and the most the geneticist could do was to help the family through the difficult time of watching their child continually get worse. Because Hurler syndrome is progressive, earlier institution of therapy is ideal. Since effective treatments now exist, there is a strong interest in whether effective newborn screening of the condition can be accomplished.

■ Board-Format Practice Questions

1. A child is born with a cleft lip and palate, a congenital heart malformation, and a missing radius. The parents ask you (the attending physician) if gene therapy is an option available for their child. You would answer:
   A. You can refer them now for gene therapy to correct the defects.
   B. Gene therapy is not quite available, but should be available in a couple of years to fix the problems.
   C. Gene therapy is not currently available, but even if it were, it would be unlikely to correct congenital malformations.
   D. Gene therapy is available but cost prohibitive.
   E. Gene therapy is ethically wrong, and you would discourage them from even considering it.

2. You are asked to speak to a civic group in your home community. They want information about "cloning." What would be good information to share with them?

   A. All forms of cloning are morally repugnant and should be outlawed.

   B. Everyone should have a clone of themselves made and preserved in case organ donation is needed in the future.

   C. The exact cloning of an individual is something that will not happen as we are more than just our genes.

   D. The cloning of Dolly the sheep was accomplished with no unexpected complications.

   E. Cloning should not be considered a controversial issue–all major religious and legal organizations have endorsed it.

3. You see a 13-year-old boy in your clinic. He is deeply upset over his size. After you assess the family you note that he has familial short stature, i.e., he is "normally" short. He and his parents ask that he be placed on growth hormone. You would tell them:

   A. Growth hormone is not licensed for normal variant short stature and you cannot treat him.

   B. They should not be worried about his size. It could be worse; he could have a bad disease.

   C. You would be glad to treat him, it is cheap, effective, and can be used for anyone who asks.

   D. It is a good idea to treat him, as it will improve his self-esteem once he gets taller.

   E. Although growth hormone has FDA approval for normal variant short stature, it is expensive, unlikely to be covered by insurance, and may not improve his self-esteem.

4. Case management has always been a part of the service that is provided by geneticists. Which of the following is a true statement about case management for persons with genetic disorders?

   A. Geneticists are the only physicians that can perform such services.

   B. In general the genetics specialist should stay out of case management and leave this function to the primary care provider.

   C. Case management is often improved by the use of interdisciplinary services.

   D. An example of case management would include performing surgery on a patient with a congenital anomaly.

   E. Case management would probably be better if it were handled by insurance companies and their medical reviewers.

5. Options available for the treatment of lysosomal storage disorders, such as Hurler syndrome, would include:

   A. Enzyme replacement therapy.

   B. Chelation of the stored glycosaminoglycans.

   C. Newborn screening.

   D. Dietary reduction of glycosaminoglycans.

   E. Gene correction.

chapter 15

Population Genetics and Genetic Diversity

CHAPTER SUMMARY

A question about inheritance usually focuses on individuals or families. That is not surprising. Individuals are the object of medical concern. Families give us information about the genes they have inherited—and which relatives might, too. But we have already seen how we can learn important information by expanding our perspective to groups of families through pedigrees. Pedigree analysis tells us things about transmission that an individual family with a small number of children might not. New information surfaces. But even single families do not explain many important factors. For example, we cannot quantify the amount of a trait's penetrance from just a single family or even a pedigree of several families. We may be able to find one, or even a few, examples of incomplete penetrance. But that does not tell us how often that event will happen in the population as a whole. Yet, it is on that population frequency that individual predictions depend. We must look at many families in which the trait is segregating. We must use "population thinking."

Every population is highly diverse, but the genetic basis of diversity is not uniformly distributed. Examples are familiar, such as the higher frequency of sickle cell hemoglobin in those with ancestry in some northern African and Mediterranean areas or the X-linked glucose-6-phosphate dehydrogenase deficiency (G6PD, or favism) in those from areas like southern Italy. As our knowledge of genetic differences between one group and another improves, so does our ability to make predictions about individuals in those groups.

Population genetics gives us a quantitative perspective on variation, and new techniques are expanding the field. Analytical approaches like genomics, proteomics, and metabolomics are beginning to make their mark. In this chapter, we will explore some of the ways that knowing about genetic makeup of a population can provide valuable predictive tools, and we will see how these new approaches promise to change the future of genetic assessment. But first, history is also important. Let's take a moment to consider the implications of population thinking in an ethical context. Our example will be a case in which, because of poor understanding of population genetics and even poorer humanitarian concern, authorities caused terrible pain for innocent people.

The story is about a woman who was ordered to undergo sterilization because she was labeled "feebleminded." Carrie Buck (Figure 15-1) was born in 1906 and became pregnant when she was 17 after being raped by a presumed member of her foster family. Perhaps from embarrassment, her foster parents had her committed to the Virginia State Colony for Epileptics and Feebleminded, which took patients for being feebleminded or for displaying unmanageable behavior or promiscuity. Her daughter, Vivian, was born in March 1924. Carrie was the first person ordered to be sterilized under a new Virginia law as part of the state's eugenics program. The case eventually ended in the United States Supreme Court. By an eight to one vote, the Virginia Sterilization Act of 1924 was found not to be in violation of the United States Constitution. There were various factors, including the contention that the Virginia Act was not a punishment and, since it was applied only to those living in a state institution, it did not deny them equal protection under the law. The Supreme Court Justice

Oliver Wendell Holmes, Jr., wrote in the decision, "It is better for all the world, if instead of waiting to execute degenerate offspring for crime, or to let them starve for their imbecility, society can prevent those who are manifestly unfit from continuing their kind. . . . Three generations of imbeciles are enough." Remember, Carrie Buck's only "crime" was being raped by a relative.

Carrie was released soon after her sterilization and eventually married. Her sister, Doris, was also sterilized without her knowledge when hospitalized for appendicitis. She did not find out until many years later, after having tried unsuccessfully to have a child for decades. Carrie's daughter, Vivian, was an average student but died of an intestinal disease when she was only eight. There is no evidence that Carrie, her daughter, or her sister were "feebleminded."

This is a sad story of an individual's mistreatment based on an erroneous understanding of the genetics of populations. When Justice Oliver Wendall Holmes declared that, "Three generations of imbeciles are enough," he implied that removal of affected individuals from the reproductive pool will have a quick, predictable, positive effect. Indeed, in the United States, as elsewhere, the eugenics movement of the late 19th and early 20th century had the goal of improving the genetic composition of our population. By 1935 more than 20,000 people had been forced to undergo "eugenic" sterilization and about 30 states had laws like the one in Virginia. In Hitler's Germany, that doctrine had terrible consequences. Using the American model, about 375,000 people were sterilized just before the start of World War II.

But the scientific logic on which these acts were based was biologically unfounded. It was mathematically wrong. Allele frequencies do not change that quickly. The proof will come in the next section. Hopefully, we can all accept this as a lesson learned, if learned the hard way. Science and medicine can never be separated from bioethical considerations. Nor should they be. None of us are ever very far from ethical questions about how information is discovered, collected, and used. And it is increasingly true that informed, intelligent people are watching and care.

Part 1: Background and Systems Integration

Some important elements of genetic analysis can only be applied when we evaluate the population as a whole. Often this must be done theoretically—at least in part. What we say about a population will seldom allow us to make a concrete prediction about a specific future individual in that population. Instead, it is an argument built on probabilities. But powerful molecular and genetic tools are beginning to help us better understand individual patients and their families. In this section, we will introduce the quantitative approach of these tools.

Allele Frequencies in a Gene Pool

In Chapter 6 on patterns of Mendelian transmission, we used the Punnett square to help visualize the events that can occur at fertilization (Figure 6-4). The Punnett square combines two independent probabilities, i.e., the genetic makeups of an egg nucleus and of a sperm. If the cross is between two heterozygotes ($A\,a$), for example, then the probability of a gamete carrying, say, the A allele is ½, and the probability of the offspring inheriting the A allele from both parents and being $A\,A$ is the product of the individual probabilities, $½ \times ½ = ¼$.

The same approach can be used to predict probabilities of each genotype in a population, with one minor generalization of the Mendelian cross assumptions. In a Mendelian cross, a heterozygous individual ($A\,a$) will have a ½ chance of producing a gamete with the A allele and ½ chance of the a allele. Thus, $p = q = ½$. But in a population, our thinking must expand from looking at the outcomes of a genotype, and instead consider the events that occur in a **gene pool**. The gene pool is a theoretical concept that represents all of the alleles in all of the individuals in the population. In a population, then, we can let p represent the proportion of all A alleles and q all of the a alleles in the gene pool. If these are the only alleles for a given gene, then

$$p + q = 1$$

Although we can expand the algebra to account for more than two alleles (e.g., $p + q + r = 1$), in most cases that is not necessary. Note that, if we know one of these frequencies, say the frequency of a recessive allele $a = 0.21 = q$, then we can directly calculate the frequency of the other, since $p = 1 - q$ and, in this example, $p = 1 - 0.21 = 0.79$. We will see the application of this idea as we explore the ways it is used to model genotype predictions.

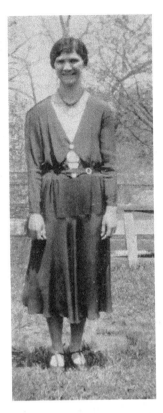

Figure 15-1. Photograph of Carrie Buck a young woman to be sterilized under a state law under the auspice of the state's eugenics program. (Reprinted from Paul B. Popenoe, "The Progress of Eugenic Sterilization," *Journal of Heredity*, 25:1 (1934), 23.)

The Hardy-Weinberg Equilibrium

From the allele frequencies in a population, it is an easy step to predicting the proportions of each genotype, assuming that nothing except normal meiosis and random fertilization are at work. We will use a simple application of the rule of multiplying independent probabilities (Figure 15-2). The assumption is

Male gametes

	R	r
R	$(p^2)\ R\,R$	$(pq)\ R\,r$
r	$(pq)\ R\,r$	$(q^2)\ r\,r$

Female gametes

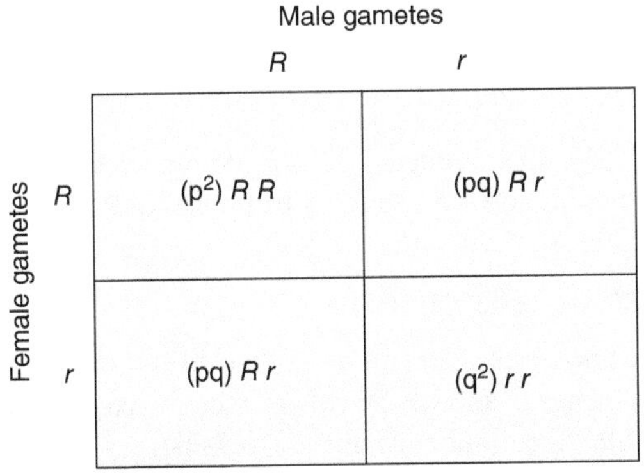

Figure 15-2. The Hardy-Weinberg equilibrium is a simple derivation from the familiar Punnett square, which summarizes all outcomes and their proportions. If we let p be the frequency of the dominant R allele and q be the frequency of the recessive r allele, random associations among gametes in the reproducing gene pool will yield the three genotypes in the proportion $p^2 + 2pq + q^2$.

that gametes with a given allele will combine as a function of the frequency of that allele in the gene pool. If, say, 10% of the alleles are R, then the likelihood that two R alleles will combine at fertilization to produce a $R\,R$ genotype is $0.1 \times 0.1 = 0.01$.

Often the application of this rule works in the reverse. If we know the frequency of a rare recessive condition in the population, the square root of that frequency (q^2) will equal the allele frequency (q). For example, let's say that a recessive condition is found in one child out of 2 500 births, a frequency of 0.0004 in the population. This is q^2, so

$$q = 0.02 \quad \text{and}$$
$$p = 1 - 0.02 = 0.98$$

Most often the frequency of interest is that for heterozygous carriers, $2pq$, since they are phenotypically normal but have a chance of passing the allele to their offspring. In this case, for this example, the frequency of heterozygotes in the population will be

$$2pq = 2\ (0.98)\ (0.02) = 0.0392$$

or about one child in 25 will be heterozygous. Hardy-Weinberg is a simple, but very powerful, predictive tool. The heterozygotes are often hidden among the homozygous dominant members of the population. But their frequency can be estimated if we know how many in the population show the recessive trait. While it is true that advances in biochemical techniques can detect heterozygotes for some important traits, these are not often employed in routine assessments of a family. To sort out these associations, the Hardy-Weinberg relationship is very useful. But it only holds if key assumptions are true.

Hardy-Weinberg Assumptions: A Null Hypothesis for Population Genetics

The Hardy-Weinberg relationship is the null hypothesis of population genetics. By "null hypothesis" we mean the predictions hold if nothing is acting to change the basic process of passing alleles to offspring. It only assumes that meiosis and fertilization are normal and random. But this model has some additional dimensions. An obvious underlying assumption is that the species reproduces sexually. One cannot, therefore, apply these ideas to a human pathogen like bacteria. Another is that individuals are diploid. Some of the consequences of this discussed earlier, such as linkage disequilibrium (Chapter 11), are also relevant when considering the composition of a gene pool. In this chapter we will primarily look at examples involving simple diploid inheritance. Here, of course, there is an important exception: X-linked genes in males. In fact, it is the exceptions to this and other assumptions that make the study of population genetics such a fascinating and complex subject. The general impacts of exceptions are summarized in Table 15-1 and are described more formally in the next several sections. But we will only develop the formal mathematics in a couple of examples.

Table 15-1.	Consequences for Exceptions to the Hardy-Weinberg Equilibrium Assumptions	
Assumption	**Effect on Gene Pool When Assumption Is Not Met**	
Random mating	Inbreeding and assortative mating increase the frequency of homozygotes	
Large population size	Small population size leads to random drift; founder effect is a case of establishing a new population with a small sample from a larger population	
No migration	Migration can bring in alleles from a population with a different frequency	
No mutation	Mutation changes one allele for another	
No selection	Selection is favoring or not favoring a genotype's contribution to the next generation; consequences depend on the strength of selection and its distribution among genotypes	

Effects of Migration

Migration is a good example to show how exceptions can change expected gene frequencies. In this case, they may not change very much. But the point is that the effect of migration can be quantified with a relatively simple mathematical model. You might think that something like migration only relates to animals and plants. But migration among human populations with their regional and ethnic genetic histories will act the same way.

Assume two populations differ in the frequency of an allele (Figure 15-3). In this example, the frequency of the A allele ($p = 0.8$) is higher in the recipient population (r) than in the group providing migrants, where $p = 0.4$. The effect of this difference in allele frequency will be a function of how many migrants (m) move to the recipient population. All of the other alleles in the recipient population ($1 - m$) represent the nonmigrants that stayed in the original population. To see the effect of migration on allele frequency in the next generation, it is traditional to focus on the recessive allele frequency, with q denoting the frequency of the a allele after one generation ($q = 0.2$ in this recipient population and $= 0.6$ in this donor population).

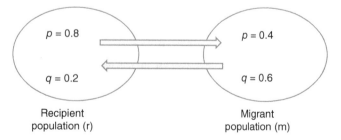

Figure 15-3. An example of migration between two partially separated gene pools, in which the recipient population (r) receives a proportion of migrants (m) from a population having a different frequency of the two alleles.

The frequency of the a allele in the recipient population, r, after migration has occurred will be symbolized q_r'. This new frequency is a function of the proportion of alleles that remain in the recipient population and their frequency, plus the proportion of migrant alleles and their frequency in the donor population:

$$q_r' = q_r (1 - m) + q_m (m) = q_r - m\,q_r + m\,q_m$$

If we let Δq (read "delta q") represent the change in allele frequency for this one generation of migration (i.e., $q_r' - q_r$ is the difference in frequency of the new generation minus the previous generation), we can substitute into the formula and derive the generalized prediction of this migration effect.

$$\begin{aligned} \Delta q &= q_r' - q_r \\ &= q_r - m\,q_r + m\,q_m - q_r \end{aligned}$$

The q_r terms cancel out, since $q_r - q_r = 0$. If we factor migration (m) out of the remaining terms and rearrange them to subtract, this reduces to:

$$\begin{aligned} &= q_r - m\,q_r + m\,q_m - q_r \\ &= -m\,q_r + m\,q_m \\ &= m\,(q_m - q_r) \end{aligned}$$

In other words, the effect of migration is a function of two things: how often does migration occur (m) and what is the difference in allele frequency between the two populations? This is logical. It also shows how relatively straightforward and precise the mathematical relation describing important population dynamics can be. We will not develop the formulae for other exceptions to the Hardy-Weinberg assumptions, except for the important case of selection. Instead, we will simply describe the consequences such processes can have. But all can be formalized in a manner like this.

To complete this specific example, we only need to substitute allele frequencies. For this demonstration, we will let the proportion of migrants, m, be high ($m = 0.10$). The new slightly elevated frequency of a in the recipient population is the original frequency plus the change introduced by the migrants:

$$q_r' = q_r + \Delta q = 0.20 + 0.10\,(0.60 - 0.20) = 0.24$$

Similarly, the frequency of the dominant allele in the recipient population will decrease from 0.80 to 0.76.

Effects of Mutation

Mutation turns one allele into another. Mutation rates vary from one gene to another based on factors like the size of the gene, i.e., the number of nucleotides that can change. So-called **back mutation** can revert a mutant back to the original allele. But back mutation is much less common than the typical **forward mutation**. This makes sense if you consider that there are many points along a gene that can alter its function if changed (i.e., forward mutation). But once changed, there are many fewer ways in which that change can be corrected back to normal.

Mutation rate is a "population" measurement. It applies to individuals, but it occurs with a rate that can only be measured from a group and that can vary due to environmental and other conditions. Even in cases like chemical- or radiation-induced mutation or the insertion of transposable elements into DNA, mutation rates for a gene must be estimated from their population frequencies. But approximations based on cumulative mutation data are generally sufficient for clinical assessments.

Many processes can mask or change a trait's phenotypic expression. That can make it hard to distinguish back mutation from processes like variable expression or incomplete penetrance unless you have DNA sequence data or understand the gene's mechanism of phenotype expression. While back mutation is an uncommon finding in typical medical situations with current assessment techniques, it may become a complicating factor to keep in mind when evaluating DNA sequences as more detailed genetic diagnostic tools become available in the future.

Population Size and Nonrandom Mating

As the size of a population gets smaller, the probability of inbreeding increases. This can have at least two important consequences. First, it can improve the likelihood that a recessive allele is inherited by both parents from some common ancestor. In that case a rare recessive trait is more likely to be expressed. Examples include about 20% of the instances of recessive albinism and xeroderma pigmentosum and 30% to 40% of the occurrences of Tay-Sachs disease in the United States in families with parents who are first cousins. The effect increases with the rarity of the recessive deleterious allele. That is because a rare allele will typically be found only as an occasional heterozygote in the population. But homozygous offspring will increase when related heterozygotes mate.

A second outcome of reduced population size is that variation due to random sampling becomes more significant. This results in genetic drift (Figure 15-4), which is caused by random variation and unpredictability in allele frequencies from one generation to the next. Drifting to complete homozygosity will occur in especially small populations, such as a bottleneck due to severe reductions in population size (Figure 15-5). Earlier, we saw a similar kind of reduction in genetic diversity when we discussed the transmission of mitochondrial mutants during cytoplasmic inheritance (Chapter 13). There a bottleneck in mitochondrial number during oogenesis can significantly change the proportions of normal and affected cells carrying an mtDNA mutation.

Deviations from random mating, such as choosing a mate based on some preferred trait, can also affect genotype frequencies. In small populations like religious enclaves or geographically-isolated groups, there is often little difference between nonrandom mating due to population size and owing to behavioral factors like mate choice. But in most large populations, nonrandom mating like positive assortative mating (mates choosing each other because of similarity in a character) can be important. Instead of changing allele frequencies, assortative mating only changes genotype frequencies. Specifically, it increases the frequencies of both homozygotes.

The effect in an extreme case of inbreeding, complete self-fertilization, is shown in Figure 15-6. The proportion of heterozygotes is halved each generation. In less extreme cases the outcome is similar, but it occurs more slowly. Inbreeding increases homozygosity without changing allele frequencies.

Consequences of Selection

Factors like inbreeding, mutation, and geographic origin may be more important than selection in their influence on many human population events. But selection is still a highly visible population phenomenon, at least theoretically. The Hardy-Weinberg equilibrium assumes no selection. Another way to say this is that each genotype will contribute equivalently to the next generation. Alleles are passed to the next generation

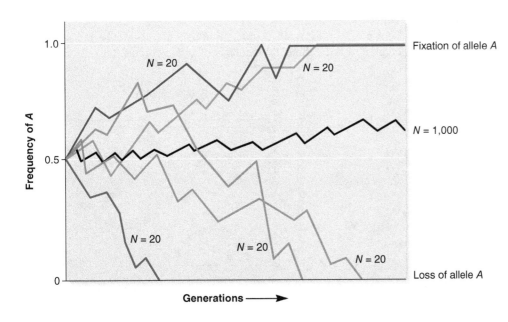

Figure 15-4. Results from a computer simulation of random sampling of alleles over time. When the number of individuals (N) is only 20, random drift changes allele frequencies and can lead to fixation of one or the other allele. When N is large, e.g., 1000, the effect of random sampling does not change the composition of the gene pool beyond minor sampling variation. (Reprinted with permission from Brooker RJ: *Genetics: Analysis & Principles*, 4th ed. New York: McGraw-Hill, 2012.)

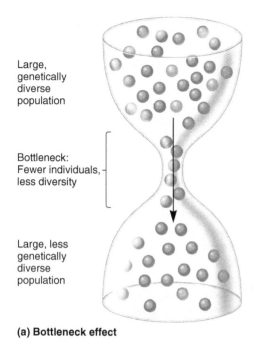

(a) Bottleneck effect

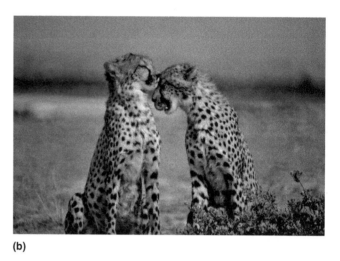

(b)

Figure 15-5. "Bottleneck effect." A decrease in genetic diversity can occur even to the point of complete homozygosity. This may occur due to severe reductions in population size. (a) Hourglass representation. (b) Cheetahs. (a: Reprinted with permission from Brooker RJ: *Genetics: Analysis & Principles*, 4th ed. New York: McGraw-Hill, 2012. b: Photo by Gary M. Stolz, U.S. Fish and Wildlife Service, via Wikimedia Commons.)

as a function of the genotype's frequency, not because it is better favored or more successful than another. But if one trait has an advantage over another, it will make a larger contribution to the next generation. There has been selection for the favored trait, and the alleles that produce it will increase in the next generation's gene pool.

We can illustrate this idea by modeling the case of a recessive lethal genotype. If the homozygous recessive individuals die before reproduction, the Hardy-Weinberg assumption of "no selection" fails to hold. In Figure 6-4, we introduced the Punnett square to show how alleles combine by the product rule to yield all genotypic outcomes in their Mendelian proportions. In Figure 15-2, we relaxed the assumption that $p = q = \frac{1}{2}$. That let us use the Punnett square to demonstrate the foundations of the Hardy-Weinberg equilibrium. Now we will make one more change: the homozygous $r\,r$ die (Figure 15-7). There is

selection in favor of the R allele, carried both in the heterozygotes and in homozygous $R\,R$ individuals.

As in earlier examples, the effect of selection can be modeled quite easily. For this example, the proportion of the three genotypes can initially be predicted from Hardy-Weinberg expectations. For this example, we will let the frequency of the normal dominant allele be 0.9 and the frequency of the recessive lethal allele be 0.1. In practice, a lethal allele would not be that high. But these beginning frequencies will let us see the effect of selection easily. If $R = 0.9$, then $p^2 = 0.81$, and so on.

$$R\,R \quad R\,r \quad r\,r$$
$$p^2 = 0.81 \quad 2pq = 0.18 \quad q^2 = 0.01$$

Now, if all $r\,r$ individuals die or at least fail to reproduce, then the frequency of heterozygotes (the only ones still

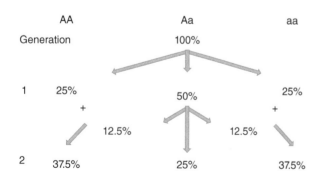

Figure 15-6. The extreme example of inbreeding (self-fertilization). Note that the proportion of heterozygotes is halved with each generation.

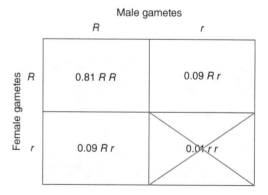

Figure 15-7. Punnett square demonstrating the case of a homozygous ($r\,r$) lethal condition.

carrying the *r* allele and that can transmit it to the next generation) will be:

$$\text{Frequency of } R\,r = 2pq/(p^2 + 2pq)$$

The new frequency of the *r* allele (q') is, therefore:

$$q' = pq/(p^2 + 2pq)$$

Note that we use *pq* here instead of *2pq*, since only half of the alleles inherited from a heterozygote (with a frequency of 2*pq*, see above) will be the recessive allele. Now, if we cancel *p* from both the numerator and denominator, this reduces to:

$$q' = q/(p + 2q)$$

But, since $p + q = 1$, it follows that $p = 1 - q$. We can substitute this value for *p*, so the change in frequency is expressed only in terms of the recessive allele, *q*.

$$q' = q/(1 - q + 2q\,) = q/(1 + q)$$

Again, this is a simple relationship that shows the predicted change in frequency of the lethal recessive allele. Substituting allele frequencies from the problem we began with, the new proportion q' is 0.1/1.1 = 0.0909, and the expected proportion of homozygous recessive individuals in a randomly-mating population the next generation will be q'^2, or 0.0083. The power of selection will rapidly decline as the frequency of the lethal allele gets smaller.

This is a demonstration of straightforward **directional selection**. The population is changed in a beneficial direction, such as increasing the frequency of an allele that gives DDT resistance to a treated agricultural pest (Figure 15-8). But other kinds of selection can also occur and may, in fact, be more common.

Not all selection acts for or against a specific allele. In fact, most traits are well fitted for the survival of the individual and the population. This means that retaining the norm is

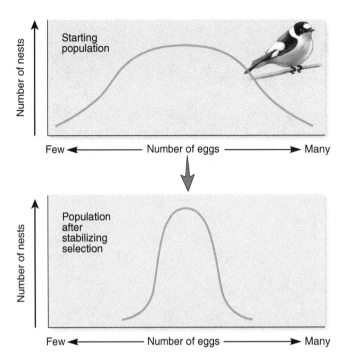

Figure 15-9. Stabilizing selection—favoring the normal or population average in which the specific trait is advantageous. Note the decreased diversity in the population after this type of selection. (Reprinted with permission from Brooker RJ: *Genetics: Analysis & Principles*, 4th ed. New York: McGraw-Hill, 2012.)

good. This kind of selection favoring the normal or population average is called **stabilizing selection** (Figure 15-9). It reduces the variation for a character, since there is selection against survival of both extremes. A classical example is birth weight in newborn babies, in which there is reduced survival of newborns who are significantly below or above the population average birth weight.

There is a slightly more complex, but still easily understood, kind of selection that can act on traits. **Diversifying selection** occurs when more than one trait is favored in a population because the habitat conditions are diverse or variable (Figure 15-10). The color changes seen for industrial melanism of moths in England is a visually concrete example. Although some discussions of this classic case describe it as directional selection, they are simply focusing attention on what occurred in a single habitat. But it is more informative to consider the different selection pressures found at different locations within the whole distribution of the species in England. Not all portions of its range were exposed to the same environmental change.

Many animals evolved melanism in response to the environmental effects of the British industrial revolution in the mid- to late-1800s. For scalloped hazel moths, the light speckled form was the most common until coal-fired factories began to dump large amounts of heavy-metal-laden smoke into the atmosphere. In the humid British climate, this rained down as heavy metal pollution and killed the light-colored lichens on tree trunks in the industrialized part of the country. The transition from light to melanic forms can, in fact, be documented

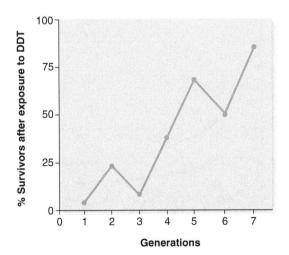

Figure 15-8. Directional selection demonstrated in survivors after DDT exposure. Note the increase in the percent of survivors with each passing generation. (Reprinted with permission from Brooker RJ: *Genetics: Analysis & Principles*, 4th ed. New York: McGraw-Hill, 2012.)

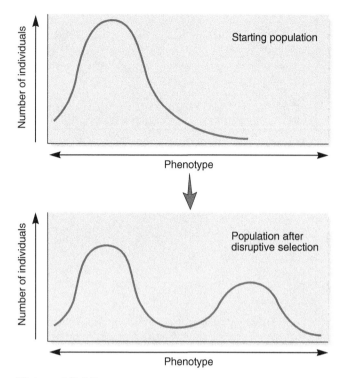

Figure 15-10. Diversifying selection occurs when more than one trait is favored in a population because the habitat conditions are diverse or variable. The bottom graph demonstrates two prevalent phenotypes after selection has occurred. (Reprinted with permission from Brooker RJ: *Genetics: Analysis & Principles*, 4th ed. New York: McGraw-Hill, 2012.)

quite accurately by looking at the moth and butterfly collections kept by wealthy landowners throughout the 19th century. A melanic mutant scalloped hazel moth was a rare prize until the industrial revolution.

Consider two contrasting habitats: tree bark covered with light-colored lichens in rural woodlands and the dark bark remaining after sensitive lichens had been killed by industrial pollution. Birds prey visually on resting moths. In clean rural forests, predators can easily see a dark moth against the lighter lichen-covered tree trunk. The spotted form is hidden and has a higher survival rate. The opposite is found in the industrialized midlands, where the loss of lichens left dark bark backgrounds exposed. Melanic moths blended better and avoided predation. Across the species range, therefore, the frequencies of the two forms differed as a function of the pollution conditions affecting lichen survival and, thus, on the differing colored backgrounds against which the moths rested and the birds hunted. No single trait was uniformly favored. It depended on environmental conditions. This, in fact, was one of the first well-documented examples of a change in allele frequency due to selection in a natural population. Many similar examples are now known. Interestingly, the light form of the scalloped hazel moth is increasing in frequency now that better air quality standards are in place and lichens are returning.

Selection is one of those genetic phenomena we are aware of intellectually. It has, of course, given us a wide range of pet dog and cat breeds. But we also tend to take it

for granted as relatively unimportant to our own species. Are humans affected by directional selection, stabilizing selection, or diversifying selection? How common are they? For us, it is hard to say. The effects of population phenomena are often measured over decades or centuries. On a more manageable scale, however, these processes have a major impact on variables like pathogen virulence. There is, in fact, a whole medical specialty devoted to exploring "evolutionary medicine." Our environment is both naturally variable each season and changing over time globally. We probably override much of the natural selection pressure on us by controlling our habitat (e.g., living in climate-controlled houses) and by promoting good health care. But as a natural process, selection is worth keeping in mind. It certainly affects the animal and plant species—and the pathogens—around us.

Diploidy and the Special Case of Sex-linked Genes

In its common form, the Hardy-Weinberg model assumes that genotypes are diploid. But there is an important exception that we discussed earlier, sex-linked genes in males. This exception actually has a mathematically simple result. Since males have only one X chromosome, the frequency of a sex-linked condition in males must equal its frequency in the gene pool (q). Its frequency in females would be the square, q^2. Thus, sex-linked recessive conditions are expressed much more often in males than in females. To be specific, the frequency in males (q) is the square root of the frequency in females (q^2).

Revisiting the Case of Carrie Buck

In the introduction to this chapter, we presented the case of Carrie Buck, one of those sterilized in an attempt to reduce the frequency of so-called "feeblemindedness" in the population.

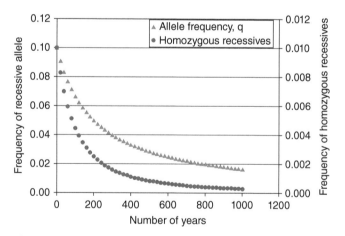

Figure 15-11. Graph demonstrating the effect over time of a recessive allele when the homozygous individuals are "genetic lethal." The proportion of homozygous recessive individuals, q^2, will become vanishingly small but eventually selection pressure fades away. However, a significant number of the targeted allele still remains for an extended time in the population gene pool.

But now applying our knowledge of allele frequencies and selection, we can make the lesson even more concrete. In the hereditary sense, sterilization is biologically equivalent to death. No offspring are produced by that genotype. Consider the analysis we did earlier for selection against a recessive lethal allele. As the frequency of the recessive, q, declines, most alleles will be carried in heterozygotes, $2pq$. The proportion of homozygous recessive individuals, q^2, will become vanishingly small and selection pressure fades away (Figure 15-11). But large numbers of the targeted allele still remain for a long time in the gene pool.

For feeblemindedness, the anticipated outcome of the eugenics movement was fundamentally flawed. While this is a mistake we hope will never happen again, we must remember that population genetics, indeed every aspect of genetics, is not just an intellectual exercise. It can have real consequences for real people.

Part 2: Medical Genetics

In this section, we will use the population perspective to explore some of its medical applications. But we will also look into the future. Advances in biotechnology are rapidly adding tools that change the way we can respond to genetic conditions. When the information about a patient includes a genetic profile, the questions and answers may become more complex. But they also become more precise. Added to this, we continue to learn a lot about our own biology from other organisms. The fruit fly, *Drosophila*, for example, has always been a centerpiece of genetic research. Some of the insights that have come from model organisms will be a key focus of the final chapter. There is no question that new insights that are coming from biotechnology and model organisms are improving our ability to understand and respond to medical questions faced by all of us.

Why Are Some Mutations So Frequent?

There are many reasons why some mutations are more frequent than others. From the population view, one of the most obvious is that a genetic difference—a "mutation" in the sense of simply being different from other common forms of the gene—may have such a minor effect on the phenotype that selection against it is relatively weak. Alternatively, one gene form may be better adapted to one environment or to one developmental context than another. Industrial melanism discussed in Part 1 is one example. Selection favors one allele in one region or at one time but favors a different allele at another.

But there are other situations that may have more direct medical or diagnostic significance. One example is a **founder effect**. Essentially, a founder effect is a form of sampling variation with consequences similar to genetic drift and bottlenecks discussed earlier. Indeed, the main difference among these processes is their cause, not so much their outcome. As the name suggests, a founder effect is due to establishing a new population with a small number of founders from a larger, more genetically diverse population. The founders will carry only a small sample of the alleles in the original gene pool and the frequency of these alleles can vary by chance. If this event is followed by some degree of inbreeding, which would be typical, then the probability of having otherwise rare recessive conditions appear in the group will be high. One example is the Kel Kummer Tuareg, a small group in the Sahara Desert that traces its origin to 156 founders about

300 years ago. Their ancestry is complex, and each pair of current members shares about 15 common ancestors. Essentially all of the current gene pool of the group traces back to just 25 individuals. Clearly, a patient's ancestral history can be valuable information.

Another mechanism for maintaining higher than expected frequencies of alternative alleles is that the heterozygote is better fit than either homozygote. **Heterozygous advantage** will cause the heterozygous individuals to make a larger contribution to the next generation gene pool than predicted by the Hardy-Weinberg equilibrium, thus maintaining both alleles.

Sickle Cell Anemia and Protection from Malaria: An Example of Heterozygous Advantage

Sickle cell anemia is a serious condition we discussed earlier. It is often found is those tracing their lineage to southern Europe and Africa. At amino acid position 6 of the β-chain of hemoglobin, the amino acid glutamic acid is replaced by valine. Those with sickle cell trait are heterozygous for the condition and can show some sickling of the red blood cells (RBCs). Those with sickle cell disease (the homozygotes) have hemoglobin that readily crystallizes in low oxygen tension, such as at high elevations or following strenuous exercise. Red blood cells become distorted and less flexible. For that reason, those with sickle cell disease have a high frequency of capillary blockages, often with devastating effects on blood supply to key organs. But this condition is also closely associated with a completely different phenomenon, malaria.

The malarial protozoan parasite, *Plasmodium falciparum*, is transferred among endothermic ("warm-blooded") hosts like humans by the mosquito, *Anopheles*. Both those homozygous and heterozygous for the sickle cell allele, $Hb\beta^S$, have a partial protection from infection, because the sickle RBCs break apart or lyse before the parasite has been able to reproduce. Those without the sickle cell gene have a 2- to 3-fold higher likelihood of becoming infected. This is an excellent example of heterozygous advantage: maintaining both alleles in the population because of the advantage of the heterozygotes due to the occurrence of malaria in the environment (selecting against the normal hemoglobin homozygotes that are more susceptible to malaria) and the sickle cell disease (selecting against those homozygous for the sickle cell allele).

Other Examples of Heterozygous Advantage

While the heterozygote advantage of malaria and sickle cell disease is one of the most cited and best understood, there are other such examples. We have discussed cystic fibrosis (CF) several times in this book (see Chapter 4 including Figure 4-21). Clinically CF is characterized by pancreatic insufficiency and chronic progressive pulmonary disease. The pathogenesis of the disorder is related to the causative gene—CFTR. The CFTR gene is a chloride transport gene that functions primarily in exocrine cells. The pancreatic and pulmonary problems are due to inspissated mucous in these organs because of hyperviscosity of the mucous secondary to increased chloride concentrations in the mucous (due to the transport defect). Homozygotes for CF have a progressive lethal condition. Cystic fibrosis occurs in a high frequency in Caucasians of northern European descent. The carrier frequency for pathogenic CF mutations in this population is around 1 in 20. This high frequency is also suspected to be due to heterozygote advantage. It has been postulated that carriers of CF (with presumably subclinical differences in ion transport) are more resistant to the severe secretory diarrhea in cholera. Thus carriers of CF were more likely to survive the great epidemics in Europe in the 19th century. This then led to an increased frequency of CF mutations in this population and their descendants. The calculated heterozygote advantage for a mutant allele to reach equilibrium at a carrier frequency of 1:20 is around 2%.

Smith-Lemli-Opitz syndrome (SLOS) is a multiple anomaly syndrome associated with a defect in the terminal stage of cholesterol synthesis (see Chapter 8 including Figures 8-5 and 8-6). The carrier frequency of SLOS is estimated to be as high as 1/30. However, the observed incidence of SLOS is between 1/20,000 and 1/60,000. Based on the carrier frequency, the incidence should be 1/3600. This discrepancy has been suggested to be due to *in utero* loss and/or unrecognized milder cases. Given the high carrier frequency of SLOS, heterozygote advantage with founder effect has been proposed. It is postulated that the advantage to carriers is due to better vitamin D synthesis.

Heterozygote Disadvantage

It is important to note that not all mutations are advantageous as heterozygotes (carriers). Homocystinuria (HC) is an autosomal recessive disorder associated abnormalities in amino acid metabolism (see Chapter 8). The condition is genetically heterogeneous. The most common cause of HC is a deficiency in the enzyme cystathione-beta-synthase (CBS). Symptoms of HC include a Marfanoid body habitus, mental retardation, and lens dislocations (Figure 8-7b). The condition is genetically heterogeneous. The common biochemical features are elevated plasma homocysteine levels with subsequent increased homocysteine in the urine, from which the condition derives its name. Elevated homocysteine in the blood is toxic to the vascular endothelium, which potentiates the lipoprotein LDL and which leads to increased platelet adhesion. Thus a major part of the pathogenesis of the condition is the occurrence of micro-emboli and the resultant problems associated with the vascular occlusion.

The carrier frequency (heterozygotes) of CBS deficiency is 0.3% to 1%. As a group, heterozygotes for CBS deficiency have normal fasting plasma homocysteine levels, but they often have increased urine concentrations. Some, but not all, will show elevated homocysteine levels in response to a methionine load. Hyper-homocysteinemia is a well-documented independent risk factor for cardiovascular disease. Likewise, increased post-load plasma homocysteine concentrations are a risk factor for vascular disease and neural tube defects. There remains significant debate in a large body of literature as to the relative overall contribution of CBS deficiency to the epidemiology of vascular disease. Regardless, the overriding concept is that carriers are at increased risk for medical problems, not at a genetic advantage.

Assessment of Human Genetic Diversity: The HapMap Example

In earlier chapters we referred to some of the initiatives that are taking place to improve genetic mapping and interpretation. One of these is the HapMap Project. It focuses on linked groups of genes, or haplotypes, that are marked by a unique single nucleotide polymorphism (SNP). Rather than trying to track the 10 million or so individual SNPs tied to all regions of the genome, the use of representative tag SNPs reduces the analysis to about 500,000 sites. This is just one example of the advances in genetic technology that will contribute to deciphering the genetic bases of heritable conditions.

The Impact of Changing Technology: Genomics-Proteomics-Metabolomics

It was not long ago that words like proteomics and metabolomics would have been nonsense. Now they are specialties with their own journals and professional organizations. Working in a field that is changing as rapidly as medicine, a physician will always be in one sense a medical student. Advances in genetic technology share a lot with the advances in population genetics. Both must think in terms of systems, not just individuals. A genome is not simply about *A* and *a* alleles or about expression of homozygotes versus heterozygotes. Instead, genotypes are at the core of a multilevel biochemical system.

The developing field of **genomics** is concerned with determining the DNA sequence of a species. The first successes were sequencing the 5368 bp genome of a virus, ϕX-174, and of a mitochondrion by Fred Sanger in the 1970s and 1980s. With this work, he and his group developed the first sequencing, data handling, and analysis tools that later work built upon. The first complete organismal genome was of *Haemophilus influenzae* in 1995. With the completion of the 13-year Human Genome Project in 2003, the technologies it developed are now being applied to sequencing genomes from other species. This allows comparisons of gene function to be made across the living spectrum.

For some the term "genomics" has now taken on a broader meaning to include not only the DNA sequence but also functions associated with it. Functional genomics focuses on the dynamics of gene and protein activities and interactions. Rather than simply annotating DNA sequences, this field explores gene transcription and translation as well as the interactions that occur between genes and proteins and in protein-protein interactions. In a similar but more medically targeted way, **pharmacogenetics** (sometimes now called pharmacogenomics) is a specialized branch of pharmacology that explores individual differences in response to drugs and environmental chemicals.

The focus of **transcriptomics** is slightly more narrow. Only a tiny percentage of the DNA in humans is transcribed. As complex as the genome is, it has the advantage of being relatively stable from one cell or one individual to another. In contrast, whereas the human genome may have 20- or 30,000 genes, there are probably more than 2 million different proteins produced during a lifetime. This is accomplished by post-translational modification and related processes we discussed in earlier chapters. Each of these proteins has a different function and participates in a wide array of catalytic reactions, as cell structural components, in trophic growth signaling, neurotransmission, defending the body against disease, and so forth. **Proteomics** is the study of these proteins and their functions.

The term "proteomics" is drawn from PROTEin and the genOME. The protein profiles differ from cell type to type and from one time in development to another. Factors that go beyond mRNA translation include various forms of post-translational modification like phosphorylation, ubiquitination, methylation, glycosylation, and other modifications. At a more complex level, each of these must be considered in terms of their protein-protein interactions. When we think of the functioning of the body, proteomics can give us a better understanding than can a study of the genome alone. By looking just at the genome, we have no idea how often a gene is transcribed or how stable will be its mRNA or its protein product. On the other hand, proteins are not easy to study, especially when present in low amounts or for short periods. At this time, therefore, proteomic studies often suffer from reproducibility problems that limit their predictive strength. Part of this limitation is, of course, the fact that proteins are being modified. So the dynamic process and its inherent limitation are intertwined.

But proteins are not end points. At a more functional level of cell biochemistry, **metabolomics** is the study of metabolites produced by cellular processes. The genome and proteome offer a profile of the controlling processes, and the metabolome documents the end products of their activity. Its tools include nuclear magnetic resonance (NMR) spectroscopy and mass spectrometry. The first metabolomics web database, METLIN, now contains information on over 40,000 human metabolites. Parallel studies are also being done in several plant species.

Metagenomics is the analysis of genomes from material collected from an environmental sample. Traditional techniques have missed many of the species living in a habitat, and this field is providing a new look at microbial diversity. Since samples are sequenced directly from natural collections, there is no requirement that an organism be cultured, a limitation that had kept the vast majority of microbial organisms from being discovered and studied. One of the earliest such projects was led by Craig Venter, a pioneer in sequencing the human genome. Analyzing samples from the Sargasso Sea, DNA was found from almost 2000 different species including almost 150 new types of bacteria. Because of the medical importance of bacteria, metagenomics is now being used to profile the microbial communities from numerous body sites in several hundred representative people in the Human Microbiome Initiative.

Personal Genomics

We carry our genetic heritage with us. For some conditions, knowing the geographic "origin" of a patient may give useful insights comparable to knowing whether a patient has traveled recently to areas where infectious disease is endemic. There is increasing availability of commercial sources for a person to gain their genome profile. Sometimes this can have a clearly beneficial outcome, such as selecting the best drug option for an individual physiology. But our knowledge of drug × physiology interactions is just in its infancy. So this is a new frontier. An associated issue is the potential for discrimination based on genetic profiles.

Let's step back for a moment. Why have we chosen to bring these developing areas of genetics into a discussion of populations? We hope the answer is fairly obvious. Population genetics and the developing fields in molecular biology all share a focus on systems. They try to understand systems of alleles or individuals in a population, systems of proteins, systems of metabolic interactions, and ultimately systems of . . . , well, systems. But as impressive as the growth of medical genetics is in understanding all these levels, the most promising realization is rather simpler. The more we know about the complexity of genetic control of development and function, the better able we are to diagnose and respond to the conditions faced by an individual patient.

Tracking Populations by Genes

The advent of molecular genetic technologies has provided powerful and exciting tools for use in tracking populations and their relationships. Many polymorphisms exist between individuals and among populations. The exclusive maternal inheritance of the mitochondrial genome provides a method for tracking maternal lineage over long periods of time. Analyses of mitochondrial polymorphisms analyses have provided fascinating insights into human populations (Figures 15-12 and 15-13). One of the most amazing observations in these studies has been how well the DNA data correlate with earlier archaeological, anthropological, and linguistic predictions.

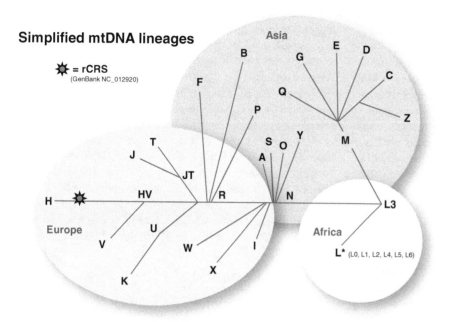

Figure 15-12. Diagram showing lineages based on mitochondrial DNA (mtDNA) polymorphisms. (Image from MITOMAP: A human mitochondrial genome database. Available at http://www.mitomap.org. Image is licensed by a Creative Commons Attribution 3.0 license.)

Similar studies have been done with polymorphisms on the Y chromosome that exclusively track paternal lineages.

DNA Sequencing of Model Organisms

One of the surprising results to come from sequencing many species is that we share a significant part of our genetic background. Population genetics was founded on the study of genes in moths, fruit flies, and snails. The genetic information from model organisms offers an insight into biology that parallels that from advances in technology. The biological similarities among animals will help us understand ourselves better. We explore this in the final chapter.

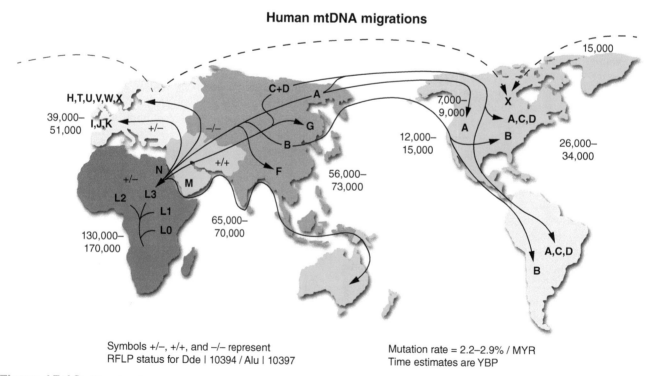

Figure 15-13. Map showing the hypothesized migration of human populations based on mtDNA analysis. (Image from MITOMAP: A human mitochondrial genome database. Available at http://www.mitomap.org. Image is licensed by a Creative Commons Attribution 3.0 license.)

Part 3: Clinical Correlation

Noonan syndrome (Figure 15-14) is an autosomal dominant syndrome characterized by dysmorphic facial features (hypertelorism, down-slanting palpebral fissures, and low-set/posteriorly rotated ears). Other features seen in Noonan syndrome include short stature, a short neck (with or without webbing), cardiac anomalies (especially pulmonic stenosis), epicanthal folds, neurosensory hearing loss, developmental delay, and a bleeding diathesis. Noonan syndrome is genetically heterogeneous with at least 11 genes now known to be associated with the condition (Table 15-2).

Neurofibromatosis type I (Figure 15-15) is an autosomal dominant disorder which exhibits complete penetrance with a wide range of variability in its expression. It is characterized by the increased propensity to develop a variety of benign and malignant tumors. Neurofibromas, from which the condition gets its name—originate from nonmyelinating Schwann cells and are among the most common tumors seen in these patients. Other tumor types reported include CNS tumors (optic gliomas and meningiomas among others), endocrine tumors, and sarcomas. Patients with neurofibromatosis I also have a variety of dermatologic findings such as hyper-pigmented macules (designated as "cafe-au-lait spots") and freckling in abnormal locations such as the axillary or inguinal regions. Other cardinal features are the presence of iris hamartomas, or Lisch

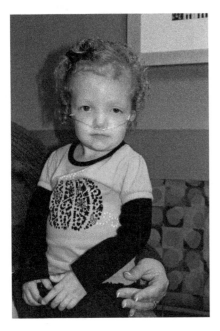

Figure 15-14. A young girl with Noonan syndrome. This child has a mutation in a gene known as KRAS. Noonan syndrome has significant genetic heterogeneity with at least 11 known genes associated with the condition.

Table 15-2.	Genes Associated with Noonan Syndrome
PTPN11 (50% of cases)	
BRAF	
CBL	
HRAS	
KRAS	
MAP2K1	
MAP2K2	
NRAS	
RAF1	
SHOC2	
SOS1	

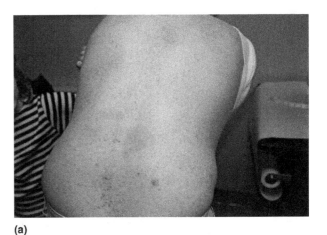

(a)

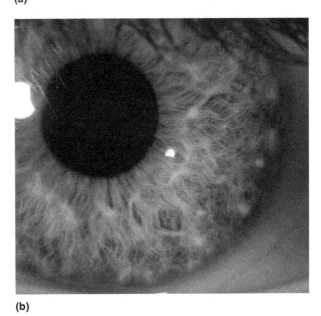

(b)

Figure 15-15. Adult male with neurofibromatosis type I. (a) Back of the patient demonstrating multiple hyperpigmented macules and tumors (neurofibromas) (b) Hamartomas of the iris (Lisch nodules) which are a characteristic feature of neurofibromatosis type I.

nodules, and bony dysplasias. Neurofibromatosis 1 is caused by mutations in the gene *neurofibromin* at chromosome location17q11.2. *Neurofibromin* functions as a tumor suppressor gene involved in the RAS signal transduction pathway.

Both Noonan syndrome and neurofibromatosis are established conditions with well-delineated phenotypes and diagnostic criteria. Over time clinicians have described a number of patients who have features overlapping both conditions. Noonan-neurofibromatosis syndrome is a condition described in patients with neurofibromatosis who also have manifestations of Noonan syndrome, such as short stature, characteristic facial features, and pulmonic stenosis (Figure 15-16). A similar condition is Watson syndrome. The two major features of Watson syndrome are pulmonic stenosis and cafe-au-lait spots. Patients with Watson syndrome may also have cognitive impairments and short stature. Most patients have macrocephaly. Many have Lisch nodules and/or neurofibromas. Molecular genetic studies have now shown that these three conditions are allelic—all being caused by mutations in the *neurofibromin* gene.

Further investigation into the relationship between Noonan syndrome and neurofibromatosis I has shown a molecular link. As mentioned earlier, the *neurofibromin* gene

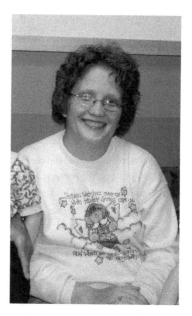

Figure 15-16. Adult female with neurofibromatosis with a confirmed *neurofibromin* mutation. Note the craniofacial features which are typical of those seen in Noonan syndrome.

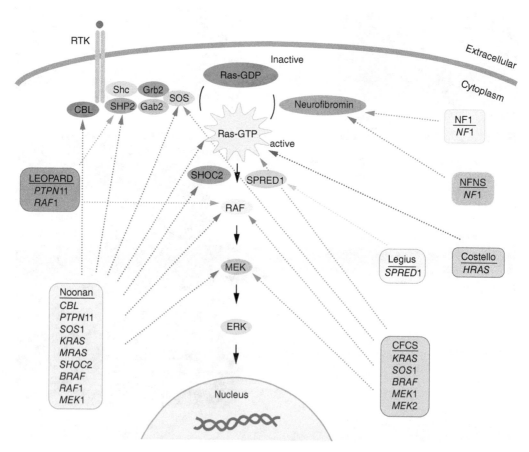

Figure 15-17. Diagram of the RAS-MAPK signal induction pathway. The multiple syndromes (RASopathies) and their associated genes are noted in the boxed areas. (Adapted from Ekvall S, Hagenas L, Allanson J, et al. "Co-occurring SHOC2 and PTPN11 mutations in a patient with severe/complex Noonan syndrome-like phenotype." *Am J Med Genet A.*, 155(6): 1217-24, 2011.)

modulates the RAS oncogene. The genes that are associated with Noonan syndrome have also been shown to be involved in the same signaling pathway. Likewise, several other conditions with phenotypes that also overlap with Noonan syndrome and/or neurofibromatosis have been shown to be involved in this pathway as well. These include Costello syndrome, cardio-facial-cutaneous syndrome, Legius syndrome, and multiple **l**entigines, **e**lectrocardiographic conduction abnormalities, **o**cular hypertelorism, **p**ulmonic stenosis, **a**bnormal genitalia, **r**etardation of growth, and sensorineural **d**eafness (LEOPARD) syndrome.

Thus at the level of metabolomics, all of these conditions are related. In fact they represent a *family* of disorders linked by their involvement in the RAS signaling pathway (Figure 15-17). Collectively they have now been termed the RASopathies based on this central shared pathogenesis. As more is understood about the molecular basis of human disorders, the list of these genetic families continues to grow accordingly.

■ Board-Format Practice Questions

1. Assume that a population is in Hardy-Weinberg equilibrium and the frequency of a rare autosomal recessive disease allele is q, then the frequency of disease carriers can be estimated as:
   A. p^2
   B. q^2
   C. $2pq$
   D. $2q$
   E. $2(1-p)$

2. Mr and Mrs Smith have come to your clinic. Mrs Smith is 9 weeks pregnant and has a sister with cystic fibrosis (CF), an autosomal recessive disease. They are concerned about whether their baby will also be born with the same disease. Mr and Mrs Smith are Caucasian (incidence for CF is 1 in 2500). What is the probability that Mrs Smith is a carrier of CF?
   A. 1/2
   B. 1/4
   C. 2/3
   D. 1/25
   E. 1/50

3. It is recognized that parents and children share ½ (half) of their genes and that siblings share ½ (half) of their genes. Which one of the following is the correct number of shared genes for first cousins?
   A. 1/8
   B. 1/16
   C. 1/32
   D. 1/64
   E. 1/128

4. Hemochromatosis is a disorder associated with iron overload. It is an autosomal recessive condition. It is caused by mutations in a gene called HFE. It is one of the most common human single gene disorders occurring in about 1 in 256 individuals of northern European descent. What then is the approximate carrier frequency of hemochromatosis in the northern European population?
   A. 1 in 2
   B. 1 in 8
   C. 1 in 50
   D. 1 in 100
   E. 1 in 256

5. One possible reason that certain mutations occur frequently in a given population would be:
   A. Heterozygote advantage.
   B. Heterozygote disadvantage.
   C. Foundation efforts.
   D. Random mating.
   E. Low mutation rate.

16 Of Fruit Flies, Mice, and Patients: Tying It All Together

CHAPTER SUMMARY

In this, the final chapter of this book, we have come full circle. The major themes that we promised we would cover have been woven throughout the chapters. To complete this process we will revisit and expand on several important themes:

1. Unity and diversity: the genetic continuity of life as evidenced in model organisms.

2. Genetic and etiological heterogeneity

3. Genotype × phenotype associations

4. Pathogenesis: how do changes in DNA translate into disease?

The Human Genome Project and developing fields like proteomics give us unprecedented detail about the primary products of genetic coding. But we have seen how hard it often is to relate protein-coding genes to phenotypes, because of posttranslational processing and other events. Studies of model organisms can help direct our understanding of this complexity. In the next section, we will describe some of the experimental advantages of a select group of model genetic organisms and identify some of the key insights that have so far come from work with them.

This chapter will, therefore, be organized a little differently than the ones before it. We begin with *Drosophila*, not because it is the simplest, but because it is one of the first and most influential non-vertebrate models of genetic organization and function. Other important model organisms will then be introduced. We will discuss different mechanisms of pathogenesis.

Finally, we will see how advances in medical genetics promise to continue altering the face of medicine and the treatment of human genetic conditions.

Part 1: Bacteria, Fruit Flies, Mice, Fish: The Value of Model Organisms

The common fruit fly was one of the first organisms used to explore the mechanisms of inheritance. It became a model for the study of transmission genetics. In fact, some of the genetic insights from work with *Drosophila* are so fundamental that it is easy to take them for granted. But research with model organisms has continued to add dramatically to understanding our own genetics and development. A model organism offers some advantages—a known or small genome, simple develop, or easy rearing for mating studies and identification of mutations. *Escherichia coli*, yeast, round worms, and even simple plants allow us to see into the common genetic processes that are shared by all forms of life.

Most of the important discoveries that are the foundation of medical genetics could not have been made in humans. Fundamental genetic mechanisms often require large numbers of replications, controlled genotypes and environments, experimental manipulation of the genome or the developmental pathways each controls, and the use of tools like mutagenesis. Even when not outright illegal, these would be far too complex and time-consuming to apply to human families and populations. Thus, to ignore the contributions that model organisms have made to understanding human genetics is very shortsighted. Simple animals allow us to study in depth the many biological processes we share with them, and for those critical insights they deserve our respect.

Table 16-1.	Some Nobel Prizes for Genetic Research Using Model Organisms With General Applicability to Humans		
Year	**Awardees**	**Organism**	**Primary Contribution**
1933	T.H. Morgan	*Drosophila melanogaster*	Discoveries concerning the role played by the chromosomes in heredity
1946	H.J. Muller	*Drosophila melanogaster*	Discovery of the production of mutations by x-ray irradiation
1958	G.W. Beadle, E.L. Tatum, and J. Lederberg	*Neurospora crassa* *Escherichia coli*	Discovery that genes act by regulating definite chemical events; Gene organization and recombination in bacteria
1965	F. Jacob, A. Lwoff, and J. Monod	*Escherichia coli*	Genetic control of enzymes and virus synthesis
1983	B. McClintock	*Zea mays*	Discovery of mobile genetic elements
1995	E.B. Lewis, C. Nüsslein-Volhard, and E.F. Wieschaus	*Drosophila melanogaster*	Genetic control of early embryonic development
2001	L.H. Hartwell, R.T. Hunt, and P.M. Nurse	*Saccharomyces cerevisiae* *Schizosaccharomyces pombe* *Arbacia* (sea urchins)	Discoveries about key regulators of the cell cycle
2002	S. Brenner, H.R. Horvitz, and J.E. Sulston	*Caenorhabditis elegans*	Genetic regulation of organ development and programmed cell death
2006	A.Z. Fire and C.C. Mello	*Caenorhabditis elegans*	Discovery of gene silencing or RNA interference by double-stranded RNA
2007	M.R. Capecchi, M.J. Evans, and O. Smithies	*Mus musculus*	Introduction of specific gene modifications in mice by embryonic stem and cells
2009	E.H. Blackburn, C.W. Greider, J.W. Szostak	*Tetrahymena*	Discovery of the way chromosomes are protected by telomeres and and telomerase
2012	J.B. Gurdon and S. Yamanaka	*Xenopus laevis* *Mus musculus*	Discovery that mature cells can become pleuripotent again after programming

Some examples of Nobel Prize winning genetic contributions using model organisms are shown in Table 16-1. The work of Thomas Hunt Morgan on basic transmission genetics earned the prize for defining the role of chromosomes in heredity. His experimental organism was *Drosophila*. Its ease of culture, special developmental characteristics like giant polytene (or **endoduplicated**) chromosomes, and the collection of mutations affecting all elements of development allowed *Drosophila melanogaster* to become the experimental model of choice. Using *Drosophila*, processes like the mutagenic effect of X-rays and the way genes control early embryonic steps in development were discovered. Similarly, the defined number of cells and the strict lineage of cell differentiation in the nematode *Caenorhabditis elegans* illustrated how science can draw general insights from the special characteristics of a model organism.

A unifying concept here, indeed in all of biology, is "homology. " This biological term refers to the similarities found in structure or function due to shared derivation from a common ancestor. What we learn from model organisms often has a revolutionary impact on our understanding of our own species. The discovery of transposable elements in maize, chromosomal telomeres in *Tetrahymena* and yeast, and even the way that the genes in bacteria and molds control biochemical pathways illustrate the importance of model organisms. It is a significant theme, because it typifies the direction that biomedical research must continue to take for the future.

Model organisms are exactly that—they are models. But models are only useful to the extent that they give an insight into general processes or to the mechanisms at work in a system of prime interest, like human biology and development. Model organisms like *Drosophila*, *C. elegans*, and the others help us understand the general rules of genetic regulation that remind us about the continuity of life. When T.H. Morgan first began to study gene organization on *Drosophila* chromosomes, he could have had no idea that a discovery like the homeobox genes, which specify key elements of body organization in *Drosophila*, would open new avenues to understanding the developmental architecture of all organisms. Indeed, the so-called "bottom line" is that experimental research on model organisms will continue to be critically important for future advances in human genetics, because we share with all organisms a major part of our biological heritage.

The Common Fruit Fly, *Drosophila melanogaster*—Historical Contributions and its Continuing Importance as a Genetic Model

A landmark in the history of genetics was the discovery of a white-eyed mutation in a culture of *Drosophila* being used by T.H. Morgan to study population growth dynamics. This event began a long history in which *Drosophila* has been used to explore many fundamental mechanisms of genetics. Genetic research is now stimulated by the extensive mutation collections of resource centers and the experimental innovation of *Drosophila* researchers. The creativity of researchers keeps opening new horizons. Of course, all of this would be essentially irrelevant were it not for the fundamental genetic similarity that *Drosophila* shares with all other species.

T.H. Morgan was awarded the Nobel Prize in 1933 for his work on the patterns of genetic transmission by chromosomes. The Nobel Prize can only be awarded to a living scientist, so Gregor Mendel was not eligible. But insights from Mendel, Morgan, and Morgan's students including the later Nobel Laureate H.J. Muller, established the foundation for understanding mechanisms of gene transmission, linkage and sex-linkage, recombination, and changes in chromosome structure. *Drosophila* offers many experimental advantages. One is that the chromosomes of the *Drosophila* larval salivary glands undergo DNA replication for many cycles without cell division, creating giant chromosomes having about 1000 matched copies of the DNA strand lying together in a cable that shows significant chromosome detail. This makes it possible to map specific gene functions to specific physical regions of a chromosome, and changes in chromosome structure can be mapped precisely.

This would be an interesting historical footnote if the story stopped there. But it did not. In the years since then, *Drosophila* has become one of the most important experimental organisms for exploring the role of genes in development, physiology, and behavior.

In part this is because many gene and special chromosome mutations have been identified over the years. These allow experiments to target processes that are difficult to match in other organisms. It also made it possible to apply the techniques of recombinant DNA when they first became available, and the discoveries from that work identified genetic mechanisms that were found to be in common with other organisms.

Drosophila has a genome of about 13,600 genes. About a quarter of its genome is made up of highly-repetitive DNA and several dozen kinds of transposable elements. Some of the earliest work on transposable elements, the P-elements of "mutator activity" or "hybrid dysgenesis," was done with *Drosophila*. P-elements have now become a powerful experimental tool for targeted mutagenesis and other genome manipulations.

At the other end of the phenotypic spectrum, research using *Drosophila* explored the genetic basis of quantitative traits. These are traits that vary in expression because the effect of each gene can be enhanced or masked by environmental factors affecting the same trait. Using carefully controlled experiments that factored out environmental effects, experiments with *Drosophila* showed that even apparently complex expression could often be explained by genetic variation in a relatively small number of contributing genes. This perspective should change a physician's approach to complex traits. Although variable in presentation, a condition may still be traced to a predictable biological process.

The International Commission on Zoological Nomenclature has moved to change the taxonomic name of this genetic landmark organism to *Sophophora melanogaster*. It is a change that may be justified taxonomically but is criticized by the genetic research community. This may be a rare example of consistency and stability of the literature being more important to the growth of science than is taxonomic precision. It is a change that is likely to be ignored by most geneticists for a long time. But do not be confused if you find this name in your future journal reading.

A Bacterium, *Escherichia coli*

Escherichia coli is one of the most important model systems for understanding simple genome organization and is central to areas like recombinant DNA technology development. On the other hand, some strains of *E coli* cause food-borne illness that can be quite serious. As a species, its genome is exceeding diverse, but the strains, like *E coli* K12, used in microbial genetics are restricted in number. A representative genome was first reported in 1997. It is a circular DNA molecule of 4.6 million base pairs with 4288 protein-coding genes, 7 rRNA genes, and 86 tRNA genes. But the number of genes varies among strains, and some genes may have come from horizontal transfer from other organisms. These variables add to the utility of *E coli* as an experimental organism for genetic study.

Joshua Lederberg and Edward Tatum discovered the process of bacterial conjugation in *E coli*, and Seymour Benzer utilized *E coli* and the T4 **bacteriophage** to study the linearity of gene structure in the genome. A foundation of modern biotechnology can be traced to work with **plasmids** and restriction enzymes in *E coli*. One early application of recombinant DNA technology was the production of human insulin from *E coli*.

Baker's Yeast, *Saccharomyces cerevisiae*

Yeast is a developmentally simple eukaryote, with a life cycle that has both haploid and diploid phases. Its short generation time allows experiments to be carried out efficiently using techniques, like plating colonies on petri dish media, that parallel some of those available for bacteria. In addition to employing mutations to dissect components of a developmental process, *Saccharomyces* is being used to study signal transduction pathways that alter cell phenotypes.

Although the *Saccharomyces* genome was completely sequenced by 1996, geneticists are still uncertain how many functional genes are present in its genome. It is likely that the number is about 6000 or so, but many hypothetical genes have functions that are not yet known. In addition to protein-coding genes, there are many noncoding RNAs, including 274 tRNA genes and RNAs for ribosome processing, intron splicing, and other cellular processes. About 20% of the loci lead to lethality when mutated. Recombination rates are higher than those for most other fungi, and good genetic maps are available for a large number of loci.

The proportion of repeated sequences is much lower than that found in most multicellular eukaryotes (see Chapter 4). About 4% of the *Saccharomyces cerevisiae* genome is composed of transposable elements. The virus-like retroelement Ty is found in about 50 copies in each genome. Intact Ty elements can pair and recombine even when they are located on different chromosomes, resulting in frequent reciprocal translocations and other chromosomal aberrations.

There are two mating types, a and α. Signal transduction pathways can be activated by pheromones that are released by cells of one mating type and then bind to receptors on the other mating type. This activates an intracellular cascade that phosphorylates, and thus activates, a transcription factor. This in turn activates the genes needed for arresting the G_1 cell cycle and for cell fusion and nuclear fusion required for mating. This type of signal transduction pathway studied in yeast is highly conserved in eukaryotes.

A Nematode, *Caenorhabditis elegans*

The nematode *Caenorhabditis elegans* is a simple eukaryote with precisely 959 cells in a female, which is a functional hermaphrodite, and 1031 cells in a male. The cell lineage relationships in both sexes are now completely mapped (Figure 3-12). Six founder cells give rise to all the cells of the adult, and mutations that alter cell lineage progression are a valuable tool for developmental analysis. Adults are about 1 mm long and can be handled with techniques that resemble those used to culture bacterial cell colonies. Since it is transparent, mutations affecting its internal anatomy and development can be studied easily. Each mating can yield hundreds of progeny, and it shares many of the experimental advantages that have benefited work with *Drosophila*. The sequence of its approximately 14,000 gene genome was completed in 1998. Insights into genetic control of development using *Caenorhabditis elegans* were recognized by the Nobel Prize to Sydney Brenner, Robert Horvitz, and John Sulston in 2002.

One special benefit of *C elegans* as an experimental model is the fact that its cell lineage during normal development is strictly defined (see Figure 3-12). The specific fate of each progenitor cell has been mapped. With this map it has been possible to define inductive signals between one cell and another, the signal transduction pathways of the recipient cell, and genetically programmed cell death events. Gene expression in *C elegans* has some unexpected elements, such

as examples of polycistronic transcription like that seen in bacteria. One process discovered in *C elegans* is RNA-mediated interference (RNAi). When used as an experimental technique, it allows researchers to study the function of targeted genes by silencing their expression.

The Zebrafish, *Danio rerio*

The zebrafish, *Danio rerio*, shares many characteristics with other model genetic systems. They have a short generation time and they lay several hundred eggs in each reproductive cycle. An important advantage for researchers is that the embryos are relatively large and transparent. This means that internal developmental changes can be observed easily. The precursors to major organs become visible through the body wall within about 36 hours after fertilization, and hatching occurs up to about 36 hours later. The genome of *D rerio* has been sequenced and many genetically-characterized strains are available to researchers. Among these are strains that allow study of diurnal sleep cycles, which are similar to those of mammals.

Using anti-sense technologies, important aspects of development can be studied. This technique uses **Morpholino oligonucleotides**. These synthetic nucleotide chains of RNA or DNA bind to complementary sequences when injected into an embryo. By binding to a complementary sequence in a cell, they effectively inactivate it and, thus, mimic a mutation. This reduces gene expression in the cell and its descendants. The technique allows the equivalent of targeted mutagenesis to explore genetic effects on development of a vertebrate with many homologies to human biology.

The House Mouse, *Mus musculus*

As a mammal that shares many aspects of physiology and development with humans, it is not surprising that our genomes are similar in size (about 3 billion bp) and content. In fact, extended regions of gene sequence similarity have been identified showing that even the organization of our genomes retains extensive homology. Gene sequence similarities are also reflected in functional parallels. Thus, homology makes the house mouse an especially valuable model for understanding human genetics. Advanced cellular and molecular techniques can be combined readily with more traditional genetic mating systems. One specific example is the use of *Mus* to develop models of many human genetic diseases.

As an experimental model, they benefit from a relative short life cycle (8 or 9 weeks), small body size, and comparatively large litters of offspring. Transgenic manipulation allows complex processes to be isolated and studied. With nuclear injection, one can add specific genes to the genome. Targeted mutagenesis can change or inactivate a locus of choice. In contrast to the defined cell lineage outcomes associated with cells of *C elegans*, cells in the early embryonic stages of *Mus* retain totipotency, or developmental flexibility. It is therefore possible to generate chimeras, composed of cells derived from two or more separate genotypes. Literally hundreds of single-gene mutations are now available in strains with well-documented genetic backgrounds, providing a rich resource for advanced experimental design. Among these are the Hox genes, homologous to the homeobox genes first described in *Drosophila*, which define critical elements of body plan in all multicellular organisms (Figures 13-19 and 13-20).

A Model Plant, *Arabidopsis thaliana*

Arabidopsis thaliana (Figure 16-1) is a small weed with no special economic importance, other than being a model plant for genetic studies. Its small size, five pairs of well-banded chromosomes, and relatively tiny genome offer an ideal organism in which to study the molecular biology and genetic control of processes like growth, biochemical pathways, and development of a plant. Its genome was published in 2000. Transposable elements that had originally been identified in corn can be introduced into *A thaliana* cells and become integrated into its genome. *Agrobacterium* is the biological agent both for this process and for transformation by plasmid DNA called T-DNA. Insertional mutagenesis is a powerful technique for generating mutations to study biochemical and developmental processes.

Genetic analysis has yielded insights into the control of development by plant hormones and in response to light, a complex of processes known as photomorphogenesis. Although plants do not contain a homeobox like that in animals, they

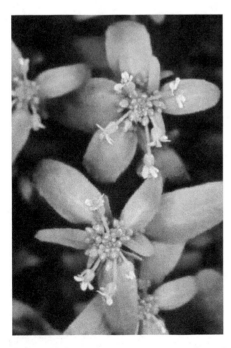

Figure 16-1. *Arabidopsis thaliana*, a model plant. This plant has no true agricultural or ecosystem value. Its importance exists in its role as a research organism. (© Jeremy Burgess/Photo Researchers.)

have a functionally equivalent group of genes that code for DNA-binding transcription factors. Surprisingly, a degree of partial homology between this plant's steroid-like gene and mammalian genes of the steroid pathway suggests that future research may uncover even more fundamental genetic connections among distantly-related organisms.

What Does This Reveal About Human Disease?

Comparative genomics hybridization is the discipline of studying genetic relationships across species. While information can be obtained in one species and applied to another, translating that information into practical applications is much more difficult. First, animal physiology is not an exact replica of that in humans. Caution has to be taken before a treatment in a model organism is verified in humans. Second, even though a particular gene may be homologous by sequence between two organisms, it is not necessarily true that the gene will perform the same function in each nor will phenotypes be predictable. For example, mutations in the *eya* gene produce a phenotype in *Drosophila* that is "eyes absent." But mutations in the homologous human gene EYA1 produces a phenotype of branchio-oto-renal syndrome—a condition associated with malformations of the branchial arch structures, kidneys, and ears/hearing. This then is a double-edged sword. While caution has the be taken in making any projections or extrapolations, it is impressive to consider that studies of the veins in fruit fly wings can give critical insights into processes like cancer, stress responses, and neural networks!

Table 16-2 lists several other such known relationships. We will describe just a few of these in more detail. Saethre-Chotzen syndrome is a disorder characterized by craniosynostosis and other craniofacial anomalies as well as digital changes (Figure 16-2 b,c). It is caused by a mutation in a gene known as TWIST which is a transcriptional regulator. The *Drosophila* homolog gene is designated *twist*. Mutations in this gene in *Drosophila* produce segmentation defects of myogenesis (Figure 16-2 a). The *hedgehog* gene in *Drosophila* gets its name from a mutation that produces short bristly hairs on the larvae that are reminiscent of a hedgehog (Figure 16-3a). The human homolog has been termed Sonic hedgehog (SHH). Mutations in SHH have been shown to cause heritable non-syndromic holoprosencephaly (Figures 16-3 b-d). The phenotypic spectrum of SHH in humans may be as mild as only showing a single central incisor (Figure 16-3 e).

Basal cell nevus syndrome (previously called Gorlin syndrome) is associated with craniofacial dysmorphisms, jaw cysts, palmar and plantar pits, and the propensity to develop basal cell carcinomas (Figure 16-4 b-d). It is caused by a gene called PTCH1. The *Drosophila* homolog is the *patched* gene. Mutations in this gene cause a variety of fly wing anomalies (Figure 16-4 a). One last example is that of Splotch mutations in mice which produce defects in neural tube development (Figure 16-5 a). The human homolog is the homeobox gene PAX3. PAX3 mutations are seen in some patients with

Drosophila Gene	Drosophila Phenotype	Mouse Gene	Mouse Phenotype	Human Gene	Human Disease	Human Signs/ Symptoms
paired	Failure of posterior segment development	Splotch (Sp)	Neural tube defects	PAX3	Waardenburg syndrome	Hearing loss, pigmentation defects, congenital anomalies
cubitus interruptus	Abnormal wing formation	Gli	Failure to thrive, early death, Hirschprung	GLI1	Glioblastoma oncogene	Brain tumors
		Gli2				
		Gli3	Malformations of GI, respiratory, renal and skeletal systems	GLI3	Greig cephalosyndactyly, Pallister Hall syndrome	Polysyndactyly, craniosynostosis, brain hamartomas
hedgehog	Larva with short curly hairs	Shh	Ventral induction defects, abnormal somites, vertebral and rib anomalies	SHH (Sonic hedgehog)	Holoprosencephaly	Non-syndromic holoprosencephaly
		Ihh	Bony defects due to abnormal chondrocyte differentiation	IHH (Indian hedgehog)	Brachydactyly	Shortened fingers
patched	Abnormal wing formation	Ptc	Hindlimb defects, brain tumors	PTCH1	Gorlin (basal cell nevus) syndrome	Basal cell tumors, jaw cysts, rib anomalies
twist	Abnormal myogenesis	Twist	Neural tube, limb and somite anomalies	TWIST	Saethre Chotzen syndrome	Asymmetric craniofacial anomalies, digital anomalies
eyes absent	Absent eyes	Eya1	Missing ears and kidneys, abnormal apoptosis of organ primordia	EYA1	Branchio-oto-renal syndrome	Branchial arch defects, ear anomalies/ deafness, renal malformations
engrailed	Abnormal development of imaginal discs	En2	Frequently lethal, cerebellar anomalies	EN2	Autism susceptibility	Autism

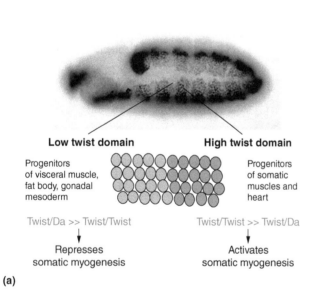

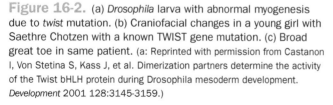

Low twist domain

Progenitors of visceral muscle, fat body, gonadal mesoderm

Twist/Da >> Twist/Twist

Represses somatic myogenesis

High twist domain

Progenitors of somatic muscles and heart

Twist/Twist >> Twist/Da

Activates somatic myogenesis

(a)

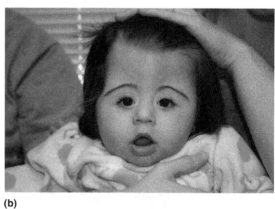

(b)

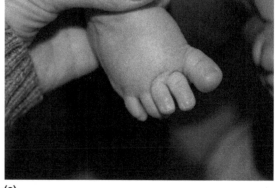

(c)

Figure 16-2. (a) *Drosophila* larva with abnormal myogenesis due to *twist* mutation. (b) Craniofacial changes in a young girl with Saethre Chotzen with a known TWIST gene mutation. (c) Broad great toe in same patient. (a: Reprinted with permission from Castanon I, Von Stetina S, Kass J, et al. Dimerization partners determine the activity of the Twist bHLH protein during Drosophila mesoderm development. *Development* 2001 128:3145-3159.)

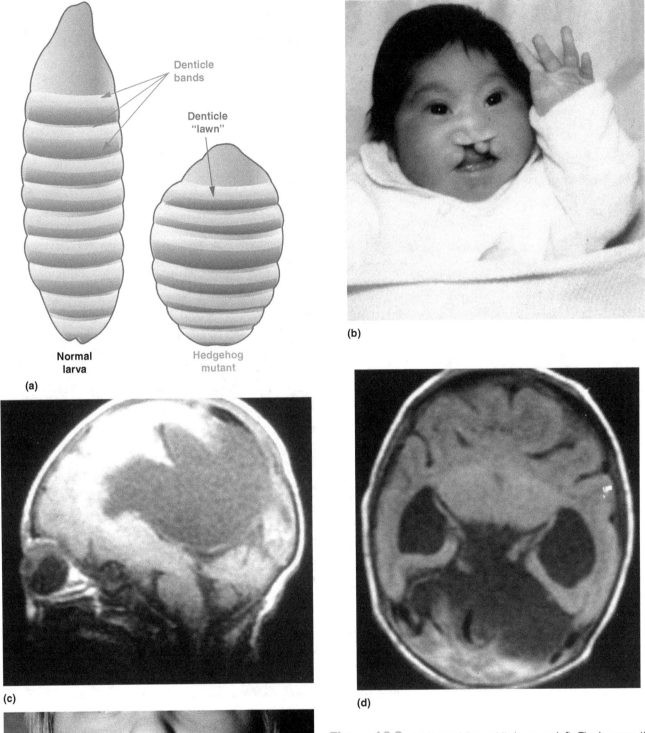

Figure 16-3. (a) Normal *Drosophila* larva on left. The larva on the right has a mutation in the *hedgehog* gene. (b) Patient with holoprosencephaly with severe bilateral cleft lip and palate. He has a positive family history with 2 half-brothers also affected. (c,d) Brain MRI of the boy in frame b showing incomplete ventral induction (separation of midline)—semi-lobar holoprosencephaly. (e) Their mother has a minor expression of the condition as a single central incisor. She and all 3 boys have an SHH mutation. (a: Reprinted with permission from van den Brink GR. Hedgehog Signaling in Development and Homeostasis of the Gastrointestinal Tract *Physiol Rev* October 2007 87:(4) 1343-1375; doi:10.1152/physrev.00054.2006.)

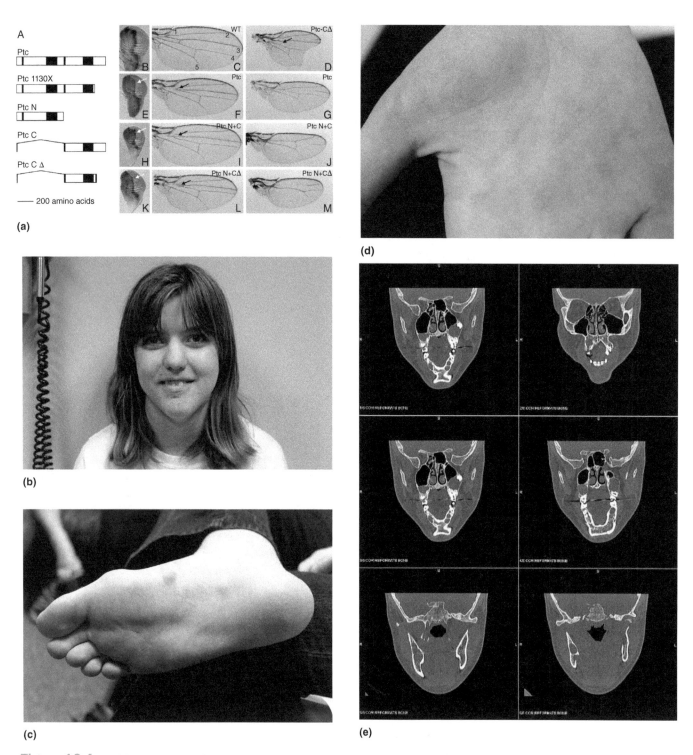

Figure 16-4. (a) Multiple wing malformations associated with *patched* mutation. (b) Adolescent girl with Gorlin (basal cell nevus) syndrome. She has a confirmed PTC mutation. Patients with Gorlin syndrome are reported to have broad facies, frontal bossing and prominent jaws. (c) Basal cell tumors on the foot. (d) Palmar pits. (e) Head CT scan demonstrating odontogenic keratocysts (in the jaw). (a: Reprinted with permission from Johnson RL, Milenkovic L, Scott MP. In Vivo Functions of the Patched Protein: Requirement of the C Terminus for Target Gene Inactivation but Not Hedgehog Sequestration, *Molecular Cell*, volume 6, issue 2, August 2000, pp 467-478, ISSN 1097-2765, 10.1016/S1097-2765 (00)00045-9.)

Waardenburg syndrome, although there is genetic heterogeneity for this condition. Waardenburg syndrome is characterized by neurosensory hearing loss and telecanthus (lateral displacement of the inner canthi of the eyes). Patients with Waardenburg syndrome also will have a variety of pigmentary changes including a characteristic "white forelock" of hair, iris heterochromia, and poliosis (patchy hypopigmentation of the hair and skin). These features are shown in Figure 16-5(b-d).

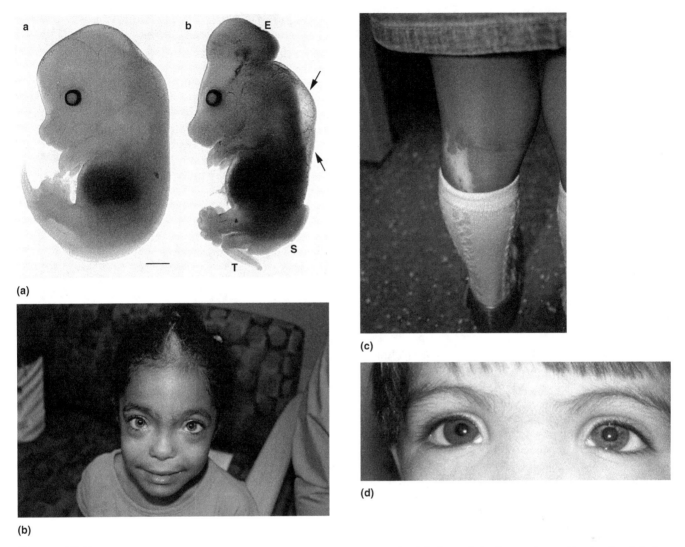

Figure 16-5. (a) Mice embryos. The one on the left is normal. The one on the right has a Splotch mutation and is showing defects of neural tube development. (b) Young girl with Waardenburg syndrome. She presented with neurosensory hearing loss. She has a known PAX 3 mutation. (Note white hair patch and dystopia canthorum). (c) Hypopigmented area of skin on her leg. (d) Young boy with Waardenburg syndrome. Note iris heterochromia. (a: Reprinted with permission from Conway SJ, Henderson DJ, Kirby ML, et al. Development of a lethal congenital heart defect in the splotch (Pax3) mutant mouse *Cardiovasc Res* (1997) 36(2): 163-173 doi:10.1016/S0008-6363(97)00172-7.)

Part 2: Pathogenesis of Disorders

From the standpoint of diagnostics, the goal is to find the etiology. **Etiology** simply means the cause of the condition. Knowing *what* the cause is, is the first step in arriving at several important conclusions about a condition. Besides simply knowing the name of a condition, an etiologic diagnosis is helpful in many ways we have already discussed, such as estimating recurrence risk, prognosis, co-morbid conditions, natural history, and other factors.

A related, but distinct, concept is that of **pathogenesis**. Pathogenesis defines the mechanism whereby changes in the genome translate into physical traits. That is, *how* does a mutation change the gene function and thus produce a recognizable phenotype? It is absolutely necessary that pathogenesis is

understood if targeted therapies are to be designed for genetic disorders.

George Beadle and Edward Tatum (after his work with Lederberg) won the Nobel Prize in Physiology or Medicine in 1958 for work they began in the early 1940s. Using mold as their model organism, they set out to identify the connection between genes and enzymes. They hypothesized a one-to-one relationship between genes and specific enzymes. They predicted that it should be possible to generate mutants in specific enzymatic reactions and thus produce a phenotypic effect. This pioneering work was among the first attempts to identify pathogenesis at a molecular level. This type of relationship makes complete sense: mutation leads to a defective enzyme, which leads to disrupted biochemical reaction, which leads to disease. If only everything were that simple! Through the course of this book we have covered many examples of genetic disorders in which the pathogenesis is not that of product insufficiency. Many other pathogenic mechanisms exist whereby disease results.

Along these lines, consider three conditions that have been previously discussed in different contexts. Wolf-Hirschhorn (WHS) is a multiple anomaly syndrome caused by a terminal deletion of the short arm of chromosome 4 (Chapter 5, Figure 5-49d). Achondroplasia is an autosomal dominant skeletal dysplasia. Patients with achondroplasia have a disproportionately short stature and macrocephaly (Chapter 6, Figure 6-18a). Huntington disease is an autosomal dominant adult-onset neurodegenerative condition that exhibits progressive dementia, involuntary movements, and neurologic decline usually beginning in the 40s or 50s (Chapter 6, Figure 6-24a).

So what is the link between these conditions? Wolf-Hirschhorn syndrome (WHS) is a chromosomal deletion syndrome (4p-). The multiple congenital anomalies in these patients are produced by absence of one of the copies of *some* of the deleted genes. Notably, the genes for achondroplasia and Huntington disease are in this same region and are typically deleted in patients with Wolf-Hirschhorn syndrome (Figure 16-6). However, patients with WHS do not have achondroplasia nor do they develop Huntington disease in adulthood—and yet these are both dominant conditions. The answer lies in the pathogenesis of the conditions.

As noted, the congenital anomalies seen in WHS are caused by the missing products of some of the genes in that region. But in achondroplasia, the bony disorder is produced not by missing protein product, but by mutations that generate a structurally abnormal protein. As mentioned, WHS patients also do not develop Huntington disease as they age. In Chapter 12 (Atypical Modes of Inheritance) we identified the pathogenesis of Huntington disease as being due to an expanding trinucleotide repeat within the gene. The expanded repeat results in excess production of molecular products that are actually cytotoxic. The result is acquired cell death of the basal ganglia and resultant progression of neurologic dysfunction. So in neither achondroplasia nor Huntington disease is the pathogenesis deficiency of product, but something completely different. In all three cases it would make sense that strategies to address therapies for each would have to take markedly different approaches!

Examples of Types of Pathogenic Changes

So it is clear that when a mutation occurs in a specific gene, it can evoke pathologic changes through a variety of different mechanisms. For illustration purposes we will discuss just a few of these in more detail here.

1. *Missing/nonfunctional protein.* This, of course, is the classic example as identified by Beadle and Tatum.

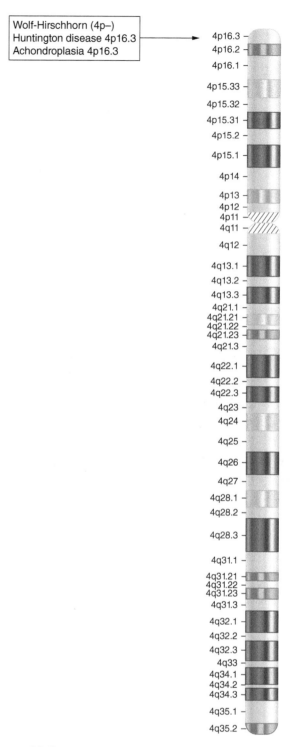

Figure 16-6. Idiogram of chromosome 4. The chromosomal location of Wolf-Hirschhorn syndrome, Huntington disease, and achondroplasia are all at the terminal end of the short arm of chromosome 4 (4p16.3).

As was discussed in Chapter 8 (Metabolism) most inborn errors of metabolism are recessive disorders. Typically enzyme systems carry a very large capacity such that it often takes enzyme levels to fall below 5% of normal for there to be clinically observable effects.

Thus the pathogenesis for inborn errors of metabolism is simply that of absent enzyme activity. Both alleles must be disabled before problems occur.

2. *Abnormal protein folding.* Sickle cell anemia was discussed in Chapter 2. In this situation, a single nucleotide change (c.20A > T) results in a single amino acid change (p.Glu6Val) of the beta globulin protein. This specific change results in abnormal folding of the hemoglobin molecule which in turn distorts the shape of the red blood cell (RBC) from a smooth "donut shaped" cell to an irregular cell that has been described as looking like a sickle (Figure 2-35). These sickled RBCs are prone to occluding the smaller blood vessels as they pass through the tight passages of the capillary beds. As such, a large part of the pathogenesis of sickle cell disease is microvasculature occlusion.

3. *Disruptive protein.* Type I collagen is a trimeric protein. It is assembled from three polypeptide chains woven into a triple helical protein. Type I collagen comprises two alpha-1: (I) chains and one alpha-2 (II) chain. Abnormalities of type I collagen are associated with phenotype of osteogenesis imperfecta (OI)–sometimes referred to as "brittle bone" disease (Figure 16-7). Pathogenic changes in any of the physiological processes of type I collagen production can result in OI. This would include problems with transcription, translation, posttranslational modification, assembly, or transport.

Mutations in either of the procollagen genes that produce structurally abnormal proteins will have an abnormal **dominant negative effect** resulting in a more severe phenotype. One interesting phenomenon in the pathogenesis of OI is that of "protein suicide". Small intragenic deletions in the pro-alpha-1collagen gene produce a shortened protein that will prevent normal folding. Not only are these molecules nonfunctional, but they are rapidly degraded. This will actually result in a milder clinical form of OI. (It should be noted that the same process happens when there is an early frameshift mutation or whole gene deletion).

4. *Gain of function.* It is intuitive that mutations can exert their effects by disabling normal gene function. But it is important to remember that biological systems occur in a balanced equilibrium. Overproduction can be as problematic as insufficient product. Indeed a number of **activating mutations** have been characterized. Albright hereditary osteodystrophy (AHO) is a recognizable syndrome that exhibits mildly shortened stature, moderate obesity, rounded facies, short neck, short metacarpals and metatarsals, subcutaneous calcium deposits, and endocrine abnormalities. Some patients with AHO will have cognitive deficits (Figure 16-8). The etiology of AHO has been shown to be due to mutations in the alpha subunit of the secondary messenger G protein (GNAS1) that decreases gene function. McCune-Albright syndrome is characterized by polyostotic fibrous dysplasia,

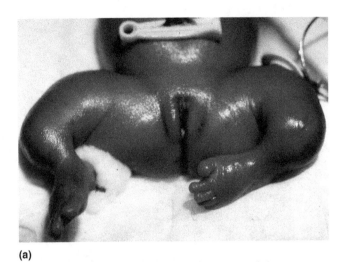

(a)

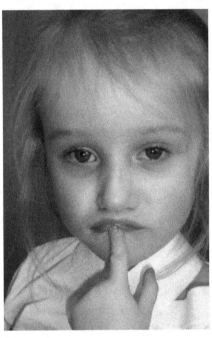

(b)

Figure 16-7. (a) Lower limbs of an infant with severe osteogenesis imperfecta. (b) Face of a young girl with milder osteogenesis imperfecta. Note the blue sclera.

clonal patches of skin hyper pigmentation, and a variety of endocrine abnormalities including isosexual precocious puberty (Figure 16-9). McCune Albright syndrome is also caused by mutations in GNAS1. What is different from this condition and AHO is that mutations in McCune Albright syndrome are *activating mutations*. Thus from a pathogenic standpoint, the two conditions are inverse disorders. It is fascinating to note that Dr. Albright described both of these conditions independently prior to molecular identification of etiology. Little did he—or anyone else—suspect that they were in fact allelic disorders! One last thing worth mentioning is that patients with McCune Albright syndrome are always

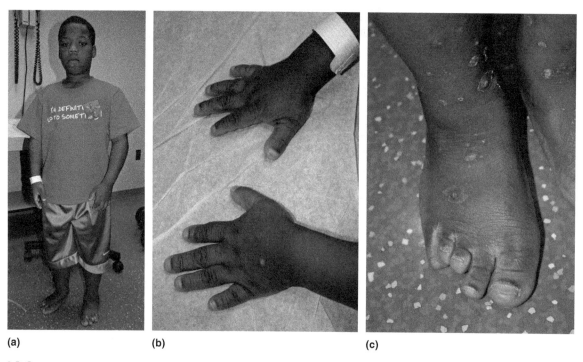

(a) **(b)** **(c)**

Figure 16-8. (a) Adolescent male with Albright hereditary osteodystrophy. He has mildly disproportionate short stature and (b, c) his hands and feet demonstrate brachydactyly. The 3/4/5 toes are especially short. This patient has a confirmed GNAS1 mutation.

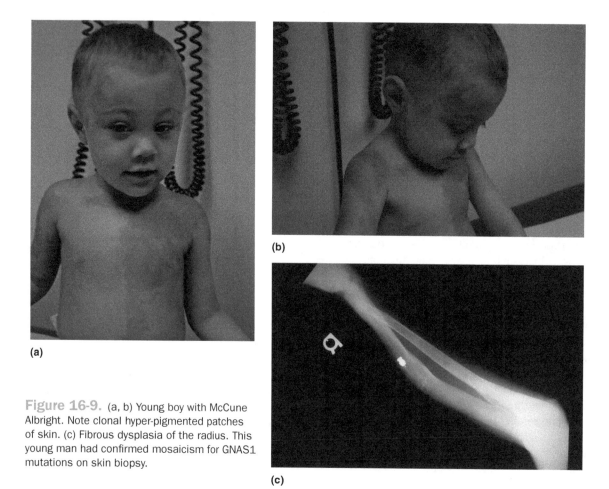

(a)

(b)

(c)

Figure 16-9. (a, b) Young boy with McCune Albright. Note clonal hyper-pigmented patches of skin. (c) Fibrous dysplasia of the radius. This young man had confirmed mosaicism for GNAS1 mutations on skin biopsy.

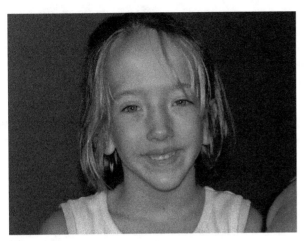

(a)

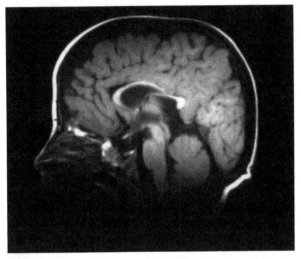

(b)

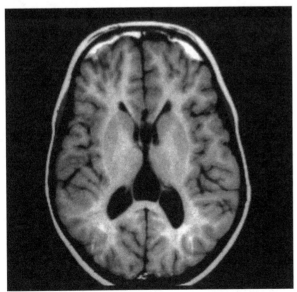

(c)

Figure 16-10. (a) Young girl with Sotos syndrome with typical facial characteristics. (b, c) Sagittal and axial MRI images of the brain of a child with Sotos syndrome showing characteristic changes.

mosaic for the mutation. This explains many things about the condition including the patchy pigmentation. It is likely then that germ line activating mutations of GNAS1 are not compatible with life.

5. *Abnormal regulation of other genes.* Sotos syndrome is a well-described multiple anomaly syndrome. The major features of Sotos syndrome are somatic overgrowth, advanced osseous maturation, characteristic facies (down-slanting palpebral fissures, triangular chin, apparent hypertelorism), relative and absolute macrocephaly, supra-nuclear (central) hypotonia, and neurodevelopmental/neurobehavioral problems (Figure 16-10a). The vast majority of patients with Sotos syndrome also have a unique pattern of changes noted on MRI scans of the brain (Figure 16-10 b, c). Over 90% of patients with Sotos are found to have a mutation in a gene designated *NSD1. NSD1* is a histone methyl-transferase implicated in transcriptional regulation. It has multiple functional domains that regulate several other genes such as the estrogen receptor, thyroid hormone receptor, retinoic acid receptor, retinoid X receptor, and nuclear receptor interaction domains. The pathogenesis of Sotos syndrome thus has to be assessed not by looking at the gene itself, but by evaluating all of the other genes it influences. Current estimates suggest that *NSD1* may directly interact with over 30 other loci.

These are just a few of the known pathogenic mechanisms. Table 16-3 lists several other types of changes.

Table 16-3.	Different Pathogenic Mechanisms (Types of Pathogenesis)

Missing/nonfunctional protein

Abnormal stereochemistry/3-dimensional protein folding

Disruptive protein

Gain of function (toxic)

Abnormal regulation of other genes

Tumor suppressor functions

Selective cell death (apoptosis)

Abnormal DNA repair

Expanded trinucleotide repeats
   loss of function
   gain of function
   dominant-negative effects

Epigenesis

Abnormal regulatory RNAs

Disorders of chromatin remodeling

Abnormalities of transcription factors

Abnormal chaperone proteins

Abnormalities of protein degradation machinery (ubiquitin-proteosome system)

By no means is this list all-inclusive, but it does provide some insight into the various possible pathogenic mechanisms to be considered. To reiterate an earlier point, the understanding of pathogenesis is central to designing targeted therapies. True personalized medicine will occur when individuals have correct clinical diagnoses coupled with a knowledge of molecular etiology and an understanding of the pathogenesis of their specific mutation. Only then can therapy be truly customized to the individual.

Part 3: How Complex Can Things Be?

Another important unifying concept to review is that genes in humans are seldom "simple." Remember that humans have about 22,000 functioning genes. This is less than some invertebrates and plants. The tremendous complexity of human biology comes from the variety of modifications that happen in gene expression beyond the genomic code itself. Also genes do not operate in isolation. As has been stressed many times before, gene × gene interactions are abundant and complex.

Take for example cystic fibrosis (CF) (see Chapter 4 including Figure 4-21). Almost everyone who has studied human genetics has heard of this condition and is aware that the condition has autosomal recessive inheritance. Few, however, understand the extreme complexity of the genetics of this condition. While it is correct that the condition does show autosomal recessive inheritance, molecular studies of the condition have revealed many different layers of understanding of its expression beyond simple Mendelian segregation.

In the current clinical setting, molecular analyses of the CF gene can provide so much more information. A complete understanding of the genetics of CF would include a description something like this:

1. Cystic fibrosis is caused by mutations at a single known locus (i.e., no locus heterogeneity). The gene is designated as *CFTR*. It is at chromosome locus 7q31.2.

2. The CFTR gene has 250,000 base pairs and 27 exons. During transcription, the introns are excised and the exons are assembled into a 6100 base pair mRNA transcript, which is translated into the 1480 amino acid sequence of the *CFTR* protein.

3. The gene codes for a protein product, the CF trans-membrane conductance regulator. This protein is a chloride channel protein found in the membranes of exocrine cells of the pulmonary epithelium, pancreas, gastrointestinal tract, and the genitourinary tract.

4. There is some predictive correlation between *CFTR* protein function and clinical symptoms (Table 16-4).

5. Although CF does not have locus heterogeneity, there is marked allelic heterogeneity. Over 1000 mutations in the CF gene have been reported to the Cystic Fibrosis Genetic Analysis Consortium as of August 2012.

6. Although there is a large degree of allelic heterogeneity, a single mutation is found in 75% of persons with CF who are of northern European descent. This mutation is a 3-bp deletion in exon 10 that results in a missing phenylalanine amino acid at position 508 of the *CFTR* protein. This is designated as deltaF508. As was discussed in Chapter 15, it is likely that the high incidence of this mutation is due to a heterozygote advantage with a resistance to cholera deaths.

7. There are multiple different pathogenic mechanisms that may cause CF. These have been grouped in five classes of mutations based on the mechanism (Table 16-5).

8. Several intragenic variants in the noncoding regions can influence gene expression. A "poly-T" tract in

Table 16-4.	Relationship Between CFTR Protein Function and Observed Symptoms
Percentage of normal	
CFTR function	**Manifestations of Cystic Fibrosis**
<1%	classic disease
<4.5%	progressive pulmonary disease
<5%	clinically demonstrable sweat abnormality
<10%	congenital absence of the vas (male infertility)
10%-49%	no known abnormality
50%-100%	no known abnormality (asymptomatic heterozygotes)

Table 16-5.	Functional Classes of Cystic Fibrosis Mutations
Class of Mutation	**Pathogenic Mechanism**
Class 1 mutations	Nonsense mutations that lead to premature termination of CFTR (little or no protein production)
Class 2 mutations	Defective transport of the CFTR protein to the cell surface membrane
Class 3 mutations	Abnormal regulation of CFTR protein function
Class 4 mutations	Abnormal ion transport through a channel which is in the normal location
Class 5 mutations	Decreased synthesis of functional CFTR

Table 16-6.	Genes reported to Modify CFTR Expression or Function
TGFβ-1	
HLA class II antigens	
Mannose binding lectin	
Alpha(1)-antitrypsin	
Alpha(1)-antichymotrypsin	
Glutathione-S-transferase	
Nitric oxide synthetase type1	
TNF-alpha	
IL-1 beta	
IL-1 Ra	

intron 8 affects gene expression by influencing splicing efficiency. Persons with 7T or 9T variants tend to have normal transcription of the *CFTR* gene. Those with the 5T variant may generate an anomalous protein product. Also, this influence can be further modified by the number of TG repeats in an adjacent region. Individuals with either 12 or 13 TG repeats are more likely to have a disease phenotype than those with only 11 TG repeats.

9. Polymorphisms in other genes may modify *CFTR* expression and function. One example is the gene for transforming growth factor beta-1 (*TGFβ-1*). *TGFβ-1* is a cytokine with multiple functions that includes roles in immune response, cell differentiation, and healing. Changes in *TGFβ-1* have been reported as modifiers of the CF phenotype. Two mutations of the *TGFβ-1* gene have been described that are associated with *increased* levels of the protein. Higher levels of *TGFβ1* are associated with a doubling of the risk of worse pulmonary disease in patients with CF. Table 16-6 lists some of the genes known to modify *CFTR* expression and function.

10. As discussed in Chapter 12 (Atypical Modes of Inheritance) a small number of patients with CF are found to have two mutations due to uniparental disomy rather than both parents being heterozygotes for the disorder.

11. Genotype: phenotype relationships have been extensively studied in CF. The best correlation between genotype and phenotype is seen in the context of pancreatic function. In contrast, genotype-phenotype correlation is generally poor for pulmonary disease in CF; other genotypes have been highly associated with a particular feature in males with CF—congenital bilateral absence of the vas deferens.

At this point the reader might be thinking, "This seems excessive. Why was all of this minutia discussed?" In our defense, this information was not provided to flood you with a lot of esoteric material. Rather we gave it to you for two key reasons. First it ties together so many of the concepts discussed in all previous chapters. Just look at the list of concepts in these facts, and all that you have now learned. Second, it is meant to highlight just how complicated clinical genetics can be. If this is what is known about a 'simple' Mendelian disorder, imagine how much more complicated things could be with other disorders that are beyond Mendelian in their inheritance. Clearly, just identifying all of the A's, T's, G's and C's of the human genome has not come close to explaining all of the factors in human disease. There will still be a need for clinicians for decades to come!

A Final Thought

Life is a gift. It is also amazingly complex. The molecular events that control development from a fertilized egg to an adult cannot help but cause awe. Yet the human mind and experimental insights yield tools to explore that complexity. Discovery of biological secrets is a testimony to the power of the human mind. Being able to appreciate how much we share with the biology of other organisms is perhaps the mark of our own uniqueness. We know that all people—and all other creatures—share a common biological heritage. All should be valued. Perhaps that is the true goal of life—to understand ourselves and our relationship to others.

A physician's job is not an easy one. But never forget to look at life from the view of the patient—especially a patient who has inherited a biological challenge that may affect their quality and length of life. Many of the questions that face biomedicine have not yet been answered. Life is still full of puzzles. That leaves us with two gradually converging paths: learning what we can about the intricacies of the genetic control of our structure and function—and then using that knowledge in creative ways to intervene for the benefit of patients. Medicine is both a science and an art. The clinical challenge to a physician may put those two dimensions in stark relief. But they work together.

■ Board-Format Practice Questions

1. You see a patient with Wolf-Hirschhorn syndrome (deletion 4p). The parents have spent a lot of time on the internet. They have read that the gene for achondroplasia is in this region. They understand that this means that their child is missing one copy of the achondroplasia gene. Thus they ask you if they should implement the surveillance recommendations for achondroplasia in their child. You would correct in telling them that:
   A. Achondroplasia surveillance should be started immediately.
   B. The first step to answer their question would be to sequence the achondroplasia gene.
   C. It is probably time to start growth hormone therapy to avoid the extreme short stature seen in achondroplasia.
   D. Forget looking on the internet for answers, this will only confuse them.
   E. The pathogenesis of achondroplasia is not haploinsufficiency, so they do not need to worry about achondroplasia related issues in their child.

2. If a condition is inherited as an autosomal recessive trait. The most likely pathogenetic mechanism would be:
   A. Haploinsufficiency.
   B. Deficiency of the protein product.
   C. Protein interference.
   D. Protein suicide.
   E. Autoregulatory dysfunction.

3. The one-gene, one enzyme hypothesis:
   A. is outdated and has no real clinical relevance.
   B. is the most common pathogenetic mechanism in human disease.
   C. explains some connective tissue disorders.
   D. explains some inborn errors of metabolism.
   E. explains some homeotic mutants.

4. Potential explanations that mutations in the same gene can produce different phenotypes would include which one of the following:
   A. Locus heterogeneity.
   B. Allelic heterogeneity.
   C. Genetic homogeneity.
   D. Homeotic modulation.
   E. Gene-gene mutagenesis.

5. All of the following mechanisms might explain autosomal dominant inheritance of a condition EXCEPT:
   A. Haploinsufficiency.
   B. Gain of function mutation.
   C. Protein interference.
   D. Protein suicide.
   E. Lyonization.

Key Genetic Diseases, Disorders, and Syndromes

As we have worked our way through this book we have used clinical examples as much as possible to highlight key points. The examples we used also were selected for their relative importance. However, not all important conditions to know were discussed in this text. (The conditions specifically mentioned in this text are in the highlighted [bold] words in the list below. For the medical student preparing for your boards, we have compiled a list of conditions we deem "key." We would suggest that you know in detail all the conditions that are bolded. For all others, you should be familiar with the condition and its key features and be able to describe the major genetic mechanism(s) involved in the disease. Of course this list is not comprehensive. It is our "top 125." There are many other conditions that may appear on your boards. This is, however, our attempt to focus on what we see as some of the conditions to highlight.

Cancer/Neoplasias

Acute lymphocytic leukemia
Ataxia-telangiectasia
Bloom syndrome
Breast cancer
Chronic myeloid leukemia (CML)—Philadelphia chromosome
Colon cancer
> **Gardner syndrome/Familial adenomatous polyposis (FAP)**
> **Lynch syndrome/Hereditary non-polypotic colorectal cancer (HNPCC)**

Dyskeratosis congenita
Ewing sarcoma
Multiple endocrine neoplasias (MEN)
Neurofibromatosis type 1
Neurofibromatosis type 2
Pancreatic cancer
Prostate cancer
Retinoblastoma
Tuberous sclerosis
von Hippel-Lindau disease

Chromosomal

1q21.1 deletion
22q.11.2 deletion (including DiGeorge syndrome and Shprintzen/velo-cardio-facial syndrome)

47 XXX
47 XYY
Cri-du-chat syndrome (5p-)
Klinefelter syndrome (XXY) and variants
Triploidy
Trisomy 13
Trisomy 18
Trisomy 21 (Down syndrome)
Turner syndrome (monosomy X)
Wolf-Hirschhorn syndrome (4p-)

Common Disorders (Single Gene or Multifactorial)

Achondroplasia
Beckwith-Wiedemann syndrome
Cystic fibrosis
Duchenne/Becker muscular dystrophy
Fragile X
Friedrich ataxia
Hearing loss (Connexin 26)
Hemochromatosis (very common genetic disease)
Hemophilia A and B
Hereditary spherocytosis
Huntington disease
Hypophosphatemic rickets
Long QT syndrome
Ehlers Danlos syndrome(s)
Marfan syndrome
Myotonic dystrophy
Neurofibromatosis type 1
Ocular albinism
Osteogenesis imperfecta type I
Polycystic kidney diseases (adult and childhood types)
Spinocerebellar ataxia/olivopontocerebellar atrophy
Thalassemia

Dysmorphology Syndromes/Malformations

Aicardi syndrome
Albright hereditary osteodystrophy
Angelman syndrome
Bardet-Biedel syndrome
CHARGE syndrome
Cleft lip with or without cleft palate
Club foot

Congenital heart disease (know the types associated with common syndromes)
Craniofrontonasal dysplasia
Ectodermal dysplasia
Gorlin syndrome
Holoprosencephaly
Joubert syndrome
Kabuki syndrome
Kartegener syndrome
McCune-Albright syndrome
Noonan syndrome and related RASopathies
Neural tube defects
Prader-Willi syndrome
Pyloric stenosis
Saethre-Chotzen syndrome
Sotos syndrome
VATER association
van der Woude syndrome
Waardenburg syndrome
Williams syndrome

Immune System Disorders

Bruton agammaglobulinemia
Severe combined immune deficiency (SCID)
Wiskott-Aldrich syndrome

Inborn Errors of Metabolism

Albinism
Alkaptonuria
Alpha 1-antitrypsin deficiency
Biotinidase deficiency
Congenital disorders of glycosylation
Fabry
Familial hypercholesterolemia
Fructosemia
Glucose-6-phosphate dehydrogenase (G6PD) deficiency
Galactosemia
Gaucher disease
Glycogen storage diseases especially **Pompe disease**
Homocystinuria (and hyper-homocysteinemia)

Hunter syndrome
Hurler syndrome
Isovaleric acidemia
Lesch-Nyhan syndrome
Maple syrup urine disease
Medium chain acyl-CoA dehydrogenase (MCAD) deficiency
Menkes disease
Phenylketonuria
Smith-Lemli-Opitz syndrome
Tay-Sachs disease
Urea cycle defects/hyperammonemia especially ornithine transcarbamylase (OTC) deficiency)
Wilson disease

Mitochondrial Disorders

Kearns-Sayre syndrome
Leber hereditary optic neuropathy (LHON)
Mitochondrial myopathy, encephalopathy, lactic acidosis, and strokelike episodes (MELAS)
Myoclonic epilepsy and ragged red fibers disease (MERRF)
Neuropathy ataxia and retinitis pigmentosa (NARP)

Polygenic and Multifactorial (Complex) Disorders

Alcoholism
Alzheimer disease
Arthrosclerosis, heart disease, and stroke
Asthma
Autism
Bipolar affective disorder
Congenital adrenal hyperplasia
Diabetes
Fetal alcohol syndrome
Fetal hydantoin syndrome
Hereditary hemorrhagic telangiectasia (Osler-Weber-Rendu syndrome)
Hypertension
Schizophrenia

Glossary

Acentric: No centromere.

Acrocentric: See chromosome.

Activating mutation: See mutation.

Activator: A protein that functions to improve gene transcription.

Affordable Care Act: Complex Federal legislation aimed at ensuring that all Americans have practical access to effective health care coverage.

Agenesis: Referring to embryonic formation. Agenesis is the failure of a specific structure to develop. (e.g., agenesis of the corpus callosum means the corpus callosum did not develop at all.)

    Hypogenesis: The underdevelopment of a specific structure. (e.g., hypogenesis of the corpus callosum refers to a smaller than normal corpus callosum.)

Allele(s): Alternative forms of a gene, or of a DNA sequence, at a given locus.

    Null allele: When applied to a gene that codes for an enzyme, the null allele changes the gene to produce zero enzyme product.

Allelic heterogeneity: See heterogeneity.

Allosteric control: The regulation of an enzyme or other metabolic function via an effector molecule at a site other than the protein's active site (e.g., an allosteric site).

Allosteric protein: A protein that alters its shape upon binding with another molecule.

Alpha-satellite: Repeating units of DNA which are about 170 bp. They are found mainly in the heterochromatic region around the centromeres.

Alternative splicing: The process of excising introns in different patterns to produce alternate DNA forms for transcription and ultimately resulting in different proteins from the same core sequence.

Anaphase: See cell cycle.

Aneuploid: Not possessing the correct number of chromosomes. There are several descriptors of such abnormalities (also see "Ploidy"). Examples would include:

    Disomy: Having two copies of one chromosome.

    Monosomy: Having one copy of one chromosome.

    Trisomy: Having three copies of one chromosome.

Anneal: The coupling of complementary strands of DNA.

    Re-anneal: The coupling of complementary DNA strands after having first been separated.

Anticipation: The apparent worsening of a heritable condition as it is passed down through generations.

Apoenzyme: See enzyme.

Apoptosis: Programmed cell death (sometimes referred to as "cellular suicide").

Array comparative genomic hybridization (aCGH): See comparative genomic hybridization.

Association: Two or more malformations, which have been found (on a population basis) to occur together more often than would be predicted by chance, but not necessarily due to a specific causal entity.

Autosome (autosomal): Referring to one of the 22 numbered (non-sex) chromosomes.

Auxology (auxologic): The study of human growth.

Auxotrophy: The inability to synthesize all of the biochemical necessary for all of the functions in an organism. (An auxotroph is an organism that exhibits auxotrophy.)

    Prototrophs: In contrast to auxotrophy, prototrophy is the ability to synthesize all of the biochemical necessary for cellular function. Prototrophs are organisms that possess these abilities.

Back mutation: See mutation.

Bacterial artificial chromosomes (BACs): Manufactured pieces of DNA derived from bacterial plasmids used as probes in DNA identification.

Bacteriophage: A virus that invades a bacteria and replicates inside it.

Banding: The appearance of bands on cytogenetic studies produced by differential staining. There are multiple types of chromosomal stains that are designed to highlight specific regions. Banding patterns allow for clear distinction of each chromosome pair from the others.

    G-banding: The most common type of banding study used in clinical settings. The "G" stands for the stain Giemsa which preferentially stains heterochromatin resulting in darker and lighter visible bands.

    High resolution banding: Cytogenetic laboratory method in which the chromosomes are induced to be more elongated, allowing much finer detection of smaller changes in the pattern of banding than usual; also called prometaphase banding.

Benign polymorphism: See polymorphism.

Biopharmaceutical: Medications derived using biotechnology.

Birth defect: A lay term that denotes an abnormality of development present at birth. The most common application of this term is to observable structural changes. (See congenital anomaly.)

Bivalent: A pair of homologous chromosomes that are coupled during meiosis.

Blaschko lines: Developmental linear patches observed in the skin. Blaschko lines do not strictly follow dermatome patterns.

Blastocyst: Early developmental stage in embryonic development characterized by an inner cell mass and a thin cellular layer enclosing a blastocyst cavity.

Blastomere: Cells derived from the cleavage of a fertilized oocyte during early embryonic development.

Blastula: A sphere of cells with a hollow core composed of blastomeres.

C value: The amount of DNA contained within a haploid (n) nucleus. This would be the equivalent of half the amount in a diploid (2n) cell.

cAMP: See cyclic AMP.

Candidate gene: See gene.

Carcinogen: An environmental factor (chemical, ionizing radiation, etc.) that can induce cancer.

Cell cycle: Interphase, prophase, prometaphase, metaphase, anaphase, then telophase.

Cellular differentiation: The process that undifferentiated (stem) cells undergo in becoming progressively more specialized in structure and function.

Centrioles: Subcellular structures that are a grouping of microtubules arranged in a characteristic pattern of 9 microtubule triplets. Centrioles play key roles in cellular division.

Centromere: A highly condensed region of the chromosome where sister chromatids are linked during cell division.

  Acentric: A chromosome having no centromere.

  Dicentric: A chromosome possessing two centromeres.

Centrosome: A subcellular organelle that serves as the primary microtubule organizing center of eukaryotic cells as well as a regulator of cell cycle.

Chaperones: Proteins that have a primary transport function to assist in the folding/unfolding or assembly/disassembly of proteins.

Chromatid: One of a pair of a duplicated chromosome bound by a single centromere. The two identical strands are called "sister chromatids."

Chromatin remodeling: Human chromosomes in the neutral state house the DNA in a highly condensed and protected state. Chromatin remodeling is the process of modifying the chromatin architecture to permit access of DNA to the transcription elements.

Chromosomal analysis (karyotype): Cytogenetic analysis to determine the number and structure of chromosomes as seen through microscopic views of prepared cells from an individual's tissue.

Chromosomal microarray: Using microchips with thousands of wells imbedded with a variety of different types of probes to screen large parts of the genome.

Chromosomes: The structures that house nuclear DNA. Chromosomes are composed of the DNA itself as well as a variety of proteins that allow for compact packaging and protection. In humans the modal (normal) number of chromosomes is 46.

  Acrocentric: A chromosome in which the centromere is positioned close to the end of the structure. This results in these chromosomes with short (p) arms.

  Telocentric: A chromosome in which the centromere is positioned at the end of the structure. This results in these chromosomes with essentially no (p) arm. Instead, all that is distal to the centromere is satellite DNA.

Chromosome abnormalities (abberations): In karyotype analysis, abnormalities of chromosome structure may be seen. Changes in whole chromosome numbers are referred to as aneuploidy. Partial changes are described as duplications, deletions, inversions, and translocations.

Chromosome painting: Using FISH probes that provide coverage of an entire chromosome to identify structural rearrangements.

Chromosome spindle: A subcellular structure upon which chromosome segregation occurs.

Cis, trans positions: When discussing the relative position of a polymorphism (allele), cis refers to the two polymorphisms being on the same allele of a given pair. Trans means they are on the two different alleles.

Clinical geneticist: A physician with special training in the clinical evaluation of patients suspected to have genetic conditions and birth defects; clinical geneticists historically came from a variety of backgrounds, such as pediatrics, obstetrics/gynecology, internal medicine, neurology, etc. but newly trained individuals may specialize in genetics alone.

Clinical genetics: See genetics.

Clinical genetics laboratory: A laboratory that performs genetic testing for clinical/diagnostic (non-research) indications.

Cloning: Making an exact copy of something. Cloning can be performed at many levels—whole organisms, individual organs, tissues, cells, or even DNA.

Coding (sense) strand: In double-stranded DNA, the coding strand is the strand that contains the actual sequence (codons) used in transcription.

  Noncoding (antisense) strand: In double-stranded DNA, the strand that contains the sequence not used in transcription (anticodons).

Co-dominance: See dominance.

Codon: A specific triplet nucleotide sequence.

  Anticodon: The triplet nucleotide sequence that is complementary to the codon found on the tRNA.

  Sense codon: The 61 triplets that bind a tRNA anticodon and result in the addition of an amino acid during translation.

  Stop codon(s): Three RNA triplets (UAG, UGA, and UAA) designate the end of a coding sequence—because there are no correlate tRNAs for these triplets. These may also be called termination codons, or in the case of mutations, nonsense codons.

Coefficient of inbreeding: A calculated value for an individual that quantifies the degree of genetic code that is shared based on common ancestry.

Coefficient of relationship: A calculated value between two individuals to determine the degree (if any) of consanguinity.

Coenzyme: See enzyme.

Cofactor: An inorganic compound that works to augment enzymatic function. In humans many cofactors are "vitamins."

Comparative genomic hybridization (CGH): Hybridizing control DNA with patient DNA in order to identify copy number variants. When performed on a microarray platform, this is referred to as array CGH (aCGH).

Compound Heterozygosity: See heterozygous.

Concordance (concordant): The occurrence of the same phenotypic feature in different individuals. Most commonly concordance is used to describe the correlation of features in twins. Discordance (discordant) then is the presence of a phenotype in one individual but not the other.

Congenital anomaly: An abnormality present at birth. The most common use of the term is in structural malformations. (See birth defects.)

Consanguinity (consanguineous): Sharing of a common ("blood") relative by two individuals.

Contiguous gene syndromes: Recognizable patterns of malformations due to loss or gain of a chromosomal segment containing several consecutive (contiguous) genes. These may be difficult or impossible to detect by routine cytogenetic analysis. Identification of the change may require high resolution chromosomal analysis, or a molecular cytogenetic test for confirmation.

Copy number variants (CNVs): Deviations from the normal expected chromosomal make up. Microdeletions or micro-duplications detected by chromosomal microarray are such examples. Identified CNVs are classified as known benign, known pathogenic, or of unknown clinical significance. Copy number variant is now the preferred term over "copy number change."

Covalent modification: Modification (regulation) of enzyme activity via a donor molecule which provides a functional moiety that alters the properties of that enzyme.

CpG island: Regions of the genome that contain high concentrations of "CpG sites." A CpG site is characterized by cytosine (C) and Guanine (G) nucleotides which are on the same strand of DNA joined by a phosphodiester (p) bond.

Crossing over: See recombination.

Cyclic AMP (cAMP): 3′5′ cyclic adenosine monophosphate. cAMP is a cell secondary messenger important in intracellular signal transduction.

Cytogenetics: Referring to the analysis of chromosomes within cells, by culturing living cells or preparing actively dividing cells from body tissues and use of various identification methods to detect individual chromosome structure.

Cytokinesis The process of physically dividing a parent cell into daughter cells by splitting the membrane and cytoplasm.

Decoding function: Ribosomal RNA provides a mechanism for decoding mRNA into amino acids. The accuracy of the codon-anticodon pairing is assisted by the decoding function associated with the 16S rRNA in the small subunit.

Deamination: The removal of an amine group.

Deformation: A congenital structural variation or abnormality which is the result of external physical forces.

Degeneracy (of code): This term refers to the fact that the RNA trinucleotides that code for amino acids in translation do not have a one-on-one correlation. Specifically more than one triplet may code for the same amino acid.

Degree(s) of relationship:

First Degree: Parents, siblings, offspring of the proband.

Second Degree: Grandparents/grandchildren, uncles/aunts, nieces/nephews.

Third Degree: Cousins, etc.

Degrees of freedom: In calculating the variance, the degree of freedom is N-1.

Deletion (deficiency): See chromosome abnormalities.

Depurination: A type of DNA mutation in which the purine base (adenine or guanine) is removed from the deoxyribose sugar between them.

Diagnostic yield: Essentially the "batting average" of a clinical genetic diagnostic evaluation. Specifically what percentage of the time does a diagnostic evaluation for a specific condition provide a known cause (etiology) for the condition?

Diandry: The mechanism of the occurrence of a triploid zygote due to a haploid ovum fertilized by a diploid sperm. The result of diandry is a triploid zygote.

Dicentric: See centromere.

Dideoxy sequencing: See sequencing.

Digenic inheritance: An inheritance pattern in which two different loci are involved in the determination of a phenotype. See also inheritance patterns.

Digyny: The mechanism of the occurrence of a triploid zygote due to diploid ovum becoming fertilized by a haploid sperm.

Diploid: See ploidy.

Discordant: See concordance.

Disease: An abnormality of function in a biologic system that results in observable signs and symptoms.

Disorder: A disease not caused by an infectious illness.

Dispersed duplication: See duplication.

Dispermy: The mechanism of the occurrence of a triploid zygote due to an oocyte being (abnormally) fertilized by two spermatozoa.

Disruption: A congenital abnormality which is the result of a destructive event or process, leading to incomplete or abnormal formation.

DNA fingerprint: A person-specific pattern of DNA obtained by a variety of methods of breaking the DNA up into small fragments.

DNA polymerase: Critical enzyme that catalyzes the addition of nucleotide chain.

DNA sequencing: See sequencing.

DNA strand: The individual runs of nucleotides in the DNA molecule. Human, nuclear DNA is double stranded possessing a coding strand and the complementary binding strand.

Coding stand: The template strand for transcription. Sometimes called the "sense" strand. The complementary strand is the anti-sense strand.

Lagging strand: Replication of the second DNA strand is more complicated. Replication of this lagging strand is in a non-continuous fashion because it is going against the unzipping of the replication fork.

Leading strand: During DNA replication, the leading strand is replicated in a relatively straightforward manner. It is the strand that is copied continuously.

Domain: See protein domain.

Dominance/dominant inheritance: Dominant conditions are those expressed in heterozygotes, i.e., individuals with one copy of a mutant allele and one copy of a normal (wild type) allele.

Co-dominance: The simultaneous expression of both alleles in a dominant fashion.

Incomplete or semi dominance: A dominant condition in which a milder phenotype is observed in heterozygotes as compared to homozygotes.

Quasi-dominance: The appearance of dominant transmission of a condition in a pedigree that is actually due to a recessive condition. This occurs when the recessive allele is sufficiently common in the general population.

True/complete dominance: True dominance is characterized by the complete (full) phenotype being seen in both heterozygotes and homozygotes. Specifically homozygotes are not more severely affected.

Dominant negative effect: In terms of pathogenesis, some dominant mutations exert their effect via the gene product adversely affecting the wild-type (normal) gene product within the same cell.

Duplication: A chromosome abnormality in which a segment of the chromosome has been abnormally replicated.

   Dispersed duplication: Chromosomal duplication in which the duplicated segments lie away from each other.

   Tandem duplication: Chromosomal duplication in which the duplicated segments lie adjacent to each other.

Dyshistogenesis: Abnormal embryonic formation at the tissue level.

Dysmorphology (dysmorphologist): A specialist trained in the recognition of physical variations and malformations and their diagnostic and clinical significance.

Dysmorphic: Literally, abnormally shaped. Dysmorphic refers to a physical feature which is sufficiently different from average as to be notable.

Dysplasia: A congenital abnormality due to abnormal development at the tissue level of organization (dyshistogenesis).

Ectoderm: See trilaminar embryo.

Ectopia: Occurring in the wrong place. In general ectopia refers to misplacement at the organ or structural level (i.e., ectopic lens). See also heterotopia.

Ethical Legal and Social Implications (of human genetics) (ELSI): This acronym refers to the complex issues surrounding genetics in clinical medicine. It is also an ongoing specifically funded federal program to address these needs.

Endoderm: See trilaminar embryo.

Endoduplicated (endoduplication): Making a copy of the nuclear genome outside the process of cell division.

Endophenotype: A defined subgroup of a specific phenotype or diagnosis.

Enzyme: A protein that functions as a catalyst in a biochemical reaction.

   Apoenzyme: The state of an enzyme that requires a cofactor when the cofactor is not bound.

   Coenzyme: Organic molecules that are needed by certain enzymes to carry out their catalytic function. (In contrast to cofactors which are inorganic compounds with the same function.)

   Holoenzyme: The active form of an enzyme when all of the components (e.g., cofactors, coenzymes) are appropriately bound.

Enzyme replacement therapy: Using enzyme replacement to treat patients with inborn errors of metabolism. The enzyme may be procured from multiple sources including biologic or engineered systems.

Epigenesis (epigenetic): Modifying gene function without changing sequence. One of the several factors (in addition to alternate splicing, opposite transcripts, posttranslational modification) that allows for the small number of functioning human genes and yet the great diversity/flexibility in human development.

Epistasis: The influence of one gene on the function of others.

Etiology: The specific cause of a disorder.

Euploid: See ploidy.

Exon: The parts of a gene that are codes for the actual protein product.

Expression (expressivity): The observed phenotype of a genetic condition.

   Variable expression: Different degrees of clinical expression given the same genotype. In describing the phenotype associated with a specific condition, variability in expression can usually be identified. In some ways variable expression may be seen as defining severity.

Familial: This simply means that a condition "runs in the family." Familial disorders may be due to genetic factors, environmental factors or both.

Family centered medical home: An important care-delivery concept in which the family (patient) is at the center of all decision making regarding their own care.

Fetal alcohol spectrum disorders: The full range of congenital anomalies due to the teratogenic effects of maternal ethanol consumption.

Field defect: A recognizable pattern of congenital anomalies due to disruption of a common primordial tissue.

Fluorescence in situ hybridization (FISH): A molecular cytogenetic method in which a molecular probe is linked to a fluorescent dye on the slide; views under a fluorescent microscope reveal presence or absence of the desired region of the chromosome through adhesion of the probe or lack thereof .

   Multi-color FISH: Using multiple different colored fluorescent labels to "mark" specific target regions of the genome

   Single locus FISH: A FISH test utilizing probes for a unique and single locus.

   Sub-telomeric FISH: A panel of 40 to 42 probes that hybridize to the sub-telomeric regions of the chromosomes.

Forward mutation: See mutation.

Founder effect: The relatively high frequency of a particular allele in the gene pool that occurs as the result of a new isolated population being founded by a small number of individuals possessing limited genetic variation.

Frameshift mutation: See mutation.

Functional mosaicism: See mosaicism.

G-banding: See banding.

G protein: Short for "guanine nucleotide-binding proteins." G proteins are a family of proteins involved signaling cascades—typically as secondary messenger. They are common mediators in post receptor-ligand binding.

Gamete: In humans, an oocyte or a spermatozoa (aka germ cells).

Gamete complementation: The phenomenon of two gametes (oocyte and sperm) possessing complementary abnormalities that essentially "fix" the other, e.g., an oocyte with no copies of a specific chromosome and the spermatozoa having 2 copies of the same chromosome.

Gastrulation: Embryologic process.

Gene: A unit of heredity. A gene refers to a specific segment of DNA that can be delineated by a start and stop position. Genes typically code for a specific product (oftentimes a protein molecule).

   Candidate gene: In research studies, a candidate gene is a gene identified in a region of interest which is deemed as possibly associated with a condition of interest.

   Gene dosage: The number of copies of a given gene in a given cell.

Structural gene: A gene that codes for a functional protein (in contrast to those genes that code for regulatory functions not mediated by proteins).

Gene dosage: See gene.

Gene pool: The total of all genes in a defined population.

Gene therapy: In the broadest sense "gene therapy" refers to treatments that are targeted at the molecular level. A stricter use of the term would be limited to those therapies that utilize molecular/DNA technologies.

Gene × environmental interactions: The current understanding of human genetic disorders involves an interaction of the individual's genome with the environment that ultimately defines the phenotype.

General population screening: See genetic screening.

Genetic: A medical condition is said to be genetic if the pathophysiology of the disorder is based in a change in the DNA.

Genetic code: The "code" in genomics refers to the particular amino acid coded for by a specific trinucleotide group.

Genetic counseling: A process by which individuals or families receive information about genetic disorders or malformations and risks for these conditions after review of family and medical history; includes analysis of diagnostic information, review of natural history of the relevant conditions, options for dealing with risks and enhancement of family decision making through nonjudgmental support .

Genetic counselor: A professional trained in counseling families about genetic conditions, genetic risks and decision making, and adapting to a genetic condition.

Genetic damage rate: See mutation.

Genetic discrimination: Use of information about genetic traits in order to identify at-risk individuals for a different selection process in employment, housing, insurance, or other usually non-medical settings; typically used to refer to an unfair selection process by which individuals are denied or presented with barriers to their application, such as much higher premiums for insurance.

Genetic heterogeneity: See heterogeneity.

Genetic Information Non Discrimination Act (GINA): Federal legislation enacted in 2008 that protects patients from having their genetic information used to their detriment (in things such as insurance and employment).

Genetic screening: The search for healthy individuals in a specified population who possess a genetic change that may cause or predispose to certain disorders. Genetic screening can be designed for "individual screening," "selected population screening," or at whole (general) "population screening."

　Sensitivity: The screening detection rate. That is, what proportion of truly affected individuals is detected by the screening?

　Specificity: The accuracy of the screening process. That is, what proportion of individuals identified by screening as a "presumptive positive" actually has the condition?

Genetic support group: A group or organization developed around a specific condition or group of conditions related to genetics or malformations, in order to provide information and support to families.

Genetic test: In the broadest sense, a genetic test is any test performed to make a diagnosis of a genetic condition. Most often it refers to testing that involves analyzing DNA or RNA in some manner.

Genetics: In the realm of medicine, genetics are the principles applied to human disorders.

　Clinical genetics: Genetics applied to direct health care practice.

　Human genetics: The genetics of humans. Encompasses all aspects (including population genetics and the genetics of non-disease traits).

　Medical genetics: Genetics of human health. Can be clinical or research.

Genomics: The discipline of genetics that focuses at the level of the genome.

Genotype: The genetic information of an individual. The genotype can be at various levels of testing (chromosomal, gene, nucleotide sequence).

　Genotype × environmental interactions: Most phenotypes are influenced by a combination of genetic and environmental factors.

Gonadal (germ-line) mosaicism: See mosaicism.

Gonadal (germ-line) mutation: See mutation.

Haploid: See ploidy.

Hemizygous: Males have a single X chromosome. Thus for most genes coded on the X-chromosome there is not a complementary allele. Males are thus hemizygous at these loci.

Hereditary: Inherited or heritable through the gametes of biological parents; commonly refers to traits related to a single gene or specific chromosome alteration.

Heterochromatin: Darkly stained regions of the chromosomes. **Heterochromatic** regions are characterized by tight packaging and increased concentrations of protective proteins.

Heteroplasmy (heteroplasmic): In reference to mitochondrial DNA, heteroplasmy denotes the status of not all mitochondria having the same DNA sequence. The opposite of heteroplasmy is homoplasmy.

Heterotopia (heterotopic): In the wrong place. In contrast to "ectopia," heterotopia is at the tissue or cellular level. (i.e., neuronal heterotopias). Heterotopias may be developmental or migrational. See also ectopia.

Heterogenous nuclear RNA (hnRNA): See RNA.

Heterodimer: See homodimer.

Heterodisomy: See uniparental disomy.

Heterogeneity: A state in which variable or divergent components exist. In medical genetics heterogeneity typically focus on genomic variability. The opposite of heterogeneity would be homogeneity.

　Allelic heterogeneity: Refers to different mutations at the same locus causing the same or similar phenotype.

　Genetic heterogeneity: Different mutations causing an identical or similar phenotype.

　Locus heterogeneity: Refers to mutations at different loci causing the same or similar phenotypes.

Heterozygote: An individual who is heterozygous for one allele at a particular locus is said to be a heterozygote for that condition.

　Advantage: The situation in which a person who is heterozygous for a mutation in a particular gene has a (population) selective advantage for reproduction.

　Compound: A person possessing two heterogeneous recessive alleles at a particular locus is said to be a compound heterozygote.

　Disadvantage: The situation in which a person who is heterozygous for a mutation in a particular gene has a (population) selective disadvantage for reproduction.

Heterozygous: Possessing a different DNA sequence at the two alleles of a particular gene.

High resolution karyotype: See banding.

High-throughput sequencing: See sequencing.

Holandric: Referring to genes on the Y chromosome.

Holoenzyme: See enzyme.

Homeobox: See homeotic genes.

Homeodomain: See homeotic genes.

Homeotic genes (HOX): Primordial genes that are primary organizers of multicellular organisms. Homeotic genes determine basic organizational templates such as sidedness, anterior versus posterior, and superior versus inferior developmental domains.

    Homeobox: A family (grouping) of homeotic genes which work in concert in the development of specific embryonic structures or regions.

    Homeodomain: A region of common sequence in a homeotic gene—usually a common string of 60 amino acid residues which are usually similar among HOX genes.

    Homeotic mutations: Simply, mutations in homeotic genes.

    Hox complex: Highly conserve clusters of homeotic genes.

Homodimer: In protein assembly, a homodimer is the result of coupling of two identical protein strands.

    Heterodimer: In protein assembly, a heterodimer is the result of coupling of two different protein strands.

Homodisomy: See uniparental disomy.

Homogeneity: A state in which uniformity exists. In medical genetics homogeneity refers to identical genetic codes.

Homologous chromosomes: In the human genome, chromosome pairs exist in the nucleus. Homologous pairs are those that are of the same type (i.e., the two chromosomes #2).

Homoplasmy (homoplasmic): See heteroplasmy.

Homozygous (homozygote): If both alleles at a locus are identical, the individual is homozygous at that locus (a homozygote for that condition).

Hox complex: See homeotic genes.

Human genetics: See genetics.

Hypogenesis: See agenesis.

Imprinting: In general terms "imprinting" means to make a mark or stamp on something. In genetics, the term applies to pre-programming of the expression of specific genes.

    Imprinting domains: Clusters of imprinted genes non-randomly distributed across the genome.

Inactivation: In its simplest form, genetic inactivation involves the "turning off" of a specific gene or set of genes. Inactivation can occur at any level including that of an entire chromosome (see X-inactivation).

Incomplete dominance: See dominant inheritance.

Incomplete penetrance: See penetrance.

Independent assortment: The random segregation of alleles on different pairs of homologous chromosomes due to the separation of these pairs during meiosis.

Individual screening: See genetic screening.

Inducible gene: A gene whose expression can "turn on" by specific external factors.

Informed consent: The process of explaining a test or a procedure to a patient that explains the details of the process including risks, benefits, and what will be done with the information. Informed consent must be understandable to the patient at his or her level of understanding and be finalized with a formal signed form.

Inheritance patterns: Observable patterns of the transmission of heritable traits as evidenced by the family history, pedigree, or gene analysis.

    Digenic inheritance: A clinical trait is expressed when mutation on two different genes (loci) are present.

    Monoallelic inheritance: A clinical trait is expressed when only one allele of a single gene pair is altered.

    Multi-locus inheritance: The expression of a condition due to the progressive accumulation of mutations in multiple genes (loci).

    Triallelic inheritance: A clinical trait is expressed only after a particular combination of 3 different alleles possess a mutation.

Initiation factors: Proteins that bind the ribosome during the start of translation (protein synthesis).

Interphase: See cell cycle.

Intron: The noncoding regions of a gene.

Inverse disorders: Genetic disorders that are reciprocal to genetic changes. For example, the deletion of a particular chromosome region may be associated with a recognizable syndrome. Likewise duplication of the same region may produce a different condition. These would be known as reciprocal or inverse disorders.

Inversion: A chromosome rearrangement that results from two breakpoints on a chromosome and the subsequent rotation of the "freed" segment along the axis of the chromosome.

    Paracentric inversion: An inversion in which both endpoints are on the same arm of the chromosome.

    Pericentric inversion: An inversion in which the endpoints are on opposite arms of the chromosome and the centromere is included.

Karyotype: See chromosomal analysis.

Krebs (citric acid) cycle: The middle component of energy generation which starts with acetyl CoA which proceeds through 8 enzyme catalyzed reactions that ultimately yields 3 NADH, 1 GTP, and 1 FADH molecules for further metabolism.

Kinetochore: A subcellular component of the chromatids which connect to the spindle fibers during cell division to aid in sister chromatids separation.

Liability (liabilities): When discussing gene × environment interactions, deleterious genetic and environmental factors that contribute to the phenotype are known as liabilities toward expression.

Linear sequencing: See sequencing.

Linkage: The tendency of alleles to segregate together based upon their proximity on the chromosome.

    Linkage disequilibrium: The co-occurrence of alleles more often than would be predicted by chance.

    Linkage group: A set of loci/alleles that segregate together during chromosome replication.

Locus (loci): A genetic locus is a specific position or location on a chromosome. Frequently, locus is used to refer to a specific gene.

Locus heterogeneity: See heterogeneity.

Long-term follow-up: A formal process of following a defined population over time with data collection on objective parameters with the primary focus being clinical outcomes.

Looped domains: The basic structural unit of eukaryotic chromatin. In the condensation of DNA nucleosomes are compacted together to form chromatin fibers. The chromatin fibers are then folded into looped domain. (The looped domains are subsequently organized into chromosomal structures.)

Lyonization: X chromosome inactivation originally described by Dr. Mary Lyon.

Lysosomal storage disorder: An inborn error of metabolism in which a lysosomal function is disrupted. The end result is normal synthesis of a biochemical, but disrupted degradation leading to accumulation (storage).

Malformation: An abnormality of development during embryogenesis. Malformation refers to structures that inherently develop abnormally.

   Major malformation or anomaly: A congenital structural abnormality which has significant effect on function or social acceptability; example: cleft lip; in its strictest definition, malformation defines a structural abnormality resulting from an abnormal developmental process, but common usage includes all structural abnormalities as malformations, regardless of cause.

   Minor malformation: Congenital structural abnormality which has little functional or societal significance on its own.

Marker chromosome: An extra piece of chromosomal material that can be detected by a karyotype that segregates with the other normal chromosomes during cell division. Marker chromosomes can be composed of almost any part and combination of the other "normal" chromosomes.

Massively parallel sequencing: See sequencing

Maternal effects: Maternal effects refer to the fact that the earliest stages of embryonic development are controlled by the maternal genome.

Mean: A statistical calculated value that is the sum of all measurements (ΣX) divided by the number of individuals in the sample (N).

Medical geneticist: A professional with a doctoral degree and special training in the relationships between genes and disease (see Clinical geneticist).

Medical genetics: See genetics.

Medical home neighbor: One role that the medical geneticist may fill in the care of patients with genetic disorders. The medical home neighbor helps the primary medical home provide the level of specialty care without disrupting the medical home relationship with the primary care provider.

Meiosis: The process of halving the chromosome number in the formation of gametes.

Mendel, Gregor: Austrian monk credited with defining the principles of independent of assortment of single alleles. The term "Mendelian inheritance" is a credit to this work.

Mendelian inheritance: Pattern of inheritance of a genetic trait due to a single gene variation which follows the classical patterns of autosomal recessive, autosomal dominant, or X-linked (dominant or recessive) inheritance.

Mesoderm: See trilaminar embryo.

Messenger: In cellular systems, messengers are compounds that facilitate communication at a variety of levels.

   Primary messenger: The initial compound involved in a communication. A hormone would be an example of a primary messenger.

   Secondary messenger: Cellular messages are often facilitated through a primary contact which initiates a subsequent

transmissible response. Compounds involved in subsequent steps are referred to as secondary messengers. Examples would include G proteins, cAMP and CREB.

Messenger RNA: See RNA.

Metabolic dietician: A health care professional with training in nutrition with special training and emphasis in working with person with inborn errors of metabolism.

Metabolomics: The study of genetic processes involving metabolites. In genetic analysis it is the study of linked proteins in chemical systems that interact around a common pathway or process.

Metagenomics: The isolation and sequencing of the DNA of microorganisms taken from the environment, without the need for culturing the organism. It is sometimes also called "community genomics" or "environmental genomics."

Metaphase: See cell cycle.

Microdeletion syndrome: A recognizable pattern of anomalies due to the deletion of multiple contiguous genes.

Microduplication syndrome: A recognizable pattern of anomalies due to the duplication of multiple contiguous genes.

Microsatellite: Repeated sequences of 2 to 6 bps of DNA. Microsatellites have proven to be important sources of genomic variability that can be used in mapping and linkage.

Microsatellite instability: Although microsatellites are quite variable between individuals, the actual number in a given person is a set number. In individuals who have mutations involving mismatch repair genes, acquired mutations in the microsatellites can alter their length. The laboratory identification of multiple lengths of microsatellites in an individual is termed "microsatellite instability" (msi).

Minisatellites: Repeating units of DNA around 15 to 100 nucleotides. Overall runs are 1 to 5 kb. Also called variable number tandem repeats (VNTRs).

Mismatch repair genes: Genes that function as biologic "spell-checkers" that identify errors in DNA replication and then initiate the process of correcting the error.

Missense mutation: See mutation.

Mitochondrial disorder: A medical condition due to disruption of mitochondrial function. A mitochondrial disorder may be due to mutations in either mitochondrial or nuclear genes.

Mitochondrial inheritance: The pattern of heritability seen with mutations in the mitochondrial DNA. Mitochondrial inheritance has several characteristics distinct from nuclear inheritance.

Mitosis: The process of duplicating chromosomes for somatic cell replication.

Modifier genes: Genes that affect the expression of other "major" genes. These may or may not have a primary function of their own.

Molecular cytogenetics: The interface of cytogenetic techniques with molecular techniques. Examples would include tests such as FISH.

Molecular decay: It is assumed that DNA replication systems will malfunction without external influence. The assumption is that over time, with enough replications, a mistake will eventually occur for no apparent reason—this is referred to as molecular decay.

Molecular (DNA) test: Laboratory analysis of an individual's genetic material for a designated piece of DNA coding for a region or gene of interest.

Monoallelic expression: A phenotype that can be explained by variances in a single gene (locus). See also inheritance patterns.

Monogenic: Due to a single gene.

Monosomy (monosomic): Possessing only one copy of a particular chromosome pair.

Morphogen: A substance directing the process of morphogenesis.

Morphogenesis: The development of form. The process of structure and organ formation in embryogenesis.

Morpholino oligonucleotides: Analogs to cDNA which are altered to be resistant to nucleases. Such nucleotide segments can bind with mRNA and can alter gene expression.

Morula: Early embryonic structure (preceding the blastula). It is a solid mass of blastomere cells. The name morula comes from its physical resemblance to a mulberry.

Mosaicism: The situation in which not all cells in an organism possess the same genotype. Mosaicism usually occurs as the result of postconceptional (acquired) changes.

    Functional mosiacism: Mosaicism that occurs as a result of differential expression of certain genes—not a change in the genetic code. (For example, X-chromosome inactivation results in functional mosaicism for females for X-linked genes).

    Gonadal (germ-line) mosaicism: Mosaicism occurring in gonadal tissue. Gonadal mosaicism involving the gametes may be heritable.

    Somatic mosaicism: Mosaicism occurring only in somatic cells.

Multi-color FISH: See FISH.

Multi-locus inheritance: A condition in which the observed phenotype can be explained by changes in more than one gene. Expression requires changes in multiple loci. See also inheritance patterns.

Multimeric protein: See protein.

Mutagen: A substance that is known to induce mutations.

Mutation: A change (deviation) of the genetic code from the normal, wild-type sequence.

    Activating mutation: A mutation which exerts its deleterious effects by actually increasing the function of that gene.

    Mutations can occur in two directions. A "forward mutation" is a change from the wild type to a mutant sequence. A "backward mutation" is a return from a mutant sequence to the wild type.

    A "point mutation" is the change in a single nucleotide. It is sometimes referred to as a single-base substitution. There are three major types of point mutations: (1) Nonsense mutations result in a premature stop codon (and thus a truncated protein product); (2) Missense mutations change the nucleotide sequence. A "transition mutation" changes a purine to another purine or a pyrimidine to another pyrimidine. A "transversion mutation" changes from a purine to a pyrimidine or vice versa; and (3) Frame shift mutations result in a shift in the reading frame. This will disrupt all of the downstream nucleotide triplets.

    Mutations can occur at any point in the ontogeny of an organism. Postconception mutations may occur in somatic (somatic mutations) or germinal cells (germ-line mutations).

    For many possible reasons, not all mutations will produce a problem. Such mutations may be referred to as "silent mutations" or "neutral mutations." Alternatively those mutations that do result in pathologic events are called "deleterious mutations" or "pathogenic mutations."

    A newly acquired mutation is called a "spontaneous mutation" in contrast to heritable (familial) mutations.

    A "mutation suppressor" is a second mutational event which alleviates or corrects the phenotypic effects of the first mutation.

    A genetic "lethal mutation" is a mutation that renders the organism incapable of passing along its genetic material.

Mutation rate: The mutation rate is the number of new mutant alleles for a given locus detected in the offspring as compared to their parents.

    Genetic damage rate: All the genetic errors that occur during a cycle of replication. (Most of these however will be corrected by DNA repair systems.)

    Mutation frequency: The ratio of mutant to normal (wild type) alleles in the population at a given time.

    Mutation hot spot: The mutation rate is not even across the genome. Certain loci have a higher than baseline rate. Such loci are termed "hotspots."

    Mutational event rate: The unrepaired genetic errors that persist after repair systems have finished their work.

Natural history: Typical course of a medical condition in the absence of specific intervention.

Noncoding RNA: See RNA.

Nonsense mutation: See mutation.

Nuclear matrix: A network of fibers located within the cell nucleus. This network is analogous to the cytoplasmic cytoskeleton.

Nuclear membrane: A membrane (double lipid bilayer) that encases the nuclear contents and defines the boundaries of the nucleus.

Nuclear lamina: A dense layer of intermediate filaments inside the nuclear membrane that provide support and regulatory functions.

Nucleolus (nucleoli): A defined subdomain of the nucleus that assembles ribosomal subunits.

Nucleosome: The basic unit of DNA packaging. It comprises a short length of DNA wrapped around a core of histone proteins.

Noncoding strand: See coding.

Nondisjunction: The failure of separation of homologous chromosome pairs during cell division.

Nucleotide: The basic unit of DNA and RNA. Nucleotides are composed of a nitrogenous base, a 5-carbon sugar (either ribose or 2-deoxyribose), and a phosphate group.

Ochronosis: A dark (blue/black) discoloration of the skin. This finding has been classically associated with the inborn error of metabolism, alkaptonuria.

Okazaki fragments: Short segments of newly synthesized DNA which are complementary to the lagging template strand.

Oligonucleotide: A small segment of connected nucleotides.

Oogenesis: The process of forming oocytes from primordial germ cells.

Operon: A grouping of associated genes that are under the control of a single regulatory signal or promoter.

Paracentric invesion: See inversion.

Parthenogenesis: Asexual reproduction which occurs with the initiation of embryogenesis without fertilization.

Paternity: Pertaining to the male parent of a child.

    Mis-assigned paternity: The situation in which the assumed father of a child is not, in fact, the biologic parent.

Pathogenesis: Physiologic process in causing disease.

Pathogenic (deleterious) mutation: See mutation.

Pattern formation: In embryogenesis, pattern formation refers to the complex predetermined organization and outcomes of cell fates spatially and temporally.

Pedigree: A formal diagram of the genetic relationships in a family using standardized symbols and nomenclature, indicating specific medical conditions, the status of each family member in relation to pertinent genetic traits (affected, unaffected, carrier, etc.) and additional relevant information necessary to discern possible patterns of inheritance and genetic risk; typically three or more generations are recorded.

Penetrance: For a given condition, the proportion of patients who show clinical signs of the disorder. Penetrance is disease specific. Some conditions are completely penetrant. Some show incomplete penetrance.

Peptidyl transfer(ase): A nuclear enzyme that catalyzes the cumulative addition of amino acid residues to a lengthening peptide chain in the ribosomes.

Pericentric inversion: See inversion.

Personalized genomics: Specific genetic testing that identifies individual risk profiles for a specific medical condition and or treatment option.

Personalized health care: Customizing diagnostics and treatments to an individual patient's specific profile.

Personalized medicine: Health care targeted to the inherent biology and physiology of an individual leading to improvements in their medical care.

Pharmacogenetics: A personalized medicine strategy that utilizes genomic data to direct the choice and dosage of medications.

Phenocopy: Similar phenotypes produced by completely different genotypes.

Phenotype: The clinical or behavioral presentation of a genetic variation in an individual.

    Expanded phenotype: The full range of phenotypes associated with a given genotype.

    Phenotype, abnormal: The clinical presentation of a genetic or malformation disorder in an individual, including associated complications and their severity.

    Phenotype, behavioral: The pattern of behavioral abnormalities and traits associated with a specific genetic or malformation disorder.

Plasmid: Circular DNA elements that replicate independent of the chromosomal DNA.

Pleiotropy (pleiotropism): Multiple clinical effects of a single gene.

Ploidy: Referring to chromosome number. One full set of human chromosomes (23) is designated as "n."

    Aneuploid: Having an incorrect number of chromosomes.

    Euploid: Having a correct number of chromosomes.

    Diploid: Having two full copies of a chromosome set (46, or 2n). This is the normal count for human somatic cells.

    Haploid: Having one full set of 23 chromosomes (n). This is the normal count for the germ cells (gametes).

    Polyploid: Having a full extra set (or multiples) of 23 beyond the usual 46 chromosomes in the human genome. This could be 69 (3n), 92 (4n), etc.

    Triploid: A polyploidy chromosome count of 69 (3n).

Pluripotent: See potency.

Point mutation: See mutation.

Polar body: During meiosis in the formation of the oocyte, all daughter cells are not equally developed. The polar body is a tiny cell containing little or no cytoplasm that is produced and ultimately eliminated.

Poly-A tail: An extended run of up to 200 adenine nucleotides added to the "tail" (3′ end) of the pre-mRNA via the process called polyadenylation catalyzed by the enzyme, polyadenylate polymerase.

Polygenic: Literally "many genes." Traditionally polygenic inheritance refers to a specific pattern of multifactorial inheritance in which multiple genes contribute in an additive fashion to a quantitative phenotype.

Polymerase chain reaction: A molecular technique of amplifying small amounts (even single copies) of DNA.

Polymorphism: As described in the text, the term polymorphism may be confusing. Population geneticists use the term for mutations that occur in the general population in at least 1% of individuals. Clinical geneticists and clinical genetic laboratory professionals often use the term synonymous with mutation (i.e., any change from the wild-type DNA code).

    Benign polymorphism: A polymorphism that does not cause clinical disease

    Single nucleotide polymorphism (SNP): A nucleotide change at a single specified locus in the genome different from the accepted "wild-type" code.

Posttranslational modification: Changes made to a transcribed protein that further defines the protein's structure and function. Such modifications would include glycosylation and acetylation of the protein.

Potency: The capacity of a cell to differentiate along various paths.

    Pluripotent cells: have the potential to differentiate in multiple different specialized cells.

    Totipotent cells: are completely undifferentiated and have the capacity to proceed down any pathway of cell specialization.

Prereplication complex (pre-RC): A multimeric protein assembled at the initiation step of DNA replication.

Primer: A short segment of nucleotides that function as the initiation point for DNA synthesis.

Proband (propositus, proposita): The first member in a family to be ascertained. If affected, the individual is the index case.

Product rule: In probabilities, the rule is to multiply "and" relationships.

Prometaphase: See cell cycle.

Prometaphase karyotype: See banding.

Promoter: The region of the DNA strand that starts the transcription of a particular gene. Promoters are typically in close proximity to the genes they promote.

Prophase: See cell cycle.

Protein: A biochemical composed of strands of amino acids.

    Regulatory protein: Specialized proteins that bind to regulatory sequences of DNA and function to regulate the gene transcription.

    Multimeric protein: A protein complex that has a specific function but which is made up of several different protein components.

Protein domain: Proteins often have multiple functions. Different parts of a given protein can perform site-specific functions.

Protein kinase: A protein that catalyzes phosphorylation of other proteins.

Proteomics: The broad study of proteins including structure, function, regulation, and interactions.

Prototroph: See Autotroph.

Pseudoautosomal regions: Complementary regions of the X and Y chromosomes which allow autosomal like activities for the sex chromosomes—including chromosomal cross-over.

Pseudodominance: See dominant inheritance.

Pseudogene: A DNA segment which shares a large amount of sequence homology to a "true" functioning gene. Pseudogenes may represent degenerate copies of previously functioning genes.

Pyrosequencing: See sequencing.

Qualitative trait: See trait.

Quantitative trait: See trait.

Quasi-dominance: See dominant inheritance.

Reanneal: See anneal.

Recessive (recessiveness): Recessive conditions are clinically manifest only in individuals homozygous for the mutant allele (or compound heterozygotes for two different mutant alleles), i.e., carrying a "double dose" of an abnormal gene.

Reciprocal translocation: See translocation.

Recombination: Also called "crossing over." During meiosis homologous chromosome pairs exchange material by physically bridging from one to another. It is likely that at least one cross-over event is necessary for normal meiosis to proceed.

Recurrence risk: See risk.

Regulation: The concept of altering gene expression without changing the code. Regulation of a gene can include turning that gene "off" or "on" or partially turning it "up" or "down."

Regulators of organelle gene expression (ROGEs): Organelles such as mitochondria possess DNA separate from the nuclear genome. These extranuclear genetic elements are coordinated and regulated by nuclear elements known as ROGEs.

Regulatory protein: See protein.

Release factor: A protein that functions to terminate translation by locating the termination (stop) codon of a gene.

Replication fork: During the process of DNA replication, the replication fork is the active site of unwinding the parent sequence and synthesizing the daughter code.

Replicative segregation: The separation of subpopulations of mitochondria within a cell by the physical process of cell division.

Replisome: The structure that carries out the activities of the replication fork. The replisome is multimeric unit composed of two DNA polymerase enzymes, primase and DNA.

Repressor (repressible): A regulatory protein that binds to the operator site and blocks transcription of the gene.

Response elements: Short DNA segments that are part of the promoter region of a gene that bind transcription factors to regulate transcription.

Restriction enzyme (point): Also called restriction endonucleases. Enzymes that cleave (cut) DNA by recognizing very specific sequences that is characteristic of that enzyme. The site at which the DNA is cut is the restriction site (point).

Reverse transcriptase: An enzyme which catalyzes the synthesis of DNA from an RNA template (the reverse of normal transcription).

Ribosomal binding site: The nucleotide sequence which signals the beginning of a gene. See Shine-Dalgarno sequence.

Ribosomal RNA: See RNA.

Risk: In clinical genetics, the "risk" identified for a patient is probability of a clinical event occurring.

Empiric risk: The risk of a condition in a defined situation ascertained from simple observational data.

Recurrence risk: The likelihood that a clinical disorder will occur in additional siblings of the same biological parents.

Relative risk: The risk of developing a disease relative to an exposure or other predisposing factor.

RNA: Ribonucleic acid. A biochemical involved in a variety of genetic processes. It is composed of long chains of nucleotides, each of which is assembled from a nitrogenous base attached to a backbone of a ribose sugar, and a phosphate molecule. Messenger RNA (mRNA), ribosomal RNA (rRNA), and transfer RNA (tRNA) are involved in the traditional understanding of transcription and translation.

Noncoding RNA: Many of the other species of RNA do not code for a product. Rather they have a primary regulatory function. Examples would include microRNAs (miRNA) which act through RNA interference (RNAi) as do small interfering RNAs (siRNA). Pri-miRNAs are the primary transcripts for miRNA which are then processed into pre-miRNAs. Nuclear RNAs include small nuclear RNAs (snRNA) whose primary function is in the processing of pre-mRNA also called heterogenous nuclear RNA (hnRNA) in the nucleus.

RNA polymerases (I-V): A family of enzymes involved in the synthesis of various forms of RNA.

Robertsonian translocation: See translocation.

Sanger sequencing: See sequencing.

Satellite DNA: Large arrays of tandemly repeating, noncoding DNA. The name "satellite" comes from a second ("satellite" band) that is adjacent to regular DNA on a density gradient.

Second(ary) messenger: See messenger.

Segmentation genes: Genes that code for embryonic organization into various "segments" (or fields) of the body.

Segregation: Separation of paired homologous chromosomes. Segregation may occur in several different ways if a translocation exists.

Adjacent segregation: The segregation of each of the structurally normal chromosomes with one of the translocated ones is said to be adjacent.

Alternate: The segregation is said to be alternate if the two normal chromosomes segregate together, as do the reciprocal parts of the translocated ones.

Selected population screening: See genetic screening.

Selection: A process that favors the survival of one kind of organism over others by a reproductive advantage.

Directional selection: When natural selection favors a single phenotype.

Diversifying selection: When natural selection favors more than one phenotype. Extreme phenotypes are favored over intermediate ones.

Stabilizing selection: Selection in which genetic diversity decreases as the population stabilizes on a particular trait value. Instead of favoring individuals with extreme phenotypes, it favors the intermediate ones.

Sense codon: See codon.

Sequence: A pattern of related malformations and/or deformations and/or disruptions such that one initial physical abnormality leads to the occurrence of additional abnormalities in a sequential manner.

Sequencing: When applied to genomics, "sequencing" means the determination of the actual order and type of nucleotides in a defined portion of the genome.

DNA sequencing: Determining the nucleotide sequence for DNA molecules.

High-throughput sequencing: A method of DNA sequencing that uses multiple modifications of regular sequencing including robotics and advanced information technology to greatly increase the possible rate of sequencing.

Linear sequencing: Sequencing a segment of genetic material in a linear fashion (i.e., from start codon to terminating sequence in order).

Massively parallel sequencing: One of the newest methods of sequencing that employs techniques of sequencing thousands of small copies (subsets) of the region to be sequenced in tandem.

Pyrosequencing: A newer method of DNA sequencing that utilizes pyrophosphate release on nucleotide incorporation.

Sanger (dideoxy) sequencing: A method of DNA sequencing developed by Frederick Sanger in 1977. The technique utilizes the selective incorporation of chain-terminating dideoxynucleotides.

Whole exome sequencing: Sequencing the entire coding region of an individual's genome.

Whole genome sequencing: Sequencing an individual's entire genetic code—both coding and noncoding parts.

Semi-dominance: See dominant inheritance.

Sensitivity: See genetic screening.

Sex (linkage, limited, influenced):

Sex-limited phenotype: The expression of a trait in only one of the sexes, due, for instance, to anatomical differences. Example: uterine or testicular defects.

Sex-influenced phenotype: A phenotype which occurs in both males and females, but with different frequencies. Example: male pattern baldness.

Sex-linked inheritance: Sex-linked genes are those located on either the X or the Y chromosome. Because few genes are known to be located on the human Y chromosome, we will focus on X-linked disorders.

Shine-Dalgarno sequence: A nucleotide sequence (AGGAGGU) that is found in 8 bps upstream of the AUG start codon of mRNA. It functions as a ribosomal binding site.

Signal transduction: The process of converting an extracellular signal into an intracellular response.

Signaling pathway: A series of biochemical reactions in an organism in which chemical signals are sequentially passed from one molecule to the next in succession.

Single nucleotide polymorphism (SNP): See polymorphism.

Tag SNP: A representative SNP in a genomic region (locus) with known high linkage disequilibrium.

Single-locus FISH: See FISH.

Sister chromatids: See chromatid.

Situs abnormalities: "Situs" refers to the place where something originates or should be (i.e., the normal place). In embryogenesis, situs refers to the location where an organ or body part should be found. There are medical descriptors of several different abnormalities of situs (e.g., laterality defects).

Dextrocardia: A situs abnormality of the heart only.

Situs abdominalis: Only the abdominal organs being on the wrong side.

Situs inversus: The description of an organ being in the opposite (mirror image) position of normal.

Situs inversus totalis: All organs being on the opposite side of normal.

Situs solitus: The normal positioning of the abdominal and thoracic organs.

Small nuclear ribonucleoproteins (snRNP): RNA-protein complexes involved in transcription. These complexes are essential to the excision of introns from mRNA.

Somatic mosaicism: See mosaicism.

Somatic mutation: See mutation.

Sorting signals: Specific amino acids in a protein sequences serve to guide the transport of that protein to specific subcellular compartments.

Southern blot: More formally referred to as a DNA blot test. Named after the British biologist Dr. Edwin Southern. The term "blot" refers to the method of transferring the DNA molecules. This process allows the separation of DNA molecules of differing sizes.

Specificity: See genetic screening.

Spermatogenesis: The embryologic process of starting with undifferentiated germ cells and proceeding to the end point of mature spermatozoa.

Spindle: See chromosome spindle.

Spontaneous mutation: See mutation.

Standard deviation: A statistical term that represents the square root of the variance.

Stop codon(s): See codon.

Structural gene: See gene.

Sub-telomeric FISH: See FISH.

Susceptibility: Genetic susceptibility refers to a genetic change (polymorphism) that renders the individual more susceptible to adverse effects from a specific environmental interaction.

Synapsis: The coupling (pairing) of two homologous chromosomes that happens during meiosis.

Synaptonemal complex: A complex multimeric (three proteins) structure that bridges across the paired chromosomes during prophase I of meiosis.

Syndrome: A recognizable recurrent pattern of malformations and/or deformations and/or disruptions with one or more specific, defined causes.

Tag SNP: See single nucleotide polymorphism.

Tandem duplications: See duplication.

Tandem repeats: Nucleotide sequences that are contiguously repeated at a given locus.

Tautomeric shift: A shift in a proton (hydrogen ion) to form a different isomer. In DNA, a tauomeric shift of a nucleotide may result in a mutation.

Telocentric: See chromosome.

Telomere: The end part of a chromosome composed of repetitive nucleotide sequences.

Telophase: See cell cycle.

Teratogen: An agent capable of inducing one or more malformations in a developing embryo. A teratogen can be environmental exposures or maternal medical conditions.

Threshold: A biologic limit which if crossed, exceeds the capability of an organism to buffer against pathologic changes.

Totipotent: See potency.

Trait: An observable feature or characteristic.

Qualitative: An observable trait.

Quantitative: A measureable trait.

Transcription: The copying of DNA to a complementary segment of mRNA.

Transcription factor: A protein that regulates the rate of DNA transcription, typically by altering RNA polymerase activity.

Transcriptomics: The transcriptome is the total set of transcripts in a given organism. This reflects all of the genes that are being actively expressed at any given time. Transcriptomics is the discipline of studying the transcriptome.

Transfer RNA: See RNA.

Transition: See mutation.

Translocation: A chromosome abnormality in which a portion of one chromosome has moved (translocated) to another location from its normal site.

> **Balanced:** A translocation in which there is no net loss or gain of chromosomal material from the normal amount and makeup.
>
> **Reciprocal:** A complementary exchange of chromosomal material between two nonhomologous chromosomes.
>
> **Robertsonian:** A special type of translocation that involves two acrocentric chromosomes. In this type of translocation the satellite material is lost on both chromosomes and the two "q arms" are joined together.
>
> **Unbalanced:** A translocation in which there is net loss (deletion) or gain (duplication) of chromosomal material.

Transposable elements (transposons): One of several classes of mobile segments of DNA.

> **Class I transposable elements:** These are called retrotransposons. Replication occurs in 2 steps: (1) DNA to RNA via transcription; and (2) From RNA back to DNA by reverse transcription. This method of duplication in retrotransposons is quite similar to retroviruses.
>
> **There are three main categories of retrotransposons:**
> - Long terminal repeats (LTRs). These encode reverse transcriptase, similar to retroviruses
> - Long interspersed elements (LINEs). These also encode reverse transcriptase but lack LTRs. They are transcribed by RNA polymerase II.
> - Short interspersed elements (SINEs). Similar to LINEs but of course shorter (<500 bp) these do not code for reverse transcriptase. They are transcribed by RNA polymerase III.
>
> **Class II transposable elements:** These are called DNA transposons. In contrast to retrotransposons, these do not involve an RNA intermediate.

Transversions: See mutation.

Trialleleic inheritance: Certain genetic conditions are caused by mutations at more than one locus (multi-locus). Triallelic inheritance refers to a condition that requires mutations in three different alleles to produce the phenotype. See also inheritance patterns.

Trilaminar embryo: In the first 2 to 3 weeks of gestation, the early embryo becomes a layered structure. The three layers (endoderm, ectoderm, and mesoderm) are the embryonic primordia for future tissue groups.

> **Ectoderm:** The embryonic layer that gives rise to the hair, skin, teeth, nails, and parts of the nervous system.
>
> **Endoderm:** The embryonic layer that gives rise to the epithelium of the abdominal and lower respiratory tracts, and associated organs such as the liver and pancreas.
>
> **Mesoderm:** The embryonic layer that gives rise to constitutional components of the body including bone, muscle, connective tissue, dermis layer of the skin, circulatory system, and the reproductive system.

Trinucleotide repeats: Repeating units of 3 nucleotides distributed in a nonrandom fashion across the genome. (See also satellite DNA.)

> **Trinucleotide repeat disorders:** Medical conditions produced by abnormal numbers (typically expansion) of trinucleotide repeats. Through pre-event mutations, transcription of regions of trinucleotide repeats can undergo sequential expansion (increase in the number of repeats beyond the normal baseline counts). Expansion of these regions can disrupt gene function and regulation through a variety of mechanisms. If the expansion exceeds tolerable threshold, human disease can occur. Typically, trinucleotide repeat disorders are neuromuscular conditions.

Triploid: See ploidy.

Trisomy (trisomic): Having a full extra copy (n = 3) of a particular chromosome (e.g., trisomy 21).

True dominance: See dominant inheritance.

Uniparental disomy (UPD): Inheriting two copies of the same chromosome number from one parent (in contrast to the normal situation of receiving one homolog from each parent).

> **Heterodisomy:** Inheriting two of the same chromosome pair from one parent.
>
> **Isodisomy:** Inheriting both copies of a homolog pair from one parent.

United States Medical Licensing Examination (USMLE): A three-part examination taken by medical students as part of the process of medical licensure.

Upstream factors: Specific proteins that bind DNA and recognize short consensus elements located upstream from the initiation of transcription.

Variability: In clinical genetics, refers to the range (severity) of a phenotype.

> **Inter-familial variability:** Clinical variation of a specific condition as observed between families.
>
> **Intra-familial variability:** Clinical variation of a specific condition as observed within a family.

Variable expression: See expression.

Variable number tandem repeats (VNTRs): See minisatellite.

Variance: A calculated statistical value which is the average squared deviation of each data point from the mean.

Whole exome sequencing: See sequencing.

Whole genome sequencing: See sequencing.

Wild type: The phenotype or genotype established as the baseline (normal) for a population.

Wobble position: The third nucleotide of a trinucleotide sequence in DNA. Because the human DNA code is degenerate (i.e., more than one trinucleotide combination can code for the same amino acid), the final nucleotide is said to be in the wobble position.

X-chromosome inactivation: Also known as Lyonization. In females—who have 2 X chromosomes–1 X chromosome is inactivated in every cell. This serves as a "balancing" mechanism because males are hemizygous—possessing only one X chromosome.

> **X-inactivation center (XIC):** The locus on the X chromosome that controls the process of X-inactivation.

Skewed X inactivation: Because X-inactivation is presumably a random process, it is predicted that on average, there will be a 50:50 split between the two X chromosomes as far as which is inactivated. There are several pathogenic mechanisms whereby one X may be preferentially inactivated over the other—leading to a skewed ratio between the two X's.

X-linked inheritance: Transmission of a condition via a gene that is on the X chromosome.

Y-linked inheritance: Sometimes called holandric inheritance. Transmission of a condition via a gene that is on the Y chromosome.

Answers to Board-Format Practice Questions

Chapter 1

1. **B** is the correct answer. The other answers are incorrect because:
   A. The genome includes DNA outside of the nucleus, such as in the mitochondria.
   C. It is the DNA content, not the protein content, of a cell that is its genome.
   D. The correlation of genomic size and the amount of information encoded has a poor correlation especially in more complex organisms.
   E. You know why.

2. **D** is the correct answer. The other answers are incorrect because:
   A. The current best estimate for humans is 22,000 functioning genes.
   B. One of the many surprises has been the marked homology of genes among species.
   C. Although the overall sequence has been identified, the actual assignment of sequences to specific genes (and diseases) is nowhere close to complete.
   E. The information from the genome project has been made widely available to the public.

3. **D** is the correct answer. The other answers are incorrect because:
   A. If diagnostics and therapies are individualized, costs should go down from less 'trial and error' complications.
   B. Personalized medicine is not a theoretical science. It has direct clinical application in current day medical practice.
   C. This should absolutely improve diagnostics—the launching point of individualized treatments.
   E. Personalized medicine is much more applicable in tertiary (and quaternary) prevention.

4. **C** is the correct answer. The other answers are incorrect because:
   A. Medical genetics interacts with all other specialties in a very real sense.
   B. Is a recognized specialty in the AMA.
   D. In the early days of medical genetics, the primary 'job' of the medical geneticist was working with multiple anomaly syndromes. In the current era, it goes into many other avenues of medicine including work with the "common" disorders.
   E. Sensational terms are not well accepted by patients and families, so care should be given to using person-friendly language.

Chapter 2

1. **A** is the correct answer. Different types of RNA play a role in an amazing breadth of functions. RNA participates in DNA replication as described in the text: "DNA polymerase III can use the 3'-OH position of an RNA nucleotide as a point for attaching the first DNA nucleotide." RNA is not involved in the other four listed processes.

2. **C** is the correct answer. Pleiotropy refers to multiple effects (consequences) of a genetic change. The other answers are incorrect because:
   A. Describes variable expression.
   B. Describes incomplete penetrance.
   D. Describes site-specific mutation expression.
   E. Describes a benign polymorphism.

3. **B** is the correct answer. The other answers are incorrect because:
   A. By definition, pseudogenes do not code for any known functional protein.
   C. Gene amplification is a function of the degree of gene expression but does not add diversity.
   D. Actually, alternative splicing is what produces increased diversity.
   E. Epimerases have nothing to do with this. Epigenetic modifications do. Just a foil with a similar sounding word.

4. **D** is the correct answer. The other answers are incorrect because:
   A. As stated earlier, pleiotropy refers to multiple effects (consequences) of a genetic change.
   B. Linkage relates to different loci, not changes in the same gene.
   C. Co-dominance is defined as the expression of both alleles independently of each other.
   E. This example refers to changes in a single gene, not changes in multiple genes that sit close to each other.

Chapter 3

1. **D** is the correct answer.
   Single transverse palmar creases would meet the definition of a "minor malformation." It is an abnormality of early (first trimester) development. It is sometimes present in normal individuals. It has no clinical significance.

2. **D** is the correct answer.
   Since porencephaly results from normal cells that are lost due to injury, this would be a disruption.

3. **E** is the correct answer.
   The fourth major category of congenital anomalies is dysplasia (abnormal histogenesis).

4. **C** is the correct answer. The other answers are incorrect because:
   A. The incidence of congenital anomalies is 5%. This is not uncommon. Every practitioner will see patients with birth defects.
   B. The overall incidence of congenital anomalies has been very stable at 4 to 6% for decades. For some of the subsets, there have been some changes. Congenital heart disease seems to be increasing. Neural tube defects seem to be decreasing.
   D. There are slight regional differences in the reported incidence of congenital anomalies. Higher rates have been reported in the South and parts of the Midwest.
   E. When a single congenital anomaly is seen, there is a 50% chance that a second anomaly exists in the same person.

5. **B** is the correct answer.
   Because the kidneys did not form, this represents a malformation (renal agenesis). With low amniotic fluid levels, the fetus is not able to move about the womb freely. The facial changes come from the face being flattened by contact with the uterus. This would be a deformation.

Chapter 4

1. **C** is the correct answer. The other answers are incorrect because:
   A. Like most early concepts in genetics, newer information has shown that the original suppositions need to be changed/updated.
   B. The concept is not completely wrong. It does hold true for selected conditions such as inborn errors of metabolism.
   D. The principles are the same in plants and animals.
   E. Few human diseases are this simple.

2. **C** is the correct answer. The other answers are incorrect because:
   A. The key theme of this chapter is that genetics is not just about protein coding.
   B. Gene-gene interactions are common.
   D. Gene expression can occur outside of the nucleus, for instance in the mitochondria.
   E. Changes in non-coding sequences can affect gene expression.

3. **A** is the correct answer. The other answers are incorrect because:
   B. The centromere is largely composed of alpha satellite material.
   C. Changes in satellite DNA can produce many different genetic syndromes.
   D. Some types of satellite DNA are classified as mini- and micro-satellites.
   E. Satellite DNA is notoriously heterogeneous. This makes it particularly attractive for marker or linkage studies.

4. **C** is the correct answer. The other answers are incorrect because:
   A. As the name implies, the gene for fragile X is on the X chromosome.
   B. Fragile X shows X-linked semi-dominant inheritance.

D. Although folate deficient media will express the fragile site, the condition is caused by an expanding tri-nucleotide repeat, not folic acid deficiency.
E. Women are also affected with fragile X.

Chapter 5

1. **C** is the correct answer. The other answers are incorrect because:
   A. Chromosome aneuploidies are not rare at conception. They occur in about 50% of all conceptions.
   B. Chromosome abnormalities are frequently lost as miscarriages. The numbers decrease as pregnancy progresses.
   C. Trisomy 13, 18 and 21 are compatible with post-natal life.
   D. A 45X karyotype is a human monosomy associated with Turner syndrome.

2. **E** is the correct answer. The other answers are incorrect because:
   The incidence of chromosome abnormalities at the time of conception is 50% (1/2).

3. **A** is the correct answer. The other answers are incorrect because:
   A. Turner syndrome is the only whole chromosome monosomy seen in live births in humans.
   B. The most common congenital heart disease in Turner syndrome is coarctation of the aorta.
   C. Turner syndrome only occurs in females.
   D. Girls with Turner syndrome condition are usually short for age.
   E. The apostrophe "s" does not go on the end of an eponym.

4. **C** is the correct answer. The other answers are incorrect because:
   A. Chromosome anomalies are common. They have tremendous clinical significance.
   B. Chromosomal anomalies show a maternal age effect.
   C. In live born infants, aneuploidies for the sex chromosomes occur more commonly than for the autosomes.
   D. Whole chromosome aneuploidies can be seen in patients for only the sex chromosomes and autosomes 13, 18, and 21.
   E. The most common clinical outcome in a chromosome abnormality is a spontaneous miscarriage.

5. **C** is the correct answer. The other answers are incorrect because:
   A. Clinical syndromes are usually associated with heterozygosity of the deletion.
   B. They usually track through a family like an autosomal dominating trait.
   C. They usually occur sporadically, but may be familial.
   D. They typically show marked variability in the phenotype.
   E. Diagnosis by FISH analysis is more sensitive and practical than chromosome testing.

Chapter 6

1. **A** is the correct answer. The condition is recessive because homozygous individuals are affected. Among the homozygotes, only males are affected. The other answers are incorrect because:
   B. Heterozygotes are not affected so it is not dominant.

C. Heterozygotes are not affected so it is not dominant.

D. Heterozygotes are not affected so it is not dominant.

E. There is nothing that suggests maternal/mitochondrial inheritance.

2. **D** is the correct answer. The increased incidence of chromosome aneuploidy seen with advanced maternal age is due to an increased rate on chromosomal non-disjunction (Chapter 5). The other answers are incorrect because:

A. Older parents have a higher incidence of congenital anomalies.

B. Older fathers have an increased incidence of single gene mutations.

C. Older mother have an increased incidence of chromosome aneuploidy (Chapter 5).

E. Transcription errors increase with advancing paternal age.

3. **C** is the correct answer. The multiple features (digital, neurologic, genital) are pleiotropic effects of the mutations in this disorder. The other answers are incorrect because:

A. Since patients tend to have a "similar" phenotype, this refers to less variability.

B. Only one gene responsible means locus homogeneity (although there is allelic heterogeneity).

D. Thresholding (incomplete penetrance) is not an issue since all recessive heterozygotes show expression.

E. Lyonization affects X-linked genes, not autosomal genes.

4. **D** is the correct answer. Males affected with an X-linked dominant condition will only transmit their Y chromosome or their only X with the mutation. Thus all of his daughters will be affected. The other answers are incorrect because:

A. Although the example of Craniofrontonasal Dysplasia in the Clinical Correlation section of this chapter is an example of an X-linked trait that has greater expression in females, this represents the rare exception. For the vast majority of X-linked conditions, males demonstrate more severe clinical expression than females.

B. Females can transmit an X chromosome to their female offspring. In X-linked dominant conditions affected mothers have a 50% chance of having affected daughters.

C. Although the degree of expression would be more in males, the number of affected males and females would be the same.

E. Mitochondrial inheritance (Chapter 13) is such that only females can transmit the condition. Clearly from answer 'D' above, descendants of affected males can be affected.

5. **B** is the correct answer. Dominant conditions typically have more variable expression than recessive disorders. The other answers are incorrect because:

A. In general, dominant conditions are more frequent than recessive conditions. As discussed in this chapter, recessive conditions may be more frequent due to phenomena such as heterozygote advantage or a founder effect. Still they are typically much less common.

C. Incomplete penetrance is typically observed with dominant conditions. This is due to the fact that recessive conditions have less variability. In theory, it is possible that a recessive condition may have incomplete penetrance. We are not aware of any such documented example.

D. Pleiotropism can be seen in dominant or recessive conditions (as per the example of SLO in question 3.

E. Holandric inheritance refers to Y-linked inheritance. There are no confirmed Y-linked disorders in humans.

Chapter 7

1. **B** is the correct answer.
DNA repair abnormalities increase the risk of cancer, but produce genome instability, premature aging, and immune deficiency. Albinism is not a common feature.

2. **C** is the correct answer.
There is a polymorphism so it is not a normal sequence. Since it has not been seen in individuals with disease it would be a known benign polymorphism. It is not pathogenic nor is it unknown. Choice E is made up.

3. **E** is the correct answer.
Mutations are common events and they are unevenly distributed across the genome (hence the term 'hot spots'). Mutations that are induced versus those that occur spontaneously are no different in their impact. As demonstrated in the clinical correlation section, therapies may be able to 'correct' a mutation.

4. **A** is the correct answer.
Mutagens may be carcinogenic and they may be teratogenic. However, the terms are not interchangeable. Man naturally occurring mutagens exist such as viruses and UV radiation from sunlight. Mutagens may be avoided. Precautions may be taken to avoid exposures to viruses; patients may be shielded from X-rays, etc. Mut^0 is a made up term.

5. **C** is the correct answer.
Mutations occur more often with unprotected DNA. Mutations may be induced by viral (not bacterial) infections. Excuse the poor sense of humor for choice D. The impact of mutations is not possible to quantify. It is simply too far reaching.

Chapter 8

1. **E** is the correct answer.
The original description of IBEMs was by Garrod in the early 1900s. Metabolic blocks produce a deficiency of product after the block and an excess of precursor before the block.

2. **E** is the correct answer.
Inborn errors of metabolism are due to monogenic abnormalities. Chromosome testing is almost always normal. The infant described most likely has galactosemia. Thus, family history, feeding history, and maybe even odors will be important clues.

3. **B** is the correct answer.
While the presentation of IBEMs is quite broad in the range of problems seen, jaundice is the only one of the symptoms listed that is a common indication of a metabolic problem (see Tables 8-4 to 8-7)

4. **A** is the correct answer.

   IBEMs not infrequently cause structural congenital anomalies. Garrod's description was in the early 1900s. Treatments work, but almost never completely "fix" things. A critical point is that IBEMs have presenting symptoms that are like so many other medical disorders.

5. **A** is the correct answer.

   In the US all states screen for PKU. Hopefully a child never slips through the process and all are picked up in the first few days of life and therapy begun quickly. Dietary therapy is effective, but by no means easy. Also therapy does not result in a completely normal outcome (IQs on average are half a standard deviation below those of sibs). It is only maternal PKU that is teratogenic.

Chapter 9

1. This pedigree shows straightforward X-linked recessive inheritance. There are only affected males. The males share common female ancestors. No male to male transmission is seen. With two affected sons, individual I-1 is a carrier of the condition. (Figure 9-11)

2. The most obvious finding is that only males are affected. The possibility of a Y-linked trait might come to mind. However, there are two females (II-2 and II-5) who have transmitted this trait that they received from their fathers. So it cannot be Y-linked. Could it be X-linked? No, as there is male-to-male transmission. You could hypothesize autosomal dominant with incomplete penetrance and it is just by chance that the females in this family were the ones that were non-penetrant. However, the correct (best) answer would be autosomal dominant with sex-limited expression. (Figure 9-12)

3. Neither parent is affected; there are two affected male children (III-3 and III-5) with the same mother (II-5). One might consider autosomal recessive inheritance. However, the two fathers (II-4 and II-6) would have to be carriers of the same disorder. If they were related, that would then be distinctly possible. However, you are not told that. You should assume that they are not related. Therefore X-linked recessive is the most likely. (Figure 9-13)

4. The correct answer is autosomal dominant with incomplete penetrance. At first glance, X-linked inheritance might be suspected. However, there is male-to-male transmission seen in this pedigree. This rules out X-linked inheritance. (Figure 9-14).

5. The best answer is autosomal recessive inheritance. In coming to this conclusion, there are several considerations. (a) This *could* be autosomal dominant with incomplete penetrance, but there are quite a few intervening meioses. The condition would have to be very weakly penetrant. (b) It is also possible that this is the chance happening of the same condition in first cousins, given that they are reasonably closely related. Chance would not be the best answer, unless this was a common condition. (c) For this to be a recessive condition the mates (II.2 and II.5) of the cousins (II.1 and II.4) would have to be carriers. The chance of this would depend on the carrier frequency in the population. (d) This is an actual pedigree from one of our clinics. The other important bit of information is not seen in the pedigree as drawn. What the cousins did not tell us at first was that their wives were sisters! This, of course, would make autosomal recessive inheritance extremely likely. (Figure 9-15).

Chapter 10

1. **E** is the correct answer.

   Different genes at different loci producing the same phenotype is genetic heterogeneity (more exactly locus heterogeneity). This is not consistent with the definitions of polygenic or multifactorial inheritance. Although the environment could obviously modify the phenotype, that is not the explanation for the three different loci.

2. **C** is the correct answer.

   Refer to the list of characteristics of multifactorial inheritance in this chapter. For choices A, B, and D the information is the opposite of what is true. Of course E is wrong, because environmental influences are central in multifactorial inheritance.

3. **B** is the best answer.

   Polygenic conditions actually have a small number of major genes that contribute to the phenotype. The offspring tend to be an average of the parents and so B would be a correct assumption. C describes a defined threshold in what is being described as a continuously distributed quantitative trait. The distribution of the phenotype is usually a single normative curve, not a bimodal curve. Sex bias could be at work, but you would not know this unless you were told so.

4. **B** is the correct answer.

   Again refer to the list of characteristics of multifactorial inheritance. The recurrence risk is higher if the least common sex is affected. More relatives affected means increased risk. Multifactorial recurrence risks are not as high as single gene disorders–often on the order of a few percent. The description is actually polygenic.

5. **D** is the correct answer.

   Please do not forget this when you visit with your patients! The other answers are incorrect. Alcohol teratogenesis is common and very important. Only one third of children with alcohol exposures *in utero* will have FAS. Of course, genetic factors do play a role.

Chapter 11

1. **D** is the correct answer.
   A. For population screening, the condition should be sufficiently common enough.
   B. For population screening, the testing modality should be easy to perform.
   C. Population screening should be reserved for conditions that are clinically serious.
   E. For population screening, the testing modality should be inexpensive to perform.

2. **A** is the correct answer.
   B. Genetic screening of necessity has to be cost effective.
   C. It is absolutely appropriate to identify specific ethnic groups in screening.
   D. The whole purpose of screening is to effect changes that prevent disease and disability.
   E. Testing can be by many different modalities (biochemical, and so forth).

3. **B** is the correct answer.
   A. After newborn screening identifies a "presumptive positive," selected biochemical studies are performed to confirm a diagnosis. This, then, is testing.
   C. This is diagnostic testing.
   D. An examination is not a genetic test.
   E. This is diagnostic testing.

4. **C** is the correct answer.
   A. The types of methodology are the same in both.
   B. The costs of doing one or the other are the same in both.
   D. The laboratories that do one or the other are the same in both.
   E. The patient can be of any age for either.

5. **C** is the closest correct answer.
   The current Uniform Screening Panel recommended by the American College of Medical Genetics is 29 (Table 11-8). Most states are in compliance with these recommendations.

Chapter 12

1. **B** is the correct answer.
   A. Uniparental disomy is inheriting two copies of the same chromosome (or locus) from the same parent.
   C. This does not describe expanding repeats or transposable elements.
   D. Anticipation is the progressive worsening of a condition through the generations.
   E. Partial expression would refer to how the trait were expressed, not the selective silencing of one allele.

2. **C** is the correct answer.
   A. Imprinting is a normal phenomenon. It is the way certain genes are supposed to be expressed.
   B. Imprinting is an epigenetic mechanism. The gene function, but not the code, is changed.
   D. The most common mechanism of imprinting is methylation.
   E. Only a small number of loci (maybe 70 or so) are imprinted. The majority of loci have typical di-allelic expression.

3. **C** is the correct answer.
   A. Females, with two X chromosomes have Barr bodies, not males.
   B. Since Lyonization is a random process, the average is around 50% for each X chromosome. However, skewing can occur and for any individual, the ratio can vary a lot from 50:50.
   D. As with most epigenetic mechanisms, the change is not permanent. It is erased in germ cells to start over in the next generation.
   E. Lyonization is an early occurring process in embryogenesis.

4. **C** is the correct answer.
   A. X-linked inheritance is due to the gene being located on the X chromosome.
   B. Semi-dominant inheritance refers to the fact that the females can be partially affected.
   D. Males are more affected than females, and this is due to fragile X being X linked.
   E. Mosaicism means a different genotype in different cells. This would not be related to trinucleotide repeats.

5. **B** is the correct answer.
   A. A chromosome translocation is not epigenetic. It is an actual physical change in the DNA location.
   C. Microsatellites are sets of repeated sequences of DNA.
   D. A mutation is an actual change in the DNA code.
   E. Expanding trinucleotide repeats are changes in the code (number of repeats).

6. **A** is the correct answer.
   B. An insertional mutation is a mechanism that a transposable element might cause.
   C. X inactivation is an epigenetic mechanism that is unrelated to trinucleotide repeats.
   D. Opposite transcripts are two different gene products from reading the same sequence on both strands of DNA.
   E. Modifier genes influence the expression of other genes. The mechanism is not related to trinucleotide repeats.

Chapter 13

1. **B** is the correct answer.
   A. Mitochondrial inheritance shows maternal transmission.
   C. Homozygous and heterozygous are terms applied to nuclear genes. Mitochondrial DNA patterns are described as showing homoplasmy or heteroplasmy.
   D. Mitochondrial genes have a higher mutation rate than the nuclear genes.
   E. The correct term is 'bottleneck' phenomenon.

2. **D** is the correct answer.
   A. Clearly she could be affected by any number of mechanisms–either nuclear gene (Mendelian) inheritance or a mtDNA mutation she inherits from her mother.
   B. Mitochondrial disorders may have adult onset.
   C. Mitochondrial disorders exhibit highly variable expression including intra-familial variation.
   E. Of course patient centered counseling would never make such a recommendation.

3. **C** is the correct answer.
   A. Respiratory problems are not a key feature of peroxisomal disorders.
   B. Performing a biopsy of a single organ in a multisystem disorder would be unlikely to reveal an answer.
   D. You cannot make any assumption at this point. A diagnosis is needed first.
   E. Of course testing may give you an answer. That's what this is all about.

4. **A** is the correct answer.
   B. Mitochondrial disorders usually present with neuromuscular symptoms.
   C. Peroxisomal disorders may have structural congenital anomalies, but not typically the types listed here.
   D. Lysosomal disorders are storage disorders not associated with structural congenital anomalies.
   E. Similar to lysosomal disorders.

5. **D** is the correct answer.
   A. A quick review of basic genetics: X-linked recessive conditions affect males.
   B. Lysosomal disorders are progressive storage disorders. The child could look normal now, but still have an emerging phenotype.
   C. Remember that screening is not perfect. All screens will have some degree of false negatives. Also, current newborn screening efforts do not include lysosomal storage disorders. However, this may change in the very near future.
   E. We are not even sure what "lysosomal transplantation" is, if it even exists.

Chapter 14

1. **C** is the correct answer.
   A. Gene therapy is currently not a standardly available mode of therapy.
   B. Congenital malformations are not likely to be helped by gene therapy–this would only work if the defects were known ahead of time and the genetic manipulation performed at or around the time of conception—in the embryo.
   D. Gene therapy is not standardly available regardless of the issue of being cost prohibitive.
   E. Of course patients should not be counseled in such a directive manner.

2. **C** is the correct answer.
   A. Cloning can be a non-controversial mode of therapy.
   B. Even if this technology were available, the ethical issues are yet to be resolved.
   D. The cloning of Dolly the sheep was accomplished, but there was the unexpected complication of early aging.
   E. Cloning is an extremely controversial issue.

3. **E** is the correct answer.
   A. Normal variant short stature is a licensed use of hGH.
   B. The patient declares their disease.
   C. hGH therapy is expensive. Just because the FDA has approved its use in normal variant short stature, most third party payers will not cover it.
   D. Self-esteem will not necessarily get better with improved height. In fact, it often will not improve at all.

4. **C** is the correct answer.
   A. Clearly other health care providers can be very well suited to help patients with case management.
   B. The geneticist can be a "medical home neighbor" in the case management of patients working with the PCP.
   D. Surgery is a direct service.
   E. Although many third part payers now offer case management services, these are primarily for common disorders (such as diabetes). It is unlikely that an insurance company will have extensive expertise or experience with genetic disorders.

5. **A** is the correct answer.
   B. Chelation of the stored glycosaminoglycans is not a therapeutic option. There is no known agent that can "pull" the GAGs out of the lysozymes in cells.
   C. Newborn screening would help detect, but not treat, these disorders.

D. Dietary reduction of glycosaminoglycan does not prevent the accumulation of these compounds.
E. Gene correction is not a currently available treatment modality. It may be in the not so distant future.

Chapter 15

1. **D** is the correct answer.
   According to the Hardy Weinberg distribution:

   $$(p^2 + 2pq + q^2 = 1)$$

   Thus the genotype frequency of a carrier (heterozygous) of the recessive allele q is $2q(1-q)$ which is approximately $2q$ when q is rare as noted in the question.

2. **C** is the correct answer.
   Mrs Smith is a healthy sibling of an affected person. Half of the siblings will be healthy and carriers. One fourth (25%) will be healthy and not carriers and the remaining one fourth will have disease. Therefore, of the healthy siblings the chance of being a carrier is 2/3. This type of question is commonly asked. Be sure you completely understand this. Drawing out a Punnett square may help you visualize the proportions; the answer refers only to the phenotypically normal individuals in the Punnett square.

3. **A** is the correct answer.
   First cousins will have one of their parents who are siblings. Siblings share ½ of the genes. Parents and children also share ½ of their genes. The chance a child from one family will share ½ × ½ of the genes = ¼ with one of their uncle or aunt. Therefore, the first cousins will share ¼ × ½ = 1/8 of the genes.

4. **B** is the correct answer.
   Since the condition is autosomal recessive, males and females are no different. If the condition occurs in 1 in 256 individuals (q^2) then the frequency of the allele (q) is the square root of 1/256 or 1/16. The carrier frequency then would be $2pq$ or $(2)(15/16)(1/16) = 30/256 = 12\%$ which is closest to 1/8.

5. **A** is the correct answer.
   B. If the heterozygous sate produces a disadvantaged situation, this would not increase the frequency of the mutation
   C. "Foundation efforts" sounds like "founder effects", but of course is nonsensical in this context.
   D. Random mating would keep specific mutations at a random (low) level.
   E. A low mutation rate would of course not increase the occurrence of a specific mutation.

Chapter 16

1. **E** is the correct answer.
   A. Achondroplasia is not caused by a missing copy of the gene.
   B. Sequencing the gene would not add any helpful information.
   C. Again, the child will not have achondroplasia (and hGH is not effective for achondroplasia anyways).
   D. Families will find their own information. There is no way to prevent or dissuade it.

2. **B** is the correct answer.
   A. Haploinsufficiency is a mechanism for dominant conditions. Only one allele has to be affected.
   C. Protein interference is likely to cause dominant disorders.

D. Likewise protein suicide will be associated with dominant conditions.

E. Autoregulatory dysfunction is a made-up term.

3. **D** is the correct answer.

A. It is not outdated, but has limited applications.

B. Is an uncommon pathogenetic mechanism in human disease.

C. Connective tissue disorders are typically dominant disorders that are problems with structural proteins, not enzymes.

E. Homeotic genes regulate other processes. They do not code for enzymes.

4. **B** is the correct answer.

A. Locus heterogeneity would involve more than one gene.

C. Genetic homogeneity would not apply as this would be the same mutation.

D. Homeotic modulation is a made-up term.

E. Gene-gene mutagenesis is another made-up term.

5. **E** is the correct answer.

All others can do so. Lyonization involves the X chromosome.

Index

Note: Page numbers followed by *t* indicate tables; those followed by *f* indicate figures.

ABO blood type, 146, 146*f*
acentric fragment, 113, 114*f*
Acetabularia, 270, 271*f*
aCGH. *See* array comparative genomic hybridization
ACMG. *See* American College of Medical Genetics
acrocentric chromosomes, 114
actin genes, 92–93
activator proteins, 50, 51*f*
AD inheritance. *See* autosomal dominant inheritance
adenosine deaminase (ADA), 303
adenosine triphosphate (ATP), 273, 275
adjacent segregation, 113–114, 115*f*
Affordable Care Act, 244
agenesis, 65
AHO. *See* Albright hereditary osteodystrophy
albinism, 1, 2*f*
Albright hereditary osteodystrophy (AHO), 335, 336*f*
alkaptonuria, 192–193, 193*t*
alleles
　gene pool frequencies of, 310
　lethal, 145, 145*f*
　multiple, 145–147, 146*f*
　null, 186
allelic heterogeneity, 148, 217
allosteric control, 184
allosteric flexibility, 174
allosteric proteins, 37
allosteric regulation, 165
alpha-satellites, 83–84, 84*f*, 93
alternate segregation, 114
alternative splicing, of introns, 28, 29*f*
American College of Medical Genetics (ACMG), 12
Ames test, 169, 169*f*
amino acids
　chemical characteristics of, 30, 31*f*, 35
　hydrophobic and hydrophilic, 28
　metabolism disorders of, 192–194, 193*t*, 194*f*
　point mutations of, 37
　protein structure and, characteristics of, 28, 31*f*
　sorting signals and, 38
　tRNA attaching, 29, 32*f*, 33*f*

anaphase, in mitosis, 103*f*, 104
aneuploid structure, of chromosomes, 105
aneuploidy, 110–111, 110*f*
　sex chromosomes and, 121–124
　syndromes of, 120, 120*t*
　trisomies and, 125–127, 126*f*, 128*f*, 129*f*, 129*t*
Angelman syndrome, 12, 13*f*, 257–258, 258*f*
anticipation, genetic, 94, 254, 262–263, 262*f*, 263*t*, 264*f*–265*f*, 265*t*
anticodon, 29, 33*f*
anti-sense transcripts, 253, 261
apoenzymes, 187, 188*f*
apoptosis, 49, 63
AR inheritance. *See* autosomal recessive inheritance
Arabidopsis thaliana, 11, 11*f*, 329, 329*f*
array comparative genomic hybridization (aCGH), 119–120, 120*f*, 232, 240
ATP. *See* adenosine triphosphate
Atrulen, 181
atypical inheritance. *See also* transposable elements
　compound heterozygosity, 259, 259*f*
　digenic inheritance, 251, 253*f*, 259, 259*f*
　epigenetic inheritance, 254, 265–266, 266*t*
　genetic anticipation, 94, 254, 262–263, 262*f*, 263*t*, 264*f*–265*f*, 265*t*
　genetic imprinting, 249, 251, 252*f*, 257–259, 258*f*, 259*t*
　medical genetics and, 254–266
　mosaicism
　　functional, 250
　　gonadal, 255–256, 256*f*
　　occurrence of, 249–250, 250*f*
　　somatic, 254–255, 255*f*, 256*f*
　multi-locus inheritance, 251, 260–261, 261*f*, 262*f*
　opposite (anti-sense) transcripts, 253, 261
　triallelic inheritance, 251
　UPD, 250–251, 250*f*, 256–257
autonomous gene expression, 115
autosomal dominant inheritance (AD inheritance)
　classical characteristics of, 150–151, 150*f*–153*f*, 151*t*, 156*t*
　recurrence risks of, 151
　special inheritance considerations with, 151–156

autosomal recessive inheritance (AR inheritance)
　classical characteristics of, 156
　frequency of, 156–157, 156*t*
　recurrence risks with, 156
　special inheritance considerations with, 156–160
auxologic studies, 224
auxotrophs, 185

back mutation, 312
bacteria. *See Escherichia coli*
bacterial artificial chromosomes, 240
bacteriophage, 327
baker's yeast. *See Saccharomyces cerevisiae*
Bardet-Biedel syndrome (BBS), 259–260, 260*f*, 294
Barr body, 111, 111*f*
Barry, Joan, 147
BBS. *See* Bardet-Biedel syndrome
Beadle, George, 40, 89
Beckwith-Wiedeman syndrome (BWS), 266–267, 267*f*
behavior genetics, 11*t*
benign polymorphisms, 92, 175
Best disease, 152, 154*f*
biochemical genetics, 11*t*
biochemical pathways, 40–42, 40*f*, 41*f*, 184–185
biogenesis, 3
bioinformatics, 41
biologic threshold, 219, 219*f*
biopharmaceuticals, 298–299, 299*t*, 302–303, 302*t*
bivalent, 105, 106*f*
Blaschko lines, 127
blastocyst, 49
blastomeres, 49
blastula, 49
bottleneck effect, 280–281, 313, 314*f*
branched-chain ketoacid dehydrogenase, 193–194, 193*t*
Buck, Carrie, 309–310, 311*f*, 316–317
BWS. *See* Beckwith-Wiedeman syndrome

C value, 102
Caenorhabditis elegans (nematode), 10*f*, 56, 59*f*, 328

cAMP. *See* cyclic-AMP
cAMP response element-binding protein (CREB protein), 54, 57*f*
cancer, 341
cancer therapeutics, 15, 15*t*
candidate genes, for type II DM, 222–223, 223*f*, 223*t*
carbohydrates, 4, 193*t*, 194, 194*f*, 195*f*
carcinogen, 177
CBS. *See* cystathione-beta-synthase
CDGs. *See* congenital disorders of glycosylation
CDKs. *See* cyclin-dependent kinases
cell division, 54. *See also* meiosis; mitosis
    activation of, 101*f*
    aneuploidy and, 110–111, 110*f*
    chromosome genetic information and, 99, 100*f*
    polyploidy and, 112
cell growth rate, in embryology, 63
cell migration, in embryology, 63
Cell theory, 3–4
cell-to-cell interactions, in embryology, 63
cellular differentiation, 49, 53–54
Central Dogma of molecular biology, 17–18, 18*f*, 77
centrioles, 102, 285, 291–292
centromere, 93
centrosome, 102
CF. *See* cystic fibrosis
CFND. *See* craniofrontonasal dysplasia
chaperone proteins, 35
Chargaff's rule, 20
CHARGE syndrome, 73, 74*f*
chromatin remodeling, 87, 89*f*
chromosomal disorders, 341
chromosomal microarray (CMA), 240–241, 241*f*
chromosomal mosaicism, 127, 130*f*
chromosome painting, 119, 238
chromosomes
    aberrations, 108, 109*f*, 110
    abnormalities
        aneuploidy, 120–127
        clinical correlation for, 136
        contiguous gene syndromes and, 131–132, 135
        Cri-du-chat syndrome and, 131, 133*f*, 134*f*, 134*t*
        frequency of, 116–117, 116*t*, 117*t*
        laboratory diagnosis of, 117–120, 117*f*–120*f*
        mosaicism, 127, 130*f*
        structure changes with, 127, 129–131, 131*f*–134*f*
        Wolf-Hirschhorn syndrome and, 131, 132*f*, 133*f*, 134*t*
    acrocentric, 114
    aneuploidy of, 110–111, 110*f*
        sex chromosomes and, 121–124
        syndromes of, 120, 120*t*
        trisomies and, 125–127, 126*f*, 128*f*, 129*f*, 129*t*

cell division and genetic information in, 99, 100*f*
    centromere of, 93
    deficiency of, 109*f*, 110
    deletion of, 108, 109*f*, 112, 112*f*, 135, 135*f*, 136, 136*f*
    dicentric, 113, 114*f*
    diploid, 7, 316
    duplication of, 109*f*, 110, 112, 112*f*
    endoduplicated, 326
    of eukaryotes, 77, 79*f*
        packing in nucleus of, 85, 86*f*–89*f*, 87
    G-banding of, 87, 89*f*
    genes in, 7, 8*f*
    haploid, 6–7
    homologous, 100
    inversion of, 109*f*, 110, 113, 113*f*, 114*f*
    karyotype and, 104, 105, 109*f*, 117, 117*f*
        in Klinefelter syndrome, 122–124, 124*f*, 125*f*
        in trisomies, 125–127, 126*f*, 128*f*, 129*f*, 129*t*
        in Turner syndrome, 122, 123*f*
        in XXX syndrome, 124, 125*f*
        in XYY syndrome, 124, 125*f*
    linkage groups in, 6–7
    marker, 119*f*, 238
    nuclear division and coiling of, 100, 102*f*
    number of, 102, 105, 108, 110
    polyploidy and, 112, 120
    scaffold formation in, 87, 88*f*
    sex, 121–124
    somatic mosaics and, 114–115
    structure of, 85, 87*f*
        aneuploid, 105
        changes in, 108, 109*f*, 110, 127, 129–131, 131*f*–134*f*
        euploid, 105
        polyploid, 105, 108
    sub-telomeric regions of, 93
    telocentric, 114
    telomere region in, 24, 25*f*, 93–94
    tetraploidy and, 121
    translocation of, 109*f*, 110, 113–114, 115*f*
    triploidy and, 120, 120*f*
    X, 111–112, 111*f*, 159, 159*f*, 160*f*
    Y, 115
cilia, 273, 283–285, 284*f*
    immotile (primary), 293–294, 294*f*–295*f*
    motile, 294–295
citric acid cycle, 275, 278*f*
cleft lip/palate, 220, 221*f*, 222, 222*f*, 261, 261*f*, 301, 301*t*
clinical genetic laboratories, 12
clinical geneticist, 297
clinical genetics, 11, 11*t*
clinical presentations, 42, 42*t*
cloning, 299–300, 304, 305*f*
CMA. *See* chromosomal microarray
CNVs. *See* copy number variants
coding strand, 27, 253
co-dominance, 152–153

codons
    in RNA translation, 29, 32*f*
    sense, 30
    start, 81*f*
    stop, 31, 81*f*
        release factors and, 34, 37*f*
coefficient of inbreeding/relationship, 157, 158*f*
coenzymes, 184, 187, 188*f*
cofactors, 187, 188*f*, 193*t*, 197–198
comparative genomic hybridization
    aCGH, 119–120, 120*f*, 232, 240
    Drosophila melanogaster and, 329, 330*f*, 330*t*, 331*f*
    model organisms and, 329, 330*f*–333*f*, 330*t*, 332
compound heterozygote, 152, 259, 259*f*
concordance, in twins, 217–218, 217*t*, 218*f*
conditional mutations, 167
congenital anomalies
    associations, 67–68, 69*f*, 73, 74*f*
    definition of, 63
    deformations, 66, 66*f*, 67*t*
    disruptions, 66, 67*f*, 68*t*
    dysmorphology and, 69–70
    dysplasia, 67, 68*f*
    epidemiology of, 63
    etiology of, 69–72
    evaluation of patient with, 72, 72*f*
    impact of, 64
    malformations, 64–65, 65*f*
    patterns of, 67–69, 69*f*, 70*f*
    sequences, 68–69, 70*f*
    syndromes, 67, 69*f*, 70, 72–73, 73*f*, 74*f*
    teratogens and, 71, 71*t*
    trends in, 64
    types of, 64–67, 64*t*, 65*f*–68*f*
congenital disorders of glycosylation (CDGs), 45–46, 45*f*–46*f*
consanguinity, 157
    family history and, 207
    pedigree analysis and, 204
contiguous gene syndromes, 118
    characteristics of, 132
    chromosome abnormalities with, 131–132, 135
    important types of, 134*t*
    microarray studies finding, 135, 135*f*
copy number variants (CNVs), 240–241
covalent modification, 184
CpG islands, 173
craniofrontonasal dysplasia (CFND), 163–164, 163*f*, 164*f*
CREB protein. *See* cAMP response element-binding protein
Crick, Francis, 18
Cri-du-chat syndrome, 131, 133*f*, 134*f*, 134*t*
crossing over, 105, 107*f*, 112*f*, 113, 114*f*
cyclic-AMP (cAMP), 54
cyclin-dependent kinases (CDKs), 37, 100
cystathione-beta-synthase (CBS), 318
cystic fibrosis (CF), 90–91, 90*f*, 180–181, 318, 338–339, 338*t*, 339*t*

cytogenetics, 11*t*, 116–135
  abnormalities in, 116–120
  aCGH and, 119–120, 120*f*
  advances in, 236–237, 237*f*
  FISH and, 118–119, 118*f*, 119*f*
  molecular, 120
cytokinesis, 103*f*, 104, 105*f*
cytoskeleton, 282–283, 283*f*, 291, 291*f*,
  292*f*

Danio rerio (zebrafish), 10*f*, 328
Darwin, Charles, 4, 203, 213
Darwin, George, 203
DC. *See* dyskeratosis congenita
deamination, spontaneous, 170, 170*f*
degeneracy, in Genetic Code, 30, 34*f*
degrees of freedom, 214–215
degrees of relationship, 157, 157*f*
deleterious mutations, 167
deoxyribonucleic acid (DNA), 1, 3. *See also*
  information flow, from DNA to
  phenotype
  benign polymorphisms and, 92
  coding sequence changes in, 91–92
  dideoxy sequencing of, 232,
    232*f*–234*f*, 234
  fingerprint of, 84, 84*f*, 93
  genetic testing and sequencing of, 229,
    230*f*, 232, 232*f*–234*f*, 233
  genome sequences of, 77, 78*f*
  mitochondrial, 275, 278, 280–282
  model organisms sequencing of, 320
  mutations of
    coding sequence and, 91–92
    medical conditions associated with,
      91, 91*t*
    outside coding sequence, 92, 92*f*
    repair and, 172, 173*f*, 178–180,
      179*f*, 179*t*, 180*f*
  packing, 85, 86*f*–89*f*, 87
  polymerases, 20
    polymerase III, 21, 23*f*
    Taq, 26
  pseudogenes and, 83, 93
  reannealing, 77–78, 79*f*
  repair of, 172, 173*f*, 178–180, 179*f*,
    179*t*, 180*f*
  repetitive sequences function with,
    83–84, 84*f*
  replication of, 5, 19–24
    in eukaryotes compared to
      prokaryotes, 21, 23–24, 24*f*
    events at fork in, 21, 23*f*
    fork in, 20–21, 22*f*, 23*f*
    leading and lagging strand in, 21, 22*f*
    Okazaki fragments in, 21, 22*f*
    PCR manipulation of, 24, 25*f*, 26
    primer in, 21, 22*f*
    products of, 20, 22*f*
    proteins responsible for, 20–21, 22*f*
    replisome in, 21, 24*f*
  response elements and, 52
  role of, 17
  satellite, 83–85, 84*f*, 93–94, 95*f*, 96*f*, 254

sequence complexity with, 77–78, 79*f*, 80*t*
structure of, 4–5, 6*f*, 17, 19–21, 21*f*
VNTRs and, 84–85, 84*f*, 85*f*
depurination, spontaneous, 169, 170*f*
development. *See also* congenital
  anomalies
  cellular differentiation in, 49, 53–54
  clinical correlation for, 73, 73*f*, 74*f*
  laterality in, 58, 60, 61*f*
  medical genetics and, 62–72
  morphogenesis in, 49, 57–58, 63
  organization of, 58, 60, 60*f*, 61*f*
    disorders in, 62*t*
  pattern formation in, 49, 56–57, 59*f*
  periods of, 62–63
  plasticity and, 55–56, 58*f*, 59*f*
  pleuripotency and, 55–56
  positional information in, 56, 59*f*
  timing and processes in, 49–50
developmental genetics, 11*t*
diabetes mellitus (DM), 222–223,
  223*f*, 223*t*
diagnostic yield, of genetic testing,
  239–240, 244, 244*t*
dicentric chromosome, 113, 114*f*
dideoxy sequencing, 232, 232*f*–234*f*, 234
digenic inheritance, 251, 253*f*, 259, 259*f*
DiGeorge, Angelo, 136
DiGeorge syndrome, 70, 70*f*, 136, 136*f*
diploids, 7, 316
directional selection, 315, 315*f*
discordant twins, 217
diseases, 12, 341–342. *See also specific*
  diseases
disorders. *See also specific disorders*
  definition of, 12–13
  in development organization, 62*t*
  inverse, 259
  key, 341–342
  nucleus and, 291–292, 293*f*
  signaling pathways linking, 43–44, 45*t*
  trinucleotide repeats causing, 262, 265*t*,
    266*f*
dispermy, 120
dispersed duplications, 112
disruptions, 66, 67*f*, 68*t*
diversifying selection, 315, 316*f*
DM. *See* diabetes mellitus
DMD. *See* Duchenne muscular dystrophy
DNA. *See* deoxyribonucleic acid
dominance, in Mendelian Rules of
  Transmission, 140
  co-dominance, 152–153
  exceptions to, 142–143, 142*f*
  incomplete, 142, 142*f*
  quasi-dominance, 156
  true complete, 151–152, 154*f*
dominant negative effect, 335
Down syndrome, 14, 117, 117*t*, 125–127,
  126*f*
Drosophila melanogaster (fruit fly), 6, 9,
  10*f*, 11, 56, 57, 59*f*, 169, 249
  comparative genomic hybridization with,
    329, 330*f*, 330*t*, 331*f*

historical advancements with, 327
Hox complexes in, 58, 61*f*
organization of embryonic development
  in, 58, 60, 60*f*, 61*f*
wing vein lengths in, 251, 253, 253*f*
Duchenne muscular dystrophy (DMD),
  159–160, 160*f*, 180–181, 291, 292*f*
duplication, of chromosomes, 109*f*, 110,
  112, 112*f*
dyandry, 120
dygyny, 120–121
dyshistogenesis, 67
dyskeratosis congenita (DC), 94, 95*f*
dysmorphic exam, 174
dysmorphology, 42, 69–70, 342
dysplasia, 67, 68*f*
dystrophin protein, 291, 291*f*

ear phenotype, 38
ectoderm, 57, 60*t*
ectopia, 65
Edwards syndrome, karyotype in trisomy
  18, 127, 129*f*, 129*t*
electron microscopy, 271–272, 275*f*
embryology, 62–63
embryonic tissue layers, 57, 60*t*
empiric risk counseling, 220
endoderm, 57, 60*t*
endoduplicated chromosomes, 326
endophenotype, 14, 15
endoplasmic reticulum (ER), 282, 282*f*, 287
endosomes, 282, 287
environment interactions. *See* genotype X
  environment interactions
enzyme replacement therapy (ERT), 199, 290
enzymes
  holoenzymes, 26, 27*f*, 187, 188*f*
  kinetics, 187, 188*f*
  repair, 165, 166*f*
  restriction, 84–85, 84*f*
Ephrin-B mutations (EPHB1 mutations),
  163–164, 163*f*
epidermolysis bullosa simplex, 291, 292*f*
epigenetic inheritance, 254, 265–266, 266*t*
epigenetic modification, 111, 111*f*
epistasis, 143–144, 143*f*
ER. *See* endoplasmic reticulum
ERT. *See* enzyme replacement therapy
Escherichia coli (bacteria), 10*f*, 11, 327
etiology, 69–72, 333
eukaryotes
  cell cycle in, 100, 101*f*, 102, 102*f*
  cell structure of, 50–51
  chromosomes of, 77, 79*f*
    packing in nucleus of, 85, 86*f*–89*f*, 87
  gene action control in, 50–53, 54*f*–56*f*
  Genetic Code of, 19
  prereplication complex in, 23
  prokaryotes compared to, 18, 19*f*
    in DNA replication, 21, 23–24, 24*f*
    in RNA transcription, 27–28, 28*f*, 29*f*
  RNA translation in, 34–35
  telomere region in, 24, 25*f*, 93–94
  transcription factors in, 51–53, 54*f*–56*f*

euploid structure, of chromosomes, 105
exome sequencing, whole, 242
exon sequencing, whole, 234
exons, 18
expanding trinucleotide repeat, 97
Experiments on Plant Hybridization
        (Mendel), 4
extracellular matrix, 273

Family Centered Medical Home, 300
family history. *See also* pedigree analysis
    case studies for, 209–210, 209*f*–211*f*
    consanguinity and, 207
    genetics and, 201
    importance of, 206, 206*t*
    interpreting, 208, 208*t*
    medical genetics and, 206–208
    mis-assigned paternity and, 207
    obtaining, in clinical setting, 206–207, 207*t*
    relationships in, 206
    responding to, 208, 208*t*
Family History Initiative, 206, 206*t*
FAS. *See* fetal alcohol syndrome
FASD. *See* fetal alcohol spectrum disorder
fatty acid oxidation disorders, 193*t*, 195
feedback inhibition, in gene action, 50, 54*f*
fetal alcohol spectrum disorder (FASD), 72
fetal alcohol syndrome (FAS), 71–72,
        72*f*, 226
fetal hydantoin syndrome (FHS), 226–227,
        226*f*, 227*f*
field defects, 136
first degree relative, 157, 157*f*, 206
FISH. *See* fluorescent *in situ* hybridization
flagella, 273, 283–284, 284*f*, 292–295
fluorescent *in situ* hybridization (FISH),
        118*f*, 231–232
    advances in, 237–240, 238*f*–240*f*, 238*t*
    micro-duplication/micro-deletion
        syndromes identified with, 238, 238*t*
    multi-color, 238, 239*f*
    sub-telomeric, 118–119, 119*f*, 239–240,
        240*f*
forensic genetics, 11*t*
forward mutation, 312
founder effect, 158–159, 217
fragile-X syndrome, 97, 97*f*, 98*f*, 262–263,
        262*f*, 263*t*, 264*f*–265*f*, 265*t*
frameshift mutations, 167
fRNA. *See* functional RNA
fruit fly. *See* Drosophila melanogaster
functional mosaicism, 250
functional multi-copy genes, 82–83, 83*f*
functional RNA (fRNA), 80, 82*t*

G protein, 54
G X E interactions. *See* genotype X
        environment interactions
GAGs. *See* glycosaminoglycans
Galton, Francis, 213
gamete complementation, 250–251
Garrod, Archibald, 187
gastrulation, 57
G-banding, 87, 89*f*, 105

gene action
    control of
        in bacteria, 50, 51*f*–53*f*
        in eukaryotes, 50–53, 54*f*–56*f*
    feedback inhibition in, 50, 54*f*
    transcription factors in, 50
gene dosage, 112
gene expression regulation, 18–19, 20*f*
gene pool, allele frequencies in, 310
general population screening, 246
genes
    actin, 92–93
    anatomy of protein-coding, 78–80,
        81*f*, 82*f*
    candidate, 222–223, 223*f*, 223*t*
    in chromosomes, 7, 8*f*
    definition of, 9
    disbursed family of, 92–93
    functional multi-copy, 82–83, 83*f*
    heterozygous, 148
    historical understanding of, 40
    holandric, 115
    homeotic, 58, 60*f*
    homozygous, 148
    in humans, 6
    inducible, 50, 53*f*
    interactions of, 143–144, 143*f*
    locus of, 147, 148*f*
    mismatch repair, 94
    modifier, 251, 260–261
    overlapping, 9, 27, 80, 81*f*
    pseudogenes, 83, 93
    repressible, 50, 53*f*
    role of, 40
    segmentation, 58
    structural, 50, 78
    structure and function of, 77–98
        medical genetics and, 89–96
genetics
    complexity of, 338–339
    definition of, 11
    family history and, 201
    functional context of, 3–4
    history linked with, 201
    milestones in, 13*t*, 14
    origin of life and, 2
    personalized medicine applications with,
        15–16, 15*t*
    unity and diversity in, 1–16
genetic anticipation, 94, 254, 262–263,
        262*f*, 263*t*, 264*f*–265*f*, 265*t*
Genetic Code, 28
    degeneracy in, 30, 34*f*
    of eukaryotes, 19
    of prokaryotes, 19
    universality of, 30
genetic counseling, 11*t*, 298, 300–301
genetic counselors, 12
genetic damage rate, 168
genetic discrimination, 244
genetic diversity, 309, 318
genetic drift, 313, 313*f*
genetic families, 43, 43*t*
genetic heterogeneity, 148, 217

genetic imprinting, 249, 251, 252*f*,
        257–259, 258*f*, 259*t*
Genetic Information Non Discrimination
        Act (GINA), 244
genetic screening
    controversy surrounding, 247
    general population, 246
    genetic testing compared to, 235, 245
    individual, 245
    principals of, 235–236
    selected profile, 245–246, 245*t*, 246*t*
    sensitivity and specificity in, 235
    timing and types of, 245, 245*t*
genetic sequencing
    dideoxy method of, 232, 232*f*–234*f*, 234
    high-throughput, 234, 241–242
    next-gen, 234, 242
    parallel, 242
    RNA, 234–235
    whole exome, 242
    whole exon, 234
    whole genome, 242–243
genetic susceptibility, 15*t*, 16, 225, 225*t*
genetic testing
    aCGH and, 119–120, 232, 240
    advances in
        CMA, 240–241, 241*f*
        cytogenetics, 236–237, 237*f*
        nucleotide sequencing determination,
            241–243, 242*f*
    diagnostic yield of, 239–240, 244, 244*t*
    DNA sequencing and, 229, 230*f*, 232,
        232*f*–234*f*, 233
    FISH and, 118–119, 118*f*, 119*f*, 231–232
        advances in, 237–240, 238*f*–240*f*, 238*t*
        micro-duplication/micro-deletion
            syndromes identified with,
            238, 238*t*
        multi-color, 238, 239*f*
        sub-telomeric, 239–240, 240*f*
    genetic screening compared to, 235, 245
    GWAS, 235
    informed consent in, 243–244, 244*t*
    karyotype images for, 231, 231*f*
    linkage disequilibrium and, 229–230, 230*f*
    medical genetics and, 236–247
    practical issues in, 243–245, 243*f*, 244*t*
    SNP analysis and, 232
    spectrum of utility in, 243, 243*f*
    types of, 230–231, 231*t*
genetic therapies. *See also* personalized
        medicine
    biopharmaceuticals, 298–299, 299*t*,
        302–303, 302*t*
    case management and, 297–298, 300
    clinical trials with, 303–304, 303*f*, 304*t*
    cloning and, 299–300, 304, 305*f*
    conventional, 297–298, 300–302
    definition of, 297, 303
    interdisciplinary specialty teams for, 298,
        298*t*, 301, 301*t*
    for LSDs, 305, 306*f*, 307, 307*f*
    medical genetics and, 300–305
    requirements for, 299, 299*t*

genome
  components of, 6–7
  definition of, 5
  DNA sequences in, 77, 78f
  mRNA correspondence with functional
     regions of, 78, 81f
  sequence complexity with, 77–78, 79f, 80t
  terminology for, 7, 9
  VNTRs and, 84–85, 84f, 85f
  whole sequencing, 242–243
genome-wide association study (GWAS), 235
genomics, 15–16, 15t, 318–319
Genomics Recommended Core Screening
    Panel, 246, 246t
genotype, 1, 14, 89
genotype X environment interactions
    (G X E interactions), 40, 144,
    144f, 217
germinal mutations, somatic mutations
    compared to, 173–174
GHD. See human growth hormone
    deficiency
GINA. See Genetic Information Non
    Discrimination Act
globular proteins, 36
glycogen storage disorders (GSDs),
    194, 194f
glycosaminoglycans (GAGs), 305, 307
glycosylation, congenital disorders
    of. See congenital disorders of
    glycosylation
Golgi complex, 282, 287
gonadal mosaicism, 255–256, 256f
GSDs. See glycogen storage disorders
guanine diphosphate, 54
guanine triphosphate, 54
GWAS. See genome-wide association study
gynandromorphs, 60

Hämmerling, Joachim, 269
haploids, 6–7
Hardy-Weinberg equilibrium, 311, 311f,
    312t, 313–314
Harvey, William, 269
hemochromatosis, 196–197
hemoglobin, 38
heritability, 215–217, 216f
heterochromatic state, 93
heterodimer, 52
heterogeneous RNA (hnRNA), 28
heteroplasmic sequence, 280
heterotopia, 65
heterozygote, 148
  advantage
    examples of, 158, 158t, 318
    SSA and, 157, 317
  compound, 152
  disadvantage, 318
heterozygous genes, 148
HGP. See Human Genome Project
high-throughput sequencing, 234, 241–242
histone proteins, 85, 87, 87f, 89f
hnRNA. See heterogeneous RNA
holandric genes, 115

holandric inheritance, 159
holoenzymes, 26, 27f, 187, 188f
homeobox, 58
homeodomain, 58
homeotic genes, 58, 60f
homeotic mutations, 58, 60f
homocystinuria, 193
homodimer, 52
homologous chromosomes, 100
homology, 326
homoplasmic sequence, 278
homozygote, 148
homozygous genes, 148
Hooke, Robert, 3, 269
house mouse. See Mus musculus
Hox complexes, 58, 61f
human genetics, 11
Human Genome Project (HGP), 9, 10f, 11,
    11f, 236, 243
human growth hormone deficiency (GHD),
    302–303, 302t
Hunter syndrome, 196, 196f
Huntington disease, 152, 154f
Hurler syndrome, 305, 306f, 307, 307f
Hutchinson-Gilford syndrome, 42–43
hypogenesis, 65

IBEMs. See inborn errors of metabolism
immotile (primary) cilia, 293–294,
    294f–295f
immune system disorders, 342
imprinting, genetic, 249, 251, 252f,
    257–259, 258f, 259t
imprinting domains, 258
inborn errors of metabolism (IBEMs), 342
  amino acid metabolism disorders,
    192–194, 193t, 194f
  basic principles of, 187, 188f
  carbohydrate metabolism disorders, 193t,
    194, 194f, 195f
  clinical importance of, 187
  diagnosis of, 192, 192t
  fatty acid oxidation disorders, 193t, 195
  key disorders in, 192–198, 193t
  LSDs, 193t, 195–196, 195f, 196f
  nucleic acid disorders, 193t, 197
  pathophysiology of, 187, 189, 189f
  presenting features of, 189–190, 190t,
    191f, 191t, 192, 192f
  sterol metabolism disorders, 193t, 198
  trace metals disorders, 193t,
    196–197, 197f
  treatment of, 198, 298, 298t, 301–302
  urea cycle disorders, 193t, 194–195
  vitamins and cofactors disorders, 193t,
    197–198
inbreeding, coefficient of, 157, 158f
incomplete dominance, 142, 142f
incomplete penetrance, Mendelian Rules of
    Transmission and, 144–145, 144f,
    155, 155f, 204, 204f
independent assortment, in Mendelian Rules
    of Transmission, 139–140, 141f
individual screening, 245

inducible genes, 50, 53f
information flow, from DNA to phenotype
  background and systems integration for,
    17–42
  CDGs and, 45–46, 45f–46f
  clinical correlation for, 45–46, 45f–46f
  interactions in, 19
  medical genetics and, 42–43, 43t
  pleiotropy and, 38, 39f, 40
informed consent, in genetic testing,
    243–244, 244t
inheritance. See atypical inheritance;
    Mendelian inheritance;
    multifactorial inheritance
initiation factors, 31, 36f
inorganic molecules, organic molecules
    compared to, 4
inter-familial variability, 154
interphase, 100, 101f
intrafamilial variability, 154
introns, 9, 18, 28, 29f
inverse disorders, 259
inversion, of chromosomes, 109f, 110, 113,
    113f, 114f

jumping genes. See transposable elements

Kabuki syndrome, 247, 247f
Kartagener syndrome, 295
karyotype, 104, 105, 109f, 117, 117f
  genetic testing with imagery of, 231, 231f
  in Klinefelter syndrome, 122–124,
    124f, 125f
  in trisomies
    trisomy 13 (Patau syndrome), 127,
      128f, 129f, 129t
    trisomy 18 (Edwards syndrome), 127,
      129f, 129t
    trisomy 21 (Down syndrome),
      125–127, 126f
  in Turner syndrome, 122, 123f
  in XXX syndrome, 124, 125f
  in XYY syndrome, 124, 125f
Kayser-Fleisher ring, 196, 197f
kinetochores, 87
Klinefelter syndrome, 122–124, 124f, 125f
Krebs cycle, 275, 278f
Kuvan, 199

lac operons, 50, 52f
lactose intolerance, 1
lagging strand, in DNA replication, 21, 22f
Lamarck, Jean-Baptiste, 18
last menstrual period (LMP), 62
laterality, in development, 58, 60, 61f
leading strand, in DNA replication, 21, 22f
Leber hereditary optic neuropathy (LHON),
    287, 288f, 289t
Lederberg, Joshua, 327
lethal alleles, 145, 145f
lethal mutations, 167
LHON. See Leber hereditary optic neuropathy
liabilities, in multifactorial inheritance,
    219, 219f

life
    gift of, 339
    origin of, 2
light microscopy, 271–272,
        273f, 274f
linear sequencing, 241
LINEs. *See* long interspersed nuclear
        elements
linkage disequilibrium, 229–230, 230f
linkage groups, 99, 111
lipids, 4
LMP. *See* last menstrual period
locus, of gene, 147, 148f
locus heterogeneity, 148–149, 149f,
        149t, 217
long interspersed nuclear elements
        (LINEs), 85, 254
looped domains, 87, 88f
LSDs. *See* lysosomal storage disorders
Lyon, Mary, 111
Lyonization, 111, 111f, 159, 159f
lysosomal storage disorders (LSDs), 193t,
        195–196, 195f, 196f, 287, 305,
        306f, 307, 307f
lysosomes, 282, 283f, 287, 289f–291f,
        290, 290t

major malformations, 65, 65f
malformations, 64–65, 65f
maple syrup urine disease (MSUD),
        193–194, 193t
Marfan syndrome, 154–155, 154f, 193,
        194f, 254–255, 255f, 256f
marker chromosomes, 119f, 238
maternal effects, 49
McClintock, Barbara, 85, 172
mean, 214
mediator transcription factor, 53, 56f
medical geneticists, 11–12
medical genetics. *See also specific
        instances*
    categories within, 11, 11t
    clinical milestones in, 14, 14t
    clinical presentations in, 42, 42t
    definition of, 11, 11t
    interdisciplinary teams in, 12t
    naming conditions in, 13–14
    technological milestones in, 13t, 14
    terminology for, 12–13
Medical Home Neighbor, 300
meiosis, 99
    crossing over, recombination in, 105,
        107f, 112f, 113, 114f
    goal of, 100
    key events in, 140, 140f
    metaphase I, 105, 106f, 108f
    prophase I in, 105, 106f, 107f
    stages of, 104–105, 106f, 107f
membranes
    composition of, 272–273, 276f
    defects of, 274–275
    functions of, 273–274
Mendel, Gregor, 4, 139–140,
        147, 213

Mendelian inheritance
    AD inheritance
        classical characteristics of, 150–151,
            150f–153f, 151t, 156t
        recurrence risks of, 151
        special inheritance considerations
            with, 151–156
    AR inheritance
        classical characteristics of, 156
        frequency of, 156–157, 156t
        recurrence risks with, 156
        special inheritance considerations
            with, 156–160
    autosomal, 149–162
    clinical aspects of, 149
    clinical correlation for, 163–164,
        163f, 164f
    sex-linked inheritance, 159–161, 159f,
        160f, 204, 204f
    X-linked inheritance, 159
        dominant, 161–162, 162f
        recessive, 161
Mendelian Rules of Transmission
    development of, 139–140
    dominance in, 140
        co-dominance, 152–153
        exceptions to, 142–143, 142f
        incomplete, 142, 142f
        quasi-dominance, 156
        true complete, 151–152, 154f
    G X E interactions in, 144, 144f
    gene interactions and, 143–144, 143f
    incomplete penetrance and, 144–145,
        144f, 155, 155f, 204, 204f
    independent assortment in, 139–140,
        141f
    lethal alleles and, 145, 145f
    multiple alleles and, 145–147, 146f
    PKU and, 144
    probabilities and recurrence rates in,
        141–142
    recessiveness in, 140, 142–143, 142f
    segregation in, 139–140, 140f
    sex-linked, sex-limited, sex-influenced
        expression and, 147
    variable expression and, 144–145,
        144f, 145f
        degree of, 153–154
        pleiotropism compared to, 154–155,
            154f
Mendelian traits, 147–162
Menkes disease, 196, 197f
mental retardation (MR), 96–97, 97f, 98f
mesoderm, 57, 60t
messenger RNA (mRNA), 3
    capping ends of, 28, 30f
    codon of, 29, 32f
    discovery of, 18
    genome functional region
        correspondence with, 78, 81f
    poly-A tail for stability of, 28
    processes of, 80, 82t
    Shine-Dalgarno sequence in, 32
metabolic dieticians, 298

metabolic pathways, 40, 40f, 184–185,
        185f, 186t
metabolism. *See also* inborn errors of
        metabolism
    basic chemistry of, 184
    medical genetics and, 187–198
    mutations and phenotypic discernment
        in, 186–187, 186t
    PKU and, 183, 184f
metabolomics, 319
metagenomics, 319
metaphase, in mitosis, 103f, 104
metaphase I, meiosis, 105, 106f, 108f
microarray studies, 135, 135f, 240–241,
        241f
micro-duplication/micro-deletion
        syndromes, 238, 238t
microRNAs (miRNAs), 9, 82, 82t, 83f, 96
microsatellite instability (MSI), 94
microsatellites, 85, 94, 96f, 254
microscopy, 269–270, 271–272, 273f–275f
microvilli, 273
Miescher, Friedrich, 4
miniature inverted-repeats transposable
        elements (MITEs), 254
minisatellites, 84–85, 93–94, 95f
minor malformations, 65, 65f
miRNAs. *See* microRNAs
mis-assigned paternity, 207
mismatch repair genes (MMR), 94
missense mutation, 167
MITEs. *See* miniature inverted-repeats
        transposable elements
mitochondria
    ATP in, 275, 276f
    disorders of, 285–287, 286t, 287t, 288f,
        289t, 342
    DNA, 275, 278, 280–282
    glucose digestion in, 275, 277f
    inheritance principles in, 275, 280t
    mutations in, 278, 280
    OXPHOS and, 275, 279f, 282
mitosis, 99
    anaphase in, 103f, 104
    errors in, 100
    goal of, 100
    growth-duplication cycle of, 100, 101f
    metaphase in, 103f, 104
    prometaphase in, 103f, 104
    prophase in, 102, 103f
    stages of, 102, 103f, 104
    telophase in, 103f, 104
MMR. *See* mismatch repair genes
model organisms. *See also specific
        organisms*
    comparative genomic hybridization and,
        329, 330f–333f, 330t, 332
    DNA sequencing of, 320
    HGP types of, 10f, 11, 11f
    medical genetic applications of, 42
    mutation rate measurement in,
        169, 169f
    value of, 325–333, 326t
modifier genes, 251, 260–261

molecular biology
    Central Dogma of, 17–18, 18f, 77
    pleiotropy and, 38, 39f, 40
molecular cytogenetics, 120
molecular decay, 177
molecular genetics, 11t
monoallelic expression, 251
monosomic linkage groups, 111
monosomy, 121
monozygotic twins (MZ twins), 217,
    218f, 304
Morgan, Thomas Hunt, 326–327
morphogenesis, in development, 49,
    57–58, 63
morphogens, 56–57, 59f
Morpholino oligonucleotides, 328
morula, 49
mosaicism
    functional, 250
    gonadal, 255–256, 256f
    occurrence of, 249–250, 250f
    somatic, 254–255, 255f, 256f
motile cilia, 294–295
MR. See mental retardation
mRNA. See messenger RNA
MSI. See microsatellite instability
MSUD. See maple syrup urine disease
Muller, H. J., 169
multifactorial disorders, 342
multifactorial inheritance
    cleft lip, cleft palate and, 220, 221f, 222,
        222f, 261, 261f, 301, 301t
    improving understanding for, 222–223
    liabilities in, 219, 219f
    major features of, 219
    medical genetics and, 218–225
    NTDs and, 220, 220f, 220t
    principles of, 219–220
    with sex bias, 220, 220t
multi-locus inheritance, 251, 260–261,
    261f, 262f
multimeric proteins, 37
multiple alleles, 145–147, 146f
Mus musculus (house mouse), 10f, 11,
    328–329
mutagens, 254
    damage by, 170, 172f, 173f
    types of, 177–178
mutations
    activating, 335
    back, 312
    causes of, 177–178
    clinical consequences of, 175
    clinical correlation for, 180–181
    conditional, 167
    deleterious, 167
    DNA
        coding sequence and, 91–92
        medical conditions associated with,
            91, 91t
        outside coding sequence, 92, 92f
        repair of, 172, 173f, 178–180, 179f,
            179t, 180f
    EPHB1, 163–164, 163f

event rate of, 168
forward, 312
founder effect and, 158–159, 317
frameshift, 167
frequency of, 167–168, 175–176, 176t, 217
genetic resource replenishment and, 174
germinal, 173–174
homeotic, 58, 60f
hot sports for, 176
impact of, 180
lethal, 167
medical genetics and, 174–180
medical perspective on, 174–175
in metabolic pathways, 184–185,
    185f, 186t
metabolism and phenotypic discernment
    with, 186–187, 186t
miRNA, 96
missense, 167
in mitochondria, 278, 280
negative association with, 175
neutral, 167
nonsense, 167
paternal age effect on, 174
pathogenic, 175
PAX3, 329, 332, 333f
phenotype affected by, 40–41
point, 37, 166–167, 167t
polymorphisms and, 165
population genetics and, 312–313
rate of, 167–168, 168f, 175–176, 176t
    model organism measurement of,
        169, 169f
repair enzymes and, 165, 166f
RNA, 94, 96
rRNA, 94, 96
silent, 166
somatic, 173–174, 176
spontaneous mechanisms of, 169–170,
    170f, 171f
spontaneous rate of, 165–166
suppressor, 167
TEs and, 94, 173
transition, 166, 167f, 167t
transversion, 166–167, 167t
tRNA, 94
TWIST, 329, 330f
types of, 166–167, 167t, 177, 178t
myotonic dystrophy, 262, 265f, 265t
MZ twins. See monozygotic twins

nematode. See Caenorhabditis elegans
neoplasias, 341
neural tube defects (NTDs), 220, 220f, 220t
neurofibromatosis, 44, 44f, 45t, 321, 321f
neutral mutations, 167
next-gen sequencing, 234, 242
Nightingale, Florence, 4
nmRNA. See non-messenger RNA
NO. See nucleolar organizer
noncoding RNA, 80, 82t
nondisjunction, 110, 110f
non-messenger RNA (nmRNA), 80, 82t
non-protein-coding RNA (npcRNA), 80, 82t

nonsense mutations, 167
Noonan syndrome, 44, 44f, 45t, 321–322,
    321f, 322f
npcRNA. See non-protein-coding RNA
NTDs. See neural tube defects
nuclear division. See also meiosis; mitosis
    accuracy of, 99
    chromosome coiling during, 100, 102f
    overview of, 99–100
    stages of, 100, 101f, 102, 102f
nuclear genome. See genome
nuclear matrix, 87, 88f
nuclear ribonucleoproteins, small, 28
nucleic acid, 4, 4f, 193t, 197
nucleolar organizer (NO), 83, 83f
nucleoli, 100
nucleosomes, 28, 85, 87f
nucleotides, 4–5, 4f, 5f
    excision repair of, 172
    in RNA transcription, 27
    sequencing determination of, 241–243,
        242f
    structure of, 19–20, 21f
nucleus, 83
    disorders with, 291–292, 293f
    eukaryotic chromosome packing in, 85,
        86f–89f, 87
    structural changes in, 285
null alleles, 186

Okazaki fragments, 21, 22f
oligonucleotides, 26, 85
On the Origin of Species (Darwin,
    Charles), 4
onchronosis, 193
1,000 Genomes Project, 9
1q21.1 deletion, 135, 135f
oogenesis, 105, 108f
operons, 50, 52f, 53f
opposite (anti-sense) transcripts, 253, 261
organelles. See also nucleus
    cilia and, 273, 283–285, 284f
        immotile (primary), 293–294,
            294f–295f
        motile, 292–295
    cytoskeleton and, 282–283, 283f,
        291, 291f, 292f
    domains of, 270, 272f
    endosomes, 282, 287
    ER and, 282, 282f, 287
    flagella and, 273, 283–284, 284f, 294–295
    function and imaging of, 269–270,
        271f, 272f
    Golgi complex and, 282, 287
    lysosomes, 282, 283f, 287, 289f–291f,
        290, 290t
    medical genetics and, 285–295
    membranes, 272–275, 276f
    mitochondria, 275, 276f–281f, 278,
        280–282, 280t, 285–287, 286t,
        287t, 288f, 289t
    ROGEs and, 295
organic molecules, inorganic molecules
    compared to, 4

origin of life, 2
ornithine transcarbamylase deficiency, 195
oxidative phosphorylation (OXPHOS), 275,
 279f, 282

paracentric inversion, 113, 113f, 114f
parallel sequencing, 242
parthenogenesis, 251
Patau syndrome, karyotype in trisomy 13,
 127, 128f, 129f, 129t
pathogenesis, 42
 examples of types of changes in
 abnormal protein folding, 335
 disruptive proteins, 335, 335f
 gain of function, 335, 336f, 337
 missing/nonfunctional protein, 334–335
 historical advancements with, 333–334
 types of, 337–338, 337f, 338t
pathogenic mutations, 175
pattern formation, in development, 49,
 56–57, 59f
PAX3 mutation, 329, 332, 333f
PCR. See polymerase chain reaction
Pearson, Karl, 213
pedigree analysis
 basics of, 203–204, 203f, 204f
 case studies for, 209–210, 209f–211f
 consanguinity and, 204
 organization of, 202–203
 of royal families, 201, 202f
 sample for, 205, 205f
 symbols in, 203
penetrance, incomplete, 144–145, 144f,
 155, 155f
peptidyltransferase, 34
pericentric inversion, 113, 113f, 114f
peroxisomes, 282, 289–290
personalized genomics, 15–16, 15t, 319
personalized medicine, 304–305
 clinical correlation with, 14–16
 genetic applications in, 15–16, 15t
 principles of, 300
pharmacogenetics, 11t, 15t, 16, 40, 319
phenocopy, 161
phenotype. See also information flow, from
 DNA to phenotype
 death as, 40
 ear, 38
 endophenotype, 14, 15
 mutations affecting, 40–41
 quantitative description of distributions
 of, 214–215, 215f
phenylalanine metabolism, 40–41, 40f
phenylketonuria (PKU), 40–41
 bacterial inhibition assay for, 185, 185f
 clinical correlation for, 198–199
 information known on, 187
 major events in history of, 198, 198t
 Mendelian Rules of Transmission and,
 144
 metabolism and, 183, 184f
 pathophysiology of, 189, 189f
 successful treatment of, 199
phosphorylation, 37

Pisum sativum, 139, 140f
PKU. See phenylketonuria
plasmids, 327
plasticity, developmental, 55–56,
 58f, 59f
pleiotropism, variable expression compared
 to, 154–155, 154f
pleiotropy, 38, 39f, 40
pleuripotency, 55–56
point mutations, 37, 166–167, 167t
polar bodies, 105, 108f
poly-A tail, 28
polygenic disorders, 342
polygenic inheritance, 215–217, 216f,
 223–225, 224f, 225f
polygenic predisposition, 203
polymerase chain reaction (PCR), 24, 25f,
 26, 112
polymerases
 DNA, 20
 polymerase III, 21, 23f
 Taq, 26
 RNA
 classes of, 51
 holoenzyme, 26, 27f, 187, 188f
 promoter binding to, 26, 26f, 81f
polymorphisms, 147. See also mutations;
 single nucleotide polymorphisms
 benign, 92, 175
 definition of, 168–169, 174
 mutations and, 165
 prevalence of identifiable, 176
polyploid structure, of chromosomes,
 105, 108
polyploidy, 112, 120
Pompe disease, 194, 195f, 287–290, 289f,
 290f
population genetics, 11t
 allele frequencies in gene pool and, 310
 ethics and individual mistreatment with,
 309–310, 316–317
 gene tracking for, 319–320, 320f
 Hardy-Weinberg equilibrium and, 311,
 311f, 312t, 313–314
 medical genetics and, 317–320
 migration effects on, 312, 312f
 mutation effects on, 312–313
 non-random mating and population size
 in, 313, 313f, 314f
 selection consequences for, 313–316,
 314f–316f
 technology impact on, 318–319
positional information, in development,
 56, 59f
posttranslation modification, 37–38, 39f
Potter syndrome, 73, 73f
Prader-Willi syndrome, 257–258, 257f
pre-miRNA, 82, 83f
prereplication complex, in eukaryotes, 23
primary cilia, 293–294, 294f–295f
primer, in DNA replication, 21, 22f
pri-miRNA, 82, 83f
proband, 203
product rule, 205

prokaryotes
 eukaryotes compared to, 18, 19f
 in DNA replication, 21, 23–24, 24f
 in RNA transcription, 27–28, 28f, 29f
 Genetic Code of, 19
prometaphase, in mitosis, 103f, 104
promoter, RNA polymerases binding to, 26,
 26f, 81f
prophase, mitosis, 102, 103f
prophase I, in meiosis, 105, 106f, 107f
proposita, 203
propositus, 203
protein kinase, 54
proteins, 4
 abnormal folding of, 335
 activation of, 19
 activator, 50, 51f
 allosteric, 37
 anatomy of protein-coding gene, 78–80,
 81f, 82f
 chaperone, 35
 CREB, 54, 57f
 disruptive, 335, 335f
 in DNA replication, 20–21, 22f
 domain structures of, 52, 55f
 dystrophin, 291, 291f
 formation of, 18–19
 function of, 35–37
 G, 54
 globular, 36
 histone, 85, 87f
 chromatin remodeling and, 87, 89f
 missing/nonfunctional, 334–335
 multimeric, 37
 in nuclear matrix, 87, 88f
 posttranslation modification of, 37–38, 39f
 regulatory, 50, 51f
 repressor, 50, 51f
 RNA translation to, 18
 sorting of, 37–38, 39f
 structure of
 amino acid characteristics in, 28, 31f
 levels in, 35, 38f
 shape and, 35–37
 synthesis of
 elongation in, 32, 36f
 initiation of, 31–32, 36f
 summary of events in, 31, 35f
 termination in, 34, 37f, 81f
proteomics, 41, 319
prototrophs, 185
pseudoautosomal regions, 115
pseudodominance, 112
pseudogenes, 83, 93
Punnett, R. C., 141
Punnett square, 141, 141f, 314, 314f
pyrosequencing, 234

qualitative traits, quantitative traits
 compared to, 213–214
quantitative trait loci, 213
quantitative traits, qualitative traits
 compared to, 213–214
quasi-dominance, 156

RAS/MAPK system, 44, 45t
recessiveness, in Mendelian Rules of
        Transmission, 140, 142–143, 142f
reciprocal translocations, 109f, 110
*Recognizable Patterns of Human
        Malformations* (Smith), 42, 69
recombination, 105, 107f, 112f, 113, 114f
recurrence risk, 151, 156, 218
regulators of organelle gene expression
        (ROGEs), 295
regulatory transcription factors, 52–53,
        56f, 57f
relationship, coefficient of, 157, 158f
release factors, stop codon and, 34, 37f
repair enzymes, mutation and, 165, 166f
repetitive sequences, DNA function of,
        83–84, 84f
replication fork, 20–21, 22f, 23f
replicative segregation, 278, 281f
replisome, in DNA replication, 21, 24f
repressible genes, 50, 53f
repressor proteins, 50, 51f
reproductive genetics, 11t
response elements, 52
restriction endonucleases, 241
restriction enzyme, 84–85, 84f
restriction point, 100
retrotransposons, 83, 85, 253–254
reverse transcriptase, 18
ribonucleic acid (RNA), 1. *See also*
        messenger RNA; microRNAs;
        ribosomal RNA; transfer RNA
    functional, 80, 82t
    heterogeneous, 28
    interference, 82, 83f
    mutations of, 94, 96
    noncoding, 80, 82t
    non-messenger, 80, 82t
    non-protein-coding, 80, 82t
    polymerases
        classes of, 51
        holoenzyme, 26, 27f, 187, 188f
        promoter binding to, 26, 26f, 81f
    posttranslation modification and, 37–38, 39f
    processing of, in nucleus
        intron alternative splicing in, 28, 29f
        mRNA capping in, 28, 30f
    protein from, 18
    "RNA World" hypothesis and, 3
    sequencing, 234–235
    small non-messenger, 80, 82t
    structure of, 4
    synthesis of, 3
    transcription of
        eukaryotes compared to prokaryotes
            in, 27–28, 28f, 29f
        factors in, 26–27, 27f
        key events in, 26–27, 27f
        nucleotides in, 27
        stages of, 26, 26f
    translation of, 28–35
        anticodon in, 29, 33f
        codon in, 29, 32f
        elongation in, 32, 36f

in eukaryotes, 34–35
        initiation in, 31–32, 36f
        overview of events in, 31, 34f
        summary of events in, 31, 35f
        termination in, 34, 37f, 81f
    types of, 80, 82t
ribonucleoproteins, small nuclear, 28
ribosomal binding sites, 32, 81f
ribosomal RNA (rRNA), 28
    composition of, 30–31, 34f
    decoding function and, 32
    mutations of, 94, 96
RISC. *See* RNA-induced silencing complex
RNA. *See* ribonucleic acid
"RNA World" hypothesis, 3
RNA-induced silencing complex (RISC),
        82
Robertsonian translocation, 114
Robin sequence, 68–69, 70f
ROGEs. *See* regulators of organelle gene
        expression
royal families, pedigree analysis of,
        201, 202f
rRNA. *See* ribosomal RNA

Saccharomyces cerevisiae (baker's yeast),
        10f, 327–328
Sanger, Frederick, 232
Sanger sequencing. *See* dideoxy
        sequencing
satellite DNA
    alpha-satellites, 83–84, 84f, 93
    microsatellites, 85, 94, 96f, 254
    minisatellites, 84–85, 93–94, 95f
SCA. *See* spinocerebellar atrophy
scanning electron microscopy (SEM),
        272, 275f
Schleiden, Matthias, 269
Schwann, Theodor, 269
SCID. *See* severe combined
        immunodeficiency
second degree relative, 157, 157f, 206
second messenger, 54
segmentation genes, 58
segregation, 105
    adjacent, 113–114, 115f
    alternate, 114
    aneuploidy errors in, 110–111, 110f
    in Mendelian Rules of Transmission,
        139–140, 140f
    nondisjunction and, 110, 110f
    replicative, 278, 281f
selected cell death, in embryology, 63
selected profile screening, 245–246,
        245t, 246t
selection, 313–316, 314f–316f
SEM. *See* scanning electron microscopy
sense codons, 30
sense strand, 27
sequence complexity, 77–78, 79f, 80t
sequences, in congenital anomalies, 68–69,
        70f
severe combined immunodeficiency
        (SCID), 303, 303f

sex chromosomes, aneuploidy and, 121–124
sex-influenced expression, 147
sex-limited expression, 147
sex-linked expression, 147
sex-linked inheritance, 159–161, 159f,
        160f, 204, 204f
Sherman paradox, 262
Shine-Dalgarno sequence, 32
short interspersed nuclear elements
        (SINEs), 85, 254
Shprintzen, Robert, 136
Shprintzen syndrome, 136, 136f
sickle cell anemia (SSA), 38, 39f, 157,
        317, 335
signal transduction, 54, 57f
signaling pathways, disorders linked by,
        43–44, 45t
silent mutations, 166
simple translocations, 109f, 110
SINEs. *See* short interspersed nuclear
        elements
single nucleotide polymorphisms (SNPs),
        9, 147–148, 148f
    analysis of, 232
    diseases associated with, 15t, 16
    tag, 232
sister chromatids, 100, 102f
situs abnormalities, 295
skewed inactivation, 250
skewed X chromosome inactivation,
        159, 160f
SLO. *See* Smith-Lemli-Opitz syndrome
small non-messenger (snmRNA), 80, 82t
small nuclear ribonucleoproteins, 28
Smith, David, 42, 69
Smith-Lemli-Opitz syndrome (SLO), 190,
        191f, 192f, 318
snmRNA. *See* small non-messenger
SNPs. *See* single nucleotide
        polymorphisms
somatic mosaicism, 254–255, 255f, 256f
somatic mosaics, 114–115
somatic mutations, 173–174, 176
sorting signals, 38
Sotos syndrome, 67, 69f, 337, 337f
Southern blotting, 85, 98f
spermatogenesis, 105, 108f
spindle, 102
spinocerebellar atrophy (SCA), 148–149,
        149f, 149t
spontaneous deamination, 170, 170f
spontaneous depurination, 169, 170f
SSA. *See* sickle cell anemia
stabilizing selection, 315, 315f
standard deviation, 215, 215f
start codons, 81f
sterol metabolism disorders, 193t, 198
stop codons, 31, 34, 37f, 81f
structural gene, 50, 78
sub-telomeric FISH, 118–119, 119f,
        239–240, 240f
sub-telomeric regions, of chromosomes, 93
suppressor mutations, 167
synapsis, 105, 107f

synaptonemal complex, 105, 107*f*
syndromes, in congenital anomalies, 67, 69*f*, 70, 72–73, 73*f*, 74*f*

tag SNP, 232
tandem duplications, 112
tandem repeats
    alpha-satellites, 83–84, 84*f*, 93
    microsatellites, 85, 94, 96*f*, 254
    minisatellites, 84–85, 93–94, 95*f*
    variable number of, 84–85, 84*f*, 85*f*, 93
Taq polymerase, 26
Tatum, Edward, 40, 89, 327
tautomeric shifts, 170, 171*f*
Tay-Sachs disease, 196, 196*f*
telocentric chromosomes, 114
telomere region, in eukaryotes, 24, 25*f*, 93–94
telophase, in mitosis, 103*f*, 104
TEM. *See* transmission electron microscopy
teratogens, 71, 71*t*, 177, 226–227, 226*f*, 226*t*, 227*f*
terminator, in RNA translation, 34, 37*f*, 81*f*
TEs. *See* transposable elements
tetraploidy, 121
TFIID, transcription factor, 53, 56*f*
third degree relative, 157, 157*f*, 206
threshold, biologic, 219, 219*f*
totipotency, 55
trace metals disorders, 193*t*, 196–197, 197*f*
tracking populations, 319–320, 320*f*
traits, 1
transcription factors
    domain structures of, 52, 55*f*
    in eukaryotes, 51–53, 54*f*–56*f*
    in gene action, 50
    mediator, 53, 56*f*
    regulatory, 52–53, 56*f*, 57*f*
    in RNA transcription, 26–27, 27*f*
    TFIID, 53, 56*f*
    upstream, 52

transcriptomics, 234–235, 319
transfer RNA (tRNA), 28
    amino acids attached to, 29, 32*f*, 33*f*
    anticodon of, 29, 33*f*
    codon of, 29, 32*f*
    initiation factors for, 31, 36*f*
    mutations of, 94
    peptidyltransferase and, 34
    processes of, 80, 82*t*
transition mutation, 166, 167*f*, 167*t*
translocation, of chromosomes, 109*f*, 110, 113–114, 115*f*
transmission electron microscopy (TEM), 272, 275*f*
transposable elements (TEs, transposons), 82, 85
    classification of, 253–254
    clinical implications of, 261, 262*t*
    discovery and types of, 85, 172–173
    mutations from, 94, 173
transversion mutations, 166, 167*t*
triallelic inheritance, 251
trinucleotide repeats, 173, 262, 265*t*, 266*f*
triploidy, 120, 120*f*
trisomic linkage group, 111
trisomies, 125–127, 126*f*, 128*f*, 129*f*, 129*t*
tRNA. *See* transfer RNA
trp operons, 50, 53*f*
Turner, Henry, 121
Turner syndrome, 121–122, 122*f*, 123*f*
22q11.2 deletions, 136, 136*f*
twins
    concordance in, 217–218, 217*t*, 218*f*
    discordant, 217
    MZ, 217, 218*f*, 304
TWIST mutation, 329, 330*f*

uniparental disomy (UPD), 250–251, 250*f*, 256–257
upstream factors, 52
urea cycle disorders, 193*t*, 194–195

VACTERL association, 67, 69*f*
van der Woude syndrome, 155, 155*f*, 261, 261*f*
variable expression, Mendelian Rules of Transmission and, 144–145, 144*f*, 145*f*
    degree of, 153–154
    pleiotropism compared to, 154–155, 154*f*
variable number of tandem repeats (VNTRs), 84–85, 84*f*, 85*f*, 93
variance, 214
Vesalius, Andreas, 269
vitamin disorders, 193*t*, 197–198
VNTRs. *See* variable number of tandem repeats

Waardenburg syndrome, 332, 333*f*
Wambaugh, Joseph, 84
Watson syndrome, 322
whole exome sequencing, 242
whole exon sequencing, 234
whole genome sequencing, 242–243
wild type sequence, 147
Williams syndrome, 132, 134*f*, 134*t*, 135, 135*f*, 237–238, 238*f*
Wilson disease, 196, 197*f*
wobble position, 30, 33*f*
Wolf-Hirschhorn syndrome, 131, 132*f*, 133*f*, 134*t*, 334, 334*f*

X-chromosomes, 111–112, 111*f*, 159, 159*f*, 160*f*
X-linked inheritance, 159, 161–162, 162*f*
XXX syndrome, 124, 125*f*
XYY syndrome, 124, 125*f*

Y chromosomes, 115
Y-linked inheritance, 159

zebrafish. *See Danio rerio*

CPSIA information can be obtained
at www.ICGtesting.com
Printed in the USA
FFHW011648210219
50620346-56002FF